Quality Control in Clinical Chemistry

Quality Control in Clinical Chemistry

Transactions of the VIth International Symposium, Geneva, April 23–25, 1975

Editors
G. Anido E. J. van Kampen
S. B. Rosalki M. Rubin

W DE G

Walter de Gruyter · Berlin · New York 1975

Editors:
G. Anido, M. D., Medical Director, State Division of AHSC, Miami, Florida, USA
E. J. van Kampen, Ph. D., Klinisch-Chemisch Laboratorium, Diakonessenhuis, Groningen, Netherlands
S. B. Rosalki, M. D., M.R.C.P., F.R.C. Path., Consultant Chemical Pathologist, St. Mary's Hospital, London W2, United Kingdom
M. Rubin, Ph. D., Director of Clinical Chemistry, Georgetown University Hospital, Washington D.C., USA

Publisher:
Walter de Gruyter
Genthiner Strasse 13
D-1 Berlin 30

Walter de Gruyter Inc.
3 Westchester Plaza
Elmsford, 10523 New York

With 196 figures

Library of Congress Cataloging in Publication Data

International Symposium on Quality Control, VIth, Geneva, 1975.
Quality Control in Clinical Chemistry.
1. Chemistry, Clinical – Quality Control – Congresses. I. Anido, G. II. Title.
[DNLM: I. Chemistry, Clinical – Congresses. II. Quality Control – Congresses. W.3 IN922PE 1975 Q/QY90 I613 1975q]
RB40 I64.I64 1975 616.07'56 75-41464
ISBN 3-11-006692-0

CIP-Kurztitelaufnahme der Deutschen Bibliothek

Quality Control in Clinical Chemistry:
Transactions of the VIth Internat. Symposium, Geneva, April 23–25, 1975 / ed. G. Anido ...
ISBN 3-11-006692-0
NE: Anido, Guillermo A. [Hrsg.]

Typesetting and Printing: Benteli AG, 3018 Bern. – Binding: Schluep, 3013 Bern. – Printed in Switzerland.

Table of Contents

Award Lectures

NAD – NADH – NADP – NADPH Characterization and Purity Assurance

Plenary Lectures

Free Communications

Hematology Symposium

Plenary Lectures

International Federation of Clinical Chemistry

The Clinical Laboratory from an International Viewpoint

Session I: Session Chairman: H. Adlercreutz
Discussion Leader: J. L. Giegel

Topic: International Criteria for Clinical Laboratory Materials

Session II: Session Chairman: H.Büttner
Discussion Leader: G.Anido

Topic: International Criteria for Diagnostic Methods

Session III: Session Chairman: E.J. van Kampen
Discussion Leader: G. Sims

Topic: International Criteria for Clinical Laboratory Instrumentation

Session IV: Session Chairman: R. Dybkaer
Discussion Leader: H. Bergmeyer

Topic: National Regulations and International Recommendations

Transactions of the VIth International Symposium on Quality Control, Geneva 1975

Foreword

The Transactions of the VIth International Symposium on Quality Control record the increasing maturity in the response of the clinical chemist and of his partners in industry to the challenges of our time, challenges of responsibility to patient, to physician and to government.

The highlights of this VIth Symposium include: the Dade Award Lectures delivered by clinical chemists selected by their National Societies in recognition of their contributions to Quality Control; the Richterich Memorial Lecture, instituted in honour of this renowned Swiss clinical chemist; the Symposium on nicotineamide dinucleotide coenzymes; the Symposium on Quality Control in Hematology; the Symposium of the International Federation of Clinical Chemistry, giving an overview of the clinical laboratory from an international standpoint; and last but not least, the lively discussions that took place throughout the Symposium and which constitute the most remarkable characteristic of the series of meetings originating with and subsequent to the original First Geneva Symposium in 1967.

The Transactions of the VIth Symposium throughout reflect the high degree of concern of the clinical laboratory worker for the well-being of the patient. Quality Control of laboratory tests, laboratory procedures, laboratory reagents, laboratory equipment and laboratory personnel were all scrutinised in an environment of frank and open exchange, and these exchanges are documented in this volume.

We feel that the Transactions of the VIth Symposium will be of immense value and interest to all clinical laboratory workers, constituting as it does, a unique record of established achievements and of the newest trends in the broad field of Quality Control.

G. Anido
E. J. van Kampen
S. B. Rosalki
M. Rubin

Opening Session
Welcome by the Chairman

Dr. *S.B.Rosalki*

It gives me great pleasure to welcome you to this VIth International Symposium on Quality Control. The Symposium continues and extends the tradition of the Geneva Quality Control Symposia which were established in 1967. This Symposium is a meeting of three days; the first of these includes a series of Award Lectures sponsored by DADE and by Merz + DADE. These lectures will be presented by outstanding clinical chemists from 14 countries, covering Europe and including also the United States, the Award Lecturers having been chosen by their own National Societies for Clinical Chemistry for their outstanding contributions to the quality of laboratory work.

Today also, will be presented, in the final part of the day, a Memorial Lecture established in memory of that outstanding clinical chemist, Professor *R.Richterich.*

Tomorrow, the morning will be devoted to a Symposium on the problems of nicotinamide-adenine coenzyme quality and purity assurance, and in the afternoon, a novel departure in this Symposium will be the introduction of lectures devoted to quality control in hematology, recognizing the links between clinical chemistry and hematology.

For the third day, we are hosts to the International Federation of Clinical Chemistry, who have organized a symposium on 'The Clinical Chemistry Laboratory from the International Viewpoint.'

Having outlined the format of the Symposium, I would like to call upon Dr. *Bürgi,* former President of the Swiss Society for Clinical Chemistry, to introduce the Symposium; at the same time I would like to welcome to our number the new President of the Swiss Society for Clinical Chemistry, Dr. *Colombo.*

Introduction

Dr. *W. Bürgi*, former President of the Swiss Society for Clinical Chemistry

Mister Chairman,
Ladies and Gentlemen,

It is a pleasure for me and a great honour to give a short introduction to the VIth International Symposium on Quality Control in Clinical Chemistry. A pleasure, because I am positive that the many personal contacts made during the previous Symposia will be renewed and new contacts made during the days ahead of us. An honour, because I have reasons to be proud to welcome as Past-President, on behalf of the Swiss Society of Clinical Chemistry, almost half a thousand scientists from Europe and all over the world, all of you being not only experts in quality control, but many of you being known as pioneers in this important part of Clinical Chemistry. Since many of you are with us for the first time, I will give a schematic retrospect on the preceding Geneva Symposia. It is interesting to note that the first conference in 1967 was the outcome of an intensive exchange of thoughts between Mrs. *Divernois-Merz* from Merz + Dade, Berne, Prof. *H. Büttner* and Prof. *D. Stamm* from Germany. Gradually, a concept emerged with the aim of obtaining a general view of what had been achieved in European countries, up to that time, in quality control, and of what could eventually be done in the future.

Mrs. *Divernois* accepted the task of organizing the first Symposium and she is the first person I am mentioning who merits our wholehearted acknowledgment for her engagement. She has been Organizer, Administrator, Secretary, Scientific and Social Program Manager and Committee Member, she has been the heart of the First Symposium and of the following ones ever since.

The idea of creating an international forum to discuss problems pertaining to quality control met with the agreement of DADE (Div. of AHSC) in Miami, U.S.A. In particular, assistance was given by Dr. *G. Anido*, who deserves being recognized as an engaged co-promotor to the Symposia. If he expressed his wishes, as stated in the proceedings of the 1967 Symposium, 'that the exchange of ideas be as casual and frank as possible', all of us, who have attended the Symposia since, can confirm that this has been reality.

Looking back to the mid-sixties, we realize that quality control was considered to be a playground for frustrated scientists by many of those ordering and consuming laboratory results. The Clinical Chemists, however, were convinced that quality control was not a special field of Clinical Chemistry but an important part of it. They knew from continuous experience that awareness of errors in laboratory results was often enough lacking. Moreover, the need for controlling analytical work in the medical laboratory was not commonly accepted by the medical staff.

It is therefore not surprising that the Proceedings of the first meeting described the situation in Europe to be somewhat alarming. Prof. *F. Gabl* from Austria estimated the number of laboratories performing some sort of quality control not to exceed 10%. In many of the 14 European countries represented, quality control in clinical chemistry was thought to be on a low or even rudimentary level. Moreover, the results of interlaboratory surveys were not meeting the required quality standards.

Although a complete quality control program with the now accepted terms was introduced in the early sixties in the German Federal Republic, Prof. *H. Büttner* nevertheless made the restriction 'that the break-through of the idea of quality control in a clinical chemical laboratory in Germany has not been achieved'.

The overall situation in Europe at that time is probably best characterized by quoting Dr. *F. Mitchell* from the U.K., who said that 'quality control in Britain varies from being non-existent in some laboratories to being comprehensive and very efficient in others'.

In the course of the past eight years, this situation as described before, has continuously changed and quality control has not only lost its opponents but is now accepted as an integral part of routine clinical chemistry, in some countries even by law. The many questions raised but not answered during the First Symposium were the subject of the program of the Second Symposium in 1968. This concept was carried on so that each Symposium to some extent can be considered a logical continuation of its predecessor.

In 1968, when the Second Symposium was held, Dr. *S. B. Rosalki,* London, U.K. and Dr. *H. Drescher,* Merz + Dade AG, Berne, joined the Symposium staff. Dr. *Rosalki* has accepted the responsibility for many functions within the Scientific Committee, beginning with the preparation of the program and ending with the publication of the Proceedings. He has been acting as President of the sessions ever since, with his personality warranting a high scientific standard. We owe him most of what the DADE Symposia have become.

Symposia One to Four, the latter of which took place in 1971, were devoted to building up and to gaining experience for how future conferences could eventually be organized. They were held with a limited number of participants. Beginning with the Fifth Symposium in 1973, the DADE Symposia on Quality Control in Clinical Chemistry came out of their exclusivity to be open to an international audience. In the meantime, they had attracted world-wide attention so that the first open Symposium had to be displaced to an auditorium of the University Medical School in Geneva, where it received most friendly acceptance. Yet, many applications had to be refused, because the lecture-room was large enough for only 200 persons.

As you notice, for the 1975 Symposium successful precautions have been taken in order to offer unrestricted participation. The program contains a great number of topics of burning actuality and deserves attention by this numerous audience.

I hope that this Symposium will be as successful as those in the past and that the exchange of ideas can again be as casual and frank as possible.

It is to be expected that, although this Symposium will certainly enlarge our present state of knowledge in quality control, a certain number of questions will be left open. These new questions arising might serve as a basis for future Symposia. If however, unexpectedly, the conference ends up with no further questions on the topics discussed here, important problems in other fields of quality control await being solved. Attention is called to quality control in Immunhematology and Blood Clotting. In addition, blood sampling, including the collection, the preservation, the transport of the specimen and the identification of patient and specimen have to be mentioned at this point. Although, many of us agree with Prof. *Rubin,* our President of the IFCC, who made the distinct statement in the last Symposium, that these activities be included in the responsibility of the laboratory, others might have a different opinion. Thus, clarifying discussions are needed to close the gap between the two front lines, the ward and the laboratory.

I wish all of you a pleasant stay here in Geneva and declare the Symposium open.

Award Lectures

Topic I: Quality Control in Relation to Determination Methods

Considerations on Bilirubin Determination

G. Ceriotti, Padova (Italy)

Key words: Accuracy
Bilirubin methods
Precision

Summary

The most important problems of free and conjugated bilirubin determination are schematically outlined.

The results of methods employing methanol or caffeine as accelerating agents are compared with those of a method using dimethylformamide.

Standard curves, absorption, spectra and reaction rate are studied.

Accuracy problems arising from the different reactivity of free and conjugated bilirubin in standard sera, patients sera, and bile under various experimental conditions are discussed.

The basic problem in serum bilirubin determination is the problem of solubility and consequently of reactivity of its different forms present in blood, namely bilirubinic acid and glucuronates. The solubility properties of these compounds depend not only on their chemical structure, but also on their binding to proteins, mainly albumin, and are not so clearly differentiated as to allow an easy, separate evaluation. This is, nevertheless, clinically indispensable because of the profoundly different physiopathological significance of the two forms, which may vary greatly in both absolute and relative concentrations in various morbid conditions.

Analytical problems that arise on these biochemical and physiopathological grounds, may be summarized as follows:

1. For direct reacting or conjugated bilirubin (bilirubinic acid), the essential problem is the need for suitable conditions for good solubilization, to make it to react rapidly and completely with the diazonium salt of sulfanilic acid; still the most commonly used reagent. The best conditions are those that avoid, as far as possible, the interference of proteins, hemoglobin and lipemia.
2. For conjugated bilirubin, it is especially necessary to avoid possible interferences from unconjugated bilirubin, due to partial solubilization of the latter. At the same time, the working conditions must allow as complete as possible a reaction within a reasonable time to determine the true value.
   All the conjugated bilirubin and none of the free bilirubin should react.
3. Standards. A prerequisite for a valid standard, is that, under the chosen conditions, it reacts quantitatively and in the same way as the serum sample.
   Furthermore it must have a good storage stability.

The presence of two differently reacting forms of bilirubin should require the use of two different standards.

However, standards of mono- and diglucuronides of bilirubin are not, at present, commonly accessible, and conjugated bilirubin has to be determined on the basis of a free bilirubin standard.

4. The range of sensitivity should be large enough to allow accurate determination both of the usual, low, and borderline values and also of the, sometimes very high, pathological ones.
5. In addition, the problem of blank values, although easily avoidable, deserves some attention because of its practical implications.
6. Finally, the application of manual techniques to automated flow analysis may present some difficulties for bilirubin measurement, and more limitations than usual with other kinds of analyses. Each one of the problems outlined briefly above requires a more detailed analysis.

For the determination of free and total bilirubin two kinds of approaches have been followed. The first one activates the reaction by the use of solvents such as ethyl-alcohol, as in the pioneer work of *Van den Bergh* and *Muller* [1], or methyl alcohol, as in the *Malloy-Evelyn* method [2].

The most important limitation of this method is interference by proteins, which frequently produces an opalescence and sometimes, in the presence of high concentrations of globulins, a pronounced turbidity. This makes it necessary to work with rather high dilutions of serum, and therefore decreases the accuracy of normal and borderline values.

The release of fine gas bubbles when methanol is added to the reaction, inhibits, in our experience, the possibility of application of this method to automated flow analysis.

In the second kind of approach, activation has been obtained in aqueous solution by the use of caffeine, theophylline, sodium benzoate, urea, acetamide, antipyrine, etc. [3, 4, 5, 6].

This avoids the formation of turbidity and allows the use of higher serum concentrations. However this method, according to *Michaëlsson* [7] and to *Simmons* [8] is complicated by some side reactions and tends to give a false value for the unconjugated bilirubin level.

The conjugated bilirubin is falsely elevated and this erroneous value is accentuated by the fact that the level is based on a free bilirubin standard.

For precise and accurate determination of total bilirubin, it is therefore necessary to find conditions that both avoid formation of turbidity and yield a rapid and quantitative reaction. For correct evaluation of the ratio of free to conjugated bilirubin, the different variables that may influence their respective reactivity must be investigated (table 1 and table 2).

Table 1. Problems regarding conjugated bilirubin reaction.

Partial reactivity and interference of unconjugated bilirubin.
Influence of different variables (pH, sulfanilic acid concentration, nitrite concentration).
Lack of a reference point to control completeness of the reaction.
Lack of specific standards.

Table 2. Problems regarding unconjugated bilirubin reactions.

Sensitivity and linearity.
Completeness or incompleteness of the reaction.
Reactivity of bilirubin in standards and patient sera.
Side reactions.
Interference of proteins (turbidity).
Interference of hemoglobin.
Interference of lipemia.
Interference of drugs.
Variability of blank interference under acid and alkaline conditions.
Different suitability of the various methods for automation.

All these various problems may be classified under two main categories, namely problems of precision and problems of accuracy.

Problems of precision are especially concerned with the various interferences with the reaction; problems of accuracy relate to the completeness of the reaction and to the validity of standards.

We investigated these by comparing the two kinds of reactions most commonly used (namely those employing methanol according to *Malloy-Evelyn* [2] or caffeine according to *Simmons* [8] as the 'accelerating' agents), and a reaction we developed and have used for several years in our laboratory, based on the use of dimethylformamide (DMFA) and isopropanol, according to the procedure outlined in table 3.

Table 3. Dimethylformamide reaction for total bilirubin determination.

Reagents:

1. Dimethylformamide 50 ml; H_2O 50 ml; isopropanol 5 ml; 15% Brij 1 ml.
2. Sulfanilic acid 10 g per liter of 0.125 N HCl.
3. Sodium nitrite 5 g per liter.
4. Diazo working solution: immediately prior to use mix 100 ml of reagent (2) with 2.5 ml of reagent (3).

A Reagent for the colour reaction:
Mix 52 ml of reagent (1) with 18 ml of reagent (4).

B Reagent for blank:
Mix 52 ml of reagent (1) with 18 ml of reagent (2).

Procedure: To 3.5 ml of reagents (A) and (B) add 0.3 ml of serum or standard. Mix. Read at 530 nm.

Here we will concentrate only on some accuracy problems; firstly on the completeness of the reaction.

When a series of dilutions of a standard serum are compared, a clear difference in extinction coefficients is observed (fig. 1); those for the DMFA are 12% and 16% higher

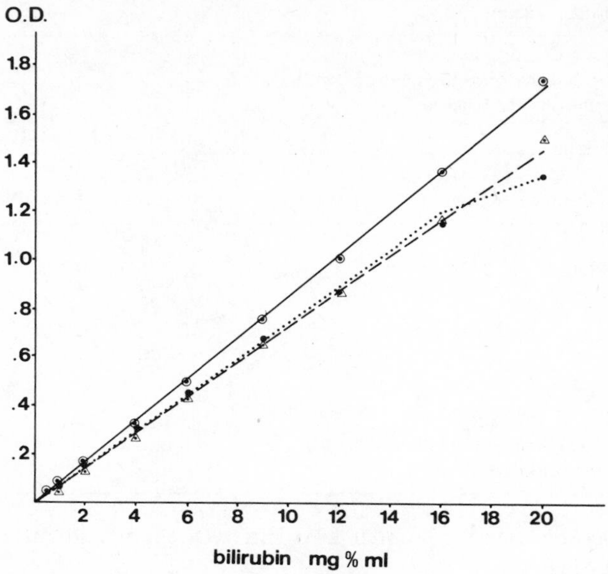

Fig. 1. Comparison of standard curves for bilirubin determination using different methods: DMFA (⊙); Malloy-Evelyn (●) and caffeine (△). Acid azobilirubin. Readings at 530 nm against the respective blanks with a double beam Optica spectrophotometer. A standard reference serum (Dade Bilirubin Control) has been used.

respectively than those for the *Malloy-Evelyn* [2] and for the *Simmons* methods [2]. These differences could be ascribed to differences in the spectrum of the colour formed, to a different reaction speed, or to a more complete reaction with the DMFA reagent.

The reaction speed of the various reactions was determined. As shown in fig. 2, the reaction with DMFA is complete in about 1 min, that with caffeine reaches a plateau in 3–4 min, while that with methanol requires at least 20 minutes to attain its equilibrium.

The readings for the curves were taken at 6 minutes after the start of the reaction for the first two methods and at 30 minutes with the *Malloy-Evelyn* method. The difference cannot therefore be ascribed to an incorrect timing of readings.

A comparison of the three absorption spectra shows complete identity between them (fig. 3).

It seems, therefore, permissible to conclude, that the higher absorption coefficient is due to a higher concentration of the azobilirubin product, namely to a more complete reaction.

Simple enhancement of the colour due to an optical effect of the solvent can be discarded on the basis of the following experiments.

When a bile solution, which is known to contain only conjugated bilirubin, is reacted both with the DMFA and the caffeine reagent, an identical absorption is obtained (fig. 2).

When a standard serum, which contains only unconjugated bilirubin, is treated with various DMFA reagents, without isopropanol or with various DMFA concentrations, the following results are obtained (fig. 4): when only isopropanol is omitted the reaction speed

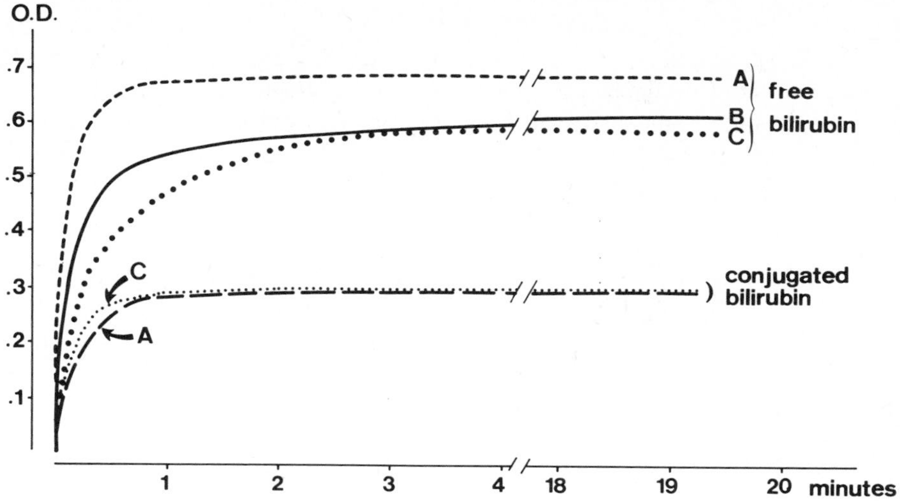

Fig. 2. Kinetics of reactions with various methods for free and conjugated bilirubin.
Upper row of curves: free bilirubin (8 mg per 100 ml) in a standard reference serum (Dade Bilirubin Control). Methods: A: DMFA; B: methanol and C caffeine.
Lower row of curves: bovine bile. Methods: A: DMFA; C: caffeine.
Tracings taken at 530 nm with an Optica double beam spectrophotometer against the respective blanks.

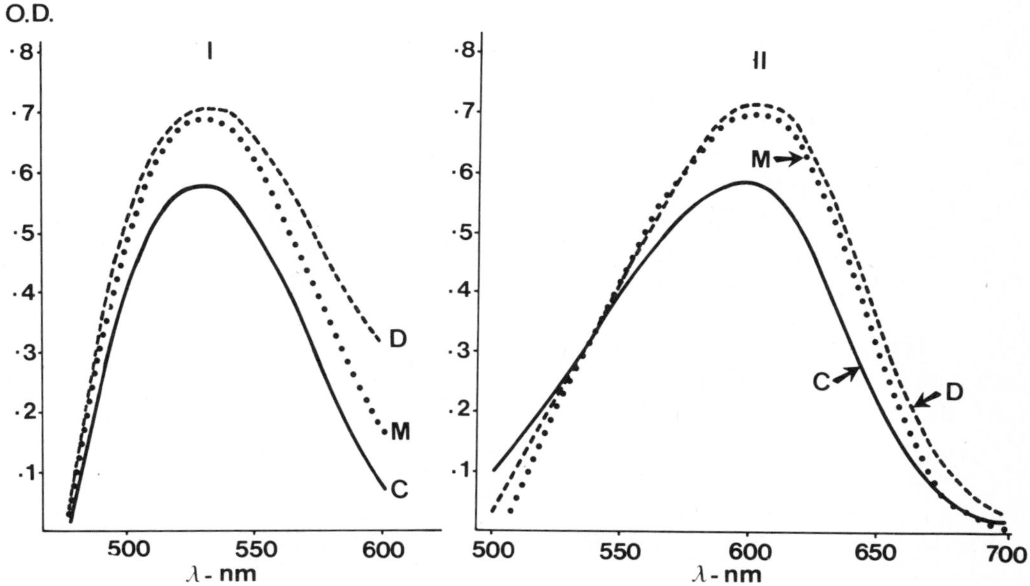

Fig. 3. Spectra at acid (I) and alkaline (II) pH for DMFA (D); Malloy-Evelyn (M); and caffeine (C) reaction. Bilirubin solutions at different concentrations.

is not changed, a plateau is rapidly reached, but the yield of colour is lower; when also the amount of DMFA is decreased, not only is there less colour, but the reaction speed is also much slower. Icteric sera from jaundiced patients behave quite differently (fig. 5); namely, the reaction speed is only slightly affected by withdrawal of isopropanol or decrease of DMFA. The colour produced is lower, however, in the latter case and does not increase with time after it has reached its plateau.

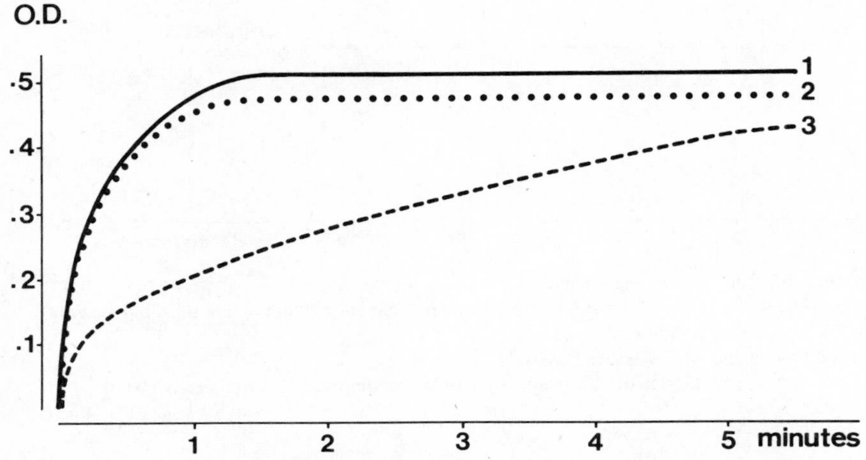

Fig. 4. Reaction of a standard serum (6.05 mg of free bilirubin per 100 ml) with various DMFA reagents: 1. Reagent with 50% DMFA + 5% isopropanol; 2. Reagent with 50% DMFA; 3. Reagent with 35% DMFA.

The above reported observations indicate:

1. That the rate of completion of the reaction is highly dependent on the reaction conditions. Those chosen for the DMFA method apparently give a more rapid reaction with unconjugated bilirubin than does the caffeine method. Increase of isopropanol concentration or the use of other solvents did not show any further colour increase, suggesting that the reaction is complete.
2. In contrast, colour production is the same for both caffeine and DMFA with conjugated bilirubin. Therefore the use of free bilirubin standards for conjugated bilirubin determination is open to question.
3. The reactivity of bilirubin in standard sera and in sera from patients appears to be quite different. Possibly, the binding of free bilirubin to proteins is not the same under natural and artificial conditions. These differences in reactivity can be overcome by appropriate determination conditions, for instance, by the addition of isopropanol in the DMFA reaction.
4. The validity of standards for bilirubin quantitation is dependent on the identity of their reaction with that of patients' sera. The caffeine reaction has been observed by

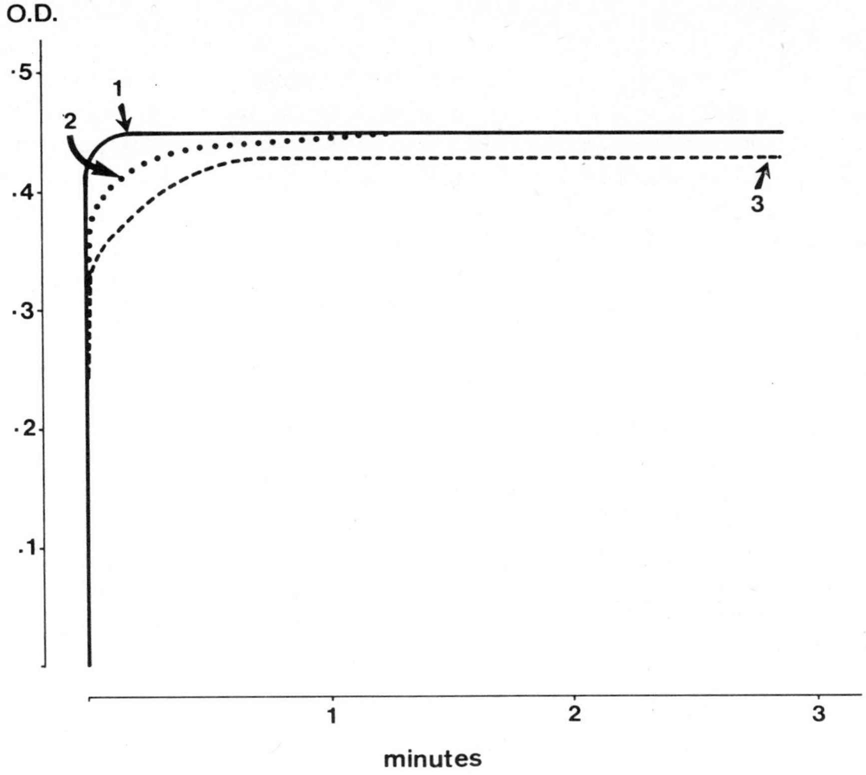

Fig. 5. Reaction of an icteric serum (5.35 mg total bilirubin per 100 ml) with various DMFA reagents.
1. Reagent with 50% DMFA + 5% isopropanol.
2. Reagent with 50% DMFA.
3. Reagent with 35% DMFA.

Michaëlsson [7] and *Simmons* [8] to give lower values for free as compared with conjugated bilirubin. If with the caffeine method the free bilirubin of patients sera reacts incompletely, as it does in standard sera, it is underestimated.
In contrast, free bilirubin is overestimated, because its concentration is calculated on the basis of an absorption coefficient lower than its actual value.

5. On the basis of the observations reported above, accurate free plus conjugated bilirubin measurement is, in principle, more likely to be attained with the DMFA than with the caffeine reaction.
Comparison of the two methods on a series of sera with various bilirubin levels gave results which were not, however, always easy to interpret.
This was presumably, largely a consequence of the different ratios of free and conjugated bilirubin in the various sera. The possible influence of differences in reactivity of

natural and standard sera, and of activators or inhibitors, must also be considered, and this deserves further investigation.

The availability of a certified conjugated bilirubin standard is an indispensable prerequisite to solving these very important and very intriguing accuracy problems, by determining its extinction coefficient by the two methods. Also a specific method, possibly that using ethyl anthranilate [9, 10] could be used to determine the true value of conjugated bilirubin present in sera and help establish the proper conditions for its accurate measurement by routinely applicable procedures.

References

[1] *Van den Bergh A.A.H. and Muller P.:* Biochem. Z. *77,* 90, 1916.
[2] *Malloy H.T. and Evelyn K.A.:* J. Biol. Chem. *119,* 481, 1937.
[3] *Jendrassik L. and Cleghorn R.A.:* Biochem. Z. *289,* 1, 1936.
[4] *Rappaport F. and Eichhorn F.:* Lancet *244,* 62, 1943.
[5] *Brückner J.:* Am. J. Clin. Pathol. *32,* 513, 1959.
[6] *Brückner J.:* Clin. Chim. Acta *6,* 370, 1960.
[7] *Michaëlsson M.:* Scand. J. Clin. Lab. Invest. *13* (Suppl. 56), 1, 1961.
[8] *Simmons N.A.:* J. Clin. Pathol. *21,* 196, 1968.
[9] *Van Roy F.P. and Heirwegh K.P.M.:* Biochem. J. *107,* 507, 1968.
[10] *Heirwegh K.P.M., Van Hees G.P., Leroy P., Van Roy F.P., Jansen F.H.:* Biochem. J. *120,* 877, 1970.

Comparison between Determination Methods

L. Havelec, Vienna (Austria)

Key words: Accuracy
Method comparison
Precision
Quality control

Summary

In survey-data from clinical chemical laboratories, the factor 'quality of laboratory' is confounded with the factor 'quality of method'. With the aim of comparison between determination methods, an attempt was made to disentangle these two factors by first estimating the working-quality of the laboratories and subsequently comparing the different methods with respect to the quality scores. For this estimation (accuracy and precision being treated separately), a ranking procedure has been developed. Allowance for missing data was also provided, by an adjustment of the ranking procedure.

An application, and comparison between determination methods is shown in the example of glucose determination using data from an Austrian survey.

In the course of introducing quality control into the work of clinical laboratories, several surveys on national and international bases have been performed. A great number of laboratories have participated, determined many components of sera and sent their results to the organizers for evaluation. As is well known, various laboratories often use different methods for the determination of a particular component. Whenever different methods are used, the question arises whether these methods are comparably good in accuracy and precision.

To find an answer to this question, when evaluating only results of surveys, is somewhat more difficult than would seem at first: laboratories are free to choose one of the existing determination methods which from then on they use routinely. Comparing the results of several laboratories using different methods we easily can establish which values come nearer to the reference-value or which laboratory has the better precision. But we cannot answer the question concerning the quality of different methods used, because the factor 'working-quality of the laboratory' is completely confounded with the factor 'quality of method'. For example, if a 'good' laboratory uses an inferior method it might not achieve accurate and precise values, nor will a sloppy laboratory obtain good results even when using the best method. Comparing the values determined, it is impossible to decide whether a bad result is due to the poor quality of the method used or to unreliable work in the laboratory.

A way to obviate the difficulties just described, is to try to assess the working-quality of the laboratories and then to compare the determination methods with respect to the quality of the laboratories.

This was done in the present report using data from an Austrian survey (*Bauer* et al., 1971) with 52 participating laboratories.

The participants got several packs of a control serum containing 27 components in 2 different lots and were supposed to analyze them on 19 consecutive working days. The reference-values for all components were known to the organizers.

Taking into account all components evaluated, the laboratories were ranked according to their accuracy and their precision.

Ranking for accuracy

As the number of determinations was not equal for both lots, for each component and each laboratory the weighted mean of the absolute differences ($\bar{d}$) between the means ($\bar{x}_1$, $\bar{x}_2$) and the reference-values (R_1, R_2) was calculated:

$$\bar{d} = \frac{|\bar{x}_1 - R_1|\, n_1 + |\bar{x}_2 - R_2|\, n_2}{n_1 + n_2} \qquad (1)$$

n_1 and n_2 being the number of determinations of lot 1 and 2. For each component the laboratories were ranked according to the size of $\bar{d}$, the one with the smallest $\bar{d}$ getting rank 1 and the one with the greatest $\bar{d}$ getting rank L (L being the number of laboratories which had determined the component). In the next step, the ranks of each laboratory were summed and ranked again to obtain a global rank score for accuracy. Table 1 shows an example for this procedure.

Table 1. Example for calculation of global rank scores for accuracy.

components	lab. no. 1		2		3		4		5	
	$\bar{d}$	rank score	$\bar{d}$	rank score	$\bar{d}$	rank score	$\bar{d}$	rank score	$\bar{d}$	rank score
sodium	5,67	**4**	11,90	**5**	0,42	**1**	1,84	**3**	0,84	**2**
potassium	0,11	**2**	0,20	**5**	0,03	**1**	0,17	**4**	0,15	**3**
glucose	4,06	**4**	8,18	**5**	1,16	**2**	3,92	**3**	0,87	**1**
bilirubin	0,05	**1**	0,38	**4**	0,10	**3**	0,48	**5**	0,06	**2**
sum of rank scores		**11**		**19**		**7**		**15**		**8**
global rank score		**3**		**5**		**1**		**4**		**2**

Ranking for day-to-day precision

For precision,the weighted mean standard deviation ($\bar{s}$) were calculated:

$$\bar{s} = \left(\frac{\sum_{1}^{n_1} (x_1 - \bar{x}_1)^2 + \sum_{1}^{n_2} (x_2 - \bar{x}_2)^2}{n_1 + n_2 - 2} \right) \qquad (2)$$

By analogy to the above described ranking procedure, a global rank score was also attained for day-to-day precision. An example is given in table 2.

Table 2. Example for calculation of global rank scores for precision.

components	lab. no.									
	1		2		3		4		5	
	$\bar{s}$	rank score	$\bar{s}$	rank score	$\bar{s}$	rank score	$\bar{s}$	rank score	$\bar{s}$	rank score
sodium	3,11	**3**	4,77	**4**	2,62	**2**	5,24	**5**	1,69	**1**
potassium	0,13	**2**	0,23	**5**	0,07	**1**	0,18	**3**	0,20	**4**
glucose	4,24	**3**	5,77	**4**	1,48	**1**	7,36	**5**	2,03	**2**
bilirubin	0,10	**3**	0,09	**2**	0,05	**1**	0,14	**5**	0,13	**4**
sum of rank scores		**11**		**15**		**5**		**18**		**11**
global rank score		**2,5**		**4**		**1**		**5**		**2,5**

The global rank scores served as indicators for the working-quality of each laboratory, separately assessed for accuracy and precision.

Missing data

Most of the laboratories were not able to analyze all components of the serum. For the intended comparison between determination methods, only those laboratories which had analyzed at least half of the components and only those components which had been analyzed by at least half of the laboratories were taken into the study. 30 laboratories from the original 52 participants and 14 components met these conditions. Figure 1 shows the components and the number of determinations made by each laboratory.

Each line represents one component. Black fields indicate which of the 30 laboratories had not determined the particular component. In the ranking procedure each laboratory had to get a rank score for each component, also for those which had actually not been

Figure 1: Components selected for evaluation of global scores for accuracy and precision and number of components determined by each laboratory.

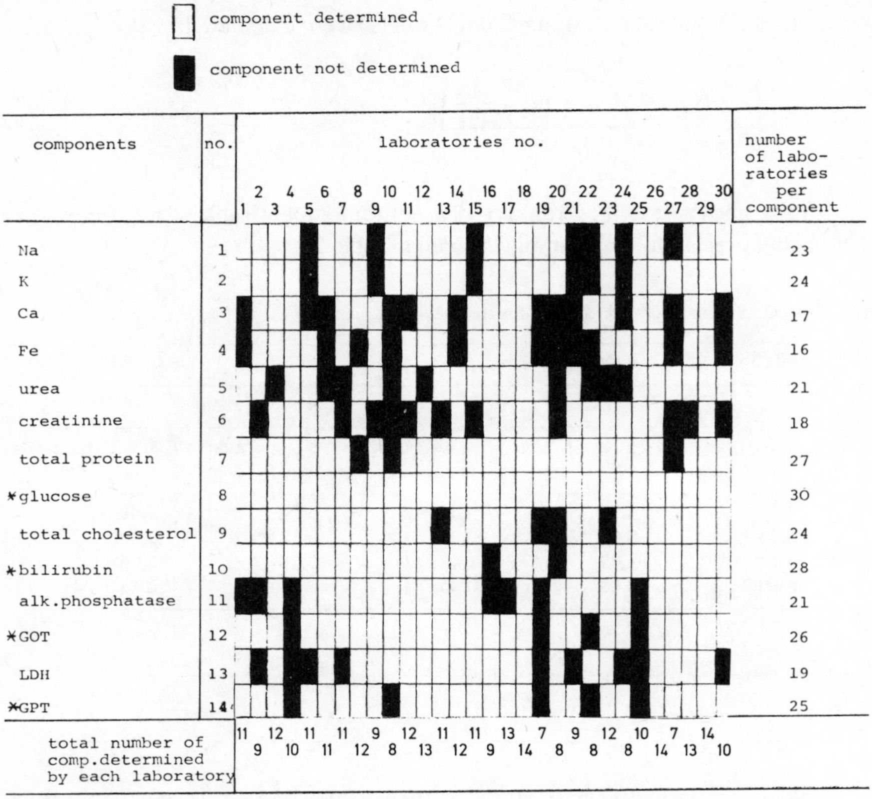

Number of laboratories per component ≧ 15.
Number of components determined by each laboratory ≧ 7.

* component selected for comparison between methods.

determined. For these components with missing determinations, the rank scores for the laboratories were calculated in the following way[1]:

L = total number of laboratories

r = number of laboratories which determined the component

The r existing $\bar{d}$ ($\bar{s}$) were ordered according to their size and given increasing rank scores:

$$\frac{L+1}{r+1}, \quad \frac{2(L+1)}{r+1}, \quad \ldots \frac{r(L+1)}{r+1}.$$

(In case of r = L these scores are the integers 1, 2 ... L).

[1] This method has been developed following a suggestion of Dr. Schreiber in our institute.

The sum of these rank scores is

$$r \frac{\frac{L+1}{r+1} + \frac{r(L+1)}{r+1}}{2} = \frac{r(L+1)}{2} \qquad (3)$$

Each of the L – r laboratories with missing determinations was given the mean score $\frac{L+1}{2}$. The sum of these scores is

$$(L-r) \quad \frac{L+1}{2} \qquad (4)$$

Formulas (3) and (4) were developed to give equal sums of rank scores for all components:

$$r \frac{L+1}{2} + (L-r) \frac{L+1}{2} = 1 \frac{L+1}{2} \qquad (5)$$

After calculation of the rank scores for all components the global score for each laboratory can be determined as is shown above in table 1 and 2.

Testing the correlation between accuracy and precision using the global rank scores the *Spearman* coefficient of correlation r_s was calculated:

$$r_s = 1 - \frac{6 \sum_{1}^{n} D^2}{n(n^2-1)} \qquad (6)$$

D = difference between the rank scores for accuracy and precision for each laboratory
n = number of laboratories

A highly significant correlation was found between overall accuracy and precision of the laboratories ($r_s = 0.57$, $n = 30$, $p < 0.001$). This result is consistent with a previously reported analysis (*Bauer* et al., 1973), which had been obtained for another group of laboratories. It should be noted, however, that a similar correlation between accuracy and precision was not found for every component when considered individually.

For the statistical evaluation, one diagram was designed for accuracy and one for precision (see fig. 2 and 3). In the diagrams, the global rank of the laboratories is given on the abscissa. Their rank for the determination of the individual component is given on the ordinate. According to its global rank and to its rank of determination, each laboratory is represented in the diagram by one mark, a dot or a triangle, depending on the method used.

Figure 2: Diagram for accuracy.

Methods used for glucose determination: ▼ non-enzymatic n = 9
● enzymatic n = 21

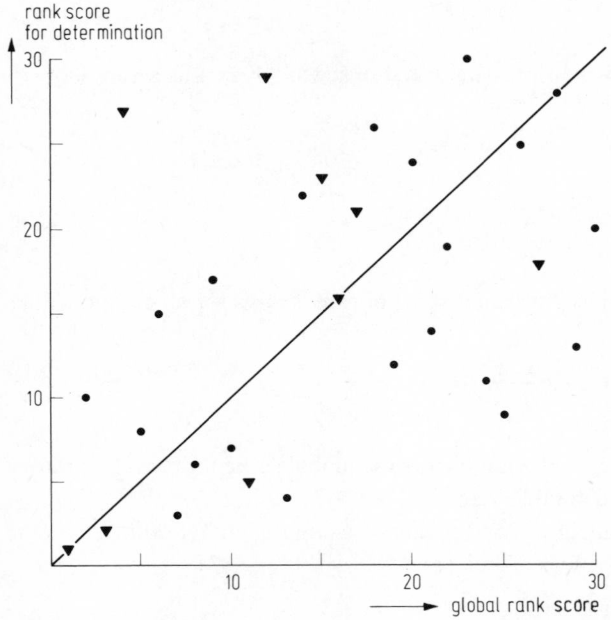

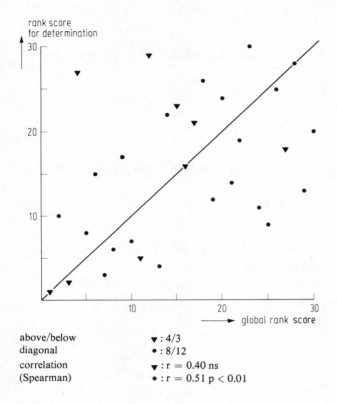

above/below diagonal	▼ : 4/3
	● : 8/12
correlation (Spearman)	▼ : r = 0.40 ns
	● : r = 0.51 $p < 0.01$

Ideally, if the accuracy or precision for the determination of an individual component would conform to the global accuracy or precision of the laboratories and if there was no difference between the methods used, all marks would fall on a 45° diagonal. Marks above the diagonal indicate worse results than those corresponding to the working-quality of the laboratories, and vice versa. A discrimination between methods can only be accomplished if the marks for different methods lie mostly on different sides of the diagonal. If, for example, dots lie mostly above and triangles mostly below the diagonal, this would indicate that the method marked by triangles is the better one, because laboratories using this method achieved better results than would be expected from their quality score. On the other hand, dots and triangles scattered equally on both sides of the diagonal or lying all near the diagonal can be taken as an indication of both methods being comparably good.

Figure 3: Diagram for precision.

Methods used for glucose determination: ▾ non-enzymatic n = 9 ● enzymatic n = 21

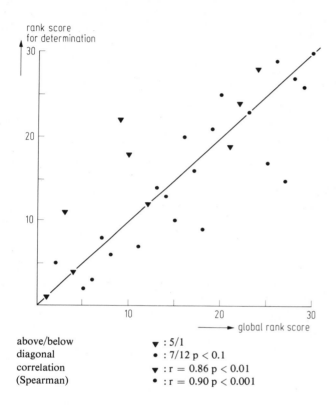

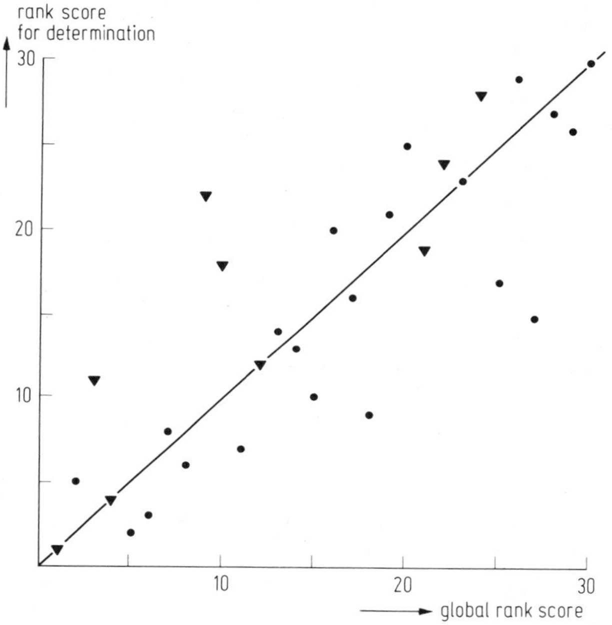

above/below diagonal	▾ : 5/1
	• : 7/12 $p < 0.1$
correlation (Spearman)	▾ : $r = 0.86$ $p < 0.01$
	• : $r = 0.90$ $p < 0.001$

Additional information about the determination methods was gained by calculating the following coefficients of correlation for each method: correlation between accuracy and global rank score for accuracy, correlation between precision and global rank score for precision, and finally correlation between accuracy and precision (fig. 4).

Figure 4: Correlation between accuracy and precision.

Methods used for glucose determination: ▲ non-enzymatic n = 9; ● enzymatic n = 21

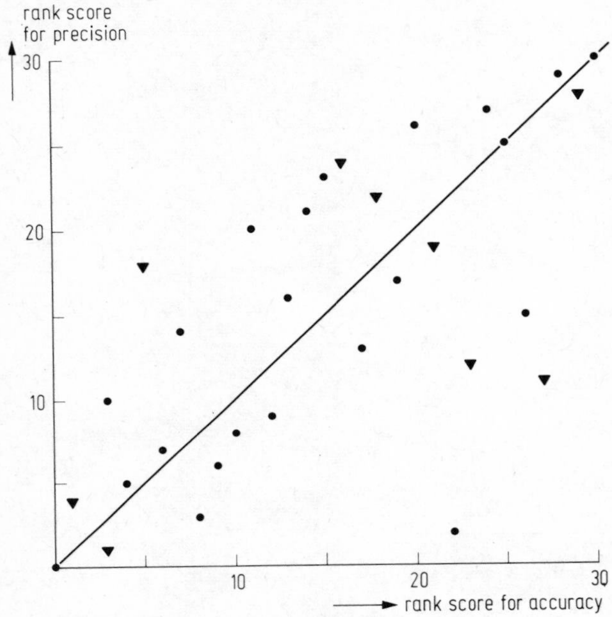

correlation (Spearman): ▼ $r = 0.50$ ns; ● $r = 0.67$ $p < 0.001$

The comparison between determination methods using the global rank scores for the working quality of the laboratories is demonstrated using the example of glucose determination.

Results

Methods used: non-enzymatic (▲) 9 laboratories
enzymatic (●) 21 laboratories

Accuracy (fig. 2): The proportion of marks above and below the diagonal is 4 : 3 for non-enzymatic and 8 : 12 for enzymatic methods. Although no statistical significance is attained, there is a fairly marked trend towards a superiority of enzymatic methods.

The coefficient of correlation between accuracy of glucose determination and global score for accuracy is significant only for enzymatic methods. This means that the statement 'the better the laboratory the better the results' holds only for enzymatic methods.

Precision (fig. 3): For precision, the proportion of marks on either side of the diagonal is 5 : 1 for non-enzymatic and 7 : 12 for enzymatic methods. The probability of this result is $p < 0.1$, indicating a superiority of enzymatic methods.

As can be judged by eye, the correlation between the precision of glucose determination and the global precision score is high for both methods, all dots and triangles lying close to the diagonal.

Summarizing the results of accuracy as well as precision, the discrimination favours enzymatic methods.

Correlation between accuracy and precision (fig. 4)

The correlation between accuracy and precision is significant for enzymatic methods only, indicating that for these methods increasing accuracy in general is also connected with increasing precision.

In the absence of a similar correlation for non-enzymatic methods, this result can be interpreted as an additional argument in favour of enzymatic methods.

Since the superiority of enzymatic methods for glucose determination is generally accepted, the results obtained support the applicability of the procedure presented in discriminating between different determination methods on the basis of surveys.

References

[1] *Bauer, P., Gabl, F., Havelec, L., Kaiser, E., Scheiber, V. and Wohlzogen, F.X.:* Vorläufiger Bericht über den österreichischen Seronorm-Rundversuch 1970. Österr. Ärztezeitung 26, p. 204 (1971).

[2] *Bauer, P., Havelec, L., Kaiser, E., Scheiber, V. and Wohlzogen, F.X.:* Ein Vorschlag zur Reihung Klinisch-Chemischer Laboratorien nach der Zuverlässigkeit ihrer Analysenergebnisse. Z. Klin. Chem. Klin. Biochem. 11, p. 174 (1973).

Interlaboratory Quality Control using the Daily Means of Patients' Results

R. Leclercq, Brussels (Belgium)

Key words: Acid-base, Daily means, Glucose, Quality Control, Sodium, Urea

Introduction

The aim of our work was to establish the validity of the daily mean of patients results as a useful tool of quality control, not only in a single laboratory, but in two laboratories, the 'Institut Médico-Chirurgical d'Anderlecht (I.M.C.A.)' and the 'Institut Edith Cavell Marie Depage (I.E.C.)', serving highly different patient populations. The use of control sera does not check more than the analytical process alone; it is evident that all the steps preceding the analytical ones are not studied by this method. Furthermore, the technicians are usually accustomed to finding the known values for the control sera and they may, consciously or not, adapt the results to the expected value. On the other hand, it is frequently impossible to obtain every day a sufficient number of control sera results to establish statistically significant values.

These limitations are not encountered with the use of patients' results. Indeed the technician cannot presume the effect of each individual result on the daily mean and furthermore all results (provided they fall between preestablished truncation limits) contribute to the mean.

However, three conditions must be met for a valid use of the daily mean of patients results as a quality control system:

1. The extreme values which markedly influence the mean must be equally distributed around the mean; this restriction can be disregarded by using truncation limits in order to eliminate these extreme values.
2. The population served must be sufficiently constant regarding age, sex, proportion of in- and outpatients, and pathology.
3. A sufficient number of patients' results must be obtained to compute a statistically significant mean. It is generally admitted that 30 specimens per day represent the minimum acceptable.

Provided these three conditions are met, the daily mean of patients' results may be used as a quality control tool, even in laboratories without a big computer's equipment. Indeed, to establish the criteria of validity, we worked only with a desk computer of 1.8 kwords capacity. The simplest programmable calculator is satisfactory to exclude the extreme values and to compute the mean and standard deviation of the remaining results.

Material and Methods

Patients' data

Results were collected in the two laboratories whose populations characteristics are described in table 1. In both laboratories, the same analytical methods were used and in most events the same batches of control sera were utilized.

Table 1.

	I.E.C.	I.M.C.A.
Patients' Mean Age	40 years	60 years
Mean Hospital Stay	5.5 days	15 days
Socio-economic Status	high	average to low
Ratio out-/inpatients	80/20	40/60
Pathology justifying hospitalization	Mostly obstetrical and surgical	70% requests for medical cases

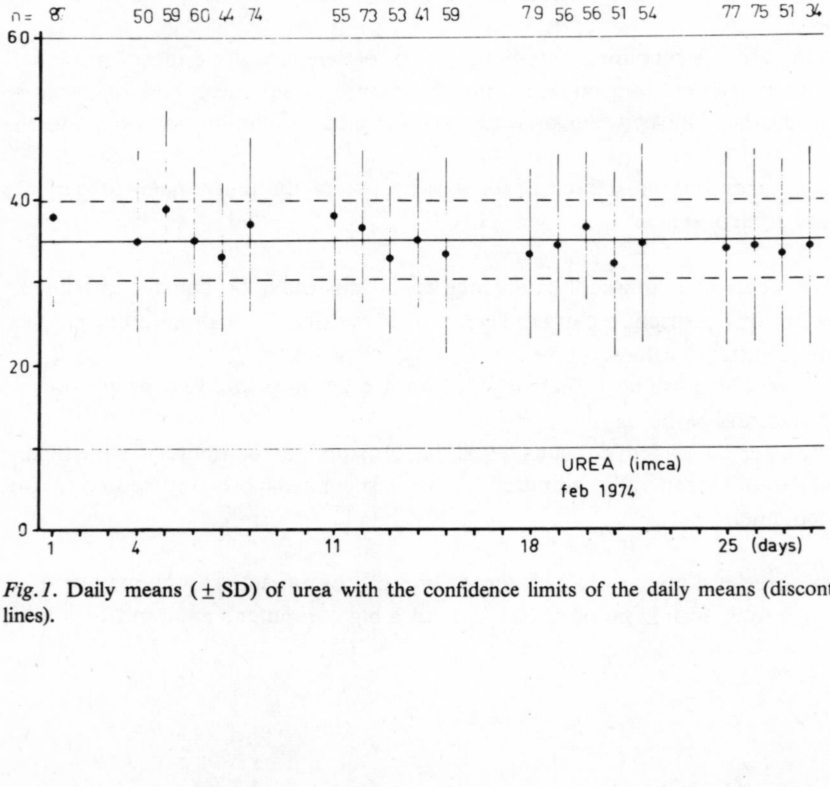

Fig. 1. Daily means (± SD) of urea with the confidence limits of the daily means (discontinuous horizontal lines).

Daily means

Every day, the daily mean of each of the 19 parameters under control is compared to the confidence interval of the daily means previously recorded (fig. 1) and every month, the monthly mean of the daily means is recorded with the confidence interval (fig. 2) and compared to the preceding value. During these computations, all patients' results within the truncation limits obtained during the month are computed together and their mean and standard deviation are recorded.

OBJET
VOORWERP

RELEVES STATISTIQUES DU LABORATOIRE

Mois de novembre 1973

ANNEXE
BIJLAGE

	MOYENNES JOURNALIERES				VALEURS INDIVIDUELLES			
Analyse	nb	moyenne	sigma	C.V.	nb	moyenne	sigma	C.V.
Sodium	16	138,384	1,071	0,8	922	138,359	4,676	3,4
Potassium	16	4,236	0,119	2,8	919	4,233	0,657	15,5
Chlore	16	101,820	1,315	1,3	922	101,729	5,249	5,2
Calcium	9	9,386	0,225	2,4	232	9,364	0,635	6,8
Phosphore	9	3,684	0,343	9,3	225	3,736	0,762	20,4
Glucose	18	99,820	2,827	2,8	1358	99,959	17,983	18,0
Urée	18	36,638	2,496	6,8	1241	36,626	10,335	28,2
Créatinine	18	1,197	0,066	5,5	1184	1,198	0,383	32,0
Ac. urique	18	5,946	0,256	4,3	1044	5,964	1,448	24,3
Prot. tot.	18	7,350	0,218	3,0	606	7,342	0,689	9,4
Albumine	18	4,277	0,187	4,4	603	4,282	0,590	13,8
pH veineux	19	7,379	0,010	0,1	855	7,370	0,042	0,6
Bicarb.Stand	19	23,321	0,406	1,7	854	23,357	2,319	9,9
pCO_2	19	39,380	2,136	5,4	854	39,566	7,129	18,0
C.P.K.	18	23,815	5,128	21,5	871	22,895	10,977	47,9
GOT	18	24,652	2,164	8,8	852	24,503	9,303	38,0
GPT	16	23,403	2,682	11,5	761	23,424	10,412	44,5
LDH	18	302,067	18,949	6,3	861	301,834	61,466	20,4
a HBDH	16	137,501	7,399	5,4	759	138,235	30,675	22,2

Fig. 2. Statistical data obtained monthly.

Left four columns: number of days, mean of the daily means, their standard deviation and coefficient of variation.

Right four columns: the same values for all results obtained during the month and falling between the truncation limits.

Validation studies

For the systematic studies, either 2000 results or all values recorded during at least one month for a given parameter are transferred onto a magnetic tape in batches corresponding to the working days during which they were obtained.

From this tape, the following computations are obtained:

1. the histogram of patients' data with or without truncation limits, simultaneously with the mean, the standard deviation and the chi square test for non normality of the distribution.
2. the daily means as a function of the various truncation limits introduced.
3. the daily means after introduction of a systematic error through addition or subtraction of either a definite amount or a percentage of each result and the subsequent use of the truncation limits.
   The addition or subtraction of a definite amount was previously studied by Dixon and Northam (1970). In our experience of the daily mean, it is much easier to detect this kind of error than a percentage error; moreover a percentage error is much more frequent as the result of a calibration error with the third generation of Technicon equipment and more generally with all methods using a 2-point calibration system. Consequently our further studies were based on a percentage error only.

Using our results and with the aid of the previous works of *Owen* and *Campbell* (1968), *Dixon* and *Northam* (1970) and *Lewis* and *Dixon* (1971), we were able to select the optimal truncation limits in order to obtain simultaneously the lowest variability in the daily mean and the highest recovery of the introduced error, which is called 'sensitivity' and is represented by the ratio of the induced change in the daily mean to the change introduced. The combination of these two values in the formula $m = t \cdot SD/R$ (where t is the value of the Student's table for the chosen probability, SD the standard deviation of the daily mean and R the sensitivity) allows one to determine m which is called the 'minimal detectable change in accuracy'. From figure 3 it can be seen that the minimal detectable change varies with the truncation limits, reaching an optimum. This operation must be repeated for each parameter studied.

Analytical methods

From the nineteen parameters under study, we selected four for detailed presentation: sodium, glucose, urea and the acid-base equilibrium.

Sodium was estimated on a flame IV photometer, glucose using an hexokinase method and urea with a diacetyl-monoxime technique, these three determinations being performed on an SMA 12/60 Technicon. Acid-base equilibrium was estimated first on an Astrup apparatus; later using direct measurement of the CO_2 by a specific electrode in the IL 413 or the Corning equipment.

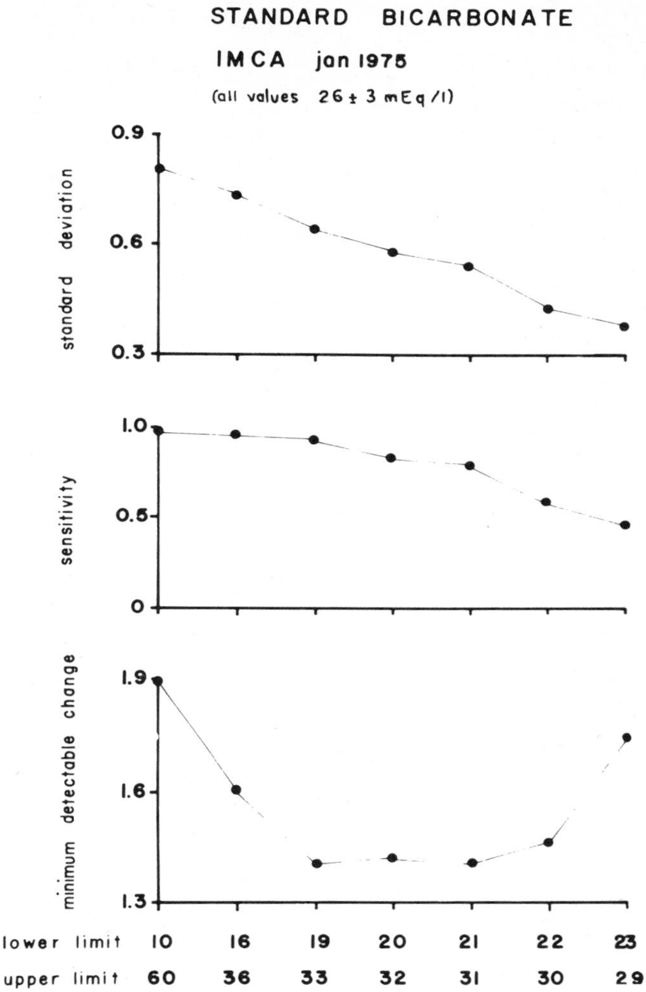

Fig. 3. Determination of the truncation limits.
Upper graph: standard deviation of the daily means as a function of the truncation limits.
Middle graph: sensitivity of the daily mean.
Lower graph: minimum detectable change.

Results and Discussion

Problems encountered being clearly different for each of the selected parameters, we will present the results and the discussion grouped by analysis.

Sodium

Sodium is evidently a very favourable determination for any quality control system; indeed the analytical variability is reduced and furthermore the inter-individual variation is generally limited. We choose truncation limits set arbitrarily at 125 and 155 mEq/l. Before beginning our study we compared the monthly means of all the control sera obtained during two consecutive months in both laboratories (fig. 4). Despite the fact that in the I.E.C. laboratory the coefficient of variation of the control sera was systematically lower than in the I.M.C.A. laboratory, the mean values were completely comparable for the 'normal' as well as for the 'pathological' serum. Furthermore, the found values were in excellent agreement with the values given by the manufacturer. Methodological differences between laboratories could thus be excluded.

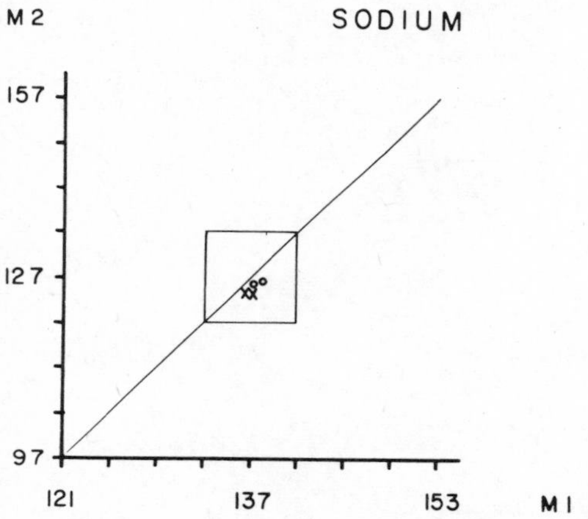

Fig. 4. Youden plot of the monthly means of 2 control sera in I.E.C. (circles) and I.M.C.A. (crosses) during 2 months.

At I.M.C.A. we worked with three control sera, the two first being commercial control sera with a known value, the third one being 'unknown' from animal origin.

Figure 5 shows the results obtained each working day for two consecutive months at I.M.C.A. with the daily means of patients' results of each of the three control sera, and the proportion of hospitalized patients. The coefficient of variation of the control sera is always greater than that of the daily mean. Moreover, we were able to confirm the statement of *Dixon* and *Northam* (1970) that the daily mean was higher when the proportion of ambulatory patients increased.

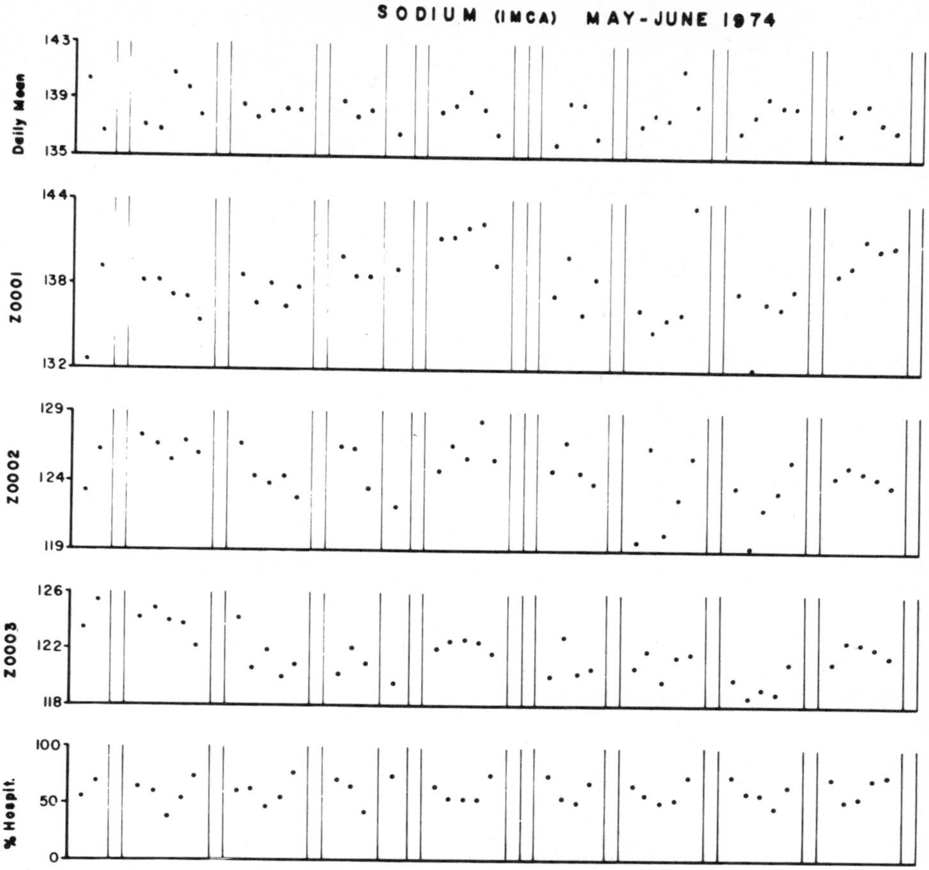

Fig. 5. Upper graph: daily means of patients results (truncation limits: 125–155 mEq/l).
Three middle graphs: daily mean values for the quality control sera.
Lower graph: % hospitalized patients in total determinations.

At I. E. C. two control sera of different origin were used (fig. 6). In this hospital, the proportion of outpatients is more important and the analytical variability is less marked. The dispersion of the daily means was strictly comparable to that of the 'normal' control serum.

The comparison of the monthly means of the daily means in both laboratories is presented in figure 7. As expected, the variation was less important in I.E.C. laboratory (circles) than in I.M.C.A. one (crosses). However, in this latter laboratory, the dispersion was dramatically reduced by including in the computations all results produced, even those corresponding to non-requested determinations (change after the discontinuous vertical line).

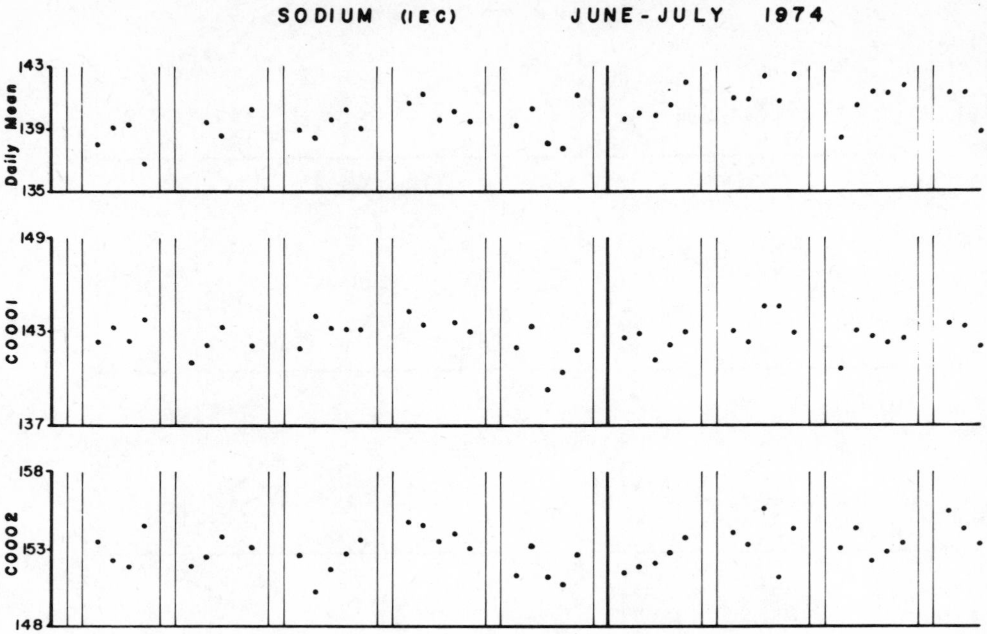

Fig. 6. Upper graph: daily means of patients results (same limits as in fig. 5).
Two lower graphs: daily mean values for the control sera.

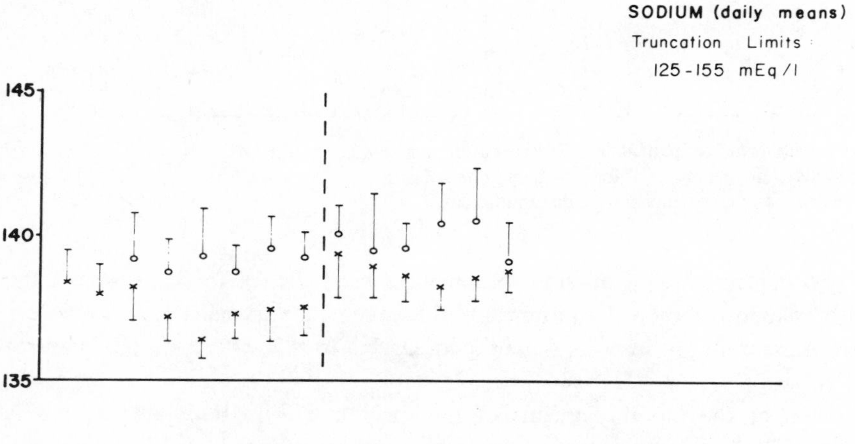

	N	D73	J74	F	M	A	M	J	J	A	S	O	N	D74
n_x =	962	994	1098	867	1075	1093	1036	1118	1364	1437	1428	1736	1225	1539
n_o =			384	347	349	338	350	337	919	910	1431	1663	1428	1723

Fig. 7. Means (± SD) of the daily means established monthly. I.M.C.A. = crosses; I.E.C. = circles.
In the lower part, number of determinations computed each month.

From the data of I.M.C.A. laboratory we tried to obtain graphically an expression of the sensitivity of the daily method mean. In this attempt we introduced a systematic error corresponding to an artefactual increase or decrease of 3% on each individual value during this 2 months' period. It can be seen from figure 8 that the statistical limits for the daily mean during this period were 136 and 141 mEq/l. The values obtained after multiplying each result by 1.03 were all largely above the mean of all the daily means and conversely all the daily means computed after the multiplication by 0.97 were below the mean. Furthermore, if we restrict the confidence limits to 137 and 140 mEq/l, we lose only one daily mean of unmodified data and all but one of the means of 'erroneous' values are detected. Thus for a laboratory having a workload of 60 samples per day and in the case of an average reproducibility (mean coefficient of variation for the control sera = 2.2%) the daily mean of patients results is a useful tool of quality control. On the other hand, in a laboratory where the coefficient of variation of control sera is only 1.2%, this is the best index.

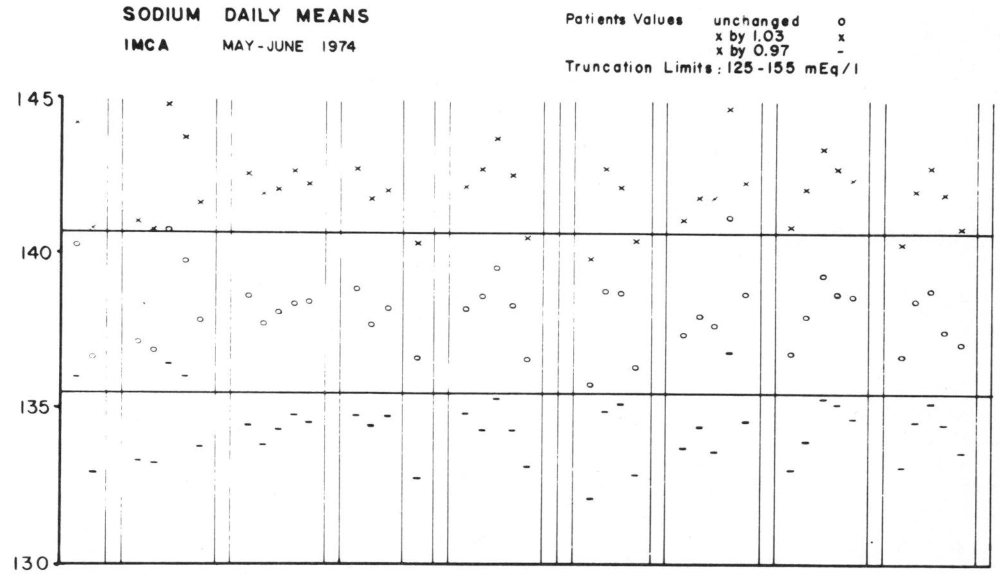

Fig. 8. Effect of multiplying each patient's result by 1.03 (crosses) or by 0.97 (horizontal bars) and computing thereafter the daily mean between truncation limits.

Comparison with data from unchanged values (circles) and with the confidence limits of the daily means (horizontal lines).

Finally, in the very favourable case of sodium, changing the truncation limits has only a limited influence on the mean and standard deviation of the daily means of patients results (table 2). It would be hazardous to imagine that the same would be true for any other parameter.

Table 2.

Limits	Month	Daily Mean	S.D.	C.V.	% determinations accounted
Sodium (mEq/l)					
none	May 74	138.1	1.2	0.87	100
	June 74	138.0	1.3	0.93	
125–155	May 74	138.3	1.1	0.83	98
	June 74	138.1	1.3	0.89	
130–146	May 74	138.5	1.0	0.70	93
	June 74	138.4	1.0	0.73	
Glucose (mg/100 ml)					
none	May 74	102.6	4.6	4.5	100
	June 74	103.8	4.9	4.7	
50–150	May 74	94.8	3.4	3.6	89
	June 74	95.1	4.0	4.2	
65–120	May 74	91.5	2.5	2.8	79
	June 74	91.9	3.3	3.6	
70–110	May 74	89.9	2.1	2.3	68
	June 74	89.9	2.3	2.6	

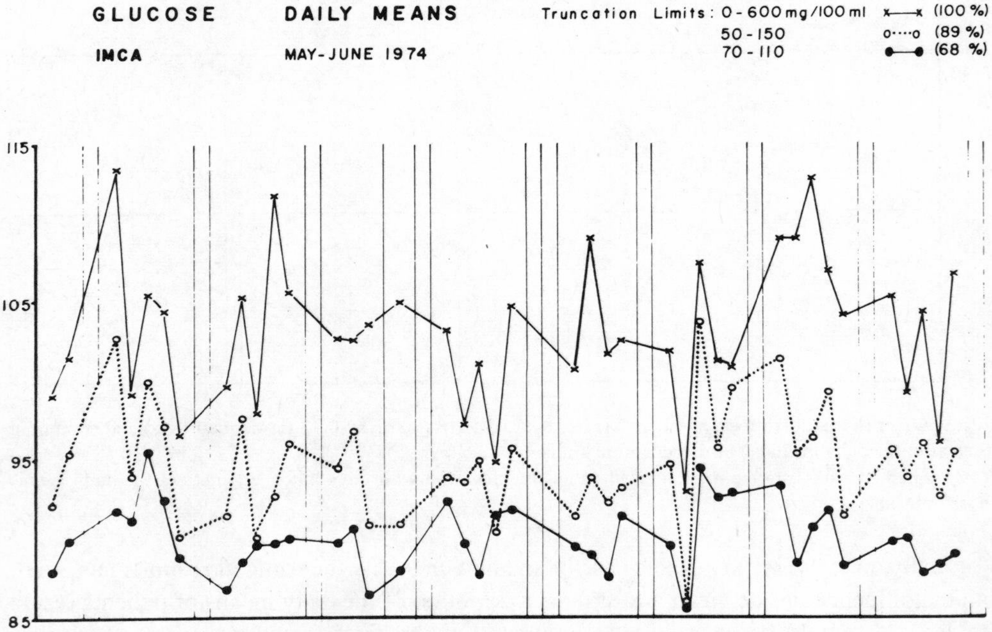

Fig. 9. Effect of change of the truncation limits on the daily mean of patients' results.

Glucose

For glucose conversely, the change of the truncation limits induces a marked change in the mean of patients' results and even more in the coefficient of variation of the daily mean, which is markedly reduced when the limits are narrowed (table 2, fig. 9).

Figure 10 illustrates the expected difference between the populations served by both laboratories; it is evident that none of these distributions can be considered as gaussian; however, restricting the limits to 50 and 150 mg/100 ml tends to reduce the deviation from normality.

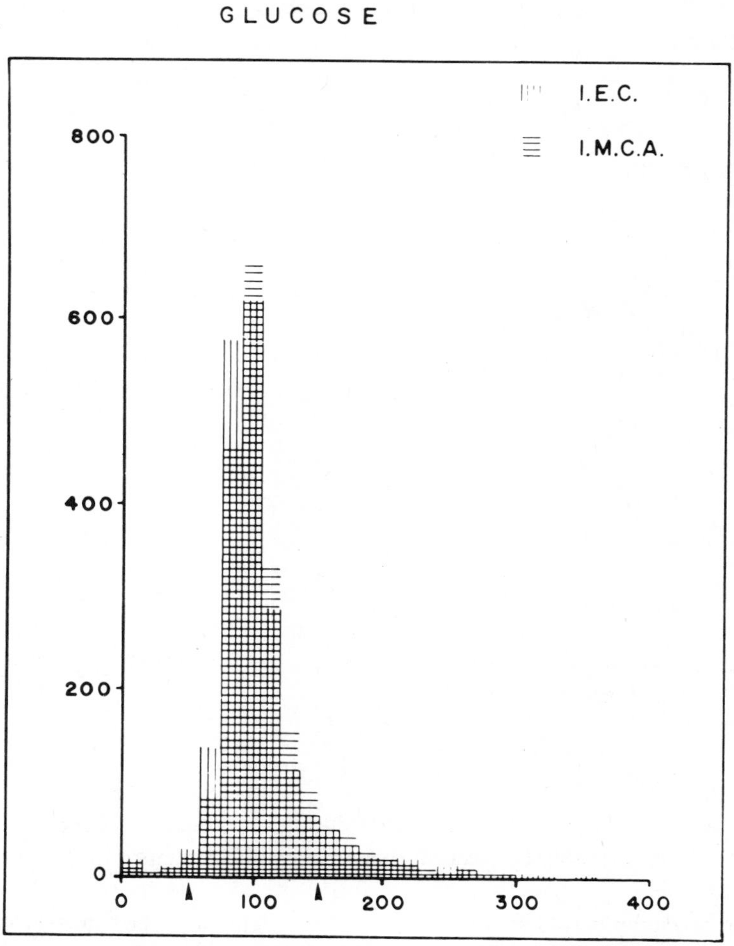

Fig. 10. Histograms of 2000 patients' results consecutively obtained at I.M.C.A. (horizontally hatched columns) and at I.E.C. (vertically hatched columns).

Values expressed in mg/100 ml.

The monthly means of the quality control sera were again compared between laboratories and in regard to the values given by the manufacturer, unfortunately not for the hexokinase method (fig. 11). It can be seen that the found values are consistently lower than those quoted: this is probably due to the difference of the methodologies. The full circle represents the value obtained. At I.E.C. in the first month of utilization of the hexokinase method, as a consequence of the adaptation to the new method, there was an abnormally high coefficient of variation for both control sera (11.9 and 9.2%); next month the situation was normalized and the coefficients of variation fell to 4.2 and 2.8%, largely below values found at I.M.C.A. (average coefficient of variation: about 7%). The mean values of the control sera were however not significantly different, allowing the comparison of patients results from both laboratories.

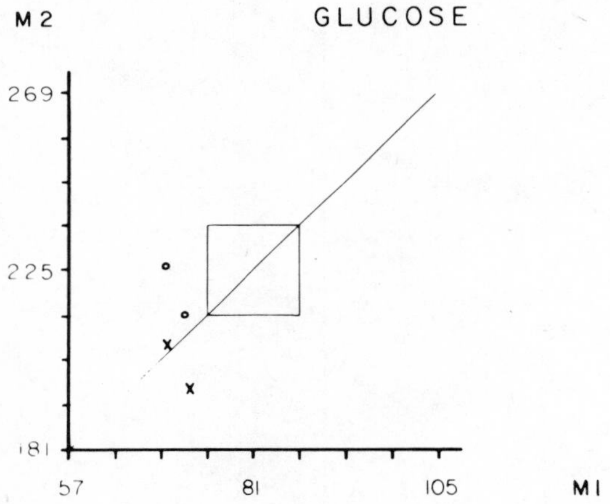

Fig. 11. Youden Plot of the monthly means of two control sera in I.M.C.A. (crosses) and at I.E.C. (first month of hexokinase utilization: full circle; second month: open circle).

Figure 12 shows the mean results obtained at I.M.C.A. during two consecutive months. We were not able to find any relationship between the percentage of inpatients and the daily mean of patients'results.

Mean values of a corresponding period at I.E.C. are shown on figure 13. The same scale was used for both the 'normal' and the 'pathological' control sera to allow a direct comparison of the results dispersion on figure 12 and 13. On figure 12, the whole scale is practically used; on figure 13, only one half to one third.

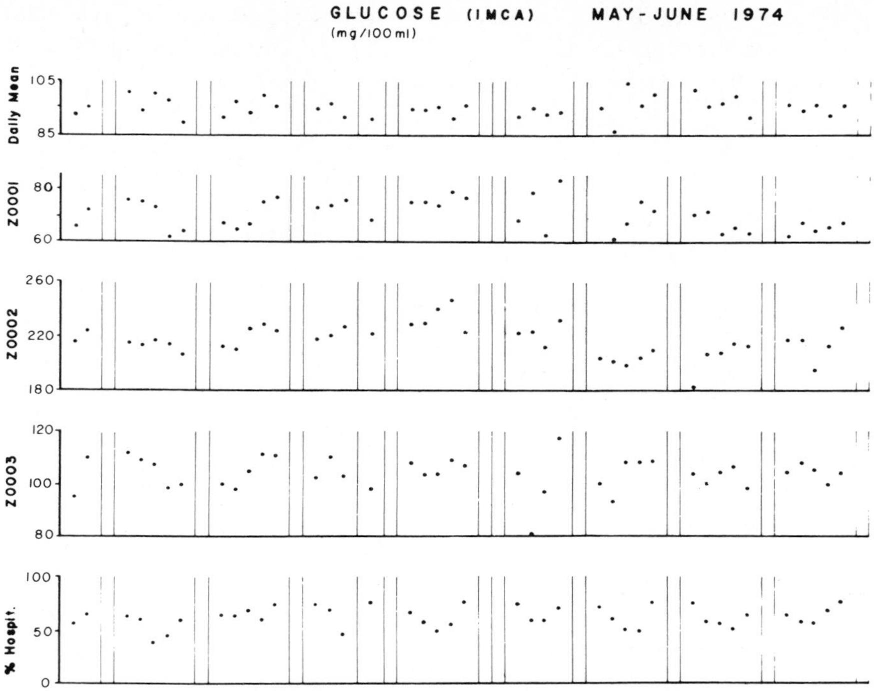

Fig. 12. Upper graph: daily means of patients' results (truncation limits: 50–150 mg/100 ml).
Three middle graphs: daily mean values for the quality control sera.
Lower graph: % hospitalized patients in total determinations.

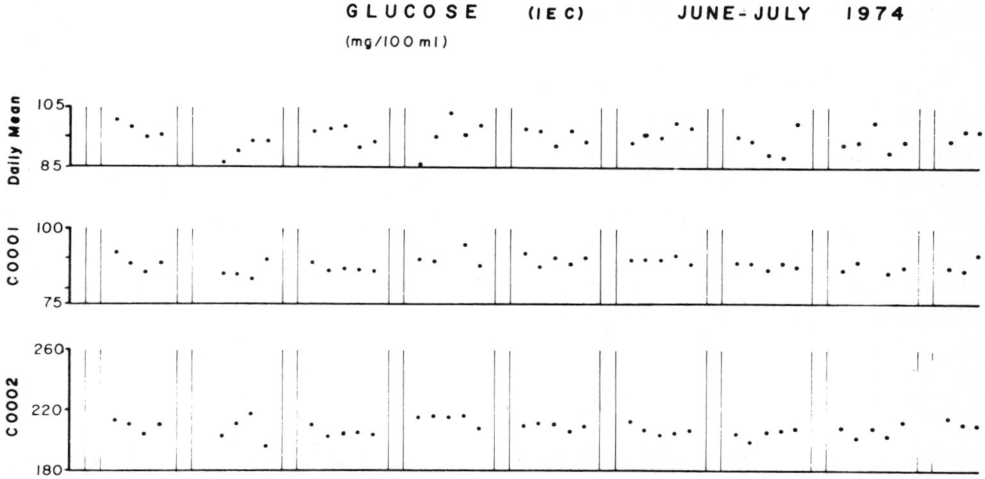

Fig. 13. Upper graph: daily means of patients' results (same limits as in fig. 12).
Two lower graphs: daily mean values for control sera.

However,this better reproducibility for control sera is not reflected in a reduced variability of the daily means of patients results. This is further illustrated in figure 14: the only evident difference is that of the populations served, giving an overall mean value higher at I.M.C.A.

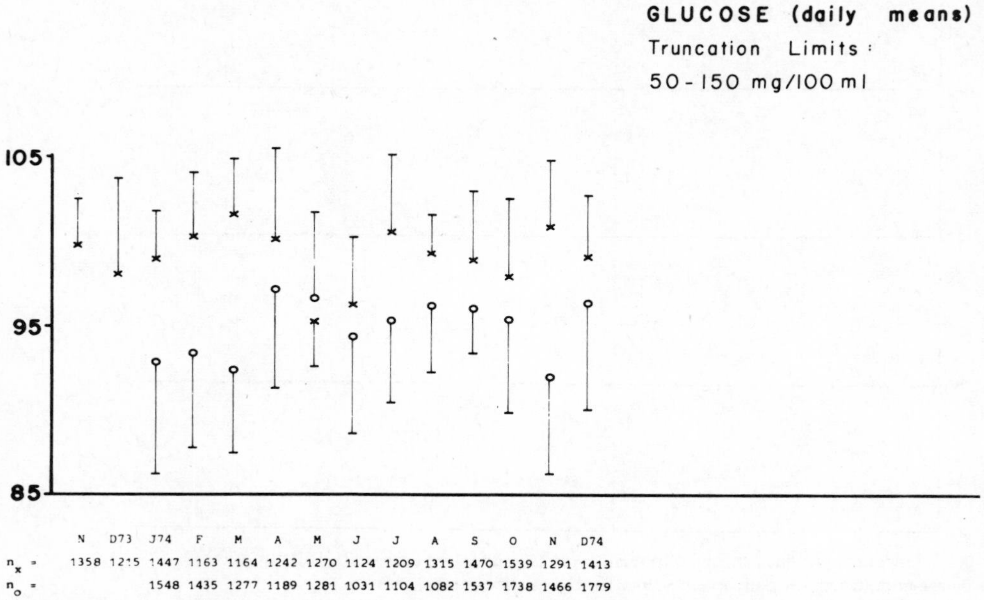

Fig. 14. Means (± SD) of the daily means established monthly. I. M. C. A. = crosses; I. E. C. = circles. In the lower part, number of determinations computed each month.

We finally introduced a 10% error either positive or negative on the results from the I.M.C.A. (fig. 15). The confidence interval for the 'unchanged' daily means is 88–102 mg/100 ml at the 95% probability level. Using these values, the discriminant power of the daily mean was poor; however, restricting our confidence interval to 90–100, we detected 65 out of 80 'erroneous' means, losing only one supplementary 'unchanged' mean. In addition, we see that the 'erroneous' values are all obviously above the overall mean with the addition of a constant percentage, and below when this percentage is subtracted. This fact alone would alarm a skilled technician.

Urea

The histogram of 2000 patients results from each laboratory (fig. 16) is characteristic of the populations served: the dispersion is much more important at I.M.C.A. where all the highest values were found.

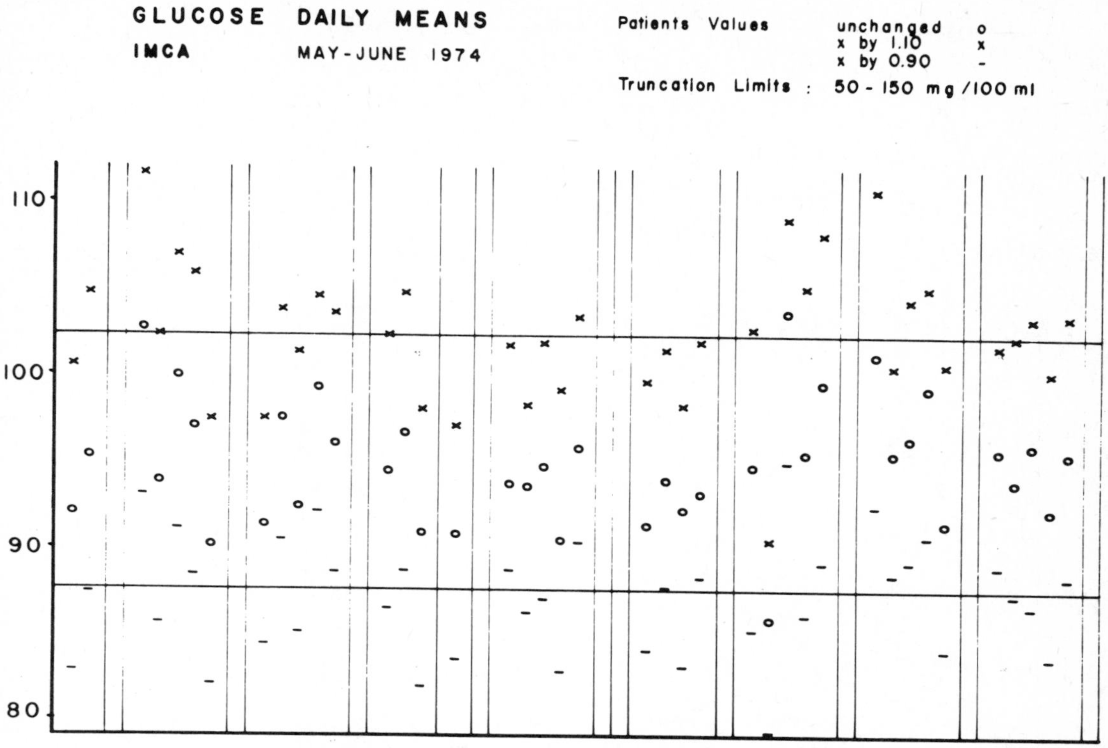

Fig. 15. Effect of multiplying each patient's result by 1.1 (crosses) or by 0.9 (horizontal bars) and computing thereafter the daily mean between truncation limits.

Comparison with data from unchanged values (circles) and with the confidence limits of the daily means (horizontal lines).

The monthly means of two control sera during a three months period fell all within the limits given by the manufacturer (fig. 17) without significant difference between laboratories.

The comparison of the monthly means of the daily means of patients results (fig. 18) does not reflect the important difference found in the histograms; this reduction is evidently related to the truncation limits selected, which almost completely eliminate the pathological cases from the populations under study.

At I.M.C.A., the coefficient of variation of the daily mean of patients results was similar to that of the control sera; at I.E.C. again, the control sera showed less variation than the daily mean of patients' results.

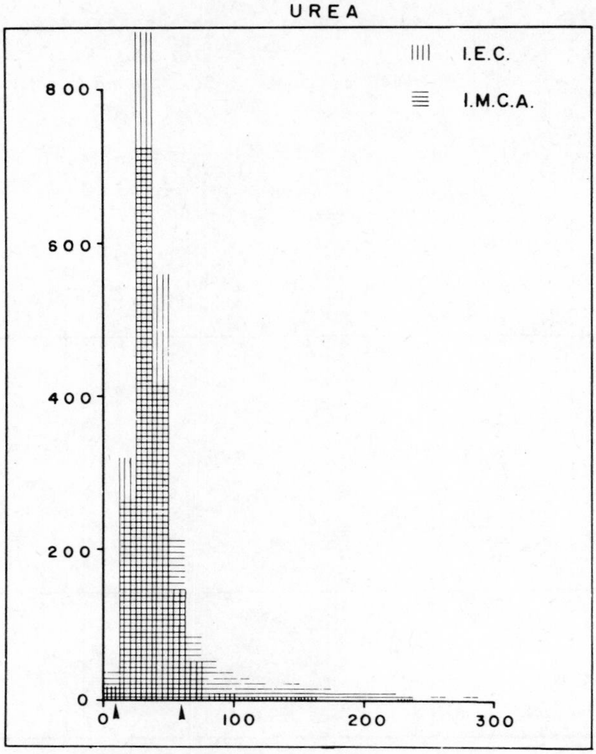

Fig. 16. Histograms of 2000 consecutive patients' results at I. M. C. A. (horizontally hatched columns) and at I. E. C. (vertically hatched columns).
Values expressed in mg/100 ml.

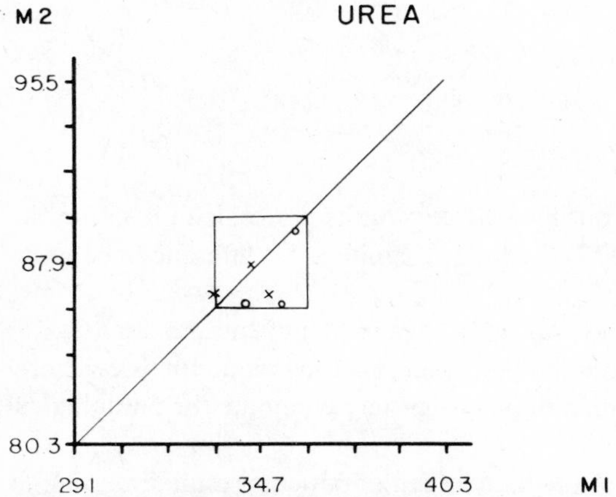

Fig. 17. Youden plot of the monthly means of 2 control sera in I. E. C. (circles) and I. M. C. A. (crosses) during 3 months. The central square represents the 95% confidence zone given by the manufacturer.

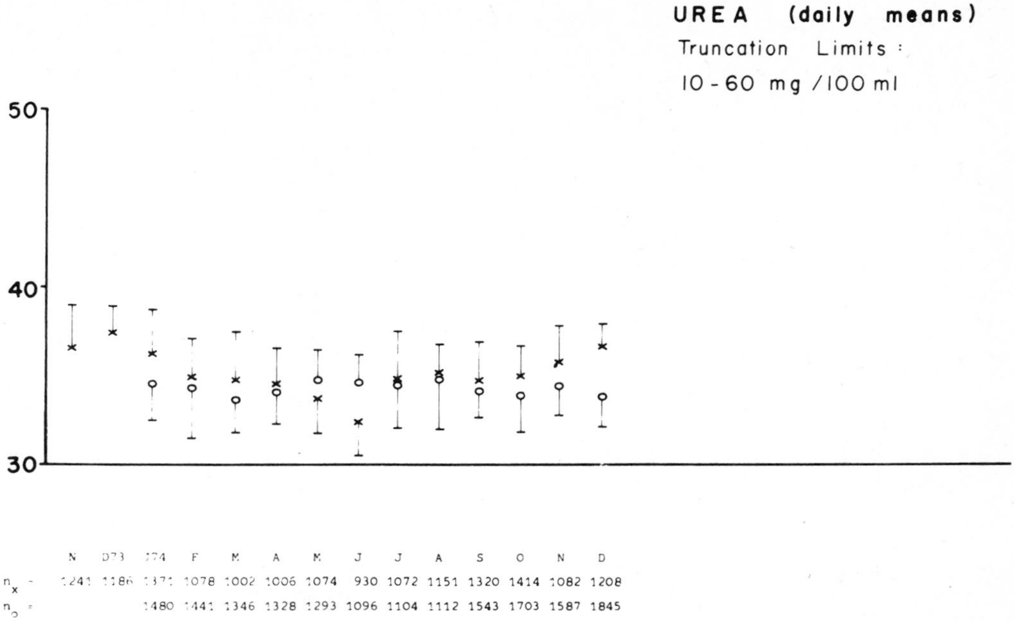

Fig. 18. Means (± SD) of the daily means established monthly. I. M. C. A. = crosses; I. E. C. = circles. In the lower part, number of determinations computed each month.

Acid-base equilibrium

At the end of December 1974 a new IL413 apparatus was delivered at I.M.C.A. We took this opportunity to make a triple comparison, taking into account the fact that the characteristics of the population served at I.M.C.A. remained stable during the last years. We collected all results obtained at I.M.C.A. in January 1975 using the direct measurement of the partial pressure of CO_2 with a specific electrode, those obtained in the same hospital in January 1974 with a tonometric method, and those from I.E.C, whose number was unfortunately too small for a valid use of the daily mean as a quality control system. We consequently limited our interlaboratory comparison to the histograms (figs. 19 and 20).

For the standard bicarbonate, computed either from 3 pH readings (tonometry) or from pH and partial pressure of CO_2, the lowest and simultaneously the most dispersed values were obtained by tonometry at I.M.C.A.; as expected the values at I.E.C. were lower than that from I.M.C.A., using similar technologies. The differences between the daily means obtained in 1974 and 1975 while the populations served were identical was 1.5 mEq/l and this difference was statistically highly significant.

For the partial pressure of CO_2, the profiles obtained at I.M.C.A. were comparable when taking into account a difference of 3 mm Hg, with also a greater dispersion of the results obtained with tonometry.

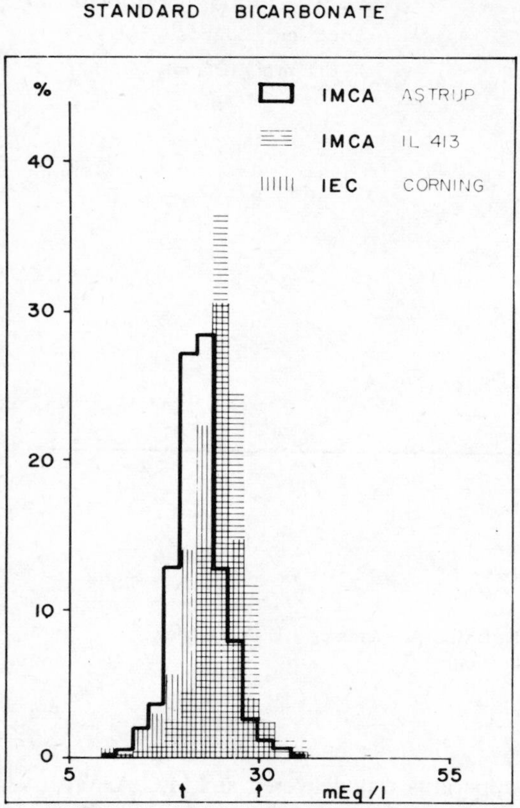

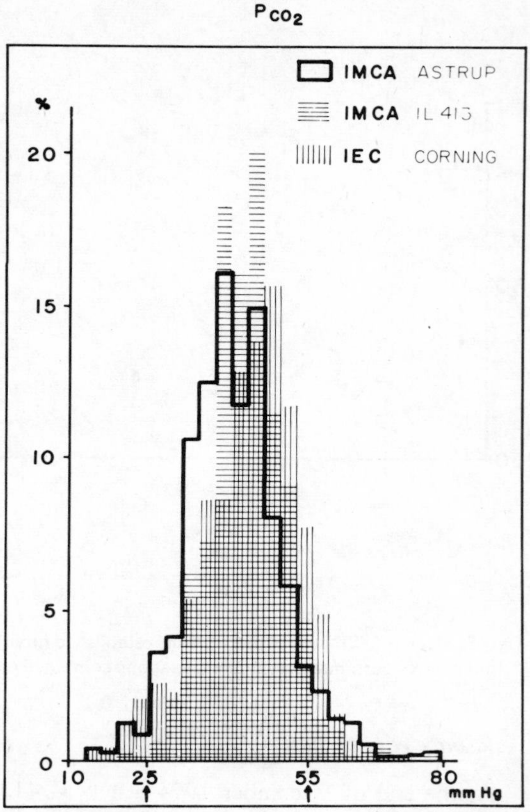

Fig. 19. Histograms of all patients' results collected in January 1974 at I. M. C. A. using a tonometric system (Astrup), in January 1975 at I. M. C. A. using specific electrode for the measurement of the partial pressure of CO_2 (IL 413) and in January 1975 at I. E. C. with a similar technique (Corning).
Fig. 20. Same legend as for fig. 19.

These changes between tonometry and measurement with a specific electrode were reflected in the first monthly mean we obtained in 1975 (fig. 21). The value of actual pH was comparable to that previously recorded with, however, a lower coefficient of variation. The mean of the standard bicarbonate daily means in Jan. 75 was clearly higher than previously, while the coefficient of variation was strongly lowered. For the partial pressure of CO_2, the mean of the daily means increased only by 1.5 mm Hg, but here again the coefficient of variation decreased significantly from more than 4% to less than 3%. It is evident that these decreased variabilities were predictable from the simple technological point of view: indeed the IL 413 gives a digital display of all results, while to obtain corresponding values with tonometry, three readings on a pH meter were necessary, though the computations were programmed on a desk computer to avoid the imprecision of the readings on the Siggaard-Andersen nomogram.

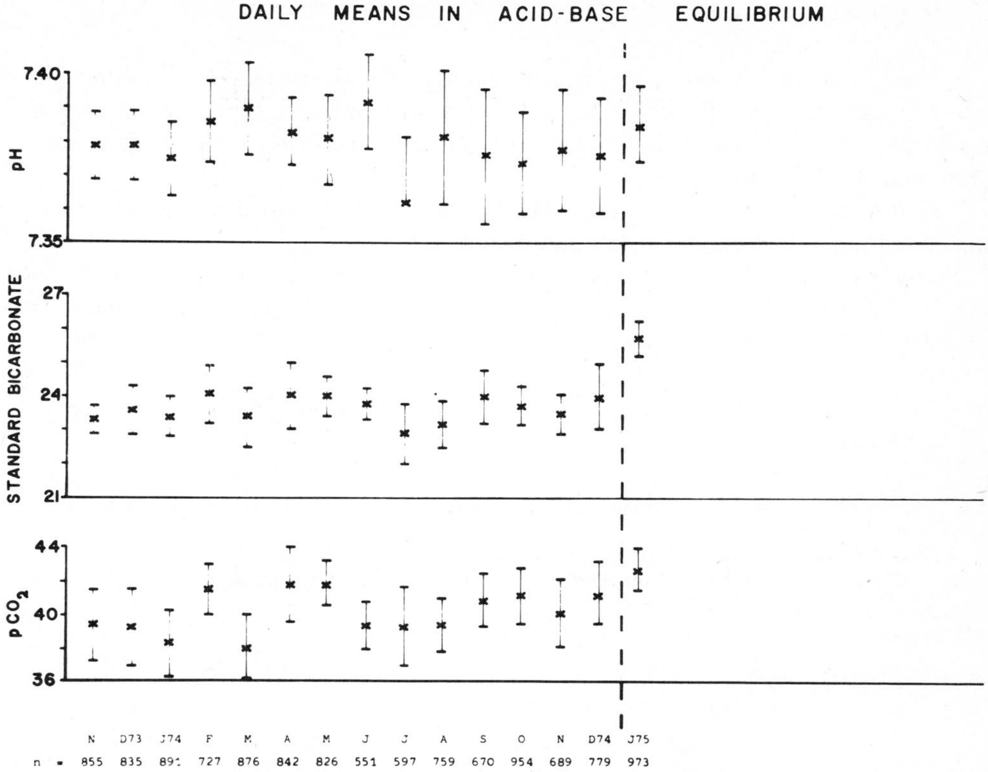

Fig. 21. Daily means of patients' results obtained at I.M.C.A. for pH (truncation limits: 7.00–8.00), for standard bicarbonate (truncation limits: 20–30 mEq/l) and for partial pressure of CO_2 (truncation limits: 25–55 mm Hg).
Lower part: number of determinations each month.
The vertical line denotes the change of method of determination.

Acid-base equilibrium is the most requested determination for which the control of the analytical steps alone is completely insufficient. Indeed the conditions of blood sampling, the temperature of storage during the transfer to the laboratory and the elapsed time between sampling and determination are all critical and not checked by the usual quality control. In the present case, the daily mean of patients data is the only method giving an overall quality control. Its usefulness was further confirmed when two analytical methodologies were compared; indeed the dramatic improvement of the daily variability after using a simpler method, demonstrates the efficiency of this quality control system in detecting subtle changes.

Conclusions

The use of the daily means of patients'results, after careful selection of truncation limits, is a useful tool for quality control. After the initial work required for the determination of truncation limits, the daily values are easily obtained and offer a control system complementary to other methods, though not replacing them.

This method is of especial interest in laboratories where reproducibility is good and can then give better information than can control sera.

Furthermore, in acid-base control, where analytical errors may not be the most important source of aberrant results, the daily mean of patients results represents a unique check on the whole process, from sampling to result.

References

J.A.Owen & D.G.Campbell: Laboratory quality control using patients results. Clin. Chim. Acta *20* (1968), 327–334.

K.Dixon & B.E.Northam: Quality Control using the daily mean. Clin. Chim. Acta *30* (1970), 453–461.

P.W.Lewis & K.Dixon: Action limits for internal quality control. Clin. Chim. Acta *35* (1971), 21–32.

Acknowledgments

I wish to express my deep gratitude to Dr. *Ph.Mascart* who initiated this work in his laboratories several years ago. He gave me at all steps of this work, helpful advice and constructive criticism; moreover he allowed me to obtain the cooperation of his whole technical staff.

Topic I
Quality Control in Relation to Determination Methods

Discussion

S. Rosalki (UK): I should like first of all to thank the speakers of this session. These papers are now open for discussion.

B. Copeland (USA): Dr. Leclercq, I wonder in your experience how satisfactory would be the use of the mode instead of the mean of truncated values?

R. Leclercq (Belgium): We examined several parameters to evaluate the usefulness of the mode rather than the daily mean. In this graph you can see that for PCO_2, for example, it may be quite difficult to obtain an exact definition of the mode. Furthermore, that in most instances the variability of the mode is greater than that of the daily mean.

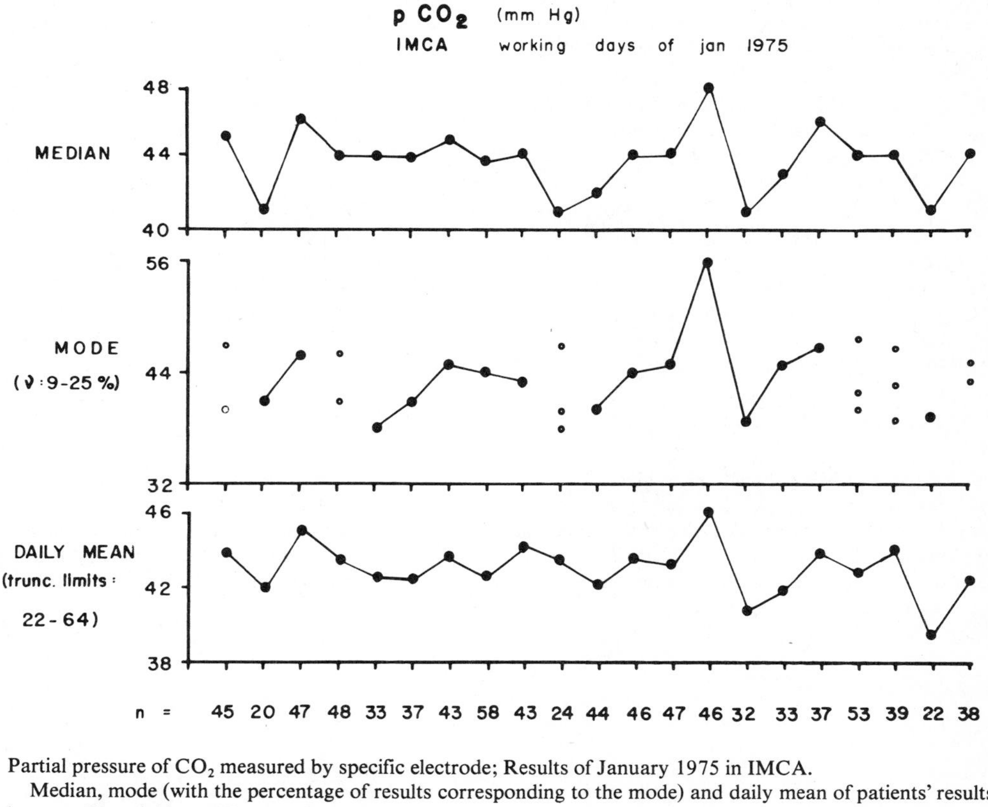

Partial pressure of CO_2 measured by specific electrode; Results of January 1975 in IMCA.

Median, mode (with the percentage of results corresponding to the mode) and daily mean of patients' results between 22 and 64 mm Hg.

At the bottom, the number of results taken into account.

K. Boroviczény (Germany): I would like to call Dr. Leclercq's attention to two other tests which are simple and also use test results; one is the median value of all values, which is very sensitive to systematic errors of the whole series, and the other is the so-called threshold. Here you calculate a factor from the number of results above and the number of results below the threshold. This is very sensitive to outliers.

I also have a comment on Dr. Havelec's lecture. We take the view that a good method should always be a fool-proof method. Therefore, if laboratories are not able to perform a method properly, it is not only the fault of the laboratories, it is also the fault of the method. We like to compare groups of similar laboratories, that is to say, hospital laboratories, or general practitioner laboratories, always comparing groups from at least 20 to 30, but preferably 50 to 100 similar laboratories. We find it is not enough to compare them within one survey, but within at least 3 or 4 surveys, because sometimes you will get dissimilar results from survey to survey. Only if you have such groups and several surveys, can you make good judgement of methods.

R. Leclercq (Belgium): To answer the first part of your question, I tested also the median and found that the variation of the median was comparable to, or worse than that of the daily mean. I will answer the second part of your question by saying that we tried to devise a quality control system which could be used as an intra-laboratory quality control. In that sense, the usefulness of the daily mean has been demonstrated.

H. Büttner (Germany): I have a question to Dr. Havelec. As I understand it, you are using a linear scale for scoring. That means the difference between the value and the reference value is used as a measure for quality. Is it possible to use non-linear scales? I think that the measure of the quality of working performance in a laboratory cannot be considered linear a priori.

L. Havelec (Austria): I will first answer the question from Dr. v. Boroviczény. Of course, you are right, but I had only data from one survey and I preferred to draw some information out of the available data rather than to wait until we had accumulated data from a series of surveys.

The answer to Dr. Büttner's question is that what I have been doing was a ranking of laboratories according to their results. The ranking scales are ordinal scales and do not imply linearity. It is possible to test the correlation between two rank-orders. For this I used the Spearman-rank-correlation, a non-parametric correlation test.

J. Izquierdo (Spain): Dr. Ceriotti, I have a question to clarify a point I did not understand from your lecture. It has to do with your experiment on using bile for bilirubin determinations. I would like to know what sort of preparation of bile you have used in your experiments. I suppose it is not one of these laborious preparations designed to yield pure conjugated bilirubin.

G. Ceriotti (Italy): We simply used human bile freshly collected during abdominal surgery.

E. Kaiser (Austria): I should like to make a comment on Dr. Havelec's paper. Statistical calculations take a long time, and the data used were gained in 1969. At the time a request was made for a general ranking of laboratories. Dr. Havelec has developed a method for doing so. The results of the four parameters are just an explanation of the usefulness of the method. If it is said that the results are not very important today, it is just because today there is no doubt about the superiority of UV tests over end-point tests for enzymes.

Award Lectures

Topic II: Quality Control in Relation to Determination Materials, Standards and Controls

Evaluation of Some Determination Materials used in the Scandinavian Recommended Methods (S. C. E.) for Determination of Four Enzymes in Blood and the Performance of Control Materials with these Methods

W. Gerhardt, Copenhagen (Denmark)

Key words: Alanine aminotransferase
Alkaline phosphatase
Aminotransferase
Aspartate aminotransferase
Catalytic activity
Lactate dehydrogenase
Scandinavian Committee on Enzymes

Summary

The recommended methods of the Scandinavian Committee on Enzymes (S.C.E.) for assessment of catalytic activity in blood of:

L-aspartate aminotransferase (E.C. 2.6.1.1, unofficial abbreviation ASAT).
L-alanine aminotransferase (E.C. 2.6.1.2, ALAT).
L-lactate: NAD oxidoreductase (E.C. 1.1.1.27, LD).
Alkaline phosphatase (E.C. 3.1.3.1, ALP).

were officially accepted in 1973 for use in Scandinavian laboratories of clinical chemistry. Some choices of components in the reagents are discussed. Problems of interpretation of the non-linear LDH reaction curves are described.

It is suggested that statements of LDH catalytic concentration in control materials be specified for a given time interval after start of the reaction.

The results of a survey of inter-lab precision among 6 Scandinavian laboratories are reported. Expressed as range of the coefficients of variation (CV, %) inter-laboratory precision with a total of 7 commercial lyophilized control materials were: LDH: 3.6–6.5%; ASAT: 0.9–4.0%; ALAT: 2.1–4.0%.

In a subsequent Nordic Survey comprising more than 20 laboratories similar precision was obtained. For ALP in this survey the CV% was about 7%.

Problems of heat-activation of ALP of lyophilized control materials are discussed.

Estimates of instrumental precision in routine reaction rate measurements with 4 enzymes are given.

Following two years of experimental work, the Scandinavian Committee on Enzymes (S. C. E.) presented to the Scandinavian laboratories of Clinical Chemistry its recommended methods for assessment of the catalytic activity of:

L-aspartate aminotransferase (E.C. 2.6.1.1, unofficial abbreviation ASAT).
L-alanine aminotransferase (E.C. 2.6.1.2, ALAT).
L-lactate: NAD oxidoreductase (E.C. 1.1.1.27, LDH).
Alkaline phosphatase (E.C. 3.1.3.1, ALP).

Criticism and suggestions from the individual laboratories were requested and considered by the S.C.E.

Subsequently, in 1973 the General Assembly of the Scandinavian Society of Clinical Chemistry and Clinical Physiology formally accepted these methods for use in Scandinavian laboratories of Clinical Chemistry.

The four recommended methods, the principles behind them, and comments have been published in detail in the Scand. J. Clin. Lab. Invest. 33, 291–306, 1974 [11]. All methods are kinetic, based on continuous monitoring of reaction rate.

The recommended methods shall serve two purposes:

a) They shall function as daily routine working methods.
b) They shall function as reference methods used for quality control in the Scandinavian reference laboratories (two in each Scandinavian country).

The description of the methods include not only statements of concentrations, but quality requirements for critical components as well.

Choice of buffer for the NADH-coupled reactions was motivated by two main concerns: The buffer should be non-inhibitory; and critical components such as NADH should be sufficiently stable in the buffer chosen. The LDH reaction is used as an example because NADH quality is most critical in this reaction.

Table 1. Reaction rates at 3 pyruvate concentrations in TRIS-EDTA-HCl and K_2HPO_4-Na_2HPO_4 buffers, 50 mmol/l, pH 7.4 (37 °C). Reaction conditions as S.C.E. LDH method, except where Tris buffer was replaced by phosphate buffer.
No significant difference in catalytic effect of human LDH H_4 and M_4 in the two buffers is seen.

	Initial reaction rate (37 °C): $\Delta A_{340\ nm}$ per minute			
	Buffer 50 mmol/l pH 7.4 (37 °C)			
	TRIS-EDTA-HCl		Phosphate (K_2HPO_4-Na_2HPO_4)	
Pyruvate	H_4	M_4	H_4	M_4
1.2 mmol/l	0.073	0.117	0.074	0.117
1.7 mmol/l	0.075	0.127	0.074	0.129
2.0 mmol/l	0.073	0.129	0.072	0.129

Table 1 shows that human LDH H_4 and M_4 enzymes function equally well in a TRIS-EDTA-HCl buffer and in a classical Sørensen KH_2PO_4-Na_2HPO_4 buffer, both 50 mmol/l, pH 7.4 (37 °C).

In contrast, NADH stability is very different in TRIS-EDTA-HCl and in phosphate buffers.

Phosphate ions accelerate the rate of destruction of NADH in solutions stored at 4 °C and at room temperature [1, 2, 4, 5, 8, 10]. The apparent first order rate constant of the decrease of 340 nm absorbance of NADH in solution has been shown to be dependent on the concentration of $H_2PO_4^-$ ion [1].

It is rarely specified even in official recommendations that the generally used term 'phosphate buffer' actually includes 4 species of buffer (table 2) with different properties.

Table 2. The four possible species of phosphate-buffer.

	'Phosphate Buffer'
1	KH_2PO_4-Na_2HPO_4
2	KH_2PO_4-K_2HPO_4
3	NaH_2PO_4-Na_2HPO_4
4	NaH_2PO_4-K_2HPO_4

On freezing a 'classical' KH_2PO_4-Na_2HPO_4 Sørensen buffer, initial pH 7.4 at 25 °C pH will decrease to below pH 5 [3]. This causes acid destruction of NADH. In contrast, pH of both KH_2PO_4-K_2HPO_4 and a TRIS-EDTA-HCl buffer increases on cooling from room temperature [3].

Figures 1 and 2 illustrate the effect of four different buffers on the stability of a high-quality NADH preparation 150 μmol/l, dissolved in TRIS-HCl buffers ± EDTA, and in KH_2PO_4-Na_2HPO_4 and KH_2PO_4-K_2HPO_4 buffers, initial pH 7.4 at 37 °C. The following properties of NADH were measured:

340 nm and 260 nm absorbance, shown as relative values (fraction of initial absorbance), and the 260 nm/340 nm absorbance ratios.

Figures 1 and 2 show that at both 4 °C and −20 °C decreases of 340 absorbance, increases of 260 nm absorbance and of the 260/340 nm absorbance ratios with time are smaller in TRIS-HCl buffer ± EDTA, than in the two phosphate buffers. At −20 °C the measured properties of NADH in the S.C.E. TRIS buffer were nearly constant over a period of 10 days. In contrast great changes of both 340 nm and 260 nm absorbance occurred in the two phosphate buffers; rapid destruction of NADH was observed by freezing in the classical Sørensen KH_2PO_4-Na_2HPO_4 buffer.

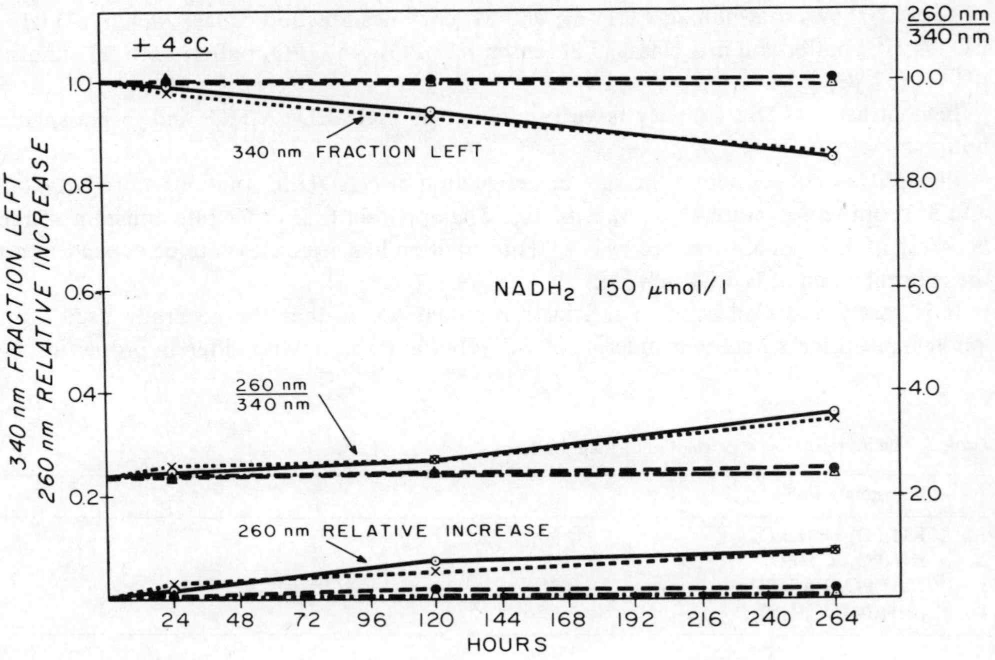

Fig. 1. Change of spectrometric properties of a high quality NADH, initial 260 nm/340 nm ratio 2.38, stored at 4 °C as 150 μmol/l solutions in two Tris and two phosphate-buffers. All values are more stable in the Tris than in the phosphate buffers.

● - - - - - - - - - - - ●	TRIS-EDTA-HCl,	50 mmol/l, pH 7.7 (25 °C)
Δ · – · – · – · Δ	TRIS-HCl,	50 mmol/l, pH 7.4 (25 °C)
⊙ ———————— ⊙	KH_2PO_4-K_2HPO_4,	80 mmol/l, pH 7.4 (25 °C)
× · · · · · · · · · · · ×	KH_2PO_4-Na_2HPO_4,	80 mmol/l, pH 7.4 (25 °C)

(From ref. 4)

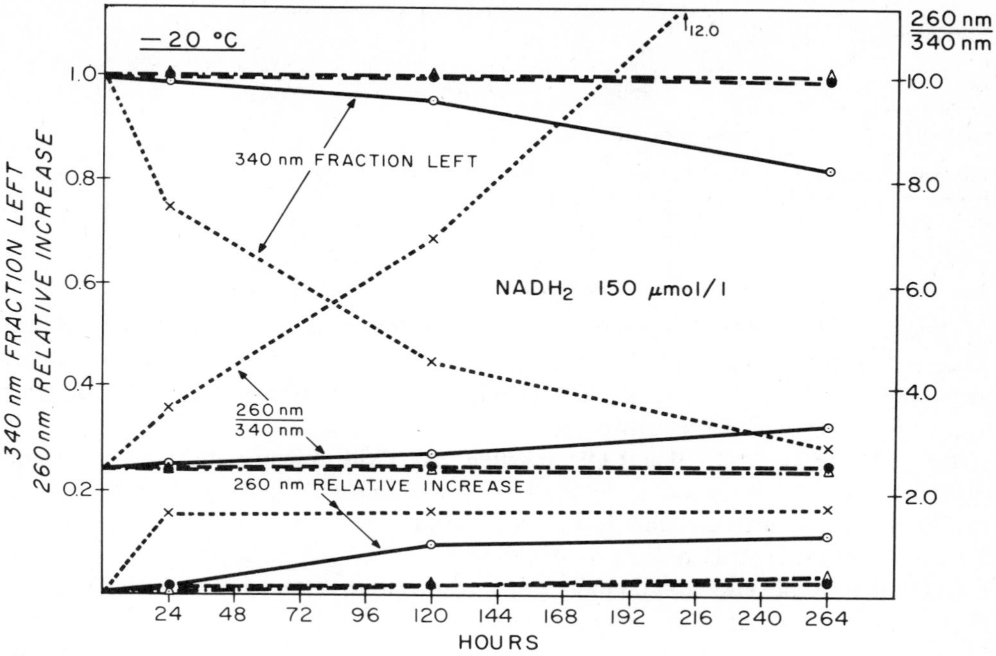

Fig. 2. See text to fig. 3.
NADH, 150 µmol/l was stored at −20 °C in the same four buffers described under fig. 3. All values are more stable in the Tris than in the phosphate buffers. Observe rapid destruction of NADH in the KH_2PO_4-Na_2HPO_4 buffer.

● - - - - - - - - - - - ●	TRIS-EDTA-HCl,	50 mmol/l, pH 7.7 (25 °C)
Δ · – · – · – · Δ	TRIS-HCl,	50 mmol/l, pH 7.4 (25 °C)
⊙ ———————— ⊙	KH_2PO_4-K_2HPO_4,	80 mmol/l, pH 7.4 (25 °C)
× · · · · · · · · · · · ×	KH_2PO_4-Na_2HPO_4,	80 mmol/l, pH 7.4 (25 °C)

(From ref. 4)

Finally, it could be shown that storage of 150 µmol/l NADH solutions in the S.C.E. TRIS-EDTA-HCl buffer at 37 °C for 5 hours and for 72 hours at 4 °C caused no decrease in reaction rate with human LDH H_4 and pyruvate. Consequently TRIS-EDTA-HCl buffers were chosen for the S.C.E. NADH-coupled methods.

In the medium for alkaline phosphatase, presence of the contaminant monoethanolamine 5 mmol/l in the 1000 mmol/l diethanolamine buffer may cause up to 20% inhibition of reaction rates (table 3).

Table 3. Inhibition of ALP reaction rate by monoethanolamine in diethanolamine buffer (data of J. Waldenstrom, Göteborg).

S.C.E. 1974
Inhibition of ALP in Serum
Monoethanolamine in Diethanolamine-HCl, 1 mol/l

Monoeth. mmol/l	Relative reaction rate
1	0.98
2	0.93
5	0.78

Quality control of the integrated function of the recommended methods with control sera requires proper interpretation of the kinetic data. The LDH reaction does not follow zero order kinetics [6, 9]. This is the case whether pyruvate or L-lactate is the substrate, and whether one or all 5 isoenzymes are present.

Figure 3 demonstrates that LDH reaction rates with a commercial control serum decrease with time after start of the reaction. For example, the average rate measured at the 30–45 second interval with this particular serum is about 85% of that observed in the 15–30 second interval. This decrease of reaction rate will still be observed if e.g. NADH concentration is increased to 200 μmol/l. It is related to the catalytic concentration and to the species of LDH in the same samples or control.

Consequently, statements of LDH catalytic concentration for any control serum must be specified for a given time interval after start of the reaction under defined conditions. Such specifications would be desirable with commercial control preparations.

In the following are reported the results of a survey of inter-lab precision with the S.C.E. methods. The data given originate from 6 Scandinavian reference laboratories (*J.H.Strømme,* Tromsø; *L.Theodorsen,* Oslo; *E.Pitkanen,* Helsinki; *N.Tryding,* Kristianstad; *M.Hørder,* Århus; *W.Gerhardt,* Copenhagen). 7 commercial control sera were used. Each serum was analyzed in at least 5 laboratories.

Each day for one working week, catalytic activity of ASAT, ALAT, LDH, and ALP was assessed on a fresh vial of each control serum. Manufacturers' directions were followed. Thus a total of 125 assessments of each enzyme, 25 in each laboratory, were made on each serum.

The mean values and coefficients of variation (CV%) for these 125 determinations of each enzyme in each of the 7 control sera are shown in tables 4–6.

The inter-laboratory precision in determination of the catalytic concentration of LDH in 5 laboratories is expressed as the range of coefficients of variation with the 7 sera: 3.6–6.5% (table 4).

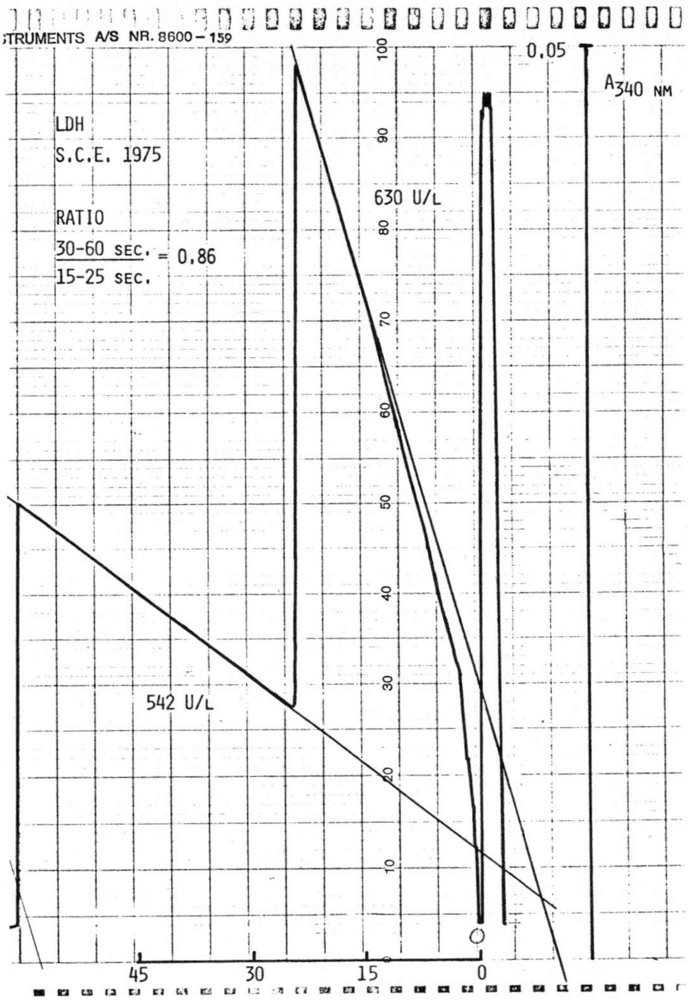

Fig. 3. Hyperbolic decrease of LDH reaction rate with time after start. S.C.E. reaction conditions; Seronorm control serum. Average early reaction rate (15–30 sec. period) is about 15% higher than that of the 30–45 sec. period.

Table 4. Mean values and variation (CV) of 125 assessments of LDH catalytic activity performed by 5 laboratories on each of 7 commercial control sera.

Note that the analytical variation shows no trend from high (1015 U/l, CV 4.2%) to low (315 U/l, CV 4.8) catalytic concentration.

LDH S.C.E. 1974 — Inter-Lab Precision, 5 Ref. Labs.

Material	U/l	CV%
Dade 39 B	1015	4.2
Dade 131 B	358	4.4
Hyland	359	6.5
Kontrollogen	922	4.8
Nyco 71	315	4.8
Precinorm E 324 A	322	5.1
Seronorm	689	3.6
Range CV%		3.6–6.5

With ASAT and 5 sera with catalytic concentrations above 75 U/l, precision was 0.9–4.0% (table 5).

2 of the 7 sera had low ASAT catalytic concentrations and showed poor signal-to-noise ratios and correspondingly poor precision: range 8–10% (table 5).

Table 5. See text to table 4. Analytical error was increased by a factor of 2 in sera with low ASAT catalytic concentration.

ASAT S.C.E. 1974 — Inter-Lab Precision, 5 Ref. Labs.

Material	U/l	CV%
Dade 39 B	84	0.9
Hyland	78	2.1
Kontrollogen	116	3.3
Precinorm E 324 A	82	2.9
Seronorm 125	215	4.0
Range CV%		0.9–4.0

Low Catalytic Activity

Material	U/l	CV%
Dade 131 B	26	8.0
Nyco 71	16	10.0
Range CV%		8.0–10.0

Inter-laboratory precision in determination of ALAT in 5 sera with catalytic concentrations above 75 U/l expressed as range of CV was 2.1–4.0% (table 6).

Table 6. See text to table 5. Analytical error was increased by a factor of 4 in sera with low ALAT catalytic concentration.

ALAT S.C.E. 1974 — Inter-Lab Precision 5 Ref. Labs.

Material	U/l	CV%
Dade 39 B	96	3.8
Hyland	78	2.1
Kontrollogen	116	3.3
Precinorm	82	2.9
Seronorm 125	215	4.0
Range CV%		2.1–4.0

Low Catalytic Activity

Material	U/l	CV%
Dade 131 B	24	11.7
Hyland	12	18.5
Nyco 71	12	4.2
Range CV%		4.2–18.5

Here too, measurement of three sera with low catalytic concentration showed poor precision with coefficients of variation in the range 4.2–18.5 (table 6).

With alkaline phosphatase, results of the first inter-laboratory test were more ambiguous. While intra-series and intra-laboratory precision were quite good, comparison of the results obtained on the seven commercial sera in five laboratories showed too high a variation. Among factors contributing to the observed variations were: the small sample volume of 10 µl; inhibitors in the diethanolamine buffer; the use of 405 nm and 410 nm filters on the LKB 8600 which necessitates that individual instruments be calibrated with standard solutions of p-nitrophenol.

A main source of variation is the well established fact that catalytic activity of alkaline phosphatases in lyophilized preparations increases after resolubilization. The extent and rate of this increase is dependent on temperature, time, and species of alkaline phosphatase [7]. The reactivation may be accelerated and with certain sera, terminated by incubation of the resolubilized serum e. g. at 37 °C for 6 hours.

Although all sera showed increases of activity by heat-incubation (table 7) only one serum was accompanied by manufacturers instructions for this purpose.

Table 7. Increases of ALP catalytic effect by incubation of sera at 37 °C for 6 hours (from 5% to nearly 30%).
S.C.E. assay method.

Relative Increase of Alkaline Phosphatase Activity (S.C.E. Methods) after Incubation of Lyophilized-Resolubilized Commercial Control Sera at 37 °C for 6 Hours.

Material	Activity before Heating (n = 20) / Activity after Heating (n = 20)
Dade (PTD 39 B)	0.84
Hyland	0.72
Kontrollogen	0.95
Nyco 71	0.75
Precinorm	0.91
Seronorm	0.71

Table 8 demonstrates the difference between results obtained with heat-activated and not-heat-activated sera, analyzed in two laboratories. Intra-series variation was about the same in these two laboratories. In contrast, intra-laboratory precision was considerably better with heat-treated than with unheated sera (CV 1.6% as compared to 5.9%).

Table 8. Difference in intra-lab precision obtained with heat-activated and untreated Seronorm control serum.
S.C.E. ALP assay method.

Alkaline Phosphatase S.C.E. Intra-Lab Precision
1974 Seronorm 125

Days	Heat Activated	(Oslo)	Not Heat Activated	(RH)
	U/l	CV%	U/l	CV%
1	308	1.1	199	1.5
2	315	0.8	185	0.0
3	317	1.7	215	0.0
4	308	1.3	199	1.7
5	–	–	186	3.5
Mean of all 25 Det.	312	1.6	200	5.9

In accordance with these results a recent Nordic screening comprising some twenty routine laboratories in Scandinavia showed an inter-laboratory precision of about 7 per cent with a heat-activated control preparation [12]. This survey also confirms the data on inter-laboratory precision with the NADH coupled methods given above. All data incorporate the variation introduced by reagents obtained from different manufacturers.

Table 9 summarizes the current estimates of instrumental, intra-laboratory routine, and inter-laboratory precision obtained with the S. C. E. methods.

Table 9. Analytical error expressed as the coefficient of variation. Instrument: (LKB 8600) under optimized conditions and with own control sera stored at −80 °C. Intra-laboratory routine quality controls during month-long periods; and inter-laboratory data described in the text.

	Error (CV %) S.C.E. Methods		
	Instrument[1]	Intra-Lab[2] Routine	Inter-Lab Comparison Material
LDH	2	2.2 (n = 142)	3.6–6.5
ASAT	1.5	1.7 (n = 50)	0.9–4.0[3]
ALAT	1.5	3.1 (n = 207)	2.1–4.0
ALP	1.5	2.4 (n = 174)	about 7[4]

[1] Own Controls (n = 50)
[2] 1–2 Month Routine Controls
[3] Sera with Values > 75 U/l
[4] Data from Nordic Screening to be published (1975).

Acknowledgment

The author expresses his gratitude toward the following members of the Scandinavian Committee on Enzymes who gave their permission to use their data of the first inter-lab comparison for this report:

J. H. Strømme, dept. of med. biology, University of Tromsø, Norway.
L. Theodorsen, det Norske Radiumhospital, Montebello/Oslo 3, Norway.
E. Pitkanen, IV clinic of Int. Med., Helsingfors, Finland.
N. Tryding, dept. Clin. Chem., Centralsjukhuset, Kristianstad, Sweden.
M. Hørder, dept. clin. chem., kommune-hospital, Århus, Denmark.

References

[1] *Alivisatos, S.G.A., Ungar, F. & Abraham, G.:* Non-enzymatic Interactions of Reduced Coenzyme I with Inorganic Phosphate and Certain Other Anions. Nature 203, 973, 1964.

[2] *Applegarth, D.A. & Eden, J.:* Deterioration of solutions of reduced nicotinamide adenine dinucleotide ($NADH_2$) during storage. Clin. Chim. Acta 13, 720, 1966.

[3] *Chilson, O.P., Costello, L.A. & Kaplan, N.O.:* Effects of freezing on enzymes. Fed. Proc. 24, 55, 1965.

[4] *Gerhardt, W.:* Quality Control of NADH. Evaluation of Methods for Detection of Inhibitors and Specifications for NADH quality. Scand. J. Clin. Lab. Invest. Suppl. 139, 1974.

[5] *Howell, B.F., Margolis, S. & Schaffer, R.:* Residual Fluorescence as an Index of Purity of Reduced Nicotinamide Adenine Dinucleotide. Clin. Chem. 19, 1280, 1973.

[6] *Ingle, J.D. & Crouch, S.R.:* Theoretical and Experimental Factors Influencing the Accuracy of Analytical Rate Measurements. Analytical Chemistry, 43, 697–701, 1971.

[7] *Landaas, S.:* Temperature-Dependence of Alkaline Phosphatase Activity in Reconstituted Control Sera. Scand. J. Clin. Lab. Invest. 31, 353–356, 1973.
[8] *Lowry, O.H., Passonneau, J.V. & Rock, M.K.:* The stability of Pyridine Nucleotides. J. biol. Chem. 236, 2756, 1961.
[9] *Moss, D.W.:* The Relative Merits and Applicability of Kinetic and Fixed-Incubation Methods of Enzyme Assay in Clinical Enzymology. Clinical Chemistry, 18, 1449–1454, 1972.
[10] *Sandifort, C.R.J.:* Some aspects of standardization in clinical enzymology. Proceedings of the 5th Int. Symp. Clin. Enzymology, Venice (ed.: A. Burlina), Edizione LAB, Milano 1974.
[11] Scandinavian Committee on Enzymes of the Scand. Soc. Clin. Chem.: Recommended Methods for the Determination of Four Enzymes in Blood, Scand. J. Clin. Lab. Invest. *33*, 291–306, 1974.
[12] *Strømme, J.:* Scand. J. Clin. Lab. Invest. (to be published 1975).

The Control of Error and Use of Standardized Reference Samples in Estimation of the True Biological Normal Range

A. Hyvärinen, Tampere (Finland)

Key words: Biological normal range
Error
Potassium
Sodium

Summary

The true biological normal ranges for serum sodium and potassium were estimated by analyzing 50 serum samples taken from healthy medical students. To achieve this, technical errors were minimized by using a stable automated technique, analyzing all samples in one single working series and using a reference serum for simultaneous measurement of the errors. Accuracy of measurement was found to be in good agreement with the results of the local regional control system which was used as a reference. The corrected true biological normal ranges, as calculated from the variances of the observed distributions and the precision errors, were 142,4–148,2 mmol/l (with corrected accuracy 142,1–147,9 mmol/l) for serum sodium and 3,91–5,07 mmol/l (with corrected accuracy 3,88–5,02 mmol/l) for serum potassium. The range for sodium was narrow and it was found to be easily affected by technical errors, extending as much as 5-fold merely with high values for errors in precision (coefficient of variation 5%) such as can be found in clinical laboratories. The normal range of serum potassium was not significantly affected by the usual technical errors. Establishment of error-free normal values and availability of internationally standardized reference sera are suggested as ways of improving normal range estimation.

In any measured laboratory value,error effects are usually present. Error may be simply described as the normal gaussian distribution of test values, found when the measurement of a true value of X is repeated several times. The mean value represents the accuracy and the standard deviation represents the precision of the technique used. These can be quite different with different methods and in different laboratories. There is also good reason to believe that such errors are not necessarily always constant with time. It is therefore necessary always to control error in all analytical work. It would also be ideal to try to guarantee reasonable error limits in order to achieve comparable results between clinical laboratories. The influence of error can then be properly considered.

Laboratory values often require eventual comparison to normal values. However, error itself gives results which are systematically too high or low, and variability additional to that due to the real differences between normal individuals. If error is properly controlled normal values should be as absolute and error-free as possible, and represent the true biological normal values of a strictly specified group of healthy individuals. This would result in basic biological data of universal significance rather than data influenced by local and temporary errors in technique at the time of measurement.

In this study an attempt was made to demonstrate the mathematical influence of error on the normal range and also to estimate the true biological normal ranges for serum sodium and potassium, these analyses being chosen to represent two extreme examples, sodium as one of the most error-sensitive and potassium as one of the least error-sensitive analyses in clinical chemistry [1, 2]. This was achieved by minimizing technical errors by using an automated technique as stable as possible, analyzing all the samples in a single working series and simultaneously using a control serum as a reference sample for error measurement to correct the final results.

Materials and Methods

Morning blood serum samples were taken from 50 fasting young medical students. The control serum was a frozen pooled human serum, as used in the Helsinki, multilaboratory regional control system previously reported [1, 2].

Serum sodium and potassium were determined in the author's laboratory (Central Laboratory, Meilahti Hospital, University of Helsinki, Central Hospital, Helsinki, Finland) by the AutoAnalyzer I 2-channel flame photometric N method (Technicon Corp.) and the results were read manually with the standard graphic comparator. Standard solution was included in every tenth cup. All samples were analyzed singly in one working series with control serum samples between all the normal serum samples (altogether 49 control samples and 50 normal samples).

Statistical study of the error was done, assuming for simplicity a normal gaussian distribution of the (N) test values X with the mean value $\bar{X}$ representing accuracy and the standard deviation SD (or here the coefficient of variation CV which is the standard deviation as percent of the mean value), representing the precision of the technique. This was also the method applied for the normal values. For calculation, the conventional formulae were used as follows:

$$SD = \sqrt{\frac{\Sigma(\bar{X}-X)^2}{N-1}}$$

$$CV = \sqrt{\frac{SD \times 100}{\bar{X}}}$$

Normality distribution was tested on probability graph paper.

Distribution of the observed serum sodium and potassium values for normal persons expressed with CV_N results from two independent sources of variability, one due to the error in precision (C_E) and another due to the true biological differences between individuals (C_B). From statistical text-books we know that the variances ($=S^2$) are additive and we have the equations as follows:

$$CV_N^2 = CV_E^2 + CV_B^2$$

$$\text{or} \quad CV_N = \sqrt{CV_E^2 + CV_B^2}$$

$$\text{or} \quad CV_B = \sqrt{CV_N^2 - CV_E^2}$$

which formulae enable us to calculate the true biological normal distribution CV_B when the error and the apparent observed normal distribution are known, or to calculate the apparent normal distribution CV_N when the true biological normal distribution and error are known.

For correction of accuracy, in other words, for any systematic bias at the time of the measurement, the mean value of the 49 control serum values observed in the present measurement was compared with *the target value* of sodium and potassium which was the average value of the long-term mean values of the laboratories in the regional control system [1, 2] using the same method. If any deviation existed the found mean value of the normal values should be corrected respectively by multiplying with their ratio as follows:

$$\text{Corrected mean value of normals} = \frac{\text{Target value of control}}{\text{Found mean value of control}} \times \text{found mean value of normals}$$

In fact, this correction means standardization of the measurement with a reference serum and not with a primary standard solution. Therefore a reference serum to be used for this purpose should be very carefully standardized, preferably with more care than the one used here.

Results and Discussion

The values of the control serum for the sodium and potassium analyses and those of the normal material for sodium followed quite well the normal type of distribution when tested on probability paper. Potassium values of the normal material followed such a distribution only approximately. This however, was not considered to have any significant effect on the conclusions made in this study.

The mean value for sodium of the control serum in the present measurement was 141,9 mmol/l as compared to the target value 141,6. The mean value for potassium 4,63 mmol/l and the target value 4,58 respectively. The differences were slight and actually without any practical significance. However, the mean values of the normal material found in this measurement for serum sodium and for serum potassium were corrected for this slight systematic bias using the formula presented before and was as follows:

Serum sodium found 145,3 mmol/l, corrected 145,0 mmol/l
Serum potassium found 4,49 mmol/l, corrected 4,44 mmol/l

Correction for accuracy as slight as this has only a theoretical meaning and here it served merely as a check that there was a good agreement in accuracy with the results in the regional control system. Standardization of the normal range estimations with a reference serum and strict control of its accuracy is an important and interesting matter for discussion. It would need a lot of international co-operation to establish normal values and produce a reference sera with true standard concentration values. Here we used as a reference point the steady average value in the regional control scheme. This is, in the author's opinion, better than no reference point at all, or one based on incompletely defined commercial serum preparations. We were limited to a regional scheme for practical reasons, though a national scheme would have been preferable. National schemes can well serve as steps to improvement in the accuracy of clinical laboratories, particularly if related to similar international activities.

Error in precision expressed as the coefficient of variation CV_E and calculated from the 49 replicates on the control serum in the present measurement series was 0,37% for serum sodium and 0,61% for serum potassium determination. The observed distribution of the normal values CV_N in the same measurement series was 1,06% for sodium and 6,49% for serum potassium. Using the previous formula we can now calculate the true biological distribution as follows:

$$\text{Serum sodium } CV_B = \sqrt{1{,}06^2 - 0{,}37^2} = 0{,}99\%$$

$$\text{Serum potassium } CV_B = \sqrt{6{,}49^2 - 0{,}61^2} = 6{,}46\%$$

The true biological ranges and limits for the mean value $\pm$ 2 standard deviations as calculated from the corrected mean values and the CV_E-values are as follows:

Serum sodium range 5,8 mmol/l
limits 142,4 – 148,2 mmol/l (found mean value)
142,1 – 147,9 mmol/l (corrected mean value)

Serum potassium range 1,15 mmol/l
limits 3,91 – 5,07 mmol/l (found mean value)
3,88 – 5,02 mmol/l (corrected mean value)

Tables 1 and 2 demonstrate the calculated influence of error on the normal range estimated in this study with some examples of errors typically found in clinical laboratories [1, 2]. The true biological normal range of sodium as calculated above is quite narrow and not easily measurable unless technical errors are effectively controlled as in this study. In sodium determination only, within a single work series and using a stable automated technique a precision is attained which is high enough not to give any practical effect on the measured range of normal sodium values. As shown in table 1, with a technical error of CV_E 2% the observed range is already doubled and with CV_E 5% it is 5-fold (130–160 mmol/l).

Table 1. Effect of analytical precision on the normal range of serum sodium as calculated from the variances. Precision values are examples as found in clinical laboratories [1, 2].
Normal range = mean value ± 2 stand. dev.
CV_E = coefficient of variation corresp. to the analytical precision
CV_N = coefficient of variation of the (gross) normal range (see text)

Precision	Normal range of serum sodium with error included (corr. mean)			Notes
CV_E %	CV_N %	Range mmol/l	Limits mmol/l	
–	0,99	5,8	142,1–147,9	True biological normal range
0,37	1,06	6,1	141,9–148,1	Observed range in present study
0,8	1,28	7,4	141,3–148,7	Day-to-day precision in routine work, limits found 140,9–148,7 (see text)
1,5	1,77	10,2	139,9–150,1	
2	2,23	12,0	138,5–151,5	
3	3,16	18,4	135,8–154,2	
5	5,09	29,6	130,2–159,8	

In contrast, the observed range of serum potassium (table 2) was practically unaffected even by a CV_E-value 2%, which was found to be the day-to-day precision in routine work. Some clearer effects were observed only with CV_E-values 5–7% but the range was still not extended more than 1,5-fold.

The same normal serum samples were also analyzed for sodium and potassium in the routine section of the laboratory using the same method, but the analyses were carried out along with the routine serum samples on different days during a period of 10 days. The day-to-day precision during that time was expressed as the coefficient of variation CV_E = 0,8% for sodium and 2,0% for potassium. The normal range with the mean value ± 2 standard deviations was found as 140,9–148,7 mmol/l for serum sodium and 3,83–4,95 mmol/l for serum potassium, which are very close to those calculated from the variances of the true normal range and the same errors presented in tables 1 and 2 (141,3–148,7 for sodium and 3,85–5,05 for potassium).

Table 2. Effect of analytical precision on the normal range of serum potassium as calculated from the variances. Precision values are examples as found in clinical laboratories [1, 2].
Normal range = mean value ± 2 stand. dev.
CV_E = coefficient of variation corresp. to the analytical precision
CV_N = coefficient of variation of the (gross) normal range (see text)

Precision	Normal range of serum potassium with error included (corr. mean)			Notes
CV_E %	CV_N %	Range mmol/l	Limits mmol/l	
–	6,46	1,15	3,88–5,02	True biological normal range
0,61	6,49	1,16	3,87–5,03	Observed range in present study
1,0	6,54	1,16	3,87–5,03	
2,0	6,76	1,20	3,85–5,05	Day-to-day precision in routine work, limits found 3,83–4,95 (see text)
3	7,12	1,27	3,82–5,08	
5	8,17	1,45	3,73–5,17	
7	9,52	1,69	3,60–5,30	

The normal range of potassium estimated here, agrees quite well with those given in literature. It seems that the establishment of the normal range for serum sodium depends much on technical errors involved. This could also explain the great variety of normal ranges suggested in literature. The ranges calculated here to correspond with a technical variation of about CV_E = 2% with limits 138–152 (table 1), are in fair agreement with those mostly referred to. It should be noted here, that this study was meant primarily to demonstrate a method of controlling the effect of errors when estimating the normal values, and not to give a well specified normal range ('50 young healthy medical students'). Such a study would need still more careful selection of normal material than here.

References

[1] *Hyvärinen A. and Saris N.E.:* Scand. J. Clin. Lab. Invest. Suppl.
[2] *Hyvärinen A.:* Ann. 1st Super. Sanita (1971) 7, 300–313.

Studies on Alkaline Phosphatases of Different Origin, with an External Quality Control Scheme

A. P. Jansen, Nijmegen (The Netherlands)

Key words: Alkaline phosphatase
Control surveys
Control serum
Isoenzymes
Method standardization
Youden plots

In 1972 the Dutch Society of Clinical Chemistry decided to recommence a national quality control program that had been initiated some 15 years before by the National Institute of Public Health.

Unfortunately, this program had ceased 5 years ago. However, a completely new program was started in 1973 with the analysis of 12 parameters in serum, including one enzyme: alkaline phosphatase. There was some discussion whether or not the determination of this enzyme should be included in the trials, because of the great differences in the results that could be expected. Yet it was decided to include the analysis of alkaline phosphatase in the scheme.

A pilot study was begun, lasting 12 months and comprising 33 laboratories, spread all over the country. Each laboratory was supplied with 2 sera for each trial. These lyophilized sera were to be reconstituted with water and the phosphatase reactivated under standard conditions. The results were presented in computer print-outs and in Youden plots.

The results for alkaline phosphatase in the first trial were amazing. The Youden plot disclosed that only systematic differences occurred, depending on buffer, temperature and so on (fig. 1).

This can also be demonstrated in a different way by taking the ratio of the alkaline phosphatase activities in the 2 sera; systematic differences are then eliminated and random errors and differences emerge in the magnitude of the relative standard deviation (synonym: coefficient of variation) of the ratios.

In the first trial this value was as low as 3% which is striking, considering that it is calculated from two determinations.

Expectations ran high for the second trial, but the results were disastrous (fig. 2). Now the relative standard deviation of the mean value for the alkaline phosphatase ratio was 22.9%!

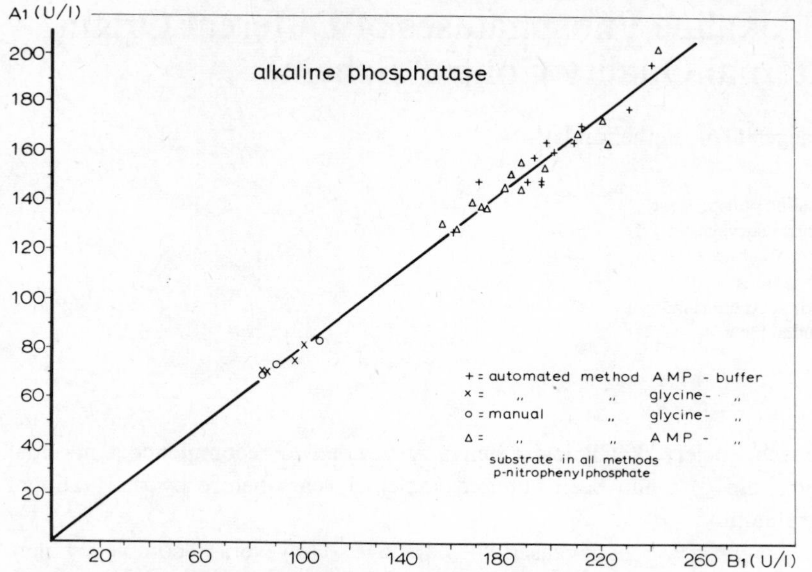

Fig. 1. Youden plot of alkaline phosphatase activities (trial 1).

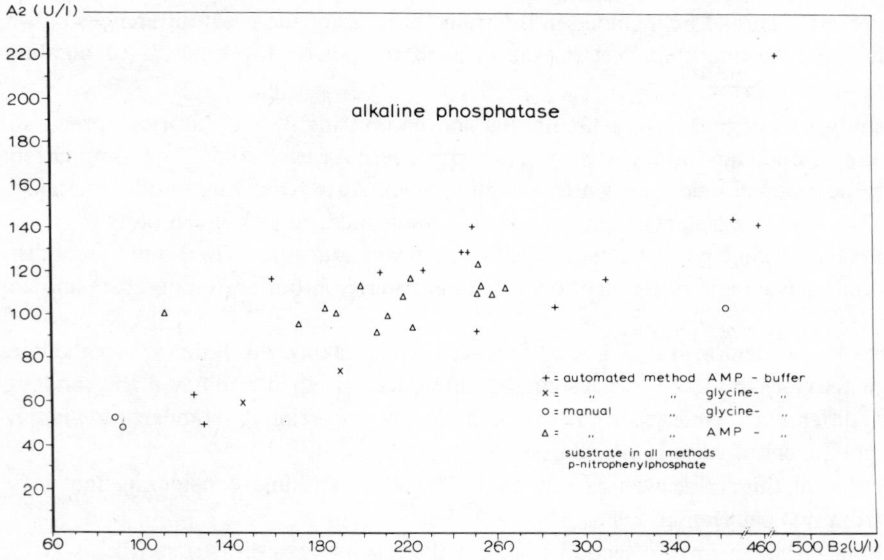

Fig. 2. Youden plot of alkaline phosphatase activities (trial 2).

In the following trials this value fluctuated from 7.4 to 16.4%. In table 1 the results of the 6 trials in the pilot study have been summarized.

Table 1. Mean ratios and relative standard deviations (cv) of alkaline phosphatase activities in 6 trials of pilot study.

ALKALINE PHOSPHATASE

mean R_1 = 1,25, coefficient of variation	2,95%
mean R_2 = 2,16, coefficient of variation	22,9 %
mean R_3 = 1,30, coefficient of variation	7,4 %
mean R_4 = 2,89, coefficient of variation	16,4 %
mean R_5 = 1,22, coefficient of variation	11,7 %
mean R_6 = 2,57, coefficient of variation	11,0 %
with standardized chemicals:	
mean R_6 = 2,52, coefficient of variation	8,2 %

R is ratio of alkaline phosphatase activity between sample B and A

We wondered what the causes of these great fluctuations might be. Now in the first trial, the same horse serum had been used at 2 different dilutions. The dilution factor was 1.25 and a mean ratio of alkaline phosphatase activity of exactly 1.25 was found. In the second trial two bovine sera were distributed; to one of them a calf intestine preparation had been added to increase the phosphatase activity. Although all participants used the same substrate – p-nitrophenylphosphate – it was possible that the different methods used gave a different response to isoenzymes of alkaline phosphatase. To test this hypothesis, the participants were provided with alkaline phosphatase preparations of different origin. Three enzyme preparations were used in the investigation: placental phosphatase of human origin (Boehringer, Mannheim GmbH), a beef liver preparation and a hog intestinal mucosa phosphatase (Sigma Chemical Company: P 5760 and P 4002 respectively).

The activity of the enzyme preparations decreased on lyophilization, unless albumin was added.

In the case of the liver preparation, enzymeactivity was lost completely on lyophilization even in the presence of albumin. The stability of the enzymes in 1% albumin solutions was satisfactory when stored at 4 °C [1].

Therefore in all investigations, except the first, liquid enzyme preparations in 1% albumin were used. The results of these studies are presented in table 2.

The following conclusions may be drawn:

1. When the same isoenzyme is analyzed in different concentrations, the relative standard deviation of the mean ratio is of the same magnitude as this value in sera to which no isoenzymes have been added.
2. The relative standard deviation of the mean ratio of different isoenzymes of alkaline phosphatase is about 2.5–3 times higher than this value for the same isoenzyme in different concentrations.

In the last trial of the pilot study the participants were provided again with 3 different specimens of alkaline phosphatase.

Table 2. Mean ratios and relative standard deviations (cv) of alkaline phosphatase activities in 3 enzyme preparations.

P_1 human placenta alkaline phosphatase

P_2 beef liver alkaline phosphatase

P_3 hog intestine alkaline phosphatase

P_4 hog intestine alkaline phosphatase, $P_4 = 3 \times P_3$

mean P_4/P_3 ratio = 3,04, coefficient of variation	9,0 %
mean P_3/P_2 ratio = 1,30, coefficient of variation	22,6 %
mean P_1/P_3 ratio = 0,75, coefficient of variation	29,5 %
mean P_1/P_2 ratio = 0,96, coefficient of variation	28,2 %

The participating laboratories were asked not only to analyze the enzyme with their own method, using their own chemicals, but also with a partially standardized method. The participants were supplied for that purpose with a buffer-solution containing 2-amino-2-methylpropanol-1 and Mg^{++}-ions and they were asked to use the same p-nitrophenyl phosphate concentration in the final solution. The results are shown in table 3.

Table 3. Mean ratios and relative standard deviations (cv) of alkaline phosphatase activities in 3 enzyme preparations, measured with own methods of participants and with standardized chemicals.

P_5 human placenta alkaline phosphatase

P_6 hog intestine alkaline phosphatase

P_7 human placenta alkaline phosphatase

P_8 beef liver alkaline phosphatase

	own method		with standardized chemicals	
ratio P_5/P_7	mean 2,40	c.v. 8,9 %	mean 2,40	c.v. 6,7 %
ratio P_7/P_6	mean 1,03	c.v. 26,6 %	mean 1,29	c.v. 12,9 %
ratio P_7/P_8	mean 1,27	c.v. 23,9 %	mean 1,44	c.v. 20,5 %
ratio P_6/P_8	mean 1,22	c.v. 21,3 %	mean 1,09	c.v. 16,7 %

From this table it can be concluded:

1. There is some improvement, it is true, if the same chemicals are used, but the improvement is less than might be expected.

2. The mean ratios are similar for the participants own methods and the so-called standard method, when sera (table 1) or human placenta preparations were analyzed. These mean ratios were not identical for both methods when different isoenzymes were compared. This means that isoenzymes demonstrate different activities when analyzed with only slightly modified methods.
3. Instability of the enzyme preparations cannot be the reason for the discrepancies observed. The fact that the magnitude of the relative standard deviations of the mean ratios is the same for all combinations of isoenzyme preparations argues against this supposition. It must be emphasized that only the same chemicals had been used in the 'standard'-method but that incubation-time and -temperature had not been standardized. In figure 3 the results of this study are shown in a Youden-plot.

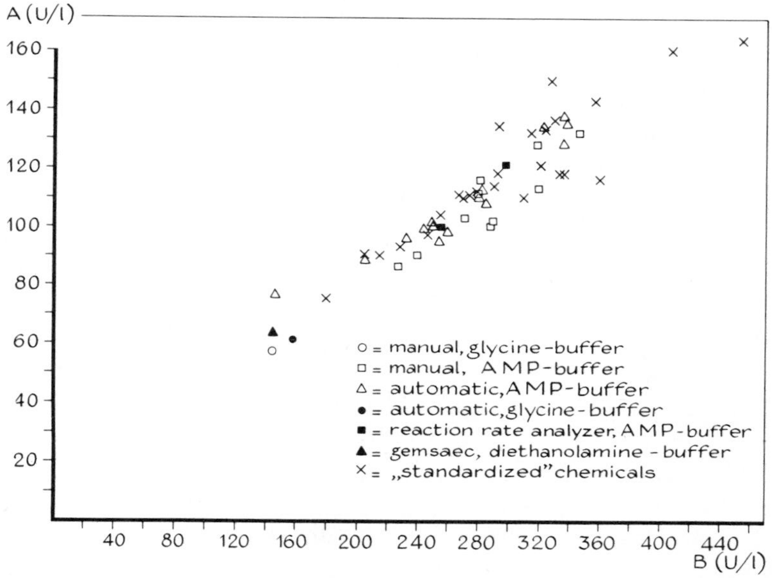

Fig. 3. Youden plot of alkaline phosphatase activities measured with own methods of participants and with standardized chemicals.

Next, the number of participants in the trials was extended to 100. The results obtained in 6 trials are presented in table 4. They are practically identical to those of the pilot study, and especially when an alkaline phosphatase preparation had been added to serum to increase the enzymatic activity, the relative standard deviation is high. Also, when enzyme preparations were distributed to the 100 participants, the results were comparable to those in the pilot study (table 5). The placenta preparation was now used at 3 different concentration levels to see if the extent of the concentration differences influenced the relative standard deviations of the mean ratios.

Table 4. Mean ratios and relative standard deviations (cv) of alkaline phophatase activities in 6 trials.

Trial 7 : R mean 1.34 coefficient of variation 10,4 %

Trial 8 : R mean 1,14 coefficient of variation 11,1 %

Trial 9 : R mean 1,23 coefficient of variation 7,3 %

Trial 10 : R mean 1,06 coefficient of variation 4,1 %

Trial 11 : R mean 1,42 coefficient of variation 13,9 %

Trial 12 : R mean 2,22 coefficient of variation 23,0 %

R is the ratio of alkaline phosphatase activity of serum A and B

Table 5. Mean ratios and relative standard deviations (cv) of alkaline phosphatase activities in different enzyme-preparations.

P_9, P_{10}, P_{11} — human placenta phosphatase (3 concentration levels)

P_{12} beef liver preparation

P_{13} hog intestinal mucosa preparation

mean	P_9/P_{10} ratio :	1,14 ,	c.v.	4,9 % ,	n = 83
mean	P_{10}/P_{11} ratio :	2,96 ,	c.v.	7,3 % ,	n = 85
mean	P_{13}/P_9 ratio :	1,80 ,	c.v.	24,2 % ,	n = 87
mean	P_{12}/P_9 ratio :	1,03 ,	c.v.	24,6 % ,	n = 89
mean	P_{13}/P_{12} ratio :	1,76 ,	c.v.	21,0 % ,	n = 89

There is at least an indication, that the closer the concentrations, the lower will be the relative standard deviations. Here again, the magnitude of the deviation is the same as in the pilot-study.

Nor is there any indication that instability of the enzyme preparations is the cause of the higher deviations of the ratios, when preparations of different origin are compared.

One may wonder if these investigations have any meaning at all, and if any conclusions can be drawn from the data available. Out of 12 trials there were 2 in which a relative standard deviation of the mean ratio of alkaline phophatase activity of 4% or less was found. In 2 other trials this value was about 7%. Now a relative standard deviation of 7% may be expected for the mean ratio, if the relative standard deviation for a single phosphatase determination is 5%.

($\sqrt{5^2 + 5^2} = 7$). A value that is found in only few non-enzymatic determinations in this type of trial.

Evidently, in some sera the isoenzyme composition is very similar, and when this composition was exactly identical and only differences in the concentrations existed, the lowest relative standard deviation was found for the ratio of the enzyme activities (trial 1). In my opinion, it has further been demonstrated that comparison of different isoenzyme preparations leads to high values for the relative standard deviations of the mean ratios of the enzyme activities. These values are much lower, when the same isoenzymes are compared in different concentrations.

Another conclusion can be that the use of reference sera for alkaline phosphatase determinations is a tricky business and may yield false results.

Comparison of pathological phosphatase values found in different laboratories is difficult, because the pathology will be caused by isoenzymes that give different results in the various methods used. The only way to get comparable results in interlaboratory trials is a very rigorous standardization of methods. The use of the same chemicals is important in the case of alkaline phosphatase, but apparently reaction temperature and perhaps other unidentified reaction conditions are of even greater importance when different isoenzymes are involved. Finally, in table 6 the results of a standard method, used by 9 laboratories, are compared with the results obtained from all methods used. It may be concluded from this table, that considerable improvement is to be expected from standardization and that the problem of different results for isoenzyme activities can be solved in this way.

Table 6. Mean values and relative standard deviations (cv) for alkaline phosphatase activities in 12 trials. Comparison of a standard method with all methods.

	standard method							all methods						
	serum A		serum B		ratio			serum A		serum B		ratio		
	mean U/l	cv %	mean U/l	cv %	mean U/l	cv %	numb. labs	mean U/l	cv %	mean U/l	cv %	mean U/l	cv %	numb. labs
trial 1	148	10,9	184	12,0	1,24	2,7	9	140	35,7	176	35,0	1,25	2,95	33
trial 2	107	7,6	212	23,0	2,10	12,6	8	115	22,9	249	33,3	2,16	22,9	32
trial 3	66	14,5	86	14,0	1,32	10,0	9	69	27,6	89	28,5	1,30	7,4	33
trial 4	48	9,2	156	19,7	3,25	14,6	9	51	29,4	145	28,4	2,89	16,4	33
trial 5	51	11,0	68	10,7	1,34	9,0	8	55	23,6	67	22,1	1,22	11,7	33
trial 6	110	12,6	289	11,4	2,63	5,7	9	108	23,4	278	28,3	2,57	11,0	31
trial 7	139	7,7	193	10,0	1,39	8,7	9	132	32,7	175	31,1	1,34	10,4	88
trial 8	71	11,0	62	11,8	1,16	12,4	8	72	30,4	65	34,5	1,14	11,1	88
trial 9	45	11,3	56	8,3	1,25	8,3	9	53	34,9	64	33,8	1,23	7,3	96
trial 10	92	9,8	98	11,2	1,06	2,2	9	94	27,0	98	26,5	1,06	4,1	95
trial 11	175	11,5	115	13,2	1,54	13,6	9	173	26,4	122	29,6	1,42	13,9	96
trial 12	52	10,4	124	13,7	2,41	13,4	8	58	23,3	126	19,5	2,22	23,0	96

Reference

[1] *J.C.M.Hafkenscheid and A.P.Jansen:* Clin. Chim. Acta 59, 63 (1975).

Evaluation of Several Commercial Controls. Correlation between them

A. Martinez, Madrid (Spain)

Key words: Accuracy
Commercial controls
Control sera
Enzyme control
Inter-, Intra-laboratory comparison
Precision
Reference sera

In my view, the main objectives of quality control in clinical chemistry should be precision and accuracy. It is important that the analytical results of a laboratory can be compared to those obtained by another laboratory.

Sometimes a given value is completely different from one laboratory to another, making it difficult for the physician to diagnose and follow up a patient.

In the 1971 Geneva Symposium, *Anido* and *Van Kampen,* showed that there was an improvement in inter-laboratory quality control, in regard to triglycerides and hemoglobin, with the introduction of a common method and standards.

In Spain (first program of Interlaboratory Quality Control – IQC) we had neither a common standard nor methods. Approximately 60–80% of serum glucose, urea, cholesterol, and calcium values were out of control. Two years later, we suggested the use of a common standard for the second program of IQC. The results then, were that the 60–70% of values were in control. Because technics were not common and intra-laboratory variability coefficients were not different from Program 1, we feel that this shows the necessity and importance of using a standard common to all laboratories. It is possible that standard values were not 'true values' in absolute terms, but a common standard permitted comparison of results obtained by several laboratories.

Here, I summarize our experiences. In the study we tried to:

1. Study commercial control sera in common use in our country.
2. Make determinations by automated methods:
   a) *SMA 6 Plus:* Total protein, calcium, phosphate, creatinine, bilirubin, and uric acid.
   b) *Vickers:* Glucose.
   c) *Beckman DSA:* Lactate dehydrogenase (LDH) and alkaline phosphatase.
   d) *Abbott ABA-100:* Aspartate Transaminase (AST) and Alanine Transaminase (ALT).

Procedure

1. Each commercial control serum was evaluated ten times, with the same number of determinations for the reference serum.
   The standard sera used were:
   For SMA, Technicon control serum; for Vickers, Primary Standard for glucose, Boehringer; for enzymes, Precinorm and Precipath, Boehringer.
2. The total number of sera (studied by several commercial laboratories) was 35.
3. During the study, the reference sera and controls were of the same batch.
4. The values obtained with commercial serum and those obtained with the standard serum using the same method were compared. It was not always possible to know if the technics we used, were exactly as originally described or were modifications.
5. We used standard serum as a 'Reference value' and not as the 'True value'.
6. The determinations were made over 8 weeks.

Results

Statistical evaluation of our results gave the following conclusions:

1. Between some commercial sera there were statistically significant differences (Student's test at 95% level).
2. These differences have been considered according to the 'actual value' of the commercial serum, and the value obtained by us using the 'Interval estimation'.

$$I = \frac{(\bar{x} \pm t_x)}{n - 1} \cdot \frac{SD}{\sqrt{n}}$$

3. With the above mentioned statistical criteria we obtained the following results:

	In control	Out of control
Glucose	44.5%	55.5%
Protein	62.0%	38.0%
Calcium	28.0%	72.0%
Phosphorus	36.0%	64.0%
Uric acid	58.0%	42.0%
Creatinine	44.8%	55.2%
Bilirubin	58.0%	42.0%

With these results, we also considered the manufacturer's acceptable range. We then had:

	Out of control (accepted range)	Out of control (Actual values)
Glucose	16.6%	55.5%
Protein	4.1%	38.0%
Calcium	14.0%	72.0%
Phosphorus	21.7%	64.0%
Uric acid	5.0%	42.0%
Creatinine	31.8%	55.2%
Bilirubin	27.7%	42.0%

These results raise problems of real concern. What is the reliability of the commercial control sera? How is it possible to accept this C. V.?

Let us consider the following example of comparison between our value and the manufacturer's values on a commercial control serum, and also the corresponding ranges:

	Uric acid	Creatinine	Bilirubin	
X =	3.87 mg %	0.98 mg %	0.99 mg %	
S. D. =	0.048	0.042	0.073	own values
C. V. =	1.24%	4.28%	7.3%	
X =	4.0 mgs%	1.2 mgs%	0.60 mgs%	
S. D. =	0.25	0.1	0.1	manufacturer's values
C. V. =	6.25%	8.33%	16.6%	

We feel from this, that the less the precision, the greater the errors in accuracy. For example, we can estimate that an automatic technic is within control if we accept the range of the commercial control serum, and it is possible that we then accept as 'normal' a 'limit' value, or an abnormal one.

Booth has pointed out the factors that are important in the differences:

1. Method used for the determination of a given constituent
2. The degree of automation involved
3. Technical skill
4. Standardization

In our present work, we believe, the factors that can influence our results are 1 and 4. If the method we used is not identical with the one recommended by the manufacturer, it is due to lack of information in this respect.

Using glucose as an example, we have reached the following conclusions, that are extensible to other parameters:

1. Of 35 commercial control sera studied with the same automatic equipment, with the same standard, 24 had an excess and 11 had a deficit, in glucose values.
2. It is not possible that inter-day variations were responsible for this, because the general standard (Technicon) fluctuations were small, and had been normalized (tables 1 and 2).

Table 1.

Control	Statistic	Glucose	T. Prot.	Ca	I. Phosph.	Uric Ac.	Creatinine	Bilirubin
1	$\bar{x}$	2.16	6.29	9.75	5.63	7.69	5.11	2.52
	S.D.	0.06	0.08	0.13	0.09	0.06	0.06	0.07
	C.V.	2.77	1.27	1.33	1.59	0.78	1.17	2.77
2	$\bar{x}$	2.18	6.45	9.42	3.69	3.60	0.86	0.63
	S.D.	0.02	0.08	0.04	0.06	0.07	0.05	0.05
	C.V.	0.91	1.27	0.44	1.52	1.83	5.90	7.70
3	$\bar{x}$	1.06	5.72	9.85	4.85	–	1.71	–
	S.D.	0.01	0.06	0.05	0.05	–	0.03	–
	C.V.	0.94	1.10	0.54	1.07	–	1.81	–
4	$\bar{x}$	2.33	6.38	9.11	5.05	7.53	5.29	2.50
	S.D.	0.02	0.15	0.06	0.05	0.08	0.06	0.01
	C.V.	0.85	2.35	0.61	1.03	1.09	1.06	0.40
5	$\bar{x}$	1.10	6.10	8.52	3.15	5.33	0.90	0.37
	S.D.	0.01	0.04	0.06	0.05	0.15	0.01	0.05
	C.V.	0.91	0.65	0.74	1.65	2.80	1.10	13.51
6	$\bar{x}$	0.88	5.95	9.52	3.07	5.70	1.17	1.44
	S.D.	0.01	0.05	0.05	0.08	0.05	0.05	0.12
	C.V.	1.13	0.84	0.48	2.67	0.82	4.10	8.33
7	$\bar{x}$	0.86	6.07	8.74	2.93	5.14	0.87	0.73
	S.D.	0.02	0.08	0.08	0.05	0.07	0.05	0.05
	C.V.	2.32	1.29	0.96	1.64	1.34	5.50	6.57
8	$\bar{x}$	1.57	6.10	7.87	5.21	5.60	7.41	3.53
	S.D.	0.01	0.04	0.05	0.06	0.08	0.06	0.09
	C.V.	0.53	0.72	0.61	1.07	1.45	0.75	2.66
9	$\bar{x}$	1.17	6.92	10.12	3.25	7.73	1.41	3.49
	S.D.	0.01	0.15	0.28	0.08	0.05	0.03	0.09
	C.V.	0.76	2.02	2.75	2.58	0.62	2.20	2.50
10	$\bar{x}$	0.80	7.09	9.44	3.23	5.58	1.00	1.68
	S.D.	0.13	0.06	0.10	0.05	0.17	0.01	0.06
	C.V.	1.02	0.79	1.06	1.49	3.01	1.00	3.75
11	$\bar{x}$	1.12	7.54	9.68	2.74	2.45	0.84	–
	S.D.	0.13	0.11	0.08	0.05	0.22	0.05	–
	C.V.	1.16	1.42	0.81	1.86	8.98	6.07	–
12	$\bar{x}$	0.83	6.62	9.49	4.20	3.31	1.51	0.77
	S.D.	0.006	0.08	0.11	0.01	0.03	0.09	0.50
	C.V.	0.72	1.18	1.15	0.24	0.94	5.76	6.23
13	$\bar{x}$	0.83	6.38	8.81	5.28	4.18	0.98	0.40
	S.D.	0.006	0.08	0.09	0.10	0.06	0.04	0.005
	C.V.	0.69	1.22	1.02	1.95	1.50	4.28	1.25

Table 1. (Continued)

Control	Statistic	Glucose	T. Prot.	Ca	I. Phosph.	Uric Ac.	Creatinine	Bilirubin
14	x̄	1.88	5.98	9.29	3.84	6.65	4.01	3.07
	S.D.	0.01	0.19	0.28	0.34	0.14	0.11	0.16
	C.V.	0.53	3.23	3.06	8.90	2.15	2.75	5.30
15	x̄	1.23	6.66	8.22	5.20	4.56	3.35	2.46
	S.D.	0.01	0.08	0.10	0.14	0.05	0.05	0.05
	C.V.	0.81	1.20	1.21	2.69	1.09	1.49	2.03
16	x̄	3.21	5.67	7.70	–	–	3.61	–
	S.D.	0.19	0.08	0.11	–	–	0.07	–
	C.V.	5.91	1.41	1.42	–	–	1.93	–
17	x̄	1.79	5.12	7.46	5.48	8.51	2.20	3.03
	S.D.	0.01	0.10	0.11	0.06	0.12	0.005	0.21
	C.V.	0.55	1.95	1.47	1.09	1.41	0.52	6.80
18	x̄	1.81	5.17	12.55	8.30	10.03	5.13	6.60
	S.D.	0.04	0.26	0.70	0.33	0.28	0.10	0.46
	C.V.	2.20	5.14	5.57	4.05	2.60	2.04	6.88
19	x̄	2.74	5.23	12.42	7.64	10.52	8.38	7.32
	S.D.	0.04	0.05	0.10	0.08	0.09	0.09	0.59
	C.V.	1.45	0.92	0.83	1.10	0.86	1.08	8.11
20	x̄	0.94	4.40	7.34	2.84	3.87	0.98	0.99
	S.D.	0.008	0.05	0.08	0.05	0.05	0.04	0.07
	C.V.	1.06	1.07	1.14	1.80	1.24	4.28	7.30
21	x̄	3.58	6.83	10.49	6.16	9.06	6.86	8.02
	S.D.	0.04	0.08	0.09	0.07	0.10	0.05	0.29
	C.V.	1.11	1.20	0.83	1.12	1.06	0.74	3.65
22	x̄	1.93	5.31	7.71	5.23	8.98	3.93	4.39
	S.D.	0.01	0.18	0.33	0.11	0.36	0.14	0.21
	C.V.	0.51	3.48	4.33	2.20	3.98	3.59	4.71
23	x̄	2.75	5.54	6.81	5.78	–	–	–
	S.D.	0.02	0.08	0.09	0.06	–	–	–
	C.V.	0.72	1.52	1.30	1.03	–	–	–
24	x̄	2.77	5.36	12.70	7.75	10.67	8.26	6.24
	S.D.	0.01	0.08	0.17	0.12	0.16	0.08	0.21
	C.V.	0.36	1.56	1.38	1.51	1.46	1.01	3.38
25	x̄	2.80	4.53	12.27	2.77	6.20	5.66	2.91
	S.D.	0.05	0.05	0.05	0.05	0.12	0.05	0.14
	C.V.	1.86	1.06	0.39	1.73	1.85	0.90	4.70
26	x̄	1.93	4.38	6.11	7.61	8.24	3.81	5.68
	S.D.	0.02	0.08	0.09	0.06	0.08	0.03	0.12
	C.V.	1.09	1.78	1.42	0.74	1.02	0.81	2.15
27	x̄	3.00	7.58	11.72	7.06	9.51	5.93	6.21
	S.D.	0.03	0.08	0.06	0.05	0.07	0.09	0.17
	C.V.	1.07	1.03	0.54	0.72	0.76	1.58	2.67
28	x̄	2.99	8.26	10.78	6.53	8.08	8.88	–
	S.D.	0.017	0.12	0.18	0.08	0.08	0.06	–
	C.V.	0.57	1.41	1.68	1.26	0.96	0.71	–

Table 1. (Continued)

Control	Statistic	Glucose	T. Prot.	Ca	I. Phosph.	Uric Ac.	Creatinine	Bilirubin
29	$\bar{x}$	0.58	4.42	5.57	2.07	2.53	0.62	0.39
	S.D.	0.006	0.09	0.23	0.07	0.05	0.04	0.08
	C.V.	1.03	2.06	4.15	3.24	1.90	6.77	20.50
30	$\bar{x}$	0.83	3.66	6.74	2.30	3.76	1.53	0.66
	S.D.	0.008	0.05	0.07	0.09	0.07	0.05	0.07
	C.V.	0.96	1.39	1.02	4.08	1.91	3.14	10.45
31	$\bar{x}$	3.17	7.06	11.67	6.81	9.60	5.90	6.37
	S.D.	0.05	0.08	0.07	0.06	0.25	0.07	0.09
	C.V.	1.57	1.19	0.57	0.82	2.64	1.12	1.47
32	$\bar{x}$	2.39	4.84	11.33	6.92	8.80	2.80	4.88
	S.D.	0.02	0.07	0.13	0.04	0.11	0.005	0.10
	C.V.	0.79	1.42	11.17	0.60	1.19	0.18	2.11
33	$\bar{x}$	0.83	5.30	9.06	3.84	4.44	1.66	1.26
	S.D.	0.017	0.06	0.20	0.13	0.25	0.05	0.16
	C.V.	2.04	1.19	2.22	3.49	5.74	3.07	12.46
34	$\bar{x}$	3.19	5.18	13.66	5.80	–	6.09	–
	S.D.	0.026	0.06	0.10	0.04	–	0.03	–
	C.V.	0.86	1.20	0.70	0.72	–	0.49	–
35	$\bar{x}$	0.86	5.94	8.78	3.09	4.93	0.94	0.73
	S.D.	0.016	0.07	0.04	0.03	0.05	0.05	0.05
	C.V.	1.85	1.16	0.48	1.00	0.97	5.42	6.57

Table 2. Glucose.

Sample	$\bar{x}$	SD	n	C.V.%	F_n	$\bar{x}$ Norm	Ac.V.	% D.
1	0.991	0.013	15	1.31	1.000	0.991	1.00	Ref. value
2	2.17	0.08	340	2.16	1.000	2.17	2.16	0.04
3	3.58	0.04	10	1.11	0.986	3.53	3.84	8.78
4	0.94	0.008	10	1.06	0.986	0.927	0.86	- 7.24
5	2.18	0.02	10	0.91	1.014	2.21	2.40	8.60
6	2.99	0.017	10	0.57	1.074	3.21	3.45	7.31
7	0.58	0.006	10	1.03	1.074	0.625	0.60	- 4.00
8	1.06	0.01	10	0.94	1.014	1.045	1.09	- 4.31
9	3.21	0.19	10	5.91	1.000	3.21	3.24	0.93
10	0.83	0.017	10	2.04	0.986	0.819	0.88	7.45
11	2.33	0.02	10	0.85	0.977	2.28	2.53	-10.96
12	1.10	0.009	10	0.81	0.977	1.25	1.14	- 8.80
13	1.81	0.04	10	2.20	1.000	1.81	2.10	16.02
14	0.88	0.01	10	1.13	0.977	0.860	0.80	- 7.00
15	1.79	0.01	10	0.55	1.000	1.79	1.88	5.03
16	1.57	0.01	10	0.53	0.964	1.514	1.74	14.90
17	0.863	0.016	10	1.85	0.927	0.800	0.88	10.00
18	2.77	0.010	10	0.36	0.986	2.732	2.85	4.32
19	0.86	0.020	10	2.32	0.964	0.829	0.83	0.12
20	2.74	0.04	10	1.45	0.986	2.702	2.88	6.59
21	1.17	0.009	10	0.76	0.964	1.128	1.08	- 4.26
22	1.88	0.010	10	0.53	1.004	1.888	2.03	7.52
23	2.99	0.032	10	1.07	1.043	3.124	3.56	13.96
24	0.83	0.006	10	0.72	1.004	0.834	0.85	1.92
25	0.85	0.006	10	0.69	1.007	0.836	0.85	1.68
26	3.11	0.049	10	1.57	0.995	3.102	3.55	14.44
27	0.881	0.008	10	0.96	0.995	0.827	0.91	10.04
28	1.925	0.021	10	1.08	1.043	2.008	1.98	- 1.39
29	2.392	0.019	10	0.79	0.995	2.381	2.31	- 2.98
30	2.80	0.052	10	1.86	1.043	2.921	3.05	4.45
31	1.12	0.13	10	1.16	0.927	1.039	1.04	- 0.096
32	0.80	0.13	10	1.62	0.927	0.742	0.86	-15.9
33	1.93	0.01	10	0.51	0.986	1.904	2.17	-13.97
34	2.75	0.02	10	0.72	0.986	2.712	2.45	9.66
35	3.19	0.06	10	0.815	0.986	3.146	3.28	- 4.26

Observations:

Normalization to make similar the daily differences of same control (Technicon), has been obtained multiplying general $\bar{x}$ = daily mean by F_n (Coefficient of normalization).

The mean normalized $\bar{x}_n$ has been calculated according to $\bar{x}_n = \bar{x} \cdot F_n$.

It is accepted the daily variations of the standard, affect in the order, the samples of the same day.

We have then these possibilities:

1. The general and the reference standard values are not correct, and the value most repeated in the histogram must be taken as glucose mean value.

2. For comparison between standards, with references, we used the deviation in % according to the formula:

$$\% \text{Deviation} = \frac{(\text{Actual value} - \text{Obtained value}) \cdot 100}{\text{Obtained value}}$$

3. The % deviations, had a range between + 16% and – 16%. In intervals of 4%, frequencies were 4, 6, 8, 4, 4, 2, 1.
4. The histogram had a bell-shape, with a mode in the excess region (fig. 1).

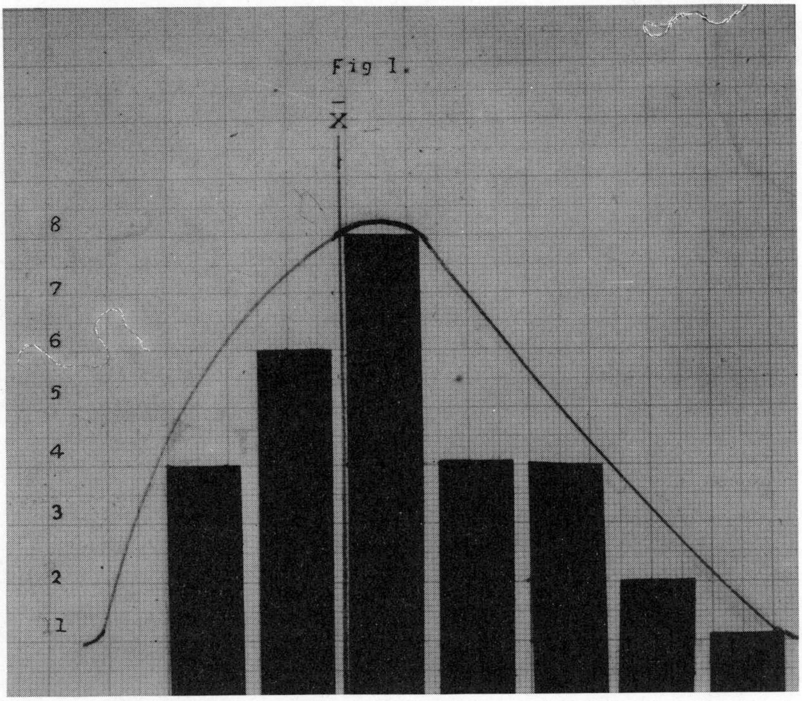

We insist, that we are not considering as absolute and true the value in the reference control used, but we would like to point out, that some commercial sera are similar to that of the reference, and others are not. Some of them must be incorrect, or they have been evaluated with a different methodology to ours.

In summary, it is not possible to obtain Quality Control if we do not have *one* control serum of reference for all the laboratories. It is also important, that the technic employed is clearly detailed.

In enzymes, as we anticipated, results have been tremendously dispersed. If precision with our methodology was 'acceptable', accuracy and comparison between different commercial sera was completely impossible (tab. 3).

Table 3. Enzymatic results.

Serum number		AST	ALT	LDH	Alkaline phosphatase
1	$\bar{x}$ =	31.3	9.4	385.4	59.2
	SD =	2.62	0.69	14.81	1.54
	CV =	8.37%	7.34%	3.84%	2.6%
2	$\bar{x}$ =	32.1	37.2	119.9	37.6
	SD =	1.72	1.35	14.01	4.4
	CV =	5.3%	3.8%	11.69%	11.7%
3	$\bar{x}$ =	3.6		59.7	15.2
	SD =	0.51		12.25	0.63
	CV =	14.16%		20.52%	4.14%
4	$\bar{x}$ =	68.5		611.9	
	SD =	1.5		17.47	
	CV =	2.19%		2.85%	
5	$\bar{x}$ =	4.3		138.5	24.0
	SD =	0.48		7.5	0.7
	CV =	11.16%		5.41%	2.91%
6	$\bar{x}$ =	30.5		352.3	67.6
	SD =	2.38		13.54	8.01
	CV =	7.8%		3.84%	11.85%
7	$\bar{x}$ =	17.45	28.4	588.25	
	SD =	0.52	0.51	16.05	
	CV =	2.97%	1.79%	2.73%	
8	$\bar{x}$ =	3.2	6.20	57.0	15.5
	SD =	0.63	0.42	11.2	1.77
	CV =	19.68%	6.77%	19.6%	11.42%
9	$\bar{x}$ =	78.0	56.5	350.9	73.54
	SD =	1.19	0.15	11.06	1.12
	CV =	1.53%	0.28%	3.15%	1.52%
10	$\bar{x}$ =			275.9	56.8
	SD =			11.3	0.78
	CV =			4.09%	1.37%
11	$\bar{x}$ =			271.1	30.3
	SD =			10.08	0.67
	CV =			3.72%	2.21%
12	$\bar{x}$ =		5.5	77.8	20.5
	SD =		0.7	9.02	0.52
	CV =		12.72%	11.6%	2.53%
13	$\bar{x}$ =	6.10			38.4
	SD =	0.56			0.51
	CV =	9.18%			1.32%

Table 3 (Contenued)

Serum number		AST	ALT	LDH	Alkaline phosphatase
14	x̄ =	31.6	14.0	535.2	107.11
	SD =	0.69	0.53	21.35	0.78
	CV =	2.18%	3.78%	3.99%	0.73%
15	x̄ =	21.9		599.0	93.44
	SD =	0.56		7.91	1.23
	CV =	2.56%		1.32%	1.32%
16	x̄ =	23.7		585.4	78.3
	SD =	0.82		6.36	1.05
	CV =	3.46%		1.08%	1.34%
17	x̄ =	103.7			125.9
	SD =	2.0			1.19
	CV =	1.93%			0.94%
18	x̄ =	36.1			83.09
	SD =	1.19			1.81
	CV =	3.09%			2.18%
19	x̄ =				9.7
	SD =				0.82
	CV =				0.74%
20	x̄ =			482.0	106.8
	SD =			11.24	0.78
	CV =			2.33%	0.74%
21	x̄ =	42.8	19.7	446	75.5
	SD =	0.92	0.67	18.72	0.75
	CV =	2.14%	3.42%	4.19%	1.28%

n = 10. Reference serums: Precipath and Precinorm (Boehringer).

In the comparison between several commercial sera we have not made any statistical study, because of the great differences between the manufacturer's and our values. To study the relations between the analyzed values we have 'normalized' the values by dividing the obtained value by the actual value. We have considered the result 'equal' when the quotient is one, and accepted the result as 'valid' with values between + 0.8 and − 1.2 (fig. 2). For some enzymes there is more dispersion than for others. We have, when possible, studied the relationship between several controls from the same manufacturer (fig. 3a and b), finding some graphic correlation.

In summary, in enzyme evaluations it is even more necessary to standardize technics for purposes of inter-laboratory comparison. Quality control based only on precision can be used for intralaboratory control, but will not be valid for comparison between interlaboratory values.

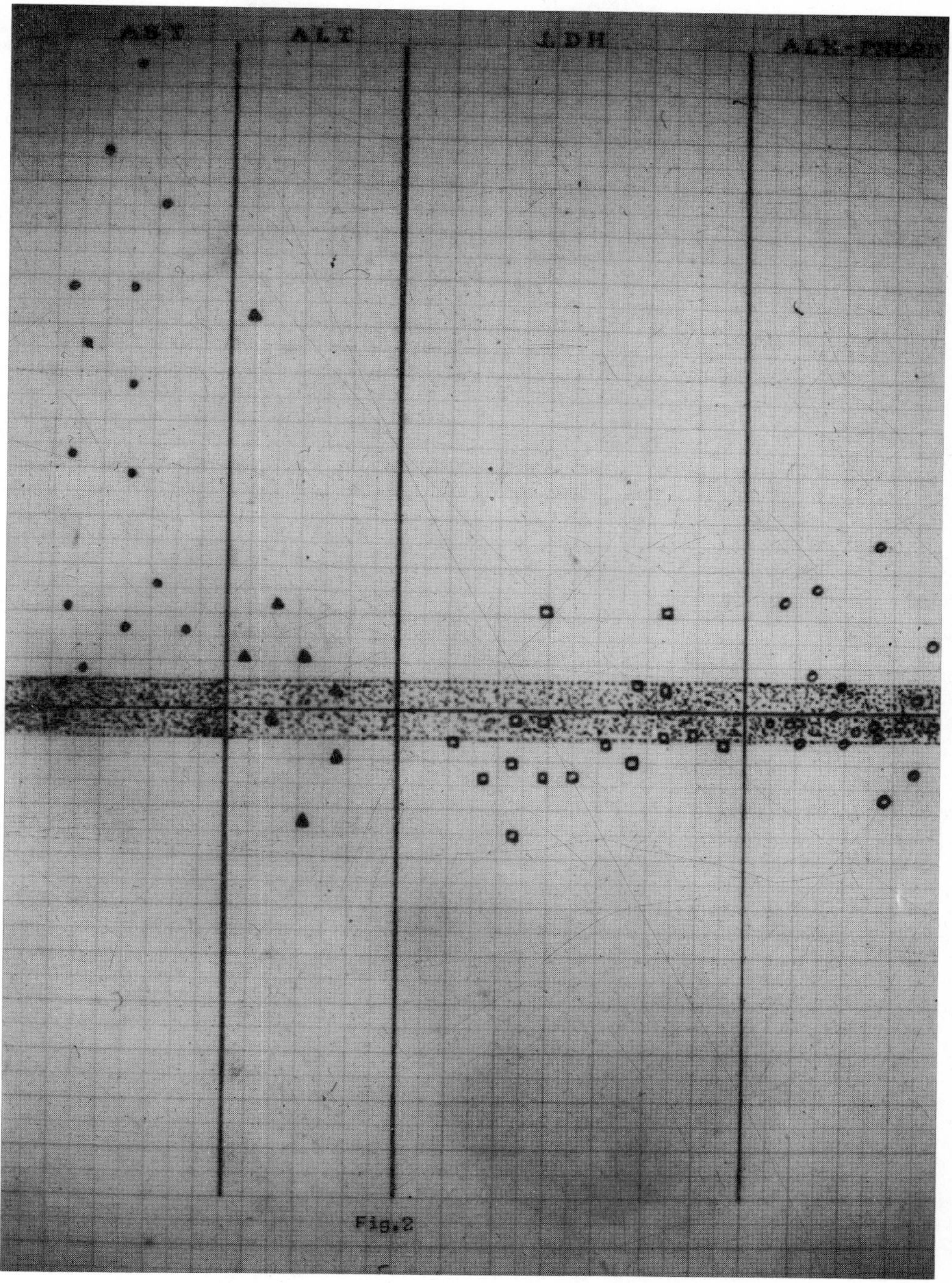

Fig.2

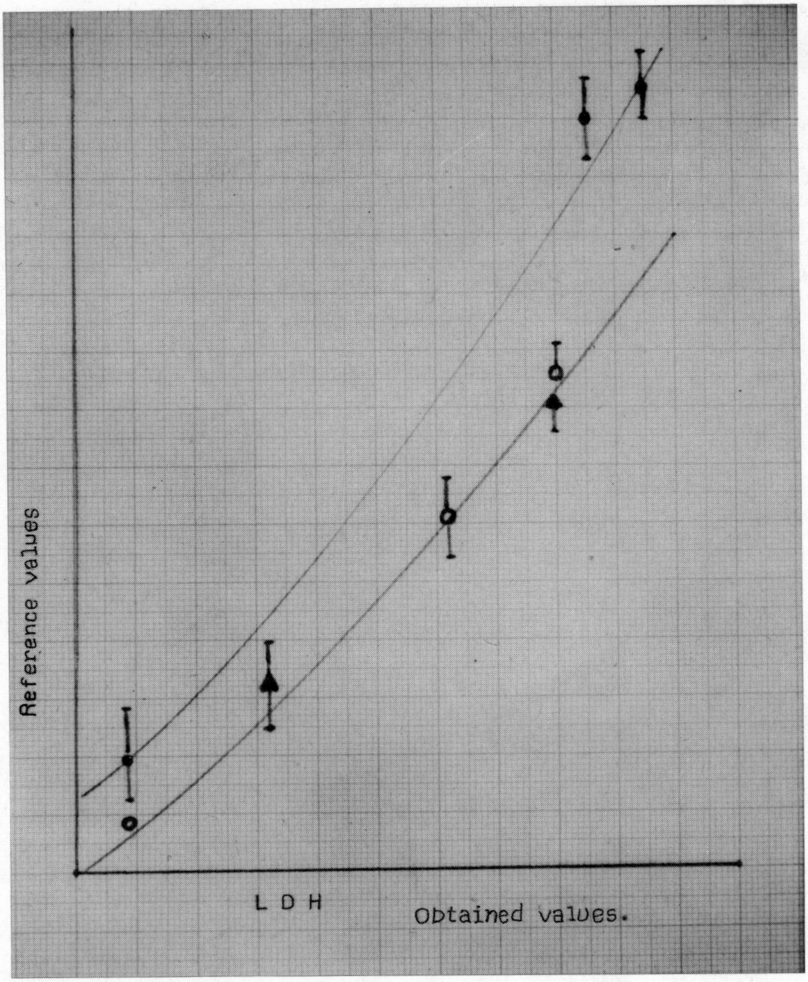

Fig. 3a.

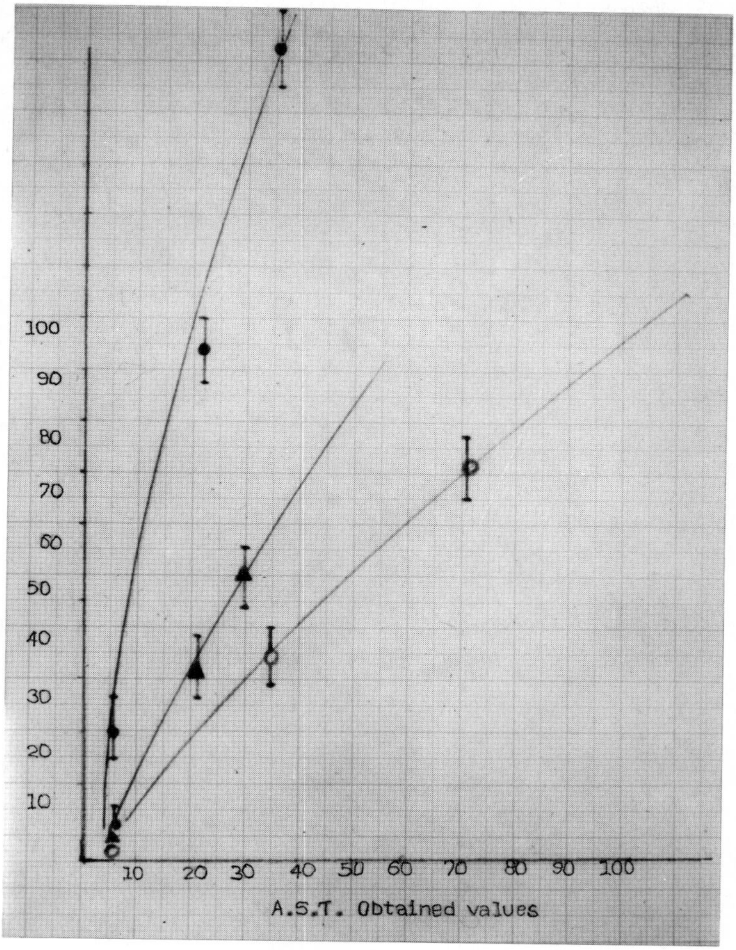
100
90
80
70
60
50
40
30
20
10
10
20
30
40
50
60
70
80
90
100
A.S.T. Obtained values

Fig. 3b.

Acknowledgment

The author wishes to acknowledge the co-operation and help of the staff of Laboratory of Clinical Chemistry of 'Ciudad Sanitaria 1° de Octubre': Drs. Hontoria, Puche, Larrumbe, Gomez-Izquierdo, Diaz-Rubio, Coca, Larrodera, Fernandez-Salas, Gomez-Segura, Muños-Rivero, Cañizares, and Hawkins.

Interlaboratory Comparison of Both Accuracy and Precision by a Two-Sample Method

R. Zender, La Chaux-de-Fonds and *A. Linder*, Geneva (Switzerland)

Key words: Accuracy
Precision
Quality control
Two-sample comparisons

Summary

A two-sample method is proposed to estimate both accuracy and precision in interlaboratory surveys. Results a_i and b_i from each laboratory on samples A and B are standardized by using a factor: $r = \bar{a} / \bar{b}$ ($\bar{a}$ and $\bar{b}$ are the mean values of all laboratories). The standardized mean location of laboratory i is $z_i = (a_i + r \cdot b_i) \cdot 0{,}5$ and its standardized variability $d_i = a_i - r \cdot b_i$. Accuracy and precision of laboratory i is estimated by comparing its z_i and d_i values to the sets of these values in the other laboratories excluding outliers. Examples are given for surveys done on sodium, glucose, creatinine and total proteins and, more particularly, laboratories are thus classified for precision in a 'blind' manner. The method can also be applied when target values α and β are different from $\bar{a}$ and $\bar{b}$.

Interlaboratory programs or surveys to evaluate the performances of test procedures or methods should be designed to estimate both accuracy and precision of each participating laboratory.

Accuracy has been defined by the International Federation of Clinical Chemistry, Expert Panel on Nomenclature and Principles of Quality Control in Clinical Chemistry [1] as: 'agreement between the best estimate of a quantity and its true value'; precision as: 'agreement between replicate measurements'. The 'numerical difference between the mean of a set of replicate measurements and the true value' is defined as inaccuracy and the 'standard deviation of the results in a set of replicate measurements' as imprecision.

It is a rather easy matter to estimate the accuracy of an individual laboratory participating in a survey concerning one or several samples, when the 'true value' is kept secret until the laboratory reports are sent back to the organisers of the survey. Assuming that the laboratories are honest and will not contact each other, the estimate of accuracy can be considered as unbiased.

Estimating the precision of an individual laboratory, however, is, in most cases, a more difficult enterprise. If one sample is sent, and the laboratory is asked to perform the same test a certain number of times, we do believe, that in many cases a large number of obviously bad results will not be reported. In such cases, the test will simply be carried out again, because the laboratory technician or the head of the laboratory genuinely feels that the poor performance registered is exceptional in his laboratory. Thus it cannot be reported in a survey in which his laboratory would be compared to others, which 'by chance', may report a better agreement between replicate measurements. This feeling is of course naïve but we have found it to be an insurmountable obstacle in surveys using the single sample method. The outcome is that precision is most often considered a minor problem in quality control even though its estimation may be highly biased.

The use of two-sample methods, as proposed by Youden (2,3), for testing laboratory performances has not been applied to estimating individual laboratory precision, even if an estimate of the 'mean' standard deviation of all laboratories is made. Youden (3) states that: '... differences in precision, between laboratories can be forgotten because, if present, they are probably minor differences anyway, ...'.

In this paper we have taken the opposite attitude and, using a two-sample method of estimation, we have attempted to distinguish between precision and accuracy for each of the reported couple of values. We also chose a unidimensional graphical display of the data since this would make it easier for laboratory technicians to comprehend the results than the Youden-plot.

Methods

1. Data

a) For one component, glucose, for example, we receive, from each of M laboratories, for the first sample *A* and the second sample *B*, a couple of results a_i and b_i. These results are elements of sets A and B.

$$A = \left\{ a_i \; ; \; i \text{ goes from } 1 \rightarrow M \right\}$$

$$B = \left\{ b_i \; ; \; i \text{ goes from } 1 \rightarrow M \right\}$$

b) For samples *A* and *B*, we have the conventional true values, or target values α and β. These target values can be established by an expert or by a group of experts; they can also be extracted from the sets and from then on be considered as constants. In the examples mentioned below,

$$\alpha = \bar{a} = \frac{1}{M} \sum_{1}^{M} a_i$$

$$\beta = \bar{b} = \frac{1}{M} \sum_{1}^{M} b_i$$

α and β can also be obtained in many other ways but it is not our intention to discuss the elaboration of so-called 'true values' here.

2. Transformations

Our purpose is to create two new sets from sets A and B, say Z and D, from which accuracy and precision can be estimated. We first calculate the ratio

$$r = \frac{\bar{a}}{\bar{b}}$$

then for each laboratory

$$c_i = r \cdot b_i$$

$$z_i = (a_i + c_i) \cdot 0,5$$

$$d_i = (a_i - c_i)$$

c_i values are thus derived from b_i values for each laboratory and it is easily understood that, if the precision of the laboratory is excellent $c_i \rightarrow a_i$.
z_i value is the standardized mean location of laboratory i in set Z.

$$Z = \left\{ z_i \; ; \; i \text{ goes from } 1 \rightarrow M \right\}$$

and the *accuracy* of each laboratory will be estimated by comparing its z_i to the standardized target value which is:

$$z^* = \left[\alpha + (r \cdot \beta)\right] \cdot 0,5$$

$$\text{when } \alpha = \bar{a} \text{ and } \beta = \bar{b}$$

$$z^* = \bar{a}$$

d_i is the standardized variability of laboratory i in set D.

$$D = \left\{ d_i \ ; \ i \text{ goes from } 1 \rightarrow M \right\}$$

and the precision of each laboratory will be estimated by comparing its d_i to zero.

3. Significance tests

On the one hand we have laboratory j with results a_j and b_j and standardized values z_j and d_j. On the other hand we have sets Z_{-j} and D_{-j} of N other laboratories (N = M−1).
We calculate the two variances for these sets, to which laboratory j does not belong:

$$S_{zz} = \sum_1^N z_j^2 - \frac{\left(\sum_1^N z_i\right)^2}{N} \qquad s_z^2 = S_{zz} / (N-1)$$

$$S_{dd} = \sum_1^N d_j^2 - \frac{\left(\sum_1^N d_i\right)^2}{N} \qquad s_d^2 = S_{dd} / (N-1)$$

We then test the difference between z^* and z_i using test FE and the value d_i using test FP. FE and FP measure accuracy and precision respectively; the corresponding probabilities are P-ex and P-pr.

$$FE = \frac{(z_j - z^*)^2}{s_z^2} \sim \text{P-ex}$$

$$FP = d_j^2 / s_d^2 \sim \text{P-pr}$$

$$\left.\right\} \quad df\,1 = 1, \quad df\,2 = N-1$$

The same tests are repeated for each laboratory, which in turn is compared to the N other laboratories.

4. Exclusion of outliers

In a first run, calculations are made for M laboratories, some of which may have results showing P-ex and/or P-pr < 0.001.

In a second run, the calculations are made again after excluding these laboratories which, by convention, do not belong to the same set as the other laboratories.

5. Graphical presentation of the results

The distributions of the results for samples *A* and *B* are illustrated by two histograms placed face to face (fig. 1). These histograms are standardized: their means coincide and their scale is in subunits of the standard deviation between laboratories.

The *accuracy* of each individual laboratory can be estimated by comparing the positions of its two results (⊛) to the target value, in our example the mean m.

The *precision* of the laboratory is best when values a_j and b_j are superposed (fig. 1 and 3) and gets worse as the horizontal distance between the two positions increases (fig. 2).

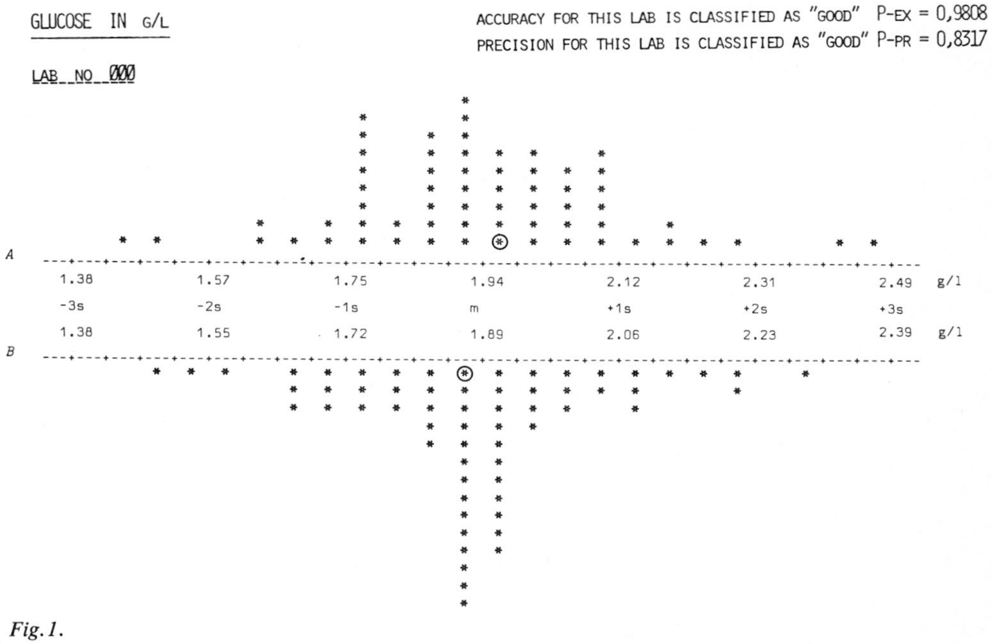

Fig. 1.

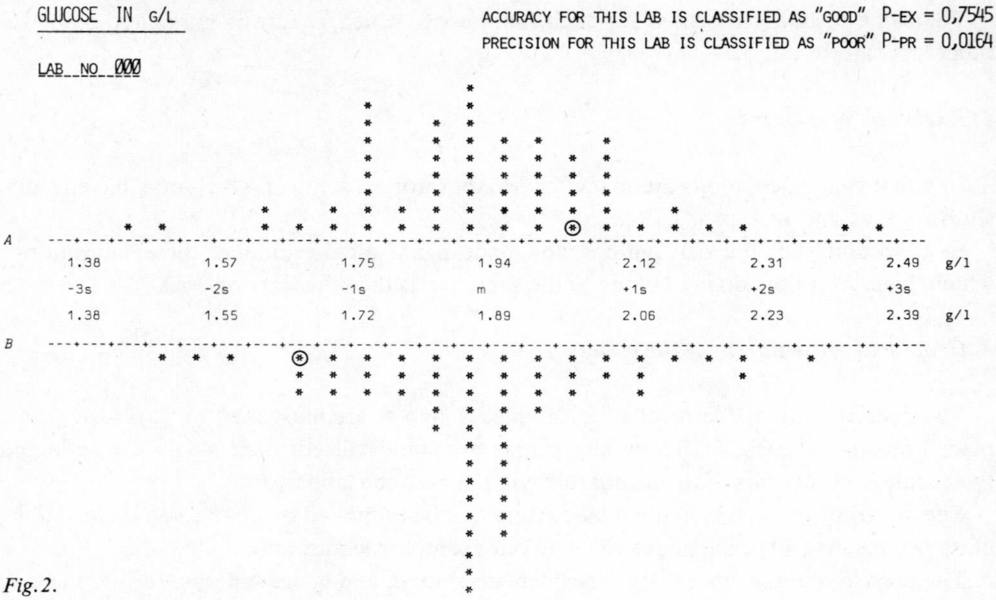
GLUCOSE IN G/L
LAB NO ØØØ
ACCURACY FOR THIS LAB IS CLASSIFIED AS "GOOD" P-EX = 0,7545
PRECISION FOR THIS LAB IS CLASSIFIED AS "POOR" P-PR = 0,0164
A
1.38 1.57 1.75 1.94 2.12 2.31 2.49 g/1
-3s -2s -1s m +1s +2s +3s
1.38 1.55 1.72 1.89 2.06 2.23 2.39 g/1
B

Fig. 2.

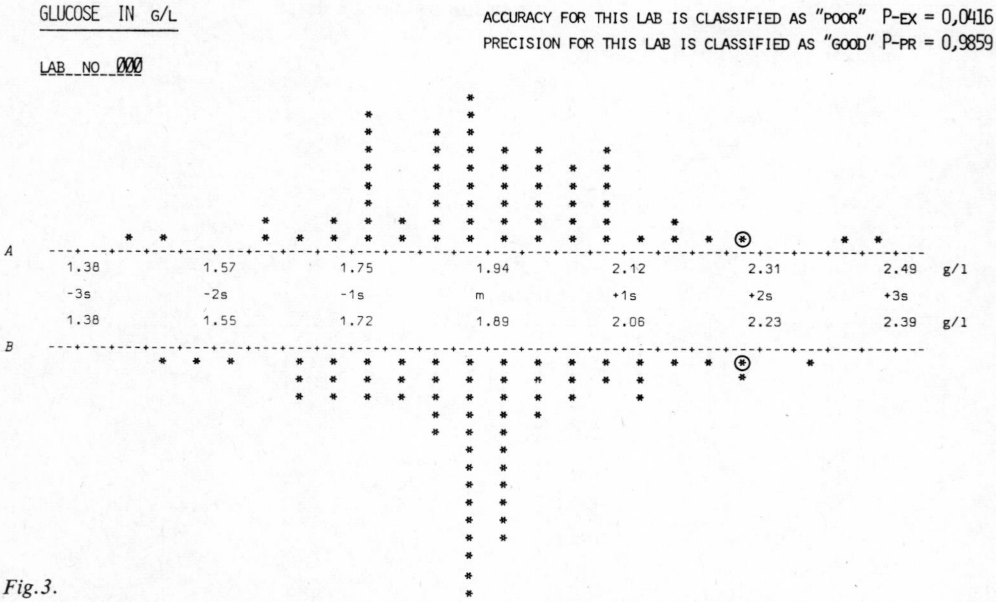
GLUCOSE IN G/L
LAB NO ØØØ
ACCURACY FOR THIS LAB IS CLASSIFIED AS "POOR" P-EX = 0,0416
PRECISION FOR THIS LAB IS CLASSIFIED AS "GOOD" P-PR = 0,9859
A
1.38 1.57 1.75 1.94 2.12 2.31 2.49 g/1
-3s -2s -1s m +1s +2s +3s
1.38 1.55 1.72 1.89 2.06 2.23 2.39 g/1
B

Fig. 3.

6. Grading the laboratories

The laboratories are classified according to the probabilities P-ex and P-pr, which are calculated for each of them.

P > 0.5 is classified as 'good'
0.5 > P > 0.25 as 'satisfactory'
0.25 > P > 0.1 as 'moderate'
0.1 > P > 0.05 as 'unsatisfactory'
0.05 > P > 0.01 as 'poor' and
0.01 > P as 'very poor'

7. Programs

The calculations and histograms are done on a IBM 3/10 computer (16 K bytes). Programs are in Fortran IV.

Results

For an experimental survey of the Swiss organisation for Quality Control in Clinical Chemistry, we have used two lots, *A* and *B* of Moni-Trol II[1]. The survey was done for four components: sodium ion, glucose, creatinine and total proteins. Target values and manufacturer's values are reported in table 1. α and β are the mean results of M laboratories *after* elimination of the outliers. The laboratories were graded and their results are summarized in table 2 for accuracy and in table 3 for precision.

Table 1.

					Producer's values	
Component	M	Outliers	$\bar{a} = z^*$	$\bar{b}$	*A*	*B*
Na (mmol/l)	57	3	128	125	126	125
Glucose (g/l)	63	1	1.94	1.89	2.03	2.03
Creatinine (mg/l)	53	1	41.5	42.3	44	41
Total Proteins (g/l)	59	2	56.5	55.5	57	57

Table 2. Accuracy.

Grading		Number of laboratories			
		Na	Glucose	Creatinine	Total Proteins
Good	P-ex > 0.5	26	38	34	36
Satisfactory	P-ex < 0.5	21	12	9	13
Moderate	P-ex < 0.25	5	6	4	4
Unsatisfactory	P-ex < 0.1	2	2	2	1
Poor	P-ex < 0.05	2	4	5	6
Very poor	P-ex < 0.01	4	2	0	1

[1] Merz + Dade Lot number 33 and 39.

Table 3. Precision.

Grading		Number of laboratories			
		Na	Glucose	Creatinine	Total Proteins
Good	P-pr > 0.5	37	43	35	42
Satisfactory	P-pr < 0.5	8	11	8	4
Moderate	P-pr < 0.25	9	4	7	7
Unsatisfactory	P-pr < 0.1	1	0	0	0
Poor	P-pr < 0.05	0	3	1	3
Very poor	P-pr < 0.01	5	3	3	5

It can be seen that precision was moderate or worse for Na in 15 laboratories (25%), for glucose in 10 laboratories (16%), for creatinine in 11 laboratories (20%) and for proteins in 15 laboratories (25%). The laboratories received a double histogram, on which their position is indicated by ◉. Comments concerning their performances are included in the same document. Three of these, for glucose, are illustrated in the included figures. Fig. 1 shows a laboratory with good accuracy and precision; fig. 2 a laboratory with good accuracy but poor precision; fig. 3 a laboratory with poor accuracy but good precision.

Comments

The method that is proposed here for the estimation of accuracy and precision for interlaboratory surveys seems to perform well and, in our tests, it has sorted out laboratories with poor accuracy and those for which precision appears to be the main problem. For instance for Na in mmol/l ($\alpha = 128.0$ and $\beta = 124.7$) laboratory i has reported results $a_j = 124$ and $b_j = 128$, the accuracy of this laboratory is good (P-ex = 0.92) but its precision is very poor (P-pr = 0.0011); but laboratory j's results were $a_j = 137$ and $b_j = 132$, giving very poor accuracy (P-ex = 0.0098) with good precision (P-pr = 0.51).

The transformation of the elements of set B is, of course, legitimate if it is assumed that the systematic error or analytical bias is proportional to the concentration of the component under study. This assumption is more likely to be right if the concentrations in samples *A* and *B* do not differ too much. It is further indispensible that neither of them is singly contaminated by substances which could interfere with the analytical procedures. These assumptions are easy to verify by using control serums.

In cases where $z^* \neq \alpha \neq \bar{a}$, the expert's target values are not equal to the mean values of sets A and B, the proposed method can still be applied but z^* will differ from the standardized mean of the two sets. We have chosen r, the transforming factor, as $\bar{a}/\bar{b}$ rather than as α/β because the latter would imply that the expert's values are of absolute precision. In contrast, the use of the former $r = \bar{a}/\bar{b}$ relates the transformation to the sets of results from all the laboratories (after excluding the outliers) and the z^* value itself is standardized with reference to the same sets. In cases where $\alpha \neq \bar{a}$ and/or $\beta \neq \bar{b}$ the d^* of the expert can be calculated as:

$$d^* = [\alpha - (r \cdot \beta)]$$

and is different from zero if $\alpha/\beta \neq \bar{a}/\bar{b}$.

We have used classical statistical tests, to grade the performances of the laboratories, on sets Z and D. It would also be possible to use, on the same sets, distribution-free tests based on the rank of the elements d_i or z_i. It would also be possible to make a supplementary transformation of the data and perform the tests on the values so obtained, for instance on log d_i. In fact this last transformation would probably be advisable as it is well known that the distribution of this type of error is very often skewed. One must stress the fact that the proposed method is, to our knowledge, the first one where precision and accuracy of individual laboratory results are both estimated in a 'blind' manner. However, the two estimations are closely linked to the confidence that we can have in the so-called target values or 'conventional true values'.

Acknowledgement

Acknowledgement is made to Miss Salma Teypar for help in the preparation of the English text and to Miss Mary-Claude Boillod for secreterial assistance.

References:

[1] Draft recommendation on Terminology and Principles of Quality Control in Clinical Chemistry; Stage 2, Draft 1; EP-NPCQ, International Federation of Clinical Chemistry (1974).

[2] *Youden, W.J.:* Graphical diagnosis of interlaboratory test results. Industrial Quality Control, *15,* 24–29 (1959).

[3] *Youden, W.J.:* The sample, the procedure and the laboratory. Analytical Chemistry, *32* / 13, 23A–37A (1960).

The World Health Organization-Center for Disease Control Lipid Standardization Program

G.R. Cooper, Atlanta (U.S.A.)

Key words: Accuracy
Cholesterol
Control sera
Control trials
Laboratory standardization
Precision
Triglycerides

Summary

Standardization of lipid analyses has been pursued on a national and international basis collaboratively by the U.S. Center for Disease Control and the World Health Organization. Activities of the WHO International Center for Lipid Determination in Cardiovascular Research are combined with those of the U.S. National Lipid Standardization Laboratory. A standardization program was first developed for the determination of cholesterol, later for triglyceride analyses, and now for combined cholesterol and triglyceride measurements. In association with the latter program, a lipid laboratory was developed to study and establish reference methods and reference materials and to help solve problems encountered in standardization projects. Results of these programs indicate that standardization requires considerable effort, not only in achievement but also in maintenance.

An international survey of cholesterol measurement in lipid laboratories is continuously being carried out collaboratively by the Cardiovascular Disease Section of the World Health Organization (WHO) in Geneva and the Lipid Standardization Laboratory of the Center for Disease Control (CDC) in Atlanta. This international cooperative program is conducted by the CDC Lipid Standardization Laboratory through its appointment as the WHO International Reference Center for Lipid Determination in Cardiovascular Research.

The operation is designed to help laboratories self-evaluate performance and, after quality performance is achieved, to offer laboratories the chance to standardize their cholesterol determinations against furnished points of reference. The major objectives of this program are to assist in the development of reference laboratories throughout the world and to help in the calibration of analyses of laboratories involved in epidemiologic studies.

Development

In 1957, the CDC agreed to serve as a neutral central laboratory to help standardize and compare the procedures for cholesterol determination used by a group of seven cardiovascular epidemiologic research laboratories in the United States. As indicated in table

1, an experimental cooperative cholesterol standardization program was designed to investigate whether (a) lyophilized human serum could be used as a reference material for total cholesterol analyses, (b) factors causing variation in results could be identified, and (c) differences in results among laboratories could be measured. The Lipid Laboratory at CDC agreed to design the project, prepare the needed reference materials, analyze the results, and report the results to the individual participating laboratories. This preliminary investigation, carried out over a 2-year period with seven lipid research laboratories, indicated that (a) lyophilized human serum specimens can serve as a satisfactory reference material for cholesterol determinations, (b) the lowest attainable average for the standard deviation of a cholesterol determination on serum among the participants was about 6 mg/dl, and (c) continuing surveillance with a system of quality control is necessary because erratic results were obtained periodically.

Table 1. CDC Lipid Standardization Program.

CCSP (Cooperative Cholesterol Standardization Program)	
Experimental	1957–60
Continuing	1960–70; 1972–73
WHO International	1962–
CTSP (Cooperative Triglyceride Standardization Program)	
Experimental	1968–70
Continuing	1970–73
CLSP (Cooperative Lipid Standardization Program)	
Continuing	1974–
WHO International	1974–
Special Lipid Standardization Programs 1972–	
National Heart & Lung Institute Clinical and Epidemiological Investigations:	
Lipid Research Clinics	
Multiple Risk Factor Intervention Trial	
Hypertension Detection & Followup Program	
Special Centers of Research in Atherosclerosis	
NHLI-VA Mild Hypertension Study	
Ileal Bypass Study	

In 1960, a national Cooperative Cholesterol Standardization Program (CCSP) was established for the United States. In 1962, a WHO International Cooperative Standardization Program, based on the design of the CCSP, was implemented to provide lipid standardization services on an international basis. A central Standardization Laboratory was designated to study and establish an accurate method as a point of reference for the determination of cholesterol; to prepare a group of serum pools of different concentrations with labeled values; to evaluate and develop techniques for preparing, storing, and shipping serum pool specimens; and to offer calibration services by distributing reference materials of known values. To the extent possible, studies were also performed to evaluate commonly used methods, reagents, and equipment. To facilitate technology, transfer and consultation, printed materials were prepared and bench training was offered.

In 1968, the standardization activity was expanded to include an experimental Cooperative Triglyceride Standardization Program (CTSP) designed to study difficulties which might be encountered in external surveillance of the triglyceride determination and to initiate standardization services, if feasible. Frozen aliquots from reference serum pools were found stable for total triglyceride content during distribution, handling, and storage. Twelve international lipid laboratories and 93 laboratories in the United States cooperated in evaluating this experimental program.

The CTSP established in 1970 was an extension of this experimental design. This program was divided into an evaluation phase (Part I), a standardization phase (Part II), and a continuing surveillance phase (Part III). Consultation on quality control and methodology was offered to laboratories that did not meet the criteria for entering the standardization phase. Supplemental serum samples of known triglyceride content and pure triglyceride primary standards were offered for checking purposes and for comparison with laboratory reference materials. Thirty-one laboratories in 17 countries have participated in this Cooperative Triglyceride Standardization Program, along with 224 laboratories in the United States.

In 1974, the cholesterol and triglyceride standardization programs were combined, and the resulting Cooperative Lipid Standardization Program (CLSP) was offered to lipid laboratories in the United States and to international lipid laboratories under the sponsorship of the WHO. The international services were offered to those laboratories not included in the region served by the Prague WHO Regional Standardization Laboratory.

In 1972, the CDC Lipids Section also became the Lipid Standardization Laboratory for several National Heart and Lung Institute epidemiological and clinical investigations which are being carried out collaboratively by 45 universities and research institutions. An intensive internal quality control and external surveillance program was designed and implemented for these groups.

Design

The objectives of the Lipid Standardization Program are (1) to assist lipid laboratories in evaluating their performance, by providing stable reference materials which have been assigned a reliable value by a reference method and (2) to provide consultation on methodology standardization and quality control.

Various designs and mechanisms to carry out these objectives have been used in developing the different standardization programs. In each of the program designs, laboratories have been given an opportunity to self-evaluate performance at an early stage in the program so that any excessive variation or deviation can be eliminated before the laboratory enters the formal standardization phase. After the laboratories have successfully completed the standardization phase, they are offered specimens for periodic checks to assure that the level of performance is maintained. The design of the original International Cooperative Cholesterol Standardization Program is described in table 2. The current

Table 2. Original Protocol of International Cooperative Cholesterol Standardization Program[1].

Part	Number of Samples Analyzed[2]	Design
1	20	This part is designed to determine a laboratory's precision within a run. Each laboratory will analyze 1 serum sample in duplicate per day for a total of 10 working days and report results. The serum samples are furnished by the individual laboratory.
2	20	This part is designed primarily to allow the laboratory to get experience in handling samples and to gain more information about the reproducibility, both within and between runs. Each laboratory will be sent 20 serum samples to be analyzed in 10 working days (2 a day).
3	96	This part is designed to study the reproducibility within and among laboratories within certain time limits and with different cholesterol concentrations. Each laboratory will be sent a set of 8 samples per month for a total of 12 months. (This schedule is sometimes changed to fit the needs of certain individual laboratories that do not perform cholesterol analyses routinely.) A single determination is made from each vial. One vial is analyzed per day; the days should be spread over a period of at least 1 month.
4	72	This part is designed as a follow-up period to determine how well the laboratories maintain their level of performance. Each laboratory will be sent a set of 18 samples 4 times during the following year. (A laboratory may continue to receive samples at 3-month intervals for as long as desired.)

[1] The parts of this program are performed in sequence.
[2] One determination per sample; hence the number of determinations equals the number of samples.

combined lipid standardization program offers a set of known samples for laboratory self-evaluation as Part I. In Part II, blind replicate specimens are provided to determine whether the accuracy and precision of the participating laboratory will permit its entering the standardization phase. During the standardization phase (Part III), reliable estimates of both short-term and long-term reproducibility are obtained, and the deviations from reference method values are determined at different cholesterol levels. If the participating laboratory meets certain performance requirements during Part III, a certificate of standardization is issued. Part IV is designed to check performance thereafter on a quarterly basis. The program design has a specified time schedule; however, this schedule is flexible, and arrangements can be made to accommodate laboratories which are unable to participate at this rate because they do not routinely perform lipid determinations.

The design permits multiple determinations to be made on aliquots of some 5 to 12 pools a year. Lyophilized samples were used at first, but problems in precisely dispensing, reconstituting, and measuring samples for analysis necessitated the use of frozen samples. Newly developed precise dispensing and sampling equipment is permitting reevaluation of use of lyophilized samples for distribution.

Participants and Methods

The number of laboratories participating in the standardization programs has usually averaged between 150 and 200. In 1970, for example, 171 laboratories were actively participating in the Cooperative Cholesterol Standardization Program, 113 of which were

Table 3. Methods used by countries participating in International Cooperative Cholesterol Standardization Program.

Country	Labs	Methods[1]
Australia	7	AK(1), AA(4), Dir(2)
Canada	1	AA(1)
Chile	1	?(1)
Czechoslovakia	2	Dir(1), SS(1)
England	2	AA(1), $FeCl_3$(1)
Finland	3	AK(2), ?(1)
France	2	Dir(1), $FeCl_3$(1)
Germany	1	AA(1)
Hong Kong	1	$FeCl_3$(1)
Hungary	1	Dir(1)
India	2	$FeCl_3$(1), SS(1)
Ireland	2	$FeCl_3$(2)
Israel	2	AK(2)
Italy	1	AK(1)
Japan	6	AK(1), Dir(1), $FeCl_3$(3), Bloor(1)
Netherlands	2	AA(1), Dir(1)
New Zealand	3	AK(2), Dir(1)
Nigeria	1	SW(1)
Philippines	1	AK(1)
Scotland	2	AK(1), AA(1)
Sweden	6	AK(1), AA(2), SW(1), ?(2)
Switzerland	2	?(2)
Taiwan	2	AK(1), Bloor(1)
Uganda	1	$FeCl_3$(1)
USA	113	AK(29), AA(33), Dir(24), $FeCl_3$(20), Bloor(2), KS(1), SS(4)
USSR	2	Dir(1), ?(1)
West Indies	1	$FeCl_3$(1)
Yugoslavia	1	AK(1)

[1] Numbers in parentheses indicate the number of laboratories using the given method in that country.
AK = Abell, Levy, Brodie, & Kendall method
AA = AutoAnalyzer method
Dir = Direct method
SS = Schoenheimer & Sperry method
$FeCl_3$ = Ferric chloride method
KS = Kingsley-Shaffert method
SW = Sperry-Webb method

Table 4. Methods used in International Cooperative Cholesterol Standardization Program by number of countries and number of laboratories.

Method	No. of Countries	No. of Laboratories
Abell-Kendall	12	43
AutoAnalyzer	8	44
Direct Methods	8	33
Ferric Chloride	9	31
Bloor	4	5
Kingsley-Shaffert	1	1
Schoenheimer-Sperry	3	6
Sperry-Webb	1	1

Table 5. Direct methods used in International Cooperative Cholesterol Standardization Program by number of countries and number of laboratories.

Method	No. of Countries	No. of Laboratories
Liebermann-Burchard	5	9
Crockett	1	1
Pearson	2	5
Huang	1	3
Drekter	1	2
Zurkowski	1	1
Hycel	1	6
Gradwohl	1	1
BMI	1	1
Dow	1	2
Rappaport-Eichorn	1	1
Miskos-Tovaneks	1	1

from the United States and 58 of which were evenly distributed among 28 other countries. The number of laboratories in each country and the methods used are shown in tables 3, 4, and 5. Most of the laboratories in this program used direct methods or the Abell-Kendall, AutoAnalyzer, or manual ferric chloride methods. Many types and modifications of direct methods are used around the world. Most of the direct methods are modifications of the Liebermann-Burchard and the ferric chloride methods (table 5).

Today, 156 laboratories are active in the CLSP, 37 of which are international laboratories. At any point in time, between 20 and 60 laboratories remain active after becoming standardized, and between 50 and 100 actively participate in the standardization phase. The number of laboratories that participate only in the self-evaluation phase varies between 50 and 100. Since most participants use the program to determine comparability of cholesterol and triglyceride results for a particular epidemiologic or clinical investigation or for a laboratory methodology development study, the period of participation often covers only 1 to 3 years. This results in a considerable turnover in participants.

Results

Cooperative Cholesterol Standardization Program, 1960–1970

The accuracy and precision of the laboratories participating in this international cooperative study were determined for any laboratory that showed stability of performance for at least 6 months. Each point on figures 1 and 2 represents an average level of accuracy or precision for a single laboratory on all pools for at least a 6-month period. The calculation of this point for each laboratory is based on 48 cholesterol determinations, each carried out on a separate day. Performance within allowable limits of accuracy was not required for participation.

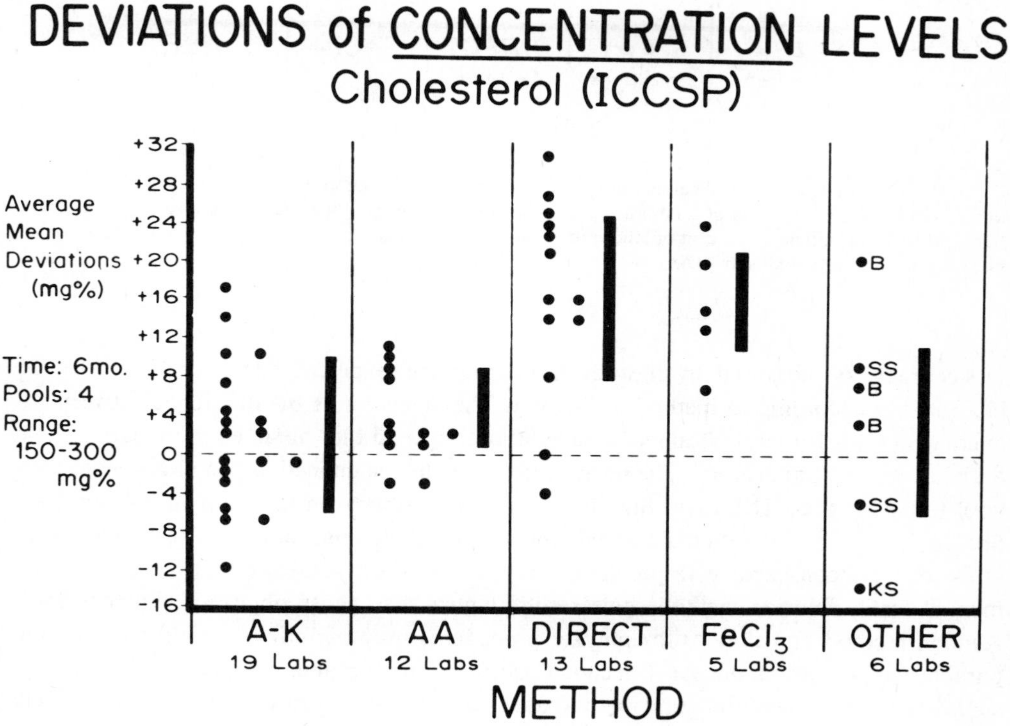

Fig. 1. Accuracy of Cholesterol Analyses in CCSP. The deviation of average level of cholesterol values from an expected value is plotted against the method of a laboratory. Abbreviations for names of methods are given in table 3. The bar represents the middle 67 percent of laboratories in each method group. No allowable limits were required for continuing participation in this program between 1960 and 1970.

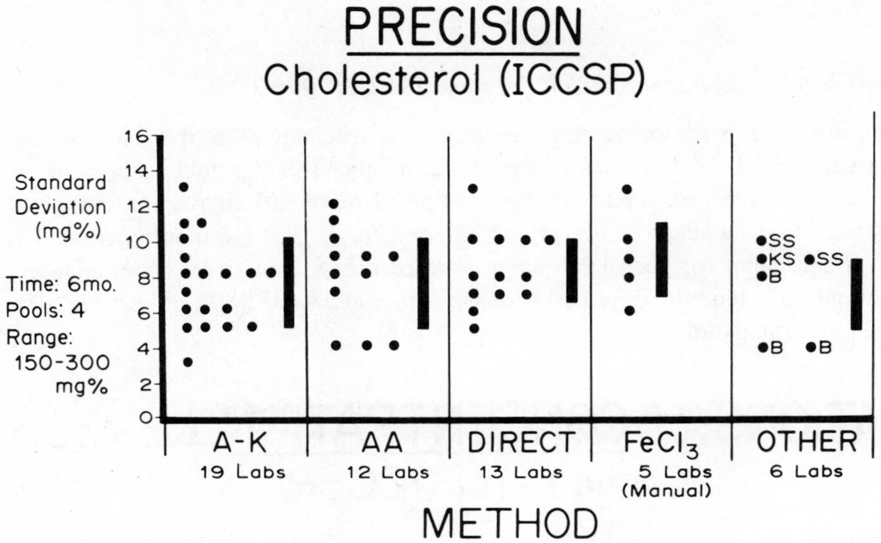

Fig. 2. Precision of Cholesterol Analyses in CCSP. The standard deviation of results averaged for pools and time is plotted against method of a laboratory. Abbreviations for names of methods are given in table 3. The bar represents the middle 67 percent of laboratories in each method group. No allowable limit was required for this program between 1960 and 1970.

Accuracy as measured by the deviation from the 'expected value' is plotted for 55 laboratories according to method in figure 1. This deviation is the difference between the average cholesterol level obtained in each laboratory and that obtained in the CDC Lipid Standardization Laboratory. The term 'expected value' is defined as the mean cholesterol level found by the CDC Lipid Standardization Laboratory on the basis of 384 analyses upon each pool by the selected manual Abell-Kendall reference method. The results shown in figure 1 are consistent with previous observations in the literature that most direct and manual ferric chloride methods give results higher than those obtained with the Abell-Kendall method and that AutoAnalyzer procedures may or may not yield results comparable with those of the Abell-Kendall method. The variability noted for all methods suggests that the use of the same method does not guarantee identical results from different laboratories.

Precision as measured by the pooled standard deviations of each laboratory is plotted according to method in figure 2. The pooled standard deviation for each laboratory, represented by a single point, includes the total variability encountered in that laboratory. The ranges of standard deviations for all methods were remarkably similar.

Examination of the standard deviation values for all methods reveals that the combined standard deviations range from 3.2 to 13.2 mg percent.

Experimental Cooperative Triglyceride Standardization Program, 1968–1970

The accuracy and precision with which serum triglyceride analyses were performed routinely in 105 laboratories were determined with 40 distributed samples from two reference serum pools that were analyzed during a period of between 5 and 12 weeks. The results of the triglyceride analyses are shown in table 6.

Table 6. Results of triglyceride analyses in Experimental Cooperative Triglyceride Standardization Program.

Pool	No. Labs	Range of Means mmol/l	Mean for 105 Labs mmol/l	Range of S.D. mmol/l
1.11 mmol/l	105	0.62–1.70	1.16	0.03–0.39
1.74 mmol/l	105	0.93–2.60	1.80	0.04–0.57

The range of means, from 0.62 to 1.70 millimoles for the 1.11 millimolar pool and from 0.93 to 2.60 millimoles for the 1.74 millimolar pool, is excessive, but the mean for all 105 participants fell close to the expected values. The range of standard deviations for both pools was also excessively wide.

The Experimental Triglyceride Standardization Program indicated that precise and accurate triglyceride values can be attained with any of the commonly used colorimetric, fluorometric, and enzymatic methods. Yet,only 25 participants of the 105, or approximately one-fourth of the laboratories, reported acceptable results for both accuracy and precision for both of the two reference serum pools. Each of the commonly used procedures for the determination of triglyceride was used by some of the 25 laboratories. This experimental study indicates the type of results and the problems that are encountered in the Part I self-evaluation phase of the lipid standardization programs.

Cooperative Lipid Standardization Program (CLSP), 1974

The accuracy and precision of the laboratories participating in the combined cholesterol and triglyceride program were determined for more than 20 laboratories that have passed the standardization phase and are currently active in the extended surveillance phase. Each point in figures 3, 4, 5, and 6 represents an average level of accuracy or precision for a single laboratory for all pools used. The calculation of each point is based on a minimum of 72 determinations made on 12 runs of 6 samples per run over a minimum time of 3 months. Replicates from 12 pools with concentrations of cholesterol varying between 125 and 375 mg/dl and concentrations of triglyceride between 50 and 275 mg/dl were analyzed according to a design permitting reports at quarterly intervals.

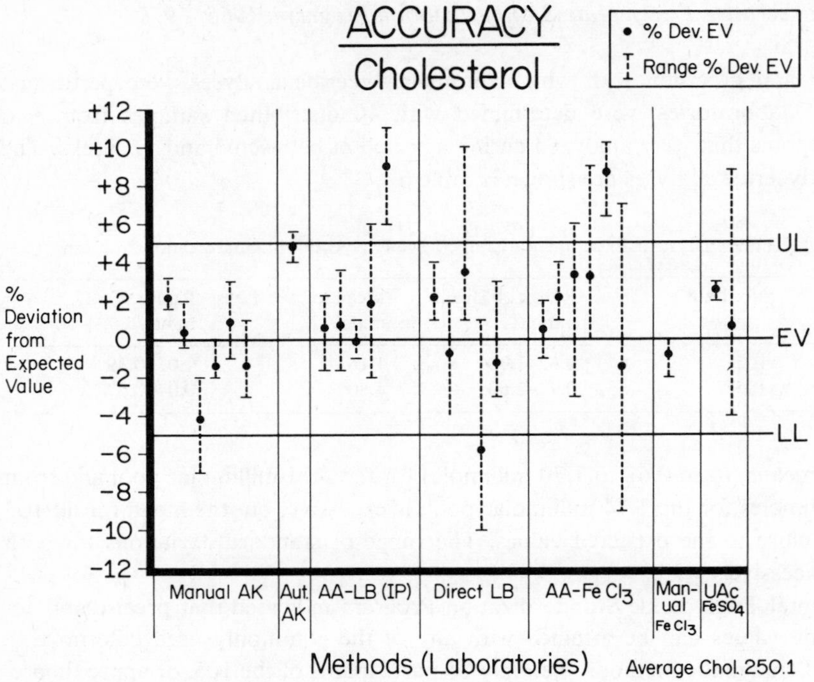

Fig. 3. Accuracy of Cholesterol Analyses in CLSP. The deviation of average level of cholesterol values from an expected value is plotted against method of a previously standardized laboratory. Points represent the average percent deviation from expected value, and the dotted bar represents the range of pool mean deviations from the expected value. Abbreviations are explained in table 3. UAc-$FeSo_4$ represents the Parekh-Jung method which uses uranium acetate and ferrous sulfate as reagents. The heading Aut. AK implies that instrumentation is used in each step of the procedure. UL and LL are allowable limits required for standardization, and EV represents the expected value determined by the CDC Lipid Laboratory.

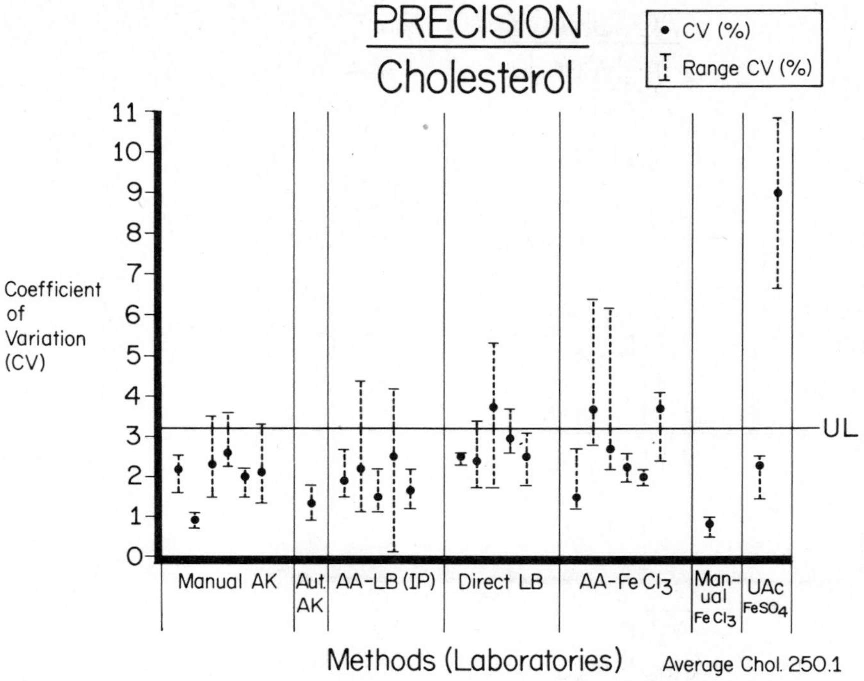

Fig. 4. Precision of Cholesterol Analyses in CLSP. The coefficient of variation (CV) of results reported in at least one 3-month period in 1974 by previously standardized laboratories is plotted against method of a laboratory. Points represent average CV (%), and the dotted bar represents the range of pool CVs. Abbreviations are explained in table 3 and figure 3. UL is the allowable CV at the average cholesterol level.

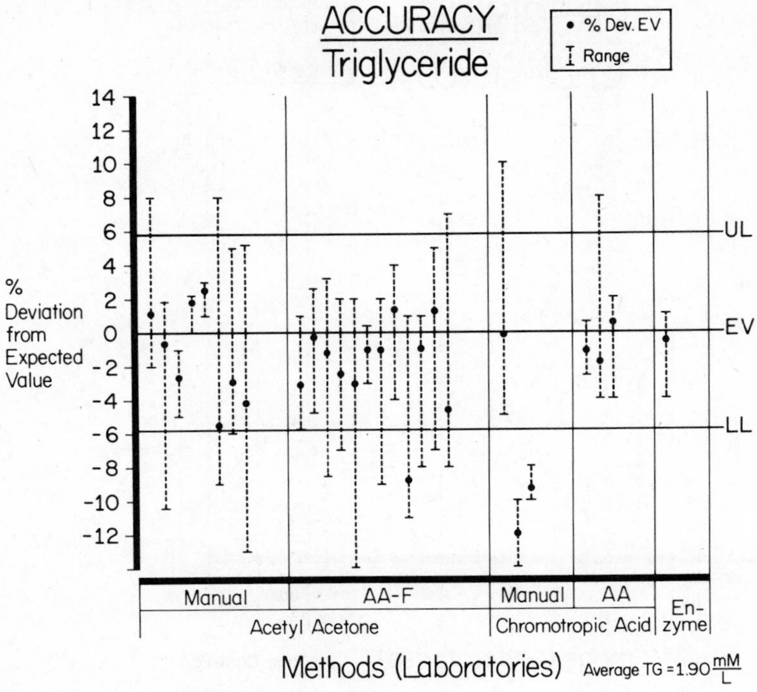

Fig. 5. Accuracy of Triglyceride Analyses in CLSP. The deviation of average level of triglyceride values from an expected value is plotted against method of a previously standardized laboratory. Points represent the average percent deviation from expected value, and the dotted bar represents the range of pool mean deviations from the expected value. AA-F represents AutoAnalyzer-Fluorometric procedure. UL and LL are allowable deviations at the average triglyceride level. EV represents the expected value determined by the CDC Lipid Laboratory.

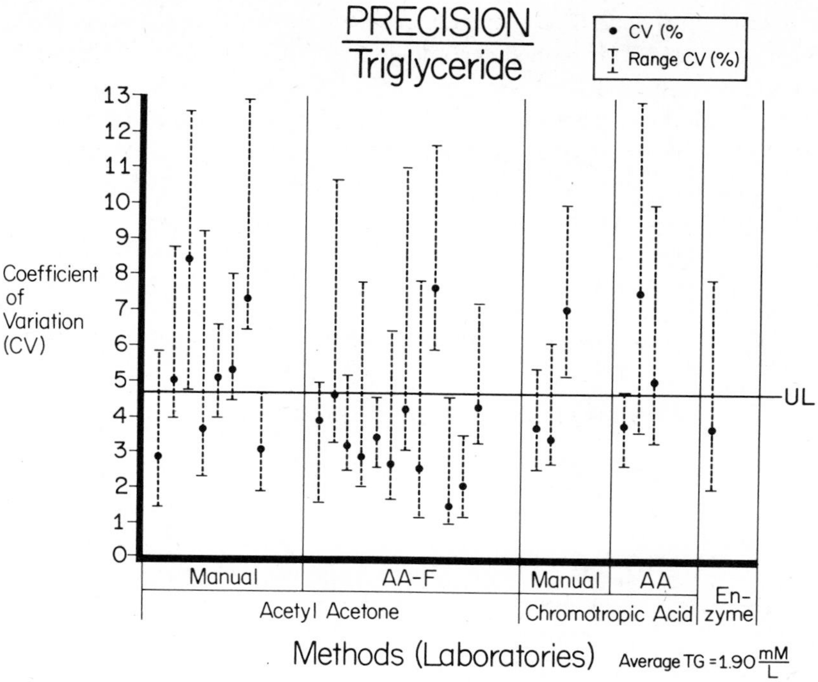

Fig. 6. Precision of Triglyceride Analyses in CLSP. The coefficient of variation (CV) of results reported in at least one 3-month period in 1974 by previously standardized laboratories is plotted against method of a laboratory. Points represent average CV (%), and the dotted bar represents the range of pool CVs. Abbreviations are the same as those in figure 5. UL is the allowable CV at the average triglyceride level.

Cholesterol External Surveillance. The average percentage deviation of the mean from the expected cholesterol value (EV) is plotted according to method in figure 3. Acceptable upper limits (UL) and lower limits (LL) of performance for accuracy are given in table 7. Acceptable levels of comparability were maintained by 23 of 26 laboratories which used seven commonly employed types of methods for the determination of cholesterol. The results obtained by three laboratories which did not come within acceptable limits of accuracy confirm that once standardization is attained, it is not permanent and requires a continuing effort for maintenance.

Table 7. Acceptable cholesterol limits on mean and overall standard deviation in International Cooperative Cholesterol Standardization Program.

Cholesterol Concentration	Acceptable Deviation of Mean from EV (5%)	Upper Limit on Overall S.D. (CV)	
mg/dl	mg/dl	mg/dl	%
100–199	5–10	7	(7–3.5)
200–299	10–15	8	(4–2.7)
300–399	15–20	9	(3–2.3)
400–499	20–25	10	(2.5–2.0)

The average coefficient of variation (CV) of each laboratory for all pools is plotted according to cholesterol method in figure 4.

Four of 26 laboratories reported values on the reference serum pools that were outside acceptable limits for precision. These were not the same laboratories that reported results outside the acceptable limits for accuracy. Seven out of 26 previously standardized cholesterol laboratories performed unsatisfactorily during the subsequent 3-month period of extended surveillance.

Triglyceride External Surveillance. The average percentage deviation of the mean of the laboratory from the expected triglyceride value (EV) is plotted according to method in figure 5. All commonly used methods were found capable of meeting the acceptable limits of performance for accuracy. Acceptable mean levels of reported values were maintained by 24 of the 27 previously standardized laboratories during the extended external surveillance phase.

The average coefficient of variation (CV) of each laboratory for all pools is plotted according to the triglyceride method in figure 6. All commonly used methods are capable of meeting the acceptable limits of performance for precision stated in table 8. Eighteen of 27 laboratories maintained acceptable performance during the continuing external surveillance phase. Results of ten laboratories out of 27 previously standardized triglyceride laboratories were not within acceptable limits either for accuracy or precision during the subsequent 3-month period of external surveillance.

Table 8. Acceptable triglyceride limits on mean and overall standard deviation in International Cooperative Triglyceride Standardization Program.

Triglyceride Concentration	Acceptable Deviation of Mean from EV (±)		Upper Limit on Overall S.D. (CV)	
mmol/l	mmol/l	%	mmol/l	%
0.25–0.99	0.10	(40–10)	0.08	(32–8.1)
1.00–1.99	0.11	(11–5.5)	0.09	(9–4.5)
2.00–2.49	0.12	(6–4.8)	0.11	(5.5–4.4)
2.50–2.99	0.13	(5.2–4.3)	0.14	(5.6–4.3)
3.00–3.49	0.15	(5–4.3)	0.16	(5–4.3)
3.50–3.99	0.17	(4.9–4.3)	0.18	(4.9–4.3)

Acknowledgment

Deep appreciation is expressed for the close collaboration of Dr. R. F. Witter, Dr. M. Kuchmak, Dr. A. Mather, Dr. E. Eavenson, Dr. C. Stewart, Miss V. Whitner, Mrs. C. L. Winn, and Mr. J. H. Williams of CDC and for the encouragement and assistance of Dr. Z. Fejfar, Dr. Z. Pisa, Dr. T. Strasser, and Dr. S. Hatano of WHO and of Dr. I. Prior of the Asian-Pacific Cardiology Association.

Topic II
Quality Control in Relation to Determination Materials, Standards and Controls

Discussion

R. Wieme (Belgium): I just want to draw attention to some more complications concerning the communication of Dr. Jansen, presented by Dr. van Kampen. Recently, it has been shown that one has not only to take into account isozymic differences between samples, but also koinozymic differences (see Clin. Chim. Acta 1975, 59, 369). This is important because in pathological sera, and most often one is concerned with analyzing the alkaline phosphatases in patients with biliary obstruction, the koinozymic structure of the alkaline phosphatase is markedly changed.

D. Stamm (Germany): I have only a short comment on Dr. Hyvärinen's paper. For theoretical and practical reasons it is preferable to avoid corrections using the results of analysis of a secondary standard.

A. Hyvärinen (Finland): Yes, I agree. Actually, the correction was very small, and it did not have any actual meaning and significance. As I mentioned, the secondary standard was not good. So if we want to use this procedure, we should have available a very carefully standardized, preferably internationally standardized reference serum for the comparisons.

H. Haug (Germany): I have a question for Dr. Gerhardt. You have measured the enzymes obviously at 37 °C. Could you please again briefly summarize the pros and cons of this? I would be interested to know if you had to repeat more often the analysis of enzymes when you used the 37 °C method. Could you also say a few words on the normal values you had to establish for the 37 °C method?

W. Gerhardt (Denmark): To summarize an answer to that question is not possible. Two questions arise regarding temperature; first is the stability of the particular enzyme and the stability of the reagents used. We did very careful studies on both. We studied whether there would be an inactivation of any of those four enzymes for which we have recommended methods, for a period of up to 15 minutes; that is, periods where we heated the samples in the reagents in the dilution used in the reaction for up to 15 minutes, from room temperature to 37 °C. We could not show that there was a significant inactivation. The second is the advantage of the higher temperature, and there we aimed at a higher signal-to-noise ratio, and we obtained that. I think you also asked about the ratio between the 37 °C assessments and perhaps the 25 °C. Of course, these will vary somewhat according to the isoenzyme composition for both LDH and alkaline phosphatase. It is more clearcut with aminotransferases. We did work out such ratios, both based on the same sera using both methods, and also simply comparing the reference ranges that we have with the reference ranges that you have. I am not quite sure of the actual figure, but it is roughly of the order of 1.5 to 2.0.

H. Haug (Germany): You have to establish new normal values for the 37 °C method. Could you say something about this?

W. Gerhardt (Denmark): Yes, we have established reference values for all four enzymes and we have done these in all six reference laboratories in Scandinavia. The idea was that we would have the same procedures, the same instruments, the same analytical and presumably the same biological error as to ethnic groups. We were able to increase the size of the reference populations of the groups and we have for alkaline phosphatase, for instance, ranges for decades down to actually prenatal values, that is, true early deliveries, and up to 80 years of age for both sexes. We also have the age groupings for the aspartate aminotransferase, whereas there is no, or at least we didn't find any, real use for age grouping for LDH or for alanine aminotransferase.

G. Vanzetti (Italy): I have a question for Dr. Hyvärinen. He has obtained rather high values for normal sodium in his subjects: I believe between 142 to 147 mmol/liter. Usually we consider normal values under basal conditions to be between 136 to 144 mmol/liter. How do you explain this difference? Did you take your specimens from ambulant patients or under basal conditions?

A. Hyvärinen (Finland): This is what this experiment showed and it seems that serum sodium determination is very sensitive to precision, and also to accuracy. I think the discrepancy is small. We have to be very careful in standardizing this determination. Anyway, this is the result which this experiment gave for these 50 ambulant medical students, which group was not very carefully standardized, and the sampling was done as we usually do every day in the routine work.

V. Schumann (Germany): I would like to comment on the Award Lecture of Dr. Zender. I find his method very interesting, but I see two difficulties. He has actually a multivariate problem, specifically a bivariate one in this case. As far as I can see, he transforms the original two component variables into two new variables: 'Z' and 'd'. Now, as far as I can judge, the theoretical distribution of 'Z' and 'd' may be quite complicated, since they are linear transformations of two correlated random variables. Moreover, I suspect that 'Z' and 'd' will also be correlated. Hence I would suggest, why not use the proper multivariate techniques? I would propose to have replicates for each laboratory, do an analysis of variance *(Anova),* take the within laboratory co-variance matrix as a measure of precision, and the between-laboratory covariance matrix as a measure of accuracy.

R. Zender (Switzerland): We could perhaps meet later and look into this, because I think this is a technical point.

L. Havelec (Austria): A question to Dr. Cooper. Which criteria did you use to set the boundaries, the upper and lower limit for the acceptability of your mean values for accuracy, and the upper limit for precision?

G. Cooper (U.S.A.): Present allowable cholesterol and triglyceride limits for the different serum reference pools were set by statistically evaluating the limits established in the laboratories participating in the first WHO-CDC Cooperative Lipid Standardization Program and those of established lipid research laboratories with respect to different methods and levels of pool concentration. Data of this WHO-CDC program were collected over a 10-year period between 1960 and 1970. For the cholesterol determination, a fixed 5% permissible deviation of reported mean from the expected value was selected as the acceptable allowable upper and lower limit of accuracy. The standard deviation selected as the upper precision limit varied from 7 mg/dl for pools with a cholesterol concentration between 100 and 200 mg/dl to 10 mg/dl for pools with cholesterol levels between 400 and 900 mg/dl. For analysis of triglyceride, variable upper und lower acceptable limits of accuracy from 0.10 mmol/l for pools with concentrations between 0.25 and 0.99 mmol/l to 0.17 for pools with expected values between 3.50 and 3.99 mmol/l were selected for evaluation of reported mean values. Upper acceptable precision limits of triglyceride results varied from 0.08 mmol/l for pools between 0.25 and 0.99 mmol/l concentration to 0.18 mmol/l for pools with concentrations between 3.50 and 3.99 mmol/l. These acceptable allowable limits which approximate to 5% for accuracy and precision for the determination of cholesterol and 10% for the determination of triglyceride for values in the 'normal' or expected range of values reflect the state of the art at this time. Tables 7 and 8 of my presentation give these acceptable allowable limits selected for precision and accuracy.

J. Lines (U.K.): May I ask one further question. Is the beta lipoprotein which you are using to fortify the cholesterol,of human origin?

G. Cooper (U. S. A.): Pooled human serum is used to prepare an alcohol-precipitated cholesterol-rich protein fraction. This fraction is added to bovine, horse, or human serum to prepare cholesterol serum reference materials of different concentrations. For the preparation of triglyceride serum pool reference materials of different concentrations, a concentrated phosphate buffer extract of egg yolk is added to serum pools of either animal or human serum. The procedure we use to prepare our serum pools of different concentrations is described in 'Preparation of hypercholesterolemic and/or hypertriglyceridemic sera for lipid determinations' by *J. H. Williams* et al. which appeared in Clin. Chim. Acta 28, 1970, pages 247–253.

Award Lectures

Topic III: Quality Control in Relation to Data Evaluation, Processing and Presentation

The Determination of Assigned Values for Control Specimens

D. Stamm, Munich (Germany)

Key words: Analytical methods
Assigned values
Control specimens
Control surveys
Internal and External control
Reference laboratories

Introduction

In West Germany, compulsory statistical quality control is currently being introduced for all quantitative clinical chemical analyses performed in the laboratories of panel doctors [1]. This is being done in a series of steps, which are the same in some *Länder* and different in others. About 20000 laboratories are involved. In the last stage, quality control must be conducted in strict accordance with the Guidelines of the Medical Society of West Germany (Guidelines MSWG) [2, 3], which were developed in connection with the Calibration Act [4, 5].

This system of quality control consists of two parts, each supplementing the other:

1. *Internal quality control*

   a. *Precision control*
   at the most frequent decision limit, by analysing samples of the same control specimen in every series of analyses.

   b. *Control of accuracy*
   over the whole clinically relevant range of measurement, by analysing an accuracy control specimen in every 4th series of analyses, the control specimen being selected from a number of different control specimens kept on hand.

2. *External quality control*

   in the form of short-term collaborative surveys, with at least two control specimens having different concentrations.

This system can serve as the basis for effective quality control in all laboratories, from those of country doctors to the central laboratories of large hospitals. The larger laboratories should undertake additional quality control measures.

This system serves to improve the comparability of analytical results from different laboratories.

For both internal control of accuracy and collaborative surveys, control specimens [6] are used, for which the assigned values have been determined by reference laboratories.

In this communication, I shall describe the procedure for assigned value determination for accuracy control specimens which has been used for several years by the reference laboratories making up the Reference Commission of the German Society for Clinical Chemistry (GSCC). This procedure follows the Guidelines of the MSWG exactly.

Some of the control specimens were used in the more than 20 collaborative surveys of the GSCC [7] before the manufacturers put them on the market for use in internal quality control.

This communication is divided into the following sections:

1. Selection of reference laboratories
2. Selection of analytical methods
3. Experimental design
4. Statistical evaluation and determination of assigned values
5. Use of assigned values in collaborative surveys of the GSCC

Selection of Reference Laboratories

In accordance with the Guidelines of the MSWG and the associated Implementation Regulations, the reference laboratories must be independent of the manufacturers and importers of equipment, reagents, standards and control specimens.

The heads of the reference laboratories are personally responsible for the results and are selected by the medical societies in cooperation with the scientific societies.

Reference laboratories must have available all such facilities and procedures as are necessary to ensure the reliability of the analytical results found by them relative to the determination of assigned values. These are:

a) comprehensive system of quality control;
b) the facilities for testing the purity of substances which are used in the making of standards and also the facilities for making standards;
c) the possibility of comparing methods according to 2.3.3 of the Guidelines;
d) continuous external control by means of comparative studies with other reference laboratories.

The head of a reference laboratory must be particularly well versed and have a great deal of experience in this field and be in a position to develop and test new methods himself.

The reference laboratories must function independently and have their own budget for personnel and equipment.

The Reference Commission of the GSCC is an association of reference laboratories, the heads of these laboratories being members of the Society. This commission negotiates with the manufacturers of control specimens, organizes the determination of assigned values and does the statistical calculations with the analytical results of the individual laboratories and the computation of assigned values. It transmits to the manufacturers or importers and to the participating reference laboratories the assigned values and related confidence limits and also the other relevant statistical measures based on the analytical results of the participating reference laboratories.

Selection of Analytical Methods

As you know, many of the analytical methods used in routine laboratory work are not completely specific. The assigned values and the associated confidence limits are thus dependent on the methods used [6].

The determination of assigned values for each constituent of interest must be made with the Selected Routine Method of the Standards Commission of the German Society for Clinical Chemistry (Methods A), insofar as such methods are available [1]. Examples of Selected Routine Methods are given in table 1.

The Standards Commission of the Society is currently developing guidelines for the description of these reference methods and for the testing of these methods by several independent laboratories. It then plans to publish tentative guidelines.

In addition, assigned values are determined for frequently used routine methods and for those methods which are reliable enough for diagnostic purposes (Methods B).

Experimental Design

The experimental design was developed in collaboration with the head of the Department of Biostatistics at the Max Planck Institute for Psychiatrie, Dr. E. Hansert, and was tested using long-term collaborative surveys [8, 9]. It is based on the following considerations:

No sufficiently reliable assumptions can be made about standard deviations from day to day or between-laboratory standard deviations [8, 9]. It has been found that the amount of variation differs from one kind of control specimen to another and often from lot to lot of the same kind of control specimen.

Table 1. Examples of Selected Routine Methods (Methods A) of the German Society for Clinical Chemistry.

Selected Routine Methods (Methods A) of the German Society for Clinical Chemistry

Constituent	Selected Method	Literature Reference
Bicarbonate	Microtechnique, Astrup-Jørgensen Equilibrate for 6 minutes	Jørgensen, K. and Astrup, P.: Scand. J. Clin. Lab. Invest. **9** (1957), 122.
Bilirubin	Photometry of the azopigment in alkaline solution after addition of an accelerator	Jendrassik, L. and Gróf, P.: Biochem. Z. **297** (1938), 81.
Calcium	Atomic absorption spectrophotometry at 422.7 nm after dilution with lanthanum chloride solution, acetylene flame	Willis, J. B.: Anal. Chem. **33** (1961), 556.
Chloride	Coulometric with silver ions	Cotlove, E.: Stand. Meth. Clin. Chem. **3** (1961), 81.
CK	Kinetic test after activation with glutathione at 25°C; Standard method of the Ger. Soc. Clin. Chem.	Z. Klin. Chem. Klin. Biochem. **10** (1972), 182.
GOT	a) Standard method of the Ger. Soc. Clin. Chem.	Z. Klin. Chem. Klin. Biochem. **10** (1972), 182.
	b) Kinetic test at 25°C, measured at 334 nm	Karmen, A., Wroblewski, F. and La Due, J. S.: J. Clin. Invest. **34** (1955), 126.
GPT	See GOT	
α-HBDH	Standard method of the Ger. Clin. Chem.	Z. Klin. Chem. Klin. Biochem. **10** (1972), 182.
LAP	Standard method of the Ger. Soc. Clin. Chem.	Z. Klin. Chem. Klin. Biochem. **10** (1972), 182.
LDH	Standard method of the Ger. Soc. Clin. Chem.	Z. Klin. Chem. Klin. Biochem. **10** (1972), 182.
AP	Standard method of the Ger. Soc. Clin. Chem. Kinetic at 25°C, measured at 405 nm	Hausamen, T.-K., Helger, R., Rick, W. and Gross, W.: Clin. Chim. Acta **15** (1967). 241. Z. Klin. Chem. Klin. Biochem. **10** (1972), 182.

In order to determine assigned values, it is, therefore, necessary to have a large enough number of analyses to ensure that the standard deviations within the individual laboratories and, based on these, the assigned value can be determined sufficiently reliable.

Taking this into account, and based on past experience, it is more practicable to determine assigned values using a small number of means with reliable standard deviations than a larger number with less reliable standard deviations.

At least three laboratories participate in the assigned value determination for each method used to quantify a particular constituent (fig. 1). These laboratories make duplicate determinations on 15 successive working days for lyophilized control specimens and on 10 successive working days for liquid control specimens. It is essential that the analyses be made under routine conditions.

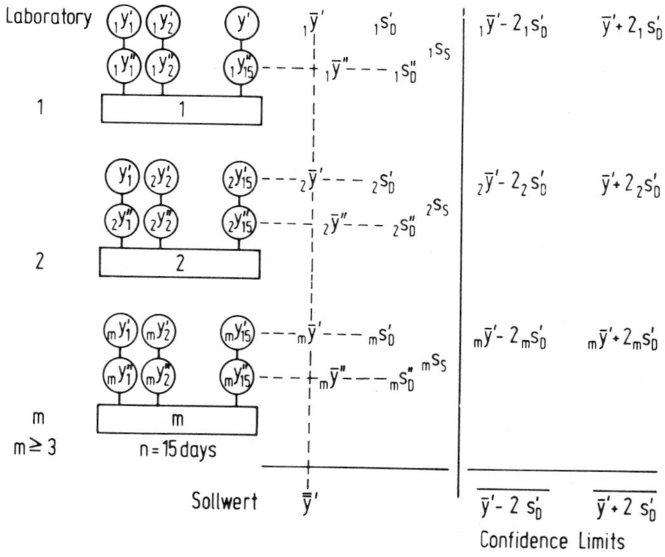

Figure 1. Method for the determination of assigned values used by the German Society for Clinical Chemistry [6].

Statistical Evaluation and Determination of Assigned Values

The data are recorded on punch cards in either conventional units or SI units [10, 11] and evaluated with the aid of a computer. The example used here is that of protein determination with the biuret method taking into consideration the blank of the sample. This example was chosen because it illustrates both the usual case and the most frequent exception (fig. 2).

GERMAN SOCIETY OF CLINICAL CHEMISTRY ** CENTRAL REFERENCE INSTITUTION ** DEPT. FOR ASSIGNED VALUES

DETERMINATION OF ASSIGNED VALUES FOR THE CONTROL OF ACCURACY

REGISTER NUMBER : 10100
TRADE MARK :
MANUFACTURER :
LOT : 433
DATE OF PRINT OUT : 15.11.74

CONSTITUENT 17 PROTEIN UNIT G/100ML

METHOD BIURET - REACTION WITH SAMPLE BLANK

	2.		6.		11.		50.		51.	
	1. RESULT	2. RESULT	1. RESULT	2. RESULT	1. RESULT	2. RESULT	1. RESULT	2. RESULT	1. RESULT	2. RESULT
	5.5 0	5.5 0	5.5 0	5.5 1	5.5 0	5.5 0	5.5 0	5.5 0	5.5 0	5.5 0
	5.6 0	5.6 0	5.6 0	5.6 1	5.6 0	5.6 0	5.6 0	5.6 0	5.6 0	5.6 0
	5.7 0	5.7 0	5.7 4	5.7 3	5.7 0	5.7 0	5.7 0	5.7 0	5.7 0	5.7 0
	5.8 0	5.8 0	5.8 4	5.8 3	5.8 0	5.8 0	5.8 0	5.8 0	5.8 0	5.8 0
	5.9 2	5.9 3	5.9 4	5.9 4	5.9 0	5.9 0	5.9 2	5.9 0	5.9 0	5.9 0
	6.0 4	6.0 5	6.0 0	6.0 0	6.0 0	6.0 0	6.0 2	6.0 1	6.0 0	6.0 0
	6.1 5	6.1 5	6.1 2	6.1 2	6.1 0	6.1 0	6.1 6	6.1 5	6.1 0	6.1 0
	6.2 4	6.2 2	6.2 1	6.2 1	6.2 2	6.2 2	6.2 4	6.2 5	6.2 0	6.2 0
	6.3 0	6.3 0	6.3 0	6.3 0	6.3 2	6.3 3	6.3 1	6.3 4	6.3 2	6.3 2
	6.4 0	6.4 0	6.4 0	6.4 0	6.4 9	6.4 8	6.4 0	6.4 0	6.4 2	6.4 1
	6.5 0	6.5 0	6.5 0	6.5 0	6.5 2	6.5 2	6.5 0	6.5 0	6.5 3	6.5 3
	6.6 0	6.6 0	6.6 0	6.6 0	6.6 0	6.6 0	6.6 0	6.6 0	6.6 3	6.6 4
	6.7 0	6.7 0	6.7 0	6.7 0	6.7 0	6.7 0	6.7 0	6.7 0	6.7 4	6.7 3
	6.8 0	6.8 0	6.8 0	6.8 0	6.8 0	6.8 0	6.8 0	6.8 0	6.8 1	6.8 2
$\bar{x}$	6.0640	6.0573	5.8667	5.8400	6.3753	6.3760	6.0933	6.1753	6.5533	6.5733
S	0.0827	0.0892	0.1589	0.1920	0.0769	0.0944	0.1081	0.0940	0.1552	0.1580
V	1.3639	1.4733	2.7079	3.2874	1.2061	1.4806	1.7748	1.5226	2.3687	2.4031
$\bar{x}$-2S	5.8986	5.8789	5.5489	5.4560	6.2215	6.1872	5.8770	5.9873	6.2429	6.2574
$\bar{x}$+2S	6.2294	6.2358	6.1844	6.2240	6.5291	6.5648	6.3096	6.3634	6.8638	6.8893
S*	0.0179		0.1653		0.0256		0.0930		0.0408	

ANZAHL DER DATEN: 15

NUMBER OF DATA

THESE DATA ARE THE PROPERTY OF THE SOCIETY AND ANY REPRODUCTION FOR PUBLICATION NEEDS A WRITTEN CONFIRMATION.

Figure 2. Computer printout showing the analytical results from the reference laboratories and evaluation of these data,for protein determination with the biuret method,taking into consideration the blank of the sample.

For each reference laboratory a computer printout with the following information is provided:

A. *For the 1st and 2nd results separately:*
   1. Frequency distribution
   2. Mean ($\bar{x}$)
   3. Standard deviation from day to day (s)
   4. Confidence limits ($\bar{x} - 2s$ and $\bar{x} + 2s$)

B. *Using the 1st and 2nd results together:*
   Standard deviation of the series (s*)

The analytical results from all the laboratories are combined using SI units, and a printout is made including the following parameters (fig. 3):

1. Frequency distribution of all analytical results, listed separately for the 1st and 2nd results;
2. Mean of all means ($\bar{\bar{x}}$) for the 1st results;
3. Mean of the standard deviations from day to day ($\bar{s}$) for the 1st results;
4. Confidence limits ($\bar{\bar{x}} - 2\bar{s}$ and $\bar{\bar{x}} + 2\bar{s}$) for the 1st results;
5. Median for the 1st results.

The printout for 2 through 5 is in both conventional and SI units.

For the protein determination, the median and the mean of the means are almost the same. So for all practical purposes we can assume a symmetrical distribution. In comparing the confidence limits calculated from $\bar{\bar{x}} \pm 2\bar{s}$ with the distributions, we see that more than 5% of the results lie outside these limits. For this reason, in such cases the 95th percentiles of all first results of the reference laboratories are used as confidence limits.

The assigned values determined in this way and the associated confidence limits are the basis for internal control of accuracy [2, 3, 12] and also for evaluation in the collaborative surveys of the GSCC. This procedure has the following advantages:

1. *Internal control of accuracy*

Since, as has already been said, the variation parameters for a given method differ from one kind of specimen to another and frequently also between lots of the same kind of specimen, it can be seen from the confidence limits what kind of results the reference laboratories attain. This makes it easier for the user to select suitable control specimens and to determine how good the results of his accuracy control are.

GERMAN SOCIETY OF CLINICAL CHEMISTRY ** CENTRAL REFERENCE INSTITUTION ** DEPT. FOR ASSIGNED VALUES

DETERMINATION OF ASSIGNED VALUES FOR THE CONTROL OF ACCURACY

REGISTER NUMBER : 10100
TRADE MARK :
MANUFACTURER :
LOT : 433
DATE OF PRINT OUT : 15.11.74

CONSTITUENT 17 PROTEIN UNIT G/100ML

METHOD BIURET - REACTION WITH SAMPLE BLANK

SUMMARY

1. RESULT		2. RESULT		
5.5	0	5.5	1	
5.6	0	5.6	1	
5.7	4	5.7	3	
5.8	4	5.8	3	
5.9	8	5.9	7	← $\bar{\bar{x}} - 2\bar{S}$
6.0	6	6.0	6	
6.1	13	6.1	12	
6.2	11	6.2	10	
6.3	5	6.3	9	
6.4	11	6.4	9	← $\bar{\bar{x}} + 2\bar{S}$
6.5	5	6.5	5	
6.6	3	6.6	4	
6.7	4	6.7	3	
6.8	1	6.8	2	

	G/100ML	G/L
$\bar{\bar{x}}$ =	6.1975	61.9746
$\bar{S}$ =	0.1209	1.2094
$\bar{\bar{x}}-2\bar{S}$ =	5.9556	59.5557
$\bar{\bar{x}}+2\bar{S}$ =	6.4393	64.3935
MEDIAN =	6.2000	62.0000

Assigned value : 62 g/l

Confidence limits: 57 - 67 g/l

NUMBER OF PARTICIPANTS: 5

THESE DATA ARE THE PROPERTY OF THE SOCIETY AND ANY REPRODUCTION FOR PUBLICATION NEEDS A WRITTEN CONFIRMATION.

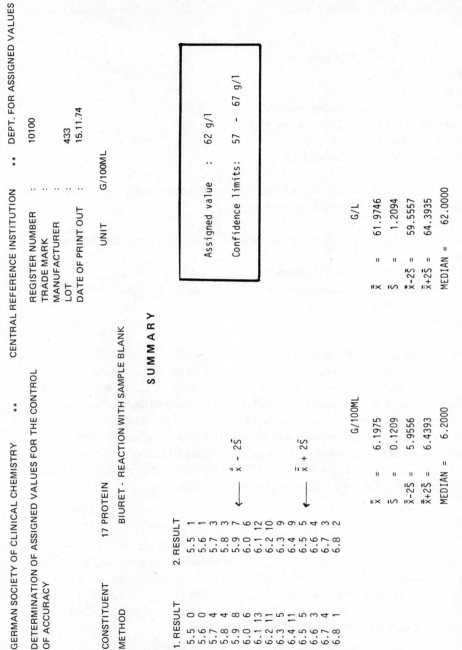

Figure 3. Computer printout summarizing the results of the reference laboratories shown in fig. 2.

2. *External control of accuracy (collaborative surveys)*

If these control specimens, in accordance with the Guidelines of the MSWG (Section 3.4), are used in collaborative surveys only after the assigned value has been determined, then there are the following advantages [7]:

1. In this way it becomes clear in good time whether the specimens are actually suitable for use in collaborative surveys.
2. The collaborative survey and the basis on which it is evaluated, i.e. the assigned value determination, are completely independent of one another.
3. The qualifications of the reference laboratories and the extensive system for assigned value determination assure the accuracy of the assigned values.
4. The determination under routine conditions provides a good level of accuracy and at the same time leads to standard deviations of a realistic order of magnitude (this is especially important because the standard deviation of the assigned value determination is the decisive factor in setting the decision limits for the collaborative survey).

Use of Assigned Values and the Associated Variation Parameters in the Collaborative Surveys of the GSCC

The assigned values and the associated variation parameters determined by the Reference Commission of the GSCC have now been used in more than 20 collaborative surveys conducted by the Society to evaluate the analytical results of the survey participants. Using the data thus collected, an interesting question may be investigated, namely, what is the relationship between the means ($mean_P$) and the standard deviations (s_P) of the participants and the assigned values ($\bar{\bar{x}}$) and standard deviations (s_R) previously determined by the reference laboratories.

The control specimen discussed above was used as Specimen A in the 20th collaborative survey of the GSCC. In the Youden Plot (fig. 4), which all participants receive, a small deviation can be seen between the assigned value and the mean of the participants. In table 2 the assigned values and participants' results are shown.

EXTERNAL QUALITY CONTROL (GERMAN SOCIETY FOR CLINICAL CHEMISTRY) 20th SURVEY OF 20.01.75

RESULTS OF BOTH SAMPLES (DIAGRAM ACC. TO YOUDEN) FOR TOTAL PROTEIN / BIURET, WITH BLANK CONSIDERATION

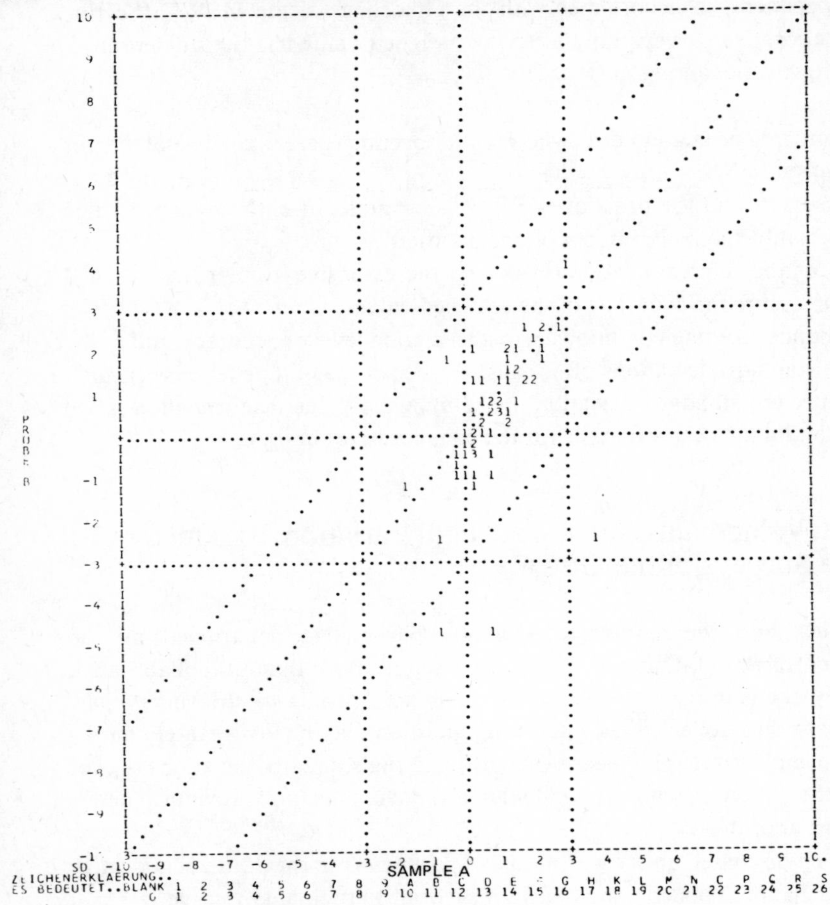

PROBE A	SC	PROBE B
83.000	10.00	87.000
82.250	9.75	86.375
81.500	9.50	85.750
80.750	9.25	85.125
80.000	9.00	84.500
79.250	8.75	83.875
78.500	8.50	83.250
77.750	8.25	82.625
77.000	8.00	82.000
76.250	7.75	81.375
75.500	7.50	80.750
74.750	7.25	80.125
74.000	7.00	79.500
73.250	6.75	78.875
72.500	6.50	78.250
71.750	6.25	77.625
71.000	6.00	77.000
70.250	5.75	76.375
69.500	5.50	75.750
68.750	5.25	75.125
68.000	5.00	74.500
67.250	4.75	73.875
66.500	4.50	73.250
65.750	4.25	72.625
65.000	4.00	72.000
64.250	3.75	71.375
63.500	3.50	70.750
62.750	3.25	70.125
62.000	3.00	69.500
61.250	2.75	68.875
60.500	2.50	68.250
59.750	2.25	67.625
59.000	2.00	67.000
58.250	1.75	66.375
57.500	1.50	65.750
56.750	1.25	65.125
56.000	1.00	64.500
55.250	.75	63.875
54.500	.50	63.250
53.750	.25	62.625
53.000	.00	62.000
52.250	-.25	61.375
51.500	-.50	60.750
50.750	-.75	60.125
50.000	-1.00	59.500
49.250	-1.25	58.875
48.500	-1.50	58.250
47.750	-1.75	57.625
47.000	-2.00	57.000
46.250	-2.25	56.375
45.500	-2.50	55.750
44.750	-2.75	55.125
44.000	-3.00	54.500
43.250	-3.25	53.875
42.500	-3.50	53.250
41.750	-3.75	52.625
41.000	-4.00	52.000
40.250	-4.25	51.375
39.500	-4.50	50.750
38.750	-4.75	50.125
38.000	-5.00	49.500
37.250	-5.25	48.875
36.500	-5.50	48.250
35.750	-5.75	47.625
35.000	-6.00	47.000
34.250	-6.25	46.375
33.500	-6.50	45.750
32.750	-6.75	45.125
32.000	-7.00	44.500
31.250	-7.25	43.875
30.500	-7.50	43.250
29.750	-7.75	42.625
29.000	-8.00	42.000
28.250	-8.25	41.375
27.500	-8.50	40.750
26.750	-8.75	40.125
26.000	-9.00	39.500
25.250	-9.25	38.875
24.500	-9.50	38.250
23.750	-9.75	37.625
23.000	-10.00	37.000

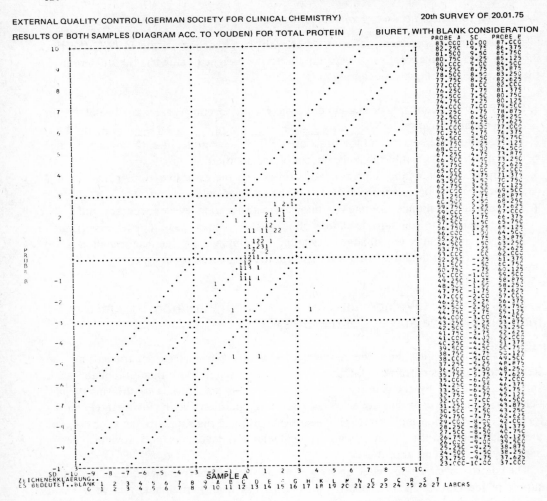

Figure 4. Youden plot from the 20th Collaborative Survey of the GSCC, January 20, 1975. Protein determination with the biuret method taking into consideration the blank of sample.

Table 2. Protein determination: 20th Collaborative Survey of the GSCC, January 20, 1975. Biuret method taking into consideration the blank of the sample.

Protein Determination
=====================

20th Collaborative Survey of the GSCC
January 20, 1975

Biuret method taking into consideration the blank of the sample

	Specimen A	Specimen B
Assigned Value Determination		
Assigned value $\bar{\bar{x}}$ (g/l)	53.0	62.0
S.D. (s_R) (g/l)	3.0	2.5
Coefficient of variation	5.6	4.0
Collaborative Survey		
Mean of the participants (g/l)	55.6	63.0
S.D. (s_P) (g/l)	2.8	3.8
Coefficient of variation	5.4	6.0
Number of participants (n)	67	67
$\frac{\text{mean - assigned value}}{\text{S.D. of the reference labs}}$	0.87	0.41

To describe the difference between the mean of the participants and the assigned value, the quotient

$$\frac{\text{mean of the participants} - \text{assigned value}}{\text{standard deviation of the reference laboratories}}$$

has proved useful. For Specimen A it is 0.87 and for Specimen B 0.41. Experience gained in the determination of assigned values and in the 20 collaborative surveys shows that at the present state of development of routine methods and taking into consideration a feasible cost factor, quotients of up to 1.0 must be accepted for assigned value determination. In table 3 such a comparison is shown for three constituents from the 20th collaborative survey; the deviation quotients lie between 0.11 and 0.77.

A summary of the deviation quotients from four collaborative surveys is given in table 4. From this summary it is seen that:

1. The means of the participants are not always the same as the assigned values.
2. In $^4/_5$ of the cases the means of the participants do not deviate from the assigned value by more than one between-laboratory standard deviation of the reference laboratories.
3. In the last 2 columns of the table,the frequency of deviation quotients greater than 1 and the constituents and methods involved are listed. The constituents and methods found here are almost exclusively ones where the limited reliability of the analytical procedure or the difficulties in use of the control specimens are already known to experts in the field.

Table 3. Comparison of the results of the assigned value determination and the 20th Collaborative Survey of the GSCC.

Comparison of the results of the assigned value determination and the 20th Collaborative Survey of the GSCC

Constituent (unit) Method	Specimen	Assigned Value	n	$\frac{\text{mean - assigned value}}{\text{S.D. of the ref. labs}}$	s_R	s_P
Bilirubin (µmol/l) Jendrassik a. Gróf	A	27.7	237	0.11	1.4	3.7
	B	27.4		0.19	1.5	3.5
Calcium (mmol/l) Atomic absorption	A	2.55	20	- 0.63	0.10	0.10
	B	2.38		- 0.20	0.08	0.09
Glucose (mmol/l) Hexokinase reaction	A	4.72	67	0.77	0.22	0.38
	B	5.00		0.73	0.20	0.35

Table 4. Deviation of the mean of the participants from the assigned value.

Deviation of the mean of the participants from the assigned value

Collab. Survey No.	Methods per 2 spec.	Deviation 0.0-0.5	0.5-1.0	>1.0	Methods
18	15	13	14	3	CK ; P
19	19	23	6	8	P ; Iron, without prec. Cholesterol Total lipids
20 I	25	24	16	10	Ca, flame photometry Creatinine, other Uric acid, other GOT, conventional; CK
20 II	18	18	12	6	Cl^-, mercurimetry Iron-binding capacity Electrophoresis β-globulins

This comparison of the results of assigned value determination and the results of the collaborative surveys, provides valuable information for the future development of routine analysis and of control specimens.

References

[1] *D. Stamm:* Introduction of quality control for all quantitative clinical chemical analyses in West Germany. Dt. Ges. f. Klin. Chemie e. V. – Mitteilungen 1974, 25–32.

[2] Richtlinien der Bundesärztekammer zur Durchführung von Massnahmen der statistischen Qualitätskontrolle und von Ringversuchen im Bereich der Heilkunde. Deutsches Ärzteblatt *68* (1971), 2228–2231.

[3] Ausführungsbestimmungen und Erläuterungen zu den Richtlinien der Bundesärztekammer zur Durchführung der statistischen Qualitätskontrolle und von Ringversuchen im Bereich der Heilkunde. Deutsches Ärzteblatt *71* (1974), 961–965.
English translations of [2] and [3] can be found in: Dt. Ges. f. Klin. Chemie e. V. – Mitteilungen 1974, 33–43.

[4] Gesetz über das Mess- und Eichwesen (Eichgesetz) vom 11. Juli 1969, Bundesgesetzblatt vom 15. Juli 1969, Teil I, 759–770.

[5] Verordnung über Ausnahmen von der Eichpflicht (Eichpflicht-Ausnahmeverordnung) vom 26. Juni 1970, Bundesgesetzblatt vom 30. Juni 1970, Teil II, 960–965.

[6] *D. Stamm:* Calibration and Quality Control Materials. Z. Klin. Chem. Klin. Biochem. *12* (1974), 137–145.

[7] *G. Röhle, H. Breuer and G. Oberhoffer:* Collaborative Surveys of the German Society for Clinical Chemistry (Deutsche Gesellschaft für Klinische Chemie). Dt. Ges. f. Klin. Chemie e. V. – Mitteilungen 1974, 43–56.

[8] *D. Stamm and H. Büttner:* Ringversuch zur Qualitätskontrolle 1968. Z. Klin. Chem. Klin. Biochem. 7 (1969), 393–403.

[9] *D. Stamm:* Ringversuche in der Klinischen Chemie. Schweiz. med. Wschr. *101* (1971), 429–437.

[10] SI Units and recommendations for the use of their multiples and of certain other units. International Standard ISO, 1000–1973.

[11] *R. Dybkaer:* Nomenclature for quantities and units. Standard Methods of Clinical Chemistry *6* (1970), 223–244.

[12] *D. Stamm:* Qualitätskontrolle klinisch-chemischer Analysen, ein Lernprogramm in 5 Lektionen für medizinisch-technische Assistentinnen, Studenten und Ärzte. Stuttgart, Georg Thieme Verlag, 1972.

The Role of External Quality Control Schemes in Improving the Quality of Laboratory Results

T.P. Whitehead, D.M. Browning and *A. Gregory*, Birmingham (U.K.)

Key words: External quality control
Variance index
Variance index score

In this paper the term *external quality control* (EQC) is used to describe surveys where portions of the same material are analysed in several laboratories and the results compared.

In clinical chemistry such surveys have a history which spans more than two decades and they have consistently shown an unsatisfactory situation in many laboratories and in different countries.

The earliest EQC surveys pre-dated the use of effective internal quality control systems. In fact, they were probably a considerable stimulus to establishing such systems.

Participation of laboratories in EQC schemes is now becoming accepted as an integral part of the assessment of the quality of analytical performance in a clinical chemistry laboratory. It has become clear in the last few years that such schemes should not merely be concerned with 'licensing' activities or a declaration of results as being 'acceptable' or 'non-acceptable'.

The possible role of EQC schemes may be summarised as follows:

1. To enable a laboratory to ascertain the effectiveness of its internal quality control systems.
2. To provide information on the analytical methods used by participating laboratories and to compare the accuracy and precision of such methods.
3. To quantitatively assess the quality of the performance of each of the participating laboratories over a wide range of substances at differing concentrations and make comparisons.
4. To provide quantitative information on the changes in the performance of the participating laboratories with time.
5. To provide a 'forum' for discussion of quality control techniques by the provision of appropriate literature.

The 420 laboratories taking part in the United Kingdom National Quality Control Scheme (UKNQCS) include virtually all laboratories in the U.K. who perform clinical chemical analyses. Distributions take place at approximately fourteen-day intervals and the print-out of results of all laboratories is received by the participants within eleven days of receipt of the specimen. The print-out, previously described by *Whitehead, Browning* and *Gregory* (1974), includes various statistical calculations. The performance of each laboratory both overall and for particular substances is quantitatively assessed by calculation of the *variance index*.

This paper describes the calculation of the variance index and illustrates how it may be used to meet some of the objectives of EQC schemes listed above.

Calculation of the Variance Index (VI)

The VI is a calculation which is carried out on the results obtained from the participating laboratories for a particular determination. First, the mean value obtained by all those laboratories classified as using the same method, is calculated. Previously the types of analytical method used by participants for individual determinations have been classified and those using the same or similar methods are grouped together for calculation of the method mean. The participant is required to agree to such classification. For some determinations, participants may use methods which cannot be classified in this way and their results cannot be used in VI calculations. More than 90% of the 420 participating laboratories use methods which can be used for VI calculation.

The calculation only uses those values which fall within the mean $\pm 3s$ for all results returned by participants. This is to avoid incorporating results which are random mistakes, such as clerical errors, into the method mean calculation and thus falsely distorting mean values.

The method mean ($\bar{x}_m$) is subtracted from the result of an individual laboratory (x) and the percentage variation from the method mean calculated.

$$\% \text{ Variation} = V = \left(\frac{x - \bar{x}_m}{\bar{x}_m} \right) \times 100$$

The VI is calculated from this figure by dividing it by the chosen coefficient of variation (CCV) given in table 1. To avoid decimal points this figure is multiplied by 100.

$$\text{Variance Index} = VI = \left(\frac{V}{CCV} \right) \times 100$$

Obviously the lower the VI the closer the result is to the method mean. The CCV values shown in table 1 are the mean value for the particular determinations over a period of several months early in the scheme. They are kept constant so that improvements in the performance of laboratories can be detected.

Table 1. Chosen coefficient of variation used in VI calculations.

Determination	Coefficient of Variation %
Sodium	1.6
Potassium	2.9
Chloride	2.2
Urea	5.7
Glucose	7.7
Calcium	4.0
Phosphorus	7.8
Iron	15.0
Uric Acid	7.7
Creatinine	8.9
Bilirubin	19.2
Total Protein	3.9
Albumin	7.5
Alk. Phos.	19.6
Cholesterol	7.6

Because the coefficient of variation is used in the calculation of VI,when the mean value falls outside the limits listed in table 2,the VI is not calculated. It is particularly important to avoid VI calculations on low mean values for serum determinations with a high variance such as bilirubin, alkaline phosphatase and iron.

Table 2. Range of values used in the variance index calculation.

Determinations	Low	High	Units
Sodium	110	160	mmol/l
Potassium	1.5	8.0	mmol/l
Chloride	65	130	mmol/l
Urea	2.5	66.7	mmol/l
Glucose	0.8	22.2	mmol/l
Calcium	1.0	4.0	mmol/l
Phosphorus	0.6	3.9	mmol/l
Iron	3.6	53.6	µmol/l
Urate	179	893	µmol/l
Creatinine	62	1770	µmol/l
Bilirubin	9	342	µmol/l
Total Protein	40	100	g/l
Albumin	15	60	g/l
Alk. Phos.	6.0	100.0	K.A. Units/100 ml
Cholesterol	1.3	12.9	mmol/l

A formal definition of variance index is 'the difference between the result obtained by a participant and calculated method mean expressed as a percentage of the mean, divided by a chosen coefficient of variation for that determination; the resultant figure is multiplied by 100'.

Variance Index Score (VIS)

The performance of an individual laboratory for several analyses of different material for the same substance may be expressed as the mean variance index. In the UKNQCS we use the term variance index score (VIS) because when VI values for a particular result is less than 50 it contributes a nil score; this is to give encouragement to those laboratories whose results are closest to the mean. To avoid incorporating high VI values in the score, possibly due to a clerical error, VI values greater than 400 are treated as 400.

The mean VIS may be calculated for different determinations and several distributions, the resultant calculation is *the overall variance index score.* In practice it has been found useful to calculate the *'running' overall variance index score.* In this,the overall variance index score for the most recent 40 analyses are calculated. Where the score for more recent results are added, the appropriate number of the earliest results are dropped out of the calculation.

Use of VI in the UKNQCS

The following is a summary of the information now provided in the UKNQCS, all calculations are performed using an IBM 1130 computer.

Normally for each distributed serum as many as eight different substances are required to be analysed. For each substance the following calculations are made:

1. The mean and the standard deviation of the results from all participating laboratories.
2. A re-calculation of the mean and standard deviation after the removal of all results falling outside $\pm 3s$.
3. A histogram of all individual results falling between this re-calculated mean $\pm 2s$ is printed. The number of results falling outside such limited is also recorded.
4. A calculation of the mean and standard deviation for the different methods used. Only results used in the re-calculation of the mean are used.
5. The VI for the results of individual laboratories is calculated and this is converted to a running overall variance index score, as described above, using the most recent forty results. Only the first fifteen types of determinations listed in table 4 are used for running overall variance index calculation.

At intervals, the running overall VIS over a period of the previous two years is prepared on the computer graph plotter. Examples are shown in figures 1–4.

Figures 1–4. Examples of Running Variance Index Score graphs for four participating laboratories. A square (□) represents the running variance index score for the most recent forty determinations following the distribution of a sera for eight or more different analyses. No line between the squares, indicates that the laboratory did not return results for the particular distribution. The time span is approximately two years. To the right of the graph the mean variance index score and limits of 90% of results either side of the mean are shown.

These graphs are prepared by computer graph plotter.

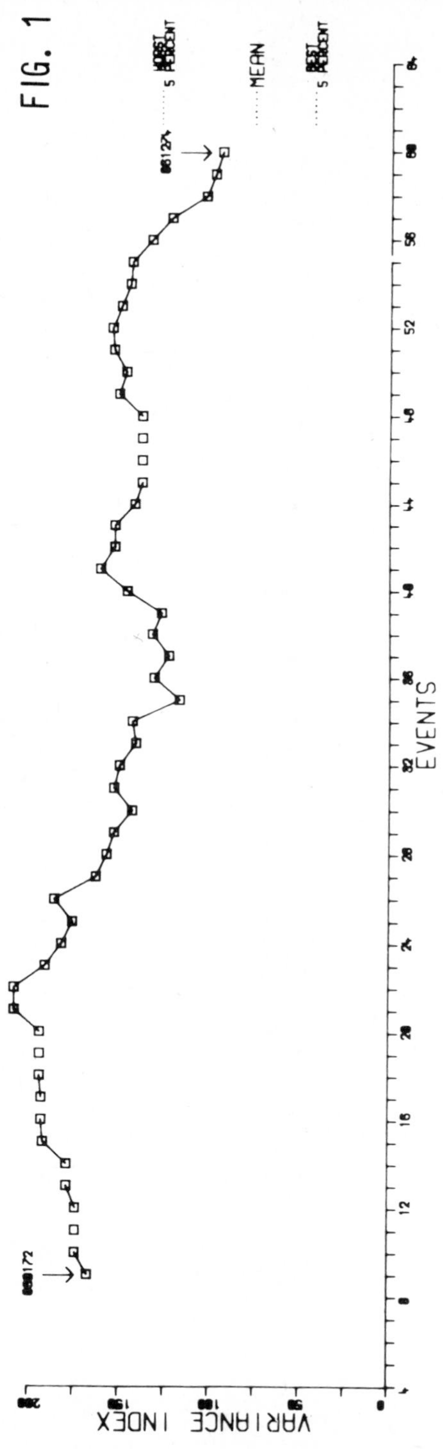
FIG. 1
VARIANCE INDEX
EVENTS
WORST 5 PERCENT
MEAN
BEST 5 PERCENT

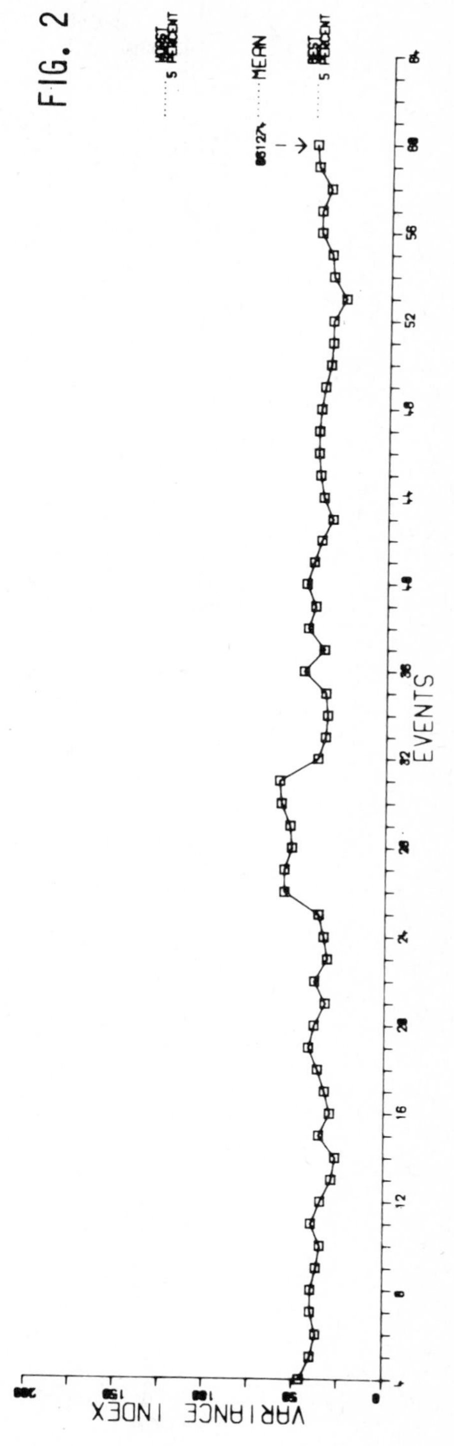
FIG. 2
VARIANCE INDEX
EVENTS
WORST 5 PERCENT
MEAN
BEST 5 PERCENT

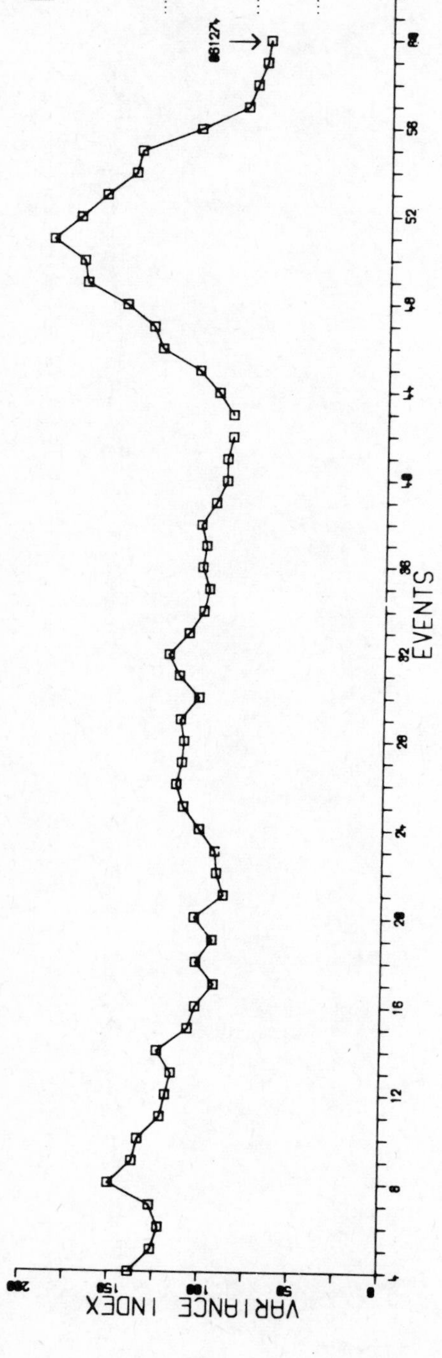

5 WORST PERCENT
MEAN
5 BEST PERCENT
061274
VARIANCE INDEX
EVENTS

FIG. 3

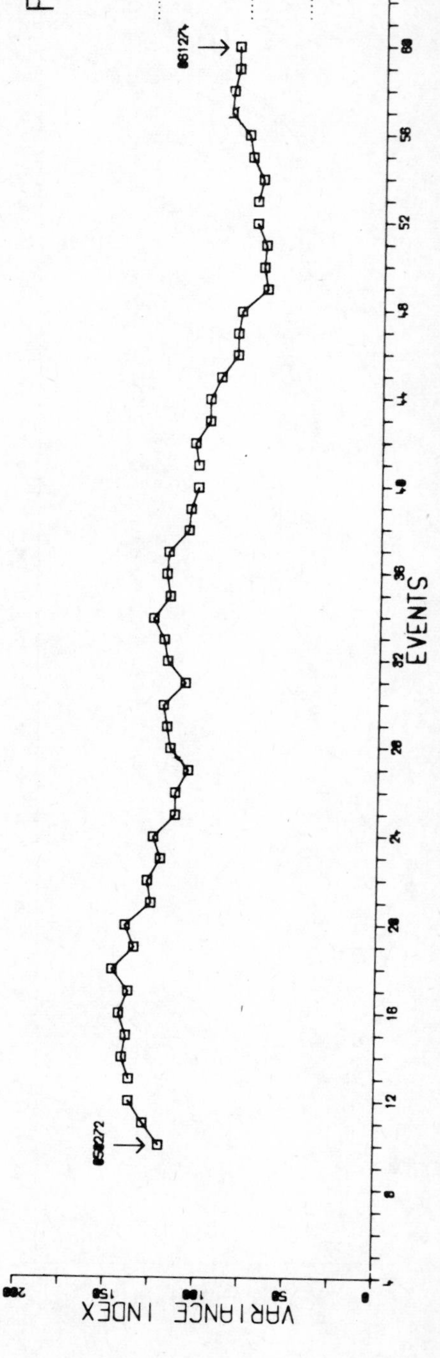

5 WORST PERCENT
MEAN
5 BEST PERCENT
061274
050272
VARIANCE INDEX
EVENTS

FIG. 4

The mean running overall VIS, and the range which includes 90% of all participants, are shown in the graph. This enables a laboratory to identify whether its performance is above or below average or whether it is included in the range associated with the best or worst performing laboratories. It is not meant to indicate 'acceptable' or 'non-acceptable' performance.

In addition, on occasions, the VIS for particular determinations are calculated and the computer print-out distributed to participants. Along with the mean VIS for the individual laboratory, the mean VIS for all laboratories for that determination is shown in table 3. These statistics enable a laboratory to assess which determinations make the most significant contribution to the overall variance index and whether their performance is above or below average.

Table 3. Example of Results of a Participating Laboratory showing the Variance Index Score for Individual Determinations compared with the Mean Variance Index Score for All Participating Laboratories.

Determination	No. of Possible Results	No. of Results returned	Mean Variance Index Score	Mean Variance Index for All Laboratories
Sodium	34	34	46	86
Potassium	29	28	42	88
Chloride	20	11	61	80
Urea	34	34	21	79
Glucose	33	33	21	85
Calcium	34	34	45	78
Phosphate	34	32	33	75
Iron	20	19	90	77
Uric Acid	33	33	28	79
Creatinine	32	32	51	98
Bilirubin	31	23	25	96
Total Protein	33	31	47	75
Albumin	33	33	17	79
Alk. Phos.	28	26	38	79
Cholesterol	33	32	56	88

These calculations based on the VI, have been accepted by all laboratories over a period of several years. The rest of this paper will be concerned with a discussion of the justification of the use of VI calculation and how it has been used to show improvement of the quality of performance of laboratories in the UKNQCS.

The Method Mean

As shown earlier, the method mean is used to calculate the VI. Is the method mean a valid calculation and should laboratories be judged by their ability to obtain results close to it?

This was a question which was difficult to answer in the early days of the UKNQCS,but confidence in the use of such values has grown during the last six years.

The accuracy of a particular result may be described as the relationship between that result and the true result. In no instance in the UKNQCS has the true result been known. We are therefore left with describing accuracy in terms of the 'best estimate' or 'most probable' result. If a particular analytical method is used in the determination of a substance in the distributed material,why should the method mean be the 'best estimate' or 'most probable' result? The evidence available is circumstantial, but, with the important exception of enzyme activity, it is in favour of the correctness of such an approach and for the following reasons:

1. Attempts to establish mean values from a group of reference laboratories have resulted in values close to, or the same as, the method mean calculated for all laboratories.
2. Surveys have shown that the mean and mode for the determinations surveyed are virtually the same,indicating equal positive and negative effects on the mean value from the results of participating laboratories.
3. Different analytical methods for determination of the same substance,give virtually the same method mean value (*Whitehead, Browning* and *Gregory* 1974).

The possible reasons why the method mean value is so useful are not understood, but they have considerable potential importance in explaining the variance in EQC surveys.

The acceptance of the method mean value for the calculation of VI by participants in the UKNQCS over a period of four years is not necessarily a scientific justification of the use of such statistics. However, none of the 420 participating laboratories have been able to show injustice in the use of such a value in assessing performance in VI calculations.

Frequency of Distribution of Material

The VI and the associated statistical calculations described above are of particular use if the distributions of material in the EQCS are frequent and the return of the results to the participating laboratories is short.

If there is too long a delay between analysis of the distributed material and the results of the survey being available in the participating laboratories, then the results will not be representative of current practice in the individual laboratories. In the UKNQCS there is a 11 day interval between receipt of material and the receipt of the computer print-out with the statistical analysis on the results of all laboratories who participated.

Material is distributed every 14 days, so that the distribution of material and statistical analysis of the results is completed for one distribution before the next distribution commences. This prevents confusion in documentation.

The frequency of distribution of material is important. It may take several distributions to convince a laboratory that their performance in some or all methods is poor compared with other laboratories, it may then take some time whilst solutions are sought and then several more distributions to check that a correct solution has been found.

The process could easily stretch over a year or more. There have been a number of requests from laboratories in the UKNQCS to increase the frequency of distributions, despite the rate of distribution being higher than other similar schemes. The number of distributions and the determinations surveyed in 1974 are given in table 4.

Table 4. The Number of Distributions Made by the U.K. National Quality Control Scheme in 1974.

Determination	No. of Times Material was distributed in 1974
Serum Sodium	11
Potassium	11
Chloride	11
Urea	11
Glucose	11
Calcium	11
Phosphate	11
Iron	11
Uric Acid	10
Creatinine	10
Bilirubin	10
Total Protein	10
Albumin	10
Alkaline Phosphatase	10
Cholesterol	10
Blood Lead	8
Serum pH	1
P_{CO_2}	1
Standard Bicarbonate	1
Serum aspartate amino-transferase	2
Buffer Solution for pH measurement	1
Total	172

Results of the Use of VI Calculations in the UKNQCS

There are several advantages to be gained from using VI calculations in EQC schemes.

First, it is possible to identify laboratories who perform extremely well, as well as those who perform badly. The high quality analytical performance that some laboratories can maintain over a period of many years has been illustrated by looking at the results from laboratories with a low overall VIS since the start of the scheme.

Showing what other laboratories are capable of, and identifying the factors in those laboratories which are important in maintaining a low overall VIS, is an essential role of EQC schemes.

Second, the running VIS graph can show the level of performance over a wide range of determinations over a long period of time.

Figure 1 shows the running VIS graph for a laboratory who, in general have performed badly but have shown considerable improvement in the last few months of 1974.

Figure 2 shows a graph for the same period of time. The results show a good performance over a long period of time.

Figure 3 shows interesting changes in performance,the general trend is to improvement, but there was a period of poor performance early in 1974.

Figure 4 shows the running VIS for a laboratory whose performance has gradually improved over a period of two years.

Third, the factors making for better performance can be assessed using the VIS. In a previous publication (*Whitehead, Browning* and *Gregory,* 1973) we have shown how the VIS can be used to illustrate that,in general, the laboratories with higher workloads have performed better in the scheme. It was also shown,that,since the introduction of the VIS, the performance of the smaller laboratories had considerably improved.

We now have evidence, that over the last three years, in many laboratories, automated methods have been adopted in place of imprecise manual methods. The changes in methods used for the determination of cholesterol and uric acid are given in tables 5 and 6.

Table 5. The Changes in the Methods used for the Determination of Serum Cholesterol 1971–1974.

Year	AutoAnalyser AAI	AutoAnalyser AAII	Manual L. Burch	Manual ZAK	Others
1971	43 (16%)		93 (34%)	49 (18%)	86 (32%)
1972	48 (17%)		98 (35%)	52 (18%)	86 (30%)
1973	87 (30%)	32 (11%)	80 (27%)	25 (9%)	68 (23%)
1974	94 (32%)	37 (13%)	76 (26%)	19 (7%)	66 (23%)

Table 6. The Changes in the Methods used for the Determination of Serum Uric Acid.

Year	AutoAnalyser AAI	AutoAnalyser AAII	Manual Col.	Manual Uricase	Others
1970	101 (41%)		109 (44%)	29 (12%)	7 (3%)
1971	112 (42%)		123 (46%)	26 (10%)	5 (2%)
1972	120 (44%)		120 (44%)	26 (10%)	5 (2%)
1973	137 (49%)	37 (13%)	83 (30%)	12 (4%)	8 (3%)
1974	142 (49%)	49 (17%)	76 (26%)	11 (4%)	9 (3%)

Conclusion

If EQC schemes are to play a part in improving the quality of performance by the participating laboratories, then quantitative information must be provided indicating

- the overall performance of individual laboratories
- the overall performance of all participating laboratories
- the factors which lead to good performance, such as adopting precise and accurate methods
- the changes in performance of individual and all laboratories with time

We suggest that the VI is a quantitative factor which is a considerable aid to such endeavours.

Acknowledgements

This work was financed by the Department of Health and Social Security. The authors are grateful to the U.K. National Quality Control Clinical Chemistry Working Party for their guidance and help in this work. The members include Dr. M. Buttolph, Dr. A. Kenny, Mr. D. Neale, Dr. P. Wilding and Professor J. H. Wilkinson.

Reference

Whitehead, T. P., Browning, D. M., and Gregory, A.: J. Clin. Path (1973) *26*, 453.

Computerized Techniques for Quality Control in the Clinical Chemistry Laboratory

H. E. Solberg, Oslo (Norway)

Key words: Acid-base control
Computerized techniques
Control techniques

Computers are now commonly used for reducing the ever increasing work load of clinical chemistry laboratories. Electronic Data Processing (EDP) may also enhance the quality of the laboratory output, both by eliminating several possible sources of human error, and by using computer-assisted quality control. Here we shall give attention to the latter aspect only. After a brief review of the application of computerized techniques for quality control in the clinical chemistry laboratory, we shall discuss in more detail some of our own routines for composite discrepancy checks of patients' results.

In the Department of Clinical Chemistry, Rikshospitalet, Oslo, we have had a laboratory computer system running since 1966. The system has been subjected to numerous revisions and in 1972 a quality control module was added. In the autumn of 1975, we hope to have completed a new real-time laboratory system, which will include a fairly broad spectrum of the quality control methods to be discussed here. We stress the importance of early detection and early reporting of errors to allow the laboratory to take the appropriate actions immediately. This is especially important for emergency tests, which constitute a great fraction of our work load.

The computer may assist in (1) the control of the performance of instruments which are on-line to the computer; (2) the evaluation of results of reference samples; and (3) the quality control of the patients' results.

1. Control of instrument performance

The computer may assure acceptable performance of instruments during on-line data acquisition by monitoring critical parameters such as temperature, carry-over contamination, base line drift etc. When the computer detects an out-of-control condition, several actions are possible, dependent on the instrument, the analysis running, and the nature of the error condition: (1) The laboratory personnel may be warned by a signal (lamp, audible alarm) or by a text message (printer, display). (2) In a real-time system, the computer may adjust the instrument by process control mechanism. (3) The program may call upon software routines correcting for the observed deviation.

2. Evaluation of reference sample results

The computer may compare the results obtained on quality control reference samples against warning or action limits stored in the computer's memory, for all relevant tests. Automatic corrections by dilution factors, which are unknown to the laboratory personnel, may easily be performed before the comparison.

In addition, the computer may store the results of reference samples, in order to plot ordinary quality control or cusum diagrams, or to update the measures of precision and the rejection limits.

3. Control of patients' results (fig. 1)

Accuracy of test series may be evaluated on the basis of the results obtained on patients' samples if the numbers of samples in the series are large enough (> 20). Usually the daily arithmetic mean of results inside truncation limits, chosen to eliminate the influence of grossly abnormal results, are used as the control parameter (e.g. the 'average of normals' method [1, 2]). Warning and/or action limits may be defined on the basis of the statistical distribution of the daily means. This method is a valuable supplement to the reference sample method [2] although it is less sensitive [3].

In contrast to the reference sample and the truncated daily mean methods, the *discrepancy check methods* aim at discovering errors in the individual test results obtained on patients' samples. When computerized, the discrepancy checks may, at least partly, substitute human supervision of all the results before reporting. These methods may be classified as simple and composite discrepancy checks.

In simple discrepancy checks, single test results are either compared with warning limits ('alert check' [4]) or with the patients' most recent previous value of the same test. Both methods may detect large analytical and entry errors. In addition, they may direct the attention of the clinical chemist to severely ill patients.

Computer Control of Patients' Results

Accuracy of test series
Discrepancy check of patients' results
  Simple discrepancy check
    Previous value
    Warning limit
  Composite discrepancy check
    Physiological consistency
    Multivariate statistics

Figure 1.

In *composite* discrepancy checks the results of at least two different tests performed on the same sample are compared for consistency. This comparison may be based upon known physiological relationship or on observed multivariate statistical distributions. In our laboratory computer system, we have had computer control of blood acid-base and electrolyte results for three years, and we are presently evaluating other possible composite control algorithms. Our acid-base and electrolyte discrepancy checks will be presented in more detail.

The blood *acid-base control* program checks whether the base excess value is consistent with the standard bicarbonate, pH and pCO_2 values [5]. Since the Henderson-Hasselbalch's equation can only be used for checking values of the simple bicarbonate

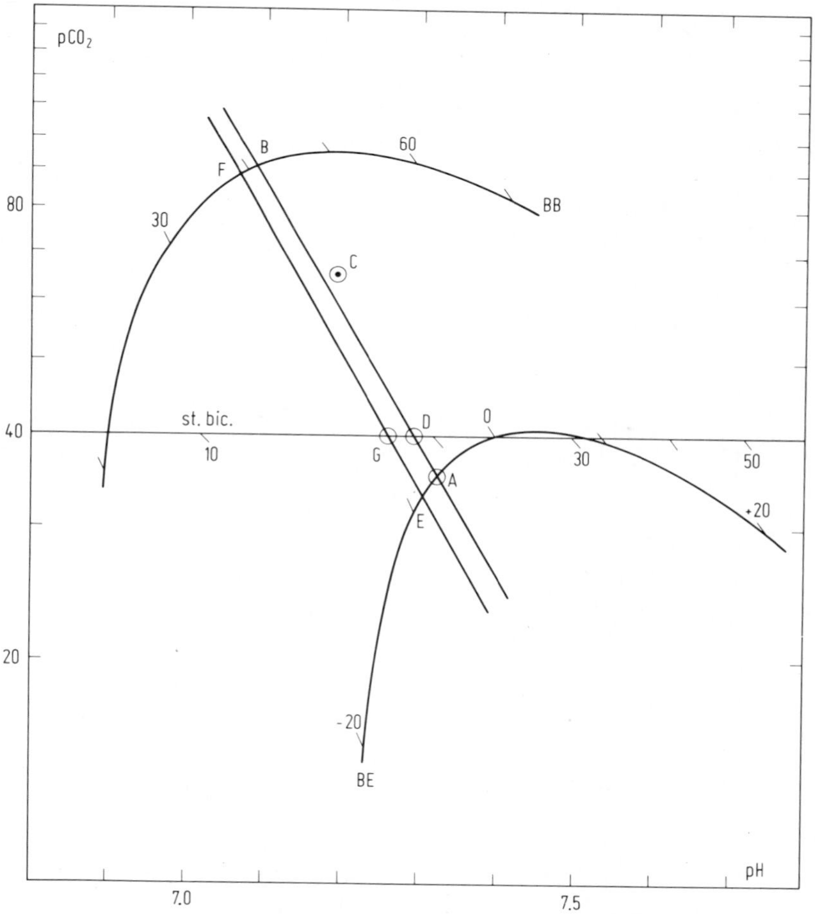

Figure 2. Graphical control procedure simulated by the computer program for quality control of blood acid-base results. See the text for explanation.

buffer system of plasma, our control algorithm for whole blood acid-base results [6] simulates a graphical control procedure [5] using the acid-base curve nomogram of *Siggaard-Andersen* [6]. The procedure is illustrated in fig. 2. The CO_2-equilibration line A-B is estimated from the base excess (A) and hemoglobin values [6]. The latter value is set to 12.6 g/100 ml if it is unknown to the control program. The standard bicarbonate value (D) may then be estimated and compared with the entered value. The difference between these two values (DSTB) is the first control parameter (should be close to zero if no errors exist). The point of actual pH and actual pCO_2 (C) should lie on or close to the line A-B if the values are internally consistent. Its perpendicular distance from the line A-B (PERP) is the second control parameter used. When the oxygen saturation of hemoglobin is below 80 per cent, the standard bicarbonate (G) and the control parameter DSTB are estimated after adjustment of the equilibration line [6] (new line: E-F).

```
1. HISTOGRAM FOR
ANALYSE NO. 201     DSTB
SPECIMEN-CODES INCLUDED - BL SE PL      AB VB

COL   NO.   FREQ.   CUM.F    CL.MIDP      . . . . V . . . . . X . . . . . V . . . . . X .

 1     27   0.52    0.52    -3.100     I*
 2      2   0.04    0.56    -2.900     I
 3      1   0.02    0.58    -2.700     I
 4      0   0.0     0.58    -2.500     I
 5      2   0.04    0.62    -2.300     I
 6      3   0.06    0.67    -2.100     I
 7      2   0.04    0.71    -1.900     I
 8      3   0.06    0.77    -1.700     I
 9      7   0.13    0.90    -1.500     I
10     11   0.21    1.12    -1.300     I
11     17   0.33    1.44    -1.100     I*
12     73   1.40    2.85    -0.900     I***
13    302   5.81    8.65    -0.700     I************
14    296   5.69   14.34    -0.500     I***********
15    475   9.13   23.48    -0.300     I******************
16    690  13.27   36.74    -0.100     I***************************
17    803  15.44   52.18     0.100     I*******************************
18   1088  20.92   73.10     0.300     I******************************************
19    360   6.92   80.02     0.500     I**************
20    299   5.75   85.77     0.700     I***********
21    197   3.79   89.56     0.900     I********
22    169   3.25   92.81     1.100     I******
23    142   2.73   95.54     1.300     I*****
24     72   1.38   96.92     1.500     I***
25     34   0.65   97.58     1.700     I*
26     16   0.31   97.88     1.900     I*
27     33   0.63   98.52     2.100     I*
28     30   0.58   99.10     2.300     I*
29     10   0.19   99.29     2.500     I
30      8   0.15   99.44     2.700     I
31      3   0.06   99.50     2.900     I
32     26   0.50  100.00     3.100     I*

     TOT.NO.    MEAN    ST.DEV

       5201    0.197    0.690
```

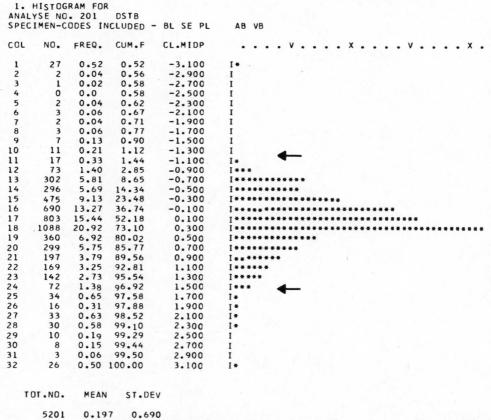

Figure 3. Distribution of the control parameter DSTB for 5201 routine blood acid-base results controlled. The arrows point at the 99 per cent confidence limits (−1.21 and + 1.55) of the distribution of DSTB for consistent acid-base results.

Figures 3 and 4 show the distribution of the two control parameters and their rejection limits. Our laboratory is very heavily loaded with acid-base determinations (daily mean number: 61.4; range: 0–198; total number controlled by the routine since 1972: approx. 55 000). The computer control has now relieved the supervising clinical chemist of the

```
 1. HISTOGRAM FOR
ANALYSE NO. 200     PERP
SPECIMEN-CODES INCLUDED  -  BL SE PL      AB VB

COL    NO.   FREQ.   CUM.F    CL.MIDP      . . . . V . . . . X

  1    309    5.94    5.94     0.0         I************
  2    529   10.17   16.11     0.001       I********************
  3    508    9.77   25.88     0.002       I********************
  4    526   10.11   35.99     0.003       I********************
  5    337    6.48   42.47     0.004       I*************
  6    423    8.13   50.61     0.005       I****************
  7    341    6.56   57.16     0.006       I*************
  8    287    5.52   62.68     0.007       I***********
  9    223    4.29   66.97     0.008       I*********
 10    205    3.94   70.91     0.009       I********
 11    190    3.65   74.56     0.010       I*******
 12    158    3.04   77.60     0.011       I******
 13    149    2.86   80.47     0.012       I******
 14     96    1.85   82.31     0.013       I****
 15    112    2.15   84.46     0.014       I****
 16     85    1.63   86.10     0.015       I***
 17     53    1.02   87.12     0.016       I**
 18     57    1.10   88.21     0.017       I**
 19     59    1.13   89.35     0.018       I**
 20     40    0.77   90.12     0.019       I**
 21     36    0.69   90.81     0.020       I*
 22     44    0.85   91.66     0.021       I**
 23     33    0.63   92.29     0.022       I*
 24     30    0.58   92.87     0.023       I*
 25     29    0.56   93.42     0.024       I*
 26     18    0.35   93.77     0.025       I*
 27     24    0.46   94.23     0.026       I*
 28     25    0.48   94.71     0.027       I*
 29     26    0.50   95.21     0.028       I*
 30      7    0.13   95.35     0.029       I
 31     16    0.31   95.65     0.030       I*
 32    226    4.35  100.00     0.031       I*********

    TOT.NO.     MEAN     ST.DEV
      5201     0.008     0.008
```

Figure 4. Distribution of the control parameter PERP for 5201 routine blood acid-base results controlled. The rejection limit (arrow) was arbitrarily set at 0.025 (the 94 percentile of the shown distribution).

heavy burden of manual checks. For long periods of time the computerized routine was compared with manual controls by clinical chemists, showing that the former control was far more reliable and sensitive to discrepancies. The computer program of the control algorithm has been published [5].

```
 1. HISTOGRAM FOR
ANALYSE NO. 202    REST
SPECIMEN-CODES INCLUDED - BL SE PL     AB VB

COL    NO.   FREQ.   CUM.F     CL.MIDP        . . . . V . . . . . X . . . . .

  1     28    0.24    0.24     -5.000     I
  2     19    0.16    0.41     -3.500     I
  3     25    0.22    0.62     -2.000     I
  4     27    0.23    0.86     -0.500     I
  5     36    0.31    1.17      1.000     I*
  6     48    0.42    1.59      2.500     I*
  7     96    0.83    2.42      4.000     I**          <--
  8    140    1.21    3.63      5.500     I**
  9    216    1.87    5.50      7.000     I****
 10    297    2.57    8.08      8.500     I*****
 11    573    4.97   13.05     10.000     I**********
 12    883    7.65   20.70     11.500     I***************
 13   1313   11.38   32.08     13.000     I***********************
 14   1536   13.32   45.40     14.500     I***************************
 15   1596   13.84   59.24     16.000     I****************************
 16   1376   11.93   71.17     17.500     I************************
 17    983    8.52   79.69     19.000     I*****************
 18    771    6.68   86.37     20.500     I*************
 19    547    4.74   91.11     22.000     I*********
 20    321    2.78   93.90     23.500     I******
 21    246    2.13   96.03     25.000     I****
 22    127    1.10   97.13     26.500     I**
 23    109    0.94   98.08     28.000     I**          <--
 24     60    0.52   98.60     29.500     I*
 25     48    0.42   99.01     31.000     I*
 26     31    0.27   99.28     32.500     I*
 27     29    0.25   99.53     34.000     I*
 28     26    0.23   99.76     35.500     I
 29      2    0.02   99.77     37.000     I
 30      8    0.07   99.84     38.500     I
 31      5    0.04   99.89     40.000     I
 32     13    0.11  100.00     41.500     I


    TOT.NO.     MEAN     ST.DEV

     11535    15.938     5.506
```

Figure 5. Distribution of the control parameter REST for 11535 blood electrolyte results controlled. The arrows point at the 99 per cent confidence limits (4.1 and 27.6) of the distribution of REST for consistent electrolyte results.

Our *control of blood electrolyte* values was also implemented in 1972. The following algorithm, very similar to that recently published by *Whitehurst* et al. [4], is used:

$$REST = [Na^+] + [K^+] - [Cl^-] - [HCO_3^-]_{standard}$$

Since we determine only standard bicarbonate [6] (set equal to 24.5 meq/l by the program if not actually entered), this value is used in the formula, even though actual plasma bicarbonate would be more appropriate. Assuming that calcium and magnesium are approximately balanced by phosphate and other non-protein anions, the control parameter REST should be close to the anion value of serum proteins (approx. 16 meq/l).

Figure 5 shows that this was the mean value actually found.

This control routine is of great value, even though its sensitivity (especially with regard to errors in the potassium value) is somewhat less than that of the acid-base discrepancy check.

Conclusion

Our three years experiences with these computer-assisted control routines are so encouraging that we are presently evaluating other possible composite discrepancy checks. Some of them will be based upon known physiological relationships, but we are also exploring the possibility of defining rejection regions by using empirical multivariate statistical distributions of test combinations where physiological relationships are unknown or difficult to define.

References

[1] *Hoffmann, R.G., and Waid, M.E.:* The 'Average of Normals' Method for Quality Control. Amer. J. clin. Path. *43,* 143 (1965).

[2] *Begtrup, H., Leroy, S., Thyregod, P., and Wallöe-Hansen, P.:* 'Average of Normals' Used as Control of Accuracy, and a Comparison with other Controls. Scand. J. clin. Lab. Invest. *27,* 247 (1971).

[3] *Amador, E., Hsi, B.P., Massod, M.F.:* An Evaluation of the 'Average of Normals' and related Methods of Quality Control. Amer. J. clin. Path. *50,* 369 (1968).

[4] *Whitehurst, O., Di Silvio, T.V., and Boyadjian, G.:* Evaluation of Discrepancies in Patients' Results – An Aspect of Computer-Assisted Quality Control. Clin. Chem. *21,* 87 (1975).

[5] *Solberg, H.E.:* A Computer Program for Quality Control of Blood Acid/Base Results. Computer Programs in Biomedicine *3,* 79 (1973).

[6] *Siggaard-Andersen, O.:* The Acid-Base Status of the Blood. Munksgaard, Copenhagen 1964.

Systems Analysis of Analytical Procedures as a Means of Improving their Performance

T. Aronsson, C.-H. de Verdier and *T. Groth,* Uppsala (Sweden)

Key words: Conceptual models
Method optimization
Simulation techniques
Systems analysis

Introduction

Problems in science and modern society have grown more complex, a circumstance that accentuates the need for new techniques for their solution. Systems analysis and, in particular, computer simulation are examples of such new techniques.

Highly complex systems may be delineated in conceptual models and expressed in symbolic form, e.g. mathematically and in terms of computer programme instructions. The major advantage of such a problem-solving approach is that systems which are hazardous, difficult or expensive to investigate by conventional methods, may be systematically analysed in a more convenient way. Provided that the model is an adequate representation of the real system, a systems analysis may help the investigator to find 'near-optimal' solutions, even though the model is not an absolutely true reproduction of reality.

Computer simulation for optimizing the function of the laboratory

A previous communication from this laboratory (*Sandblad* et al. 1974) described a simulation study of a clinical chemical laboratory. The study was made as an attempt to achieve a more optimized overall function of the laboratory. The broad concepts of the laboratory functions are outlined in figure 1. The effectiveness of the laboratory is measured in terms of speed of performance (report – request time), quality, and cost.

For the clarification of certain questions, it is necessary to have a more detailed description of the laboratory, including series of analytical channels, each one representing an existing analytical method. The overall performance of the laboratory is dependent on the flows along these channels, on bottle-necks in front of, or within, jointly used resources such as computers or transport systems.

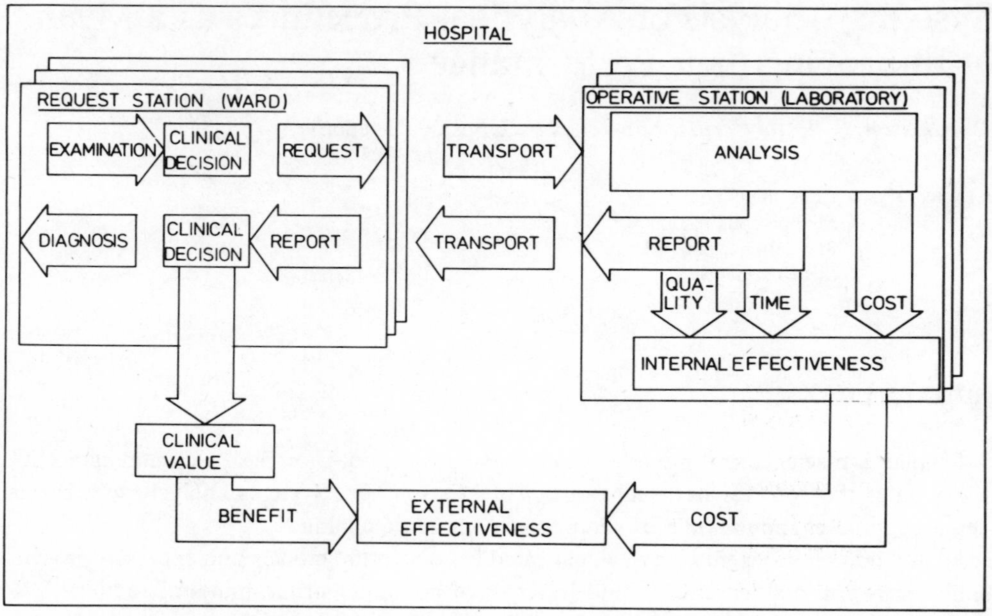

Figure 1. A conceptual model showing the interrelations between wards and the clinical chemical laboratory within the hospital.

Computer simulation for optimizing an analytical method

An investigation for a specific method regarding cost and speed of performance in relation to quality, calls for a high degree of resolution, so that the details of the analytical series can be taken into account. A simulation study on this level was published recently (*Aronsson, De Verdier* and *Groth,* 1973, 1974).

The analytical method may be functionally separated into four different procedures (fig. 2). The measuring of calibration samples generates raw values that can be used for calculating the calibration function. The raw values from the analytical samples can be transformed to concentration values with use of the calibration function. In an analytical system with high contamination, special samples with known concentrations may be inserted in the analytical series and used for determining the contamination factor, in order to more accurately estimate the calibration function and the concentrations of the analytical samples.

The outcome is influenced by random and systematic errors in the system. These are listed above the quadrangles. The outcome of results is also dependent on the choice of correction procedures and on the design of the analytical series, i.e., the number and the

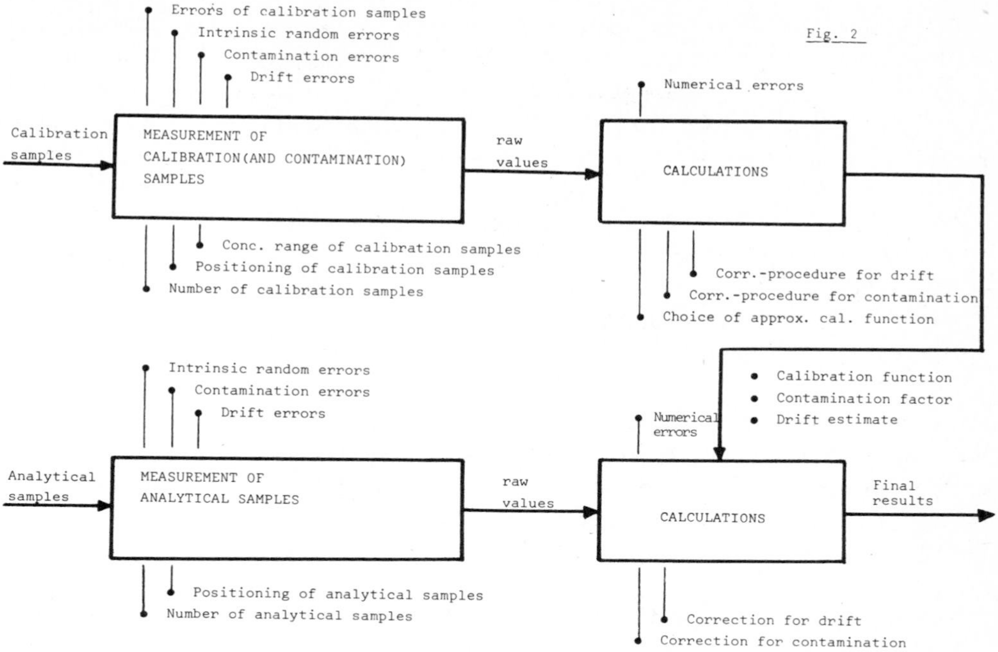

Figure 2. The conceptual model describing the relation between the calibration and the measurement of analytical samples in an analytical method. The final results are influenced by different types of errors affecting the system (indicated above the quadrangles) and by the design of the analytical method (below).

position of the calibration samples, the length of the segment of the series containing a set of calibration samples and analytical samples.

Such design parameters are indicated below the four quadrangles in figure 2.

Systems analysis was performed in order to evaluate the influence of the various error components and their relative significance for the overall performance. Our aim was also to point out how their effect could be minimized by using an appropriate design of the analytical series in combination with suitable connection procedures. In the simulation, the analytical procedure was described in a 'black-box' manner, i.e., for a given input (concentration) an output (raw value) was produced from an assumed descriptive function. The various random and systematic errors were simulated and combined as they appear in the phases of calibration and determination of analytical samples. To obtain sufficient statistics in the simulation, the calibration procedure and the concentration determination were repeated a large number of times (500) in the computations, using different random numbers (Monte Carlo simulation). The quality of the analytical method was expressed as an 'error on the 95% confidence level' and used as an objective function in the systems analysis and in the optimizations. This quantity was calculated from the dispersion and location of the simulated concentration values in relation to the 'true reference value'.

The benefit of systems analysis for a critical evaluation of analytical methods *on this level* is obvious. It increases the possibilities of understanding which factors are of major importance for improving the performance of the method. Whether or not an actual improvement of the method can be achieved by using information from simulation procedures mainly depends on:

1. The ratio between the total error of the method and the intrinsic error. This ratio has to be well above 1, since the benefits of redesigning the analytical series will otherwise be only marginal.
2. The stability of the method. This must be high enough to ensure that the parameter values used in the simulation procedure are estimated with sufficient confidence.

Our investigation of some routine analytical methods indicated that these prerequisites for using the simulation procedure are met for most methods.

What type of guidance can be obtained from the simulation procedure for the design of the analytical series or for the performance of the method? Points 1–3 give some rules of thumb:

1. The precision of the concentrations of calibration solutions does not need to be higher than the intrinsic random error.
2. Increase of the number of calibration samples per segment above a certain number ($\simeq$ 4) has only a marginal effect on the quality.
3. It is advantageous that the calibration samples are extended over a range that is somewhat wider than the intended measuring range.

The simulation procedure may also be used:

1. To indicate the level of the random intrinsic error at which it is better to use a linear calibration function instead of a more true second-order polynomial.
2. For an appropriate judgment of different correction procedures for baseline or sensitivity drift.
3. For a comparison between different procedures for a precise estimate of a contamination factor and a judgment of the usefulness of this factor.
4. For an economic optimization of a method with fixed quality specifications.

Computer simulation for the evaluation of different ways of expressing analytical quality

Many different designs for the positioning of control samples in the analytical series have been suggested for the internal quality control. These designs are mainly based on simple statistical considerations, but the actual levels of systematic, within-day random and between-day (among) errors for the specific method are generally not considered. Likewise, there are many ways for the statistical treatment of the data and for the presentation of the results for quality control within the laboratory. Objective methods for the evaluation of different procedures are not available. Naturally, such evaluation methods must take into account many prerequisites and conditions of the laboratory.

In the clinical chemical laboratory, the quality of an analytical method is, in general, expressed in terms of accuracy and precision. As emphasized by *Dybkaer* et al. (1974), these terms have little meaning for the clinician who wants to compare a given value from a patient with a value obtained from the same patient a month or a year earlier, or with reference values from a healthy reference population and from a reference group of patients with similar symptoms. Calibration of a method and quality control must be kept strictly separate. This fact, however, does not prevent a discussion about the usefulness for the clinician of obtaining selected information about the quality control data generated within the laboratory. The choice of an adequate measure of analytical quality is, however, a problem that requires consideration of several complex chains of interacting functions. The construction of a conceptual model and the use of computer simulation procedures may facilitate a discussion, without too many misunderstandings, and can eventually give rational solutions to the problems.

Figure 3 gives the conceptual model summarizing the basic functional parts and single factors which must be taken into account in the simulation of the different laboratory activities mentioned above. For the study of suitable procedures for internal quality control, a number of control samples in a specific design are simulated as sampled from batches of control samples with specified variation within- and between-batches. The concentration values, as determined by the analytical procedure, are generated by adding random (TRE) and systematic errors (TSE). In passing may be mentioned, that this quadrangle represents the system in figure 2 in a more lumped form. The influence of the design of the analytical series and of the applied correction procedures are included in the symbols TRE (total random error) and TSE (total systematic error). These total errors may very well be expressed as within-day random error, between-day random error, and a between-day systematic error. By applying different statistics to the synthetic set of control data, alternative strategies for quality control may be elevated directly by comparison with the 'true' values entered into the simulation. The importance of internal quality control for the establishment of reference values may also be advantageously studied by simulation methods.

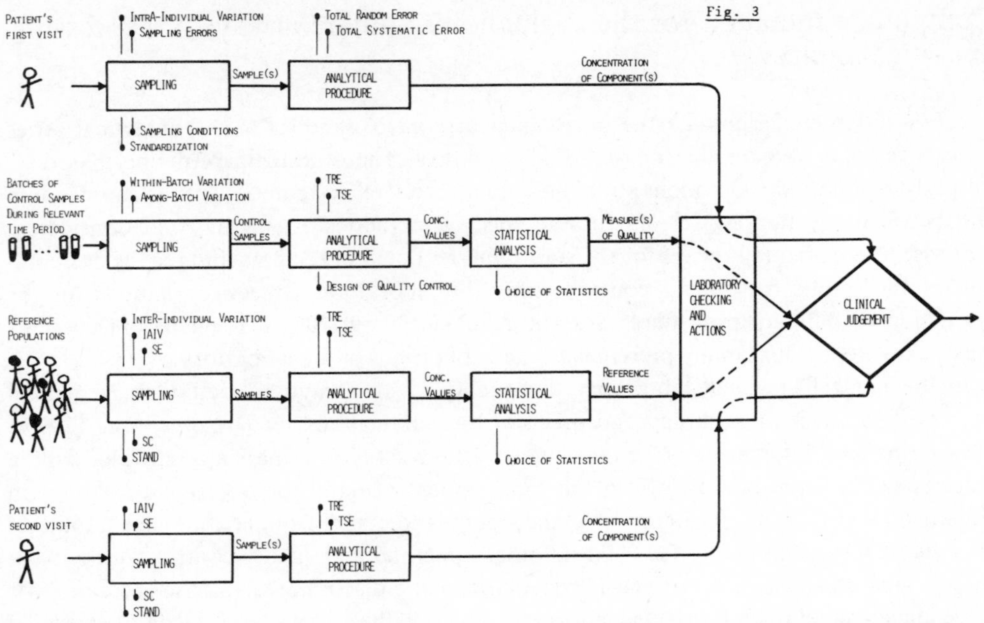

Figure 3. The basic conceptual model for the investigation of various problems concerning quality control and estimation of measures of quality and reference values. It may be noted that the detailed conceptual model in figure 2 has been lumped in one functional unit labelled 'Analytical procedure'.

The problem of choosing and estimating a suitable measure of analytical quality to be used by the clinician may be approached by studying the basic situation of comparing a patient value with a given 'discriminatory level'. The factors involved in the simulation are given in the two upper chains in figure 3.

Starting from an assumed true patient value and a corresponding intra-individual variation, the concentration value as determined in the analytical procedure may be simulated by adding random-number generated error components due to sampling, within-, and between-day random errors and a between day systematic error. Different measures of quality may then be evaluated (by Monte Carlo simulation) in terms of probability of misclassification of the patient value as compared to the given discriminatory level. The influence of other factors, such as,for instance, the design of the quality control, can then be studied in a more complete context. To make the simulation more realistic with regard to the uncertainty of an estimated discriminatory level, the third chain in figure 3 should be included. In this case, the uncertainty of a reference value depends on the choice of statistics and the number of individuals in the reference population sets (*Lindberg* and *Watson,* 1974). These sets may be simulated by assuming certain values for inter-individual, intra-individual variation, sampling errors and the location as well as the relative sizes of the reference populations.

Several previous studies have dealt with the special problem of estimating reference values. The main idea behind the simulation approach is to study this problem in relation to other procedures, and their single factors influencing the clinical judgment. In this way, it should be possible, at least for some typical situations, to optimize different laboratory functions (e.g. design of quality control, collection of reference population data and choice of statistics) in a more overall fashion.

In general, a clinical judgment is based on concentration determinations of more than one component and sometimes results from different laboratories have to be considered. The simulation model can be extended to cover also this more complex situation, by considering suitable methods for discrimination analysis and data from external laboratory quality control.

References

Aronsson, T., de Verdier, C.-H., and Groth, T.: A simulation procedure for optimizing analytical methods. Prog. in Quality Control in Clinical Chemistry. Transactions of the V. International Symposium. Geneva, April 10–11, 1973. Eds.: G. Anido, E. J. van Kampen, S. B. Rosalki, p. 288–291. Hans Huber Publishers, Bern, Stuttgart and Vienna 1973.

Aronsson, T., de Verdier, C.-H., and Groth, T.: Factors influencing the quality of analytical methods – A systems analysis, with use of computer simulation. Clin. Chem. *20,* 738–748 (1974).

Dybkaer, R., Jørgensen, K., and Nyboe, J.: Personal communication (1973).

Lindberg, D.A.B., and Watson, Fr.R.: Imprecision of Laboratory Determinations and Diagnostic Accuracy: Theoretical Consideration. Meth. Inform. Med. *13,* 151–158 (1974).

Sandblad, B., Östling, G., Schneider, W., Schütt, T., and de Verdier, C.-H.: Mathematical modelling for efficiency studies of clinical chemical laboratories. Medinfo 74. Reprints from I. World Conference on Medical Informatics. Stockholm, August 5–10, 1974. Eds.: J. Anderson and J. M. Forsythe, p. 983–987. North Holland Publishing Co., Amsterdam 1974.

Discussion of the Options followed in Processing Quality Control Data

M. Bailly, Paris (France)

Key words: Control surveys
Data presentation
Multidimensional factorial analysis
Youden plots

I, and my staff of biologists, have now been involved in interlaboratory quality control for some 6 years, most of our time being devoted to the organization of quarterly national quality control surveys with 1500 laboratories, and daily interlaboratory quality control with about 100 laboratories.

Classical statistical technics are used for the data processing, and most of our efforts have been focused on the presentation of the reported results. We were very soon aware that though statistics and computers are necessary, the psychological aspect cannot be neglected. A good understanding of a reported result can only be achieved by something additional to numbers which indicate the degree of quality of results. We observed that numbers did not sufficiently stimulate the participants, whereas added comments led to improvement when results were not acceptable. For all these reasons, individual messages are printed by the computer. They state clearly the degree of quality, and, whenever possible, the likely error, whether of accuracy, precision, reconstitution of sera etc. ... Figure 1 shows an example of an individual message. After each quarterly control survey, a longer report is produced, which comments extensively on the possible causes of error in relation to types of method, standards or instruments.

In addition, we thought it useful to add graphical presentations for quick and easy understanding. Our coding system gives us the ability to plot histograms displaying individual results, represented by a pair of code letters according to the method, standard or instrument used (fig. 2).

Société Française de Biologie Clinique
Quality Control Commission

Laboratory: XXX Month: 1274

Constituent	Serum	Un.[1]	Tech.[2]	App.[3]	Stand.[4]	All methods Result	Overall mean	100 R/M	1st code letter	Overall mean	100 R/M
Bilirubin	GG	F	AX	J	XX	11.90 (6.96)	7.177 (4.20)	165.80%$^{+++}$	A	7.736 (4.53)	153.82%$^{++}$
Bilirubin	JA	F	AX	J	XX	34.20 (20.01)	28.131 (16.46)	121.57%$^{+}$	A	28.591 (16.73)	119.61%$^{+}$
			Factors influencing accuracy to be controlled						Factors influencing accuracy to be controlled		
Calcium	GG	E	AX	J	PE	2.49 (100.00)	2.172 (87.23)	114.64%$^{++++}$	A	2.197 (88.23)	113.33%$^{++++}$
Calcium	JA	E	AX	J	PE	2.61 (104.82)	2.671 (107.27)	97.71%	A	2.687 (107.91)	97.13%
			Poor reproducibility Factors influencing accuracy to be controlled						Factors influencing accuracy to be controlled		
Glucose	GG	E	EX	J	PE	6.67 (1.20)	6.135 (1.10)	108.72%	E	6.210 (1.12)	107.40%
Glucose	JA	E	EX	J	PE	8.34 (1.50)	8.134 (1.46)	102.53%	E	8.042 (1.45)	103.70%
			Acceptable results						Acceptable results		
Magnesium	GG	E	AA	J	PE	1.19 (29.02)	0.786 (19.17)	151.39%$^{+++}$	A	0.792 (19.32)	150.25%$^{+++}$
Magnesium	JA	E	AA	J	PE	1.10 (26.83)	1.097 (26.76)	100.27%	A	1.087 (26.51)	101.19%
			Poor reproducibility Factors influencing accuracy to be controlled						Factors influencing accuracy to be controlled		
Potassium	GG	E	VB	J	PE	5.00 (5.00)	4.807 (4.81)	104.01%	V	4.684 (4.68)	106.74%
Potassium	JA	E	VB	J	PE	4.90 (4.90)	4.588 (4.59)	106.80%	V	4.469 (4.47)	109.64%$^{+}$
			Acceptable results								

For this survey, your results differ from those of the other participants. A check and control on your part will be necessary.
A regional group, or failing that, the National Commission will be at your disposal to improve your results.

[1] Unit
[2] Technic
[3] Apparatus
[4] Standard

Fig. 1

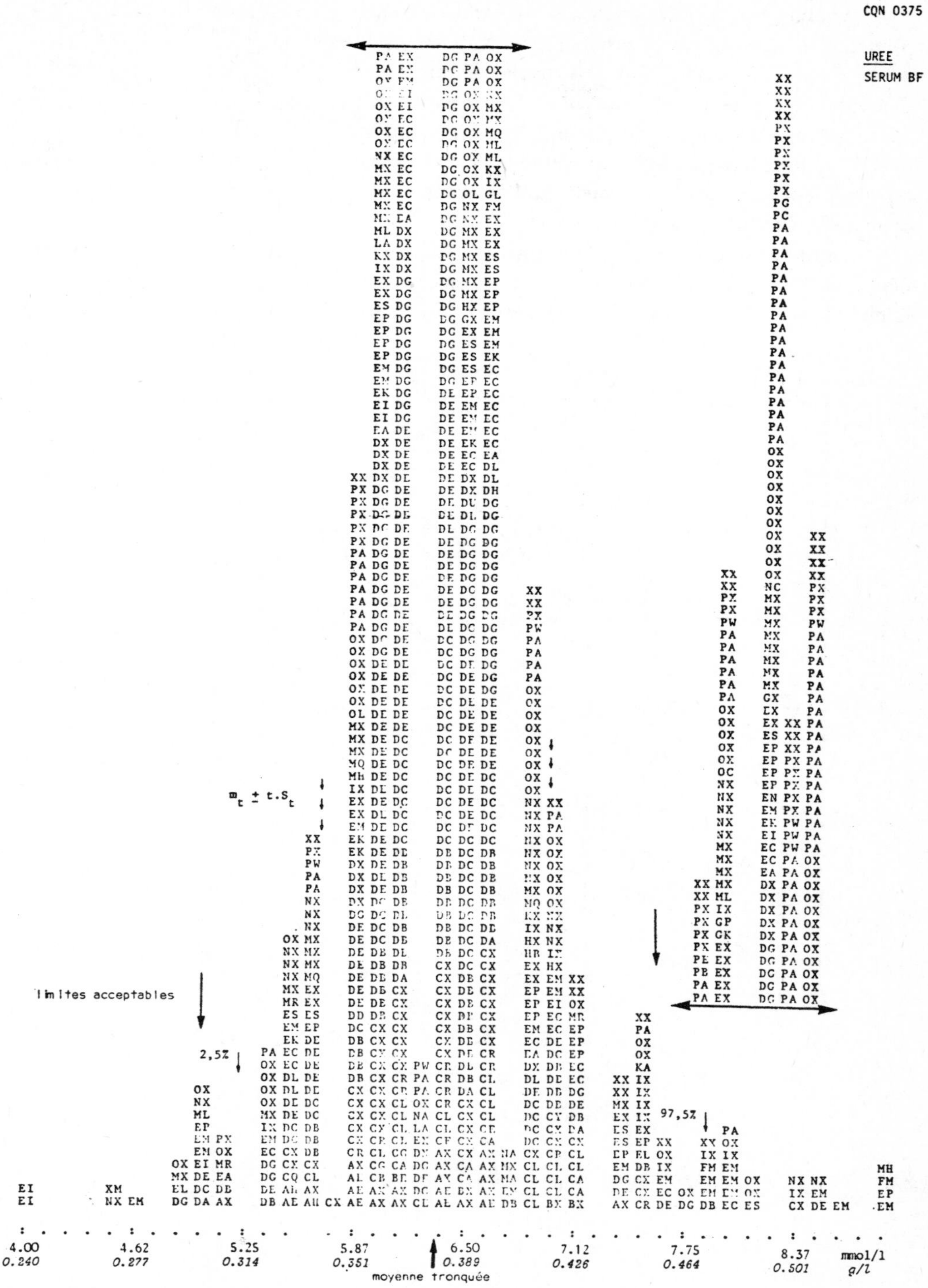
CQN 0375
UREE
SERUM BF
$m_t \pm t.s_t$
limites acceptables
2,5%
97,5%
4.00 0.240
4.62 0.277
5.25 0.314
5.87 0.351
6.50 0.389
7.12 0.426
7.75 0.464
8.37 0.501
mmol/l
g/l
moyenne tronquée

By sending two sera for each control survey, Youden plots of individual results can be printed out. The number of results in a class is represented by the density of points disposed on a spiral. We think that this display is more readily understood than a number indicating the frequency of the class. On these Youden plots the acceptable limits are narrower than the ones corresponding to each serum taken independently. They have been usually represented as circles or ellipses. This representation is not valid, since the errors on the sera are not completely independent. Therefore the theorem of composed probabilities cannot be applied.

When the concentrations of each sera are very close, we draw two parallel lines to the diagonal passing through the mean, for the acceptable limit of precision. These lines are joined together by two half-circles centered on the acceptable limits of accuracy (fig. 3 and 4).

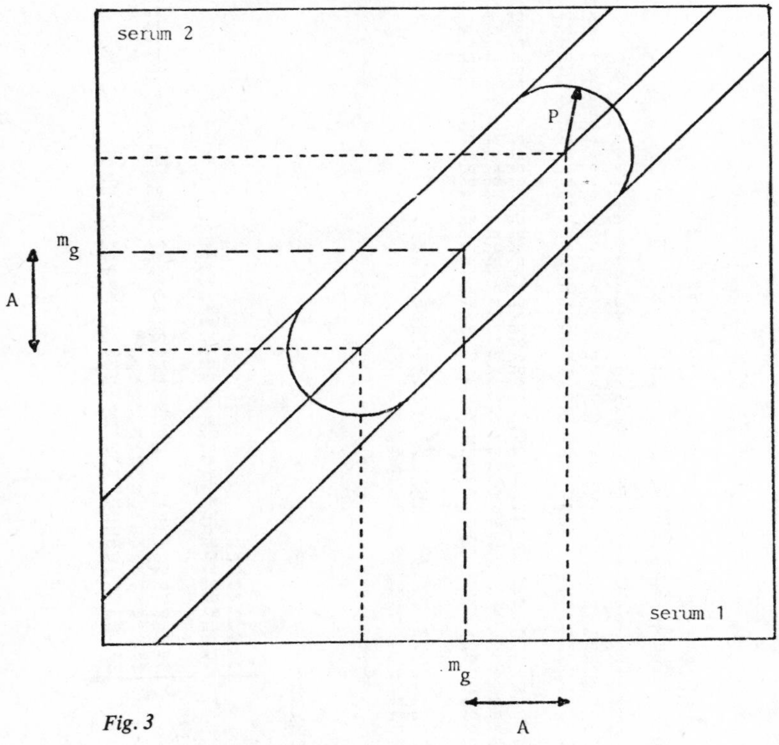

Fig. 3

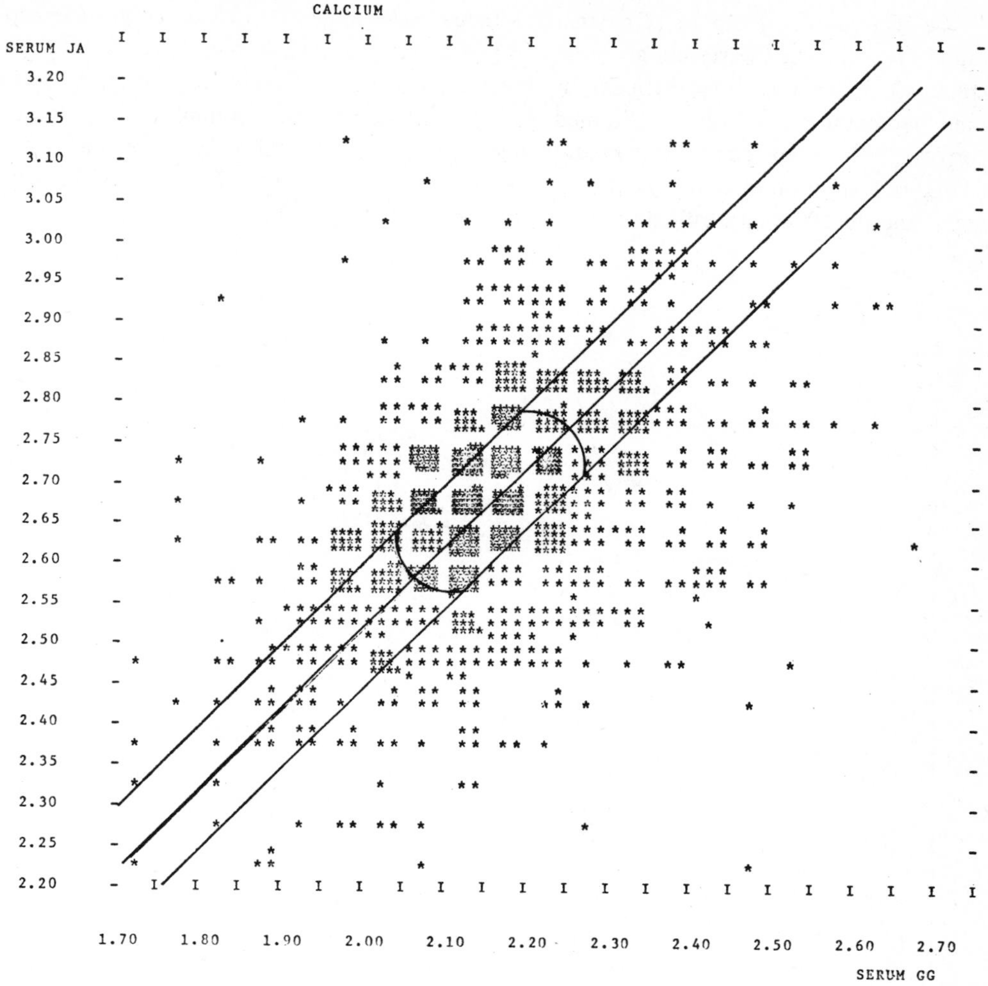
CALCIUM
SERUM JA
3.20
3.15
3.10
3.05
3.00
2.95
2.90
2.85
2.80
2.75
2.70
2.65
2.60
2.55
2.50
2.45
2.40
2.35
2.30
2.25
2.20
1.70
1.80
1.90
2.00
2.10
2.20
2.30
2.40
2.50
2.60
2.70
SERUM GG

Fig. 4

We also use Youden plots of means with their confidence limits. These means are computed after sorting the results according to one or several criteria, which can be method, standard, instruments, deproteinization, direct determination, dialysis or a combination of these. Sometimes two-step conditioned sorting is necessary. For example, all results are sorted in a first step according to method, and in a second step according to the standard.

Figure 5 shows the combined influence of the treatment of serum prior to color development, and the effect of purification, in the Jaffé method for creatinine.

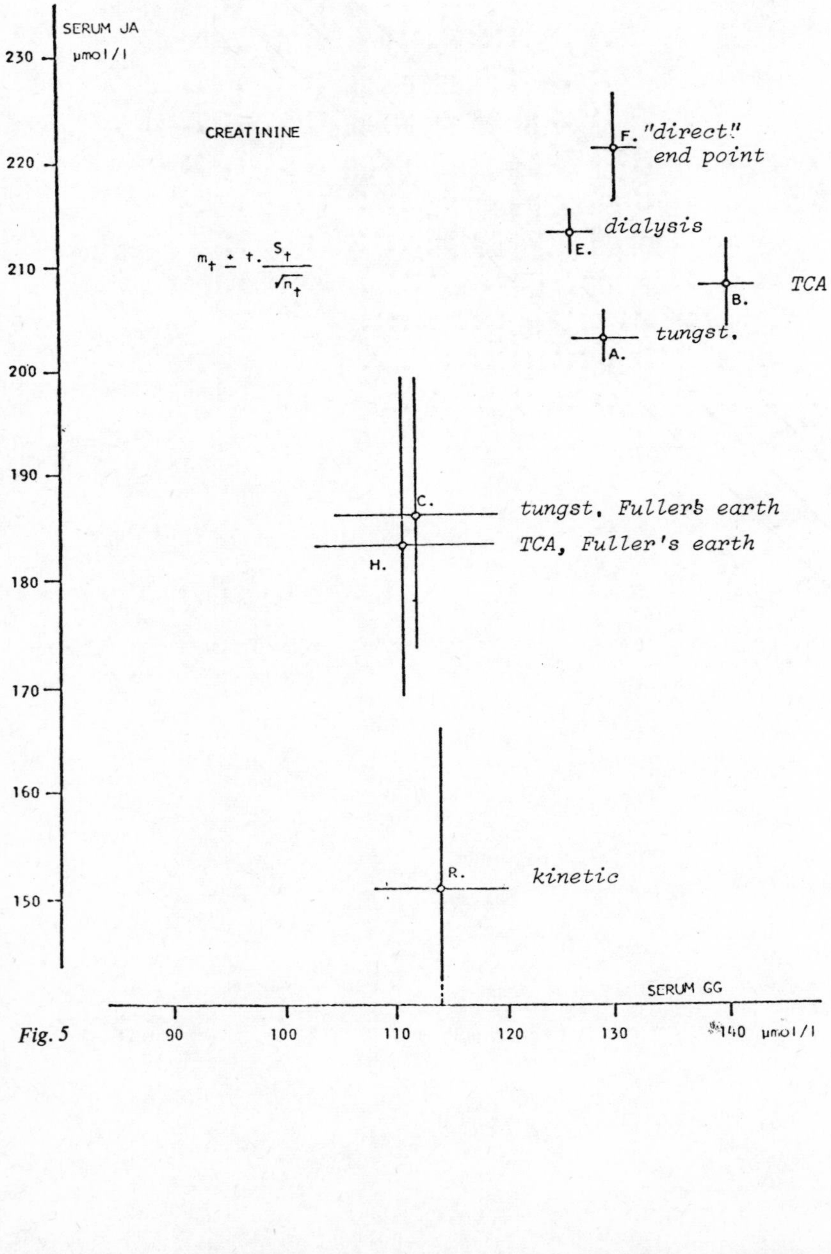

Fig. 5

Figure 6 shows that, for bilirubin determination, the type of standard makes a major contribution to the scatter of the results unlike the type of method (fig. 6).

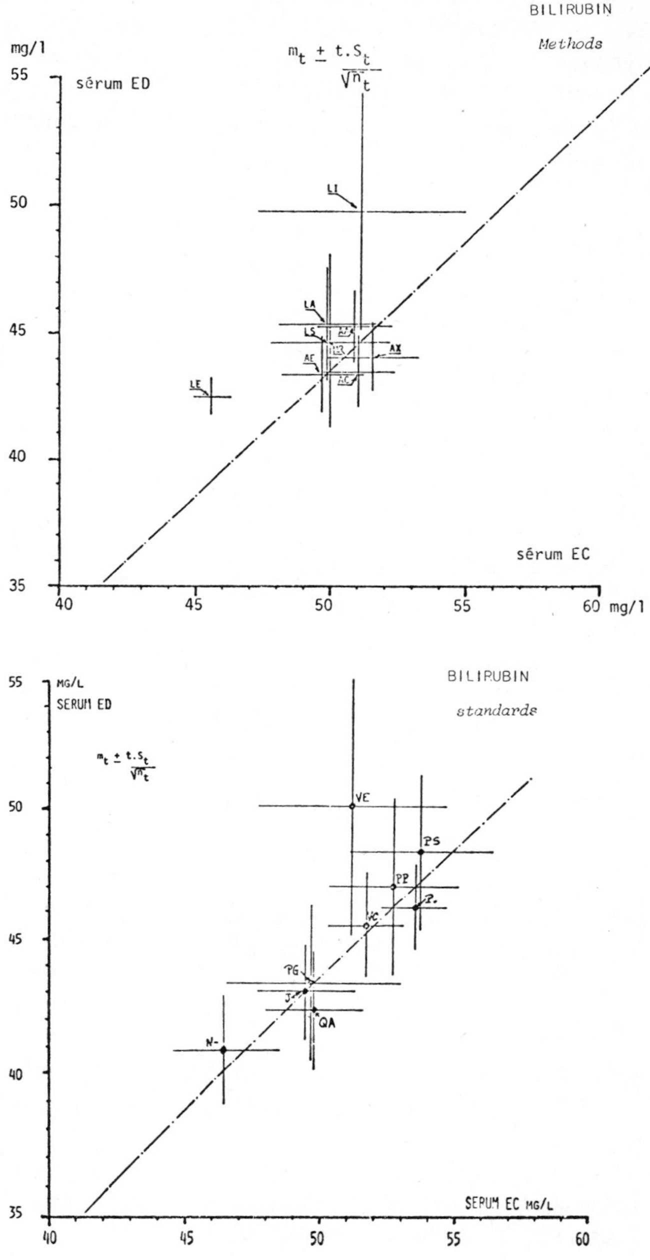

Fig. 6

Sometimes these diagrams cannot be of help in finding the causes of error, because of the numerous combinations of factors, which, by decreasing the number of results in each class, hinder a conclusive classical statistical approach. Therefore, we investigated the possibilities of a more sophisticated statistical technique: multidimensional factoral analysis of correspondances. This new tool displays clusters or discrepancies a long certain axes, the significance of which is sometimes difficult to understand.

We also applied this technique to the examination of the relative behaviour of quality control sera versus the different sorts of methods (fig. 7).

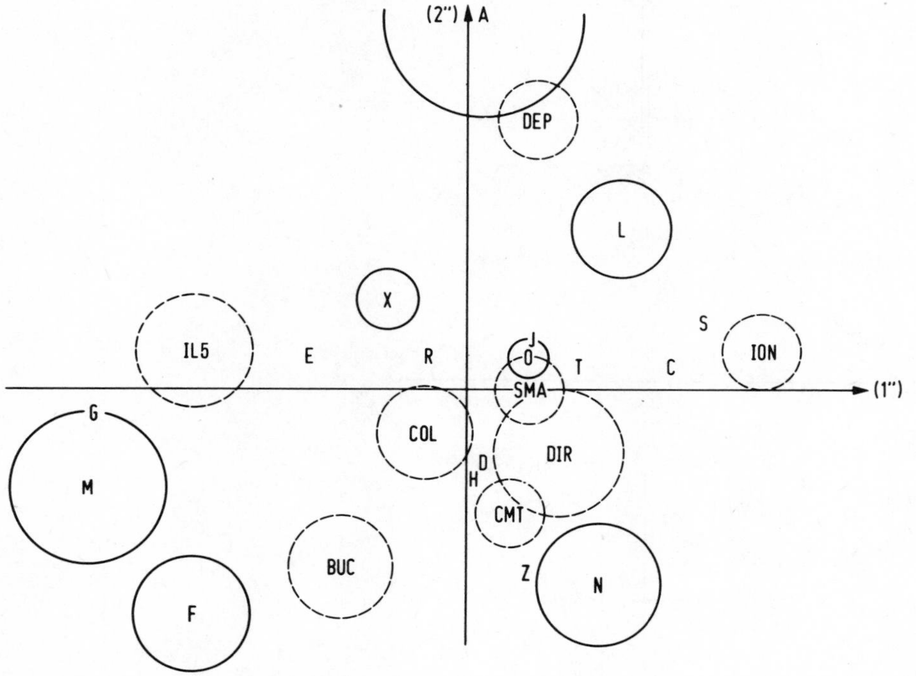

Figure 7. A, C, E ... = control sera, BUC = Büchler coulometer, CMT = Radiometer CMT 10 coulometer, DEP = mercurimetric with deproteinisation, DIR = mercurimetric without deproteinisation, COL = colorimetry thiocyanate-Gemsaec, IL 5 = colorimetry thiocyanate-IL 279, SMA = colorimetry thiocyanate-SMA 6 60.

Although a theoretical statistical approach is necessary for the interpretation of results, the data processing is frequently jeopardized by some problems I would like to discuss now.

– Coding errors, gross analytical errors, or inversion of results for the two sera,can lead either to rejection of the results by the computer or to their classification in a wrong group. This latter possibility gives rise to confusion in statistical calculations.

We decided to check all the forms before data processing. This cumbersome but vital job is made by biologists, who correct the errors when they are obvious,or put them aside when they are suspect.

– With the processing of data,it is frequently necessary to write a new program to solve particular problems which arise. This necessity is mostly felt during the writing of the detailed report sent with each survey.

This efficiency has only been achieved since the purchase of a mini-computer, easy to program and available to any member of the staff. With this policy, anybody can understand the processing and improve the programs. This situation of constant evolution, due to the accessability of the computer and the facility of its programming by biologists, is the only way to progress to a better understanding of quality control records.

Topic III
Quality Control in Relation to Data Evaluation, Processing and Presentation

Discussion

H. Büttner (Germany): I have two remarks to the paper of Dr. *Solberg*. The first is that we have a similar system of discrepancy checks as you have shown; that is, the sum of anions and cations in serum. We have additionally included calcium, protein and phosphate, and then we get a difference (Anion – Cation) which is smaller than yours and which has a normal distribution similar to yours. This figure can be used for controlling the SMA 12/60's. We can control certain of the 12 channels of our SMA 12/60 by this procedure.

The other point is, computerized laboratories give us the possibility easily to control quality; but in most laboratories and most papers, quality means only an accurate and precise result. Did you try to control the processing time in the laboratories? The laboratory result must be back on the ward within a short period of time. I think this is part of quality too. In the computerized laboratory you can control the processing time within the laboratory by means of the computer. This should be included in all computerized laboratories as a very important part of quality control.

H. Solberg (Norway): First, I think it is very interesting to hear your extended type of balancing of electrolytes. Of course, quality is also what you mentioned, and that is one of the reasons why we are now changing from a batch-oriented system to an on-line real time system because then we can monitor such things and have all the parameters immediately.

J. Henry (U.S.A.): I am wondering if anyone of the panel would comment on the impact of quality control on workload in the chemical laboratory. The emphasis on quality control in terms of accuracy and precision is acceptable within the laboratory context, but when I talk to my clinical colleagues, I often hear from them that their reaction to an abnormal value is to re-order the test. In other words, as Dr. *de Verdier* mentioned, and I have heard others suggest, we have to do something to emphasize the translation of quality control to the clinician, for if his reaction is simply to re-order a measurement in which the numerical value is suspicious, but without any appreciation of what represents a change in the laboratory versus a change in the patient, I suspect the impact of quality control could extend well beyond the limits of the laboratory, and indeed affect all of the workload in chemical laboratories throughout the world.

T. Whitehead (U.K.): There are countries where it is common for physicians to divide a specimen and send it to three laboratories and then calculate the mean value. I think that this is an example of excessive workload both in terms of the number of analyses performed and the fees paid. In my own Group, we are trying to carry out studies along these lines, because we are keen on knowing what is the motive behind many laboratory investigations. It is interesting to ask a physician, 'why did you ask for that test?' 'Because I wanted to check the previous result,' is a relatively common answer. Therefore, it is an important factor in the expanding workload.

P. Lous (Denmark): I have two questions. The first is for Dr. *Stamm*. Is it human serum or serum from another animal that you are using in your German surveys?

D. Stamm (Germany): It doesn't make much difference if you have human serum or animal serum.

P. Lous (Denmark): May I continue?

Do you agree that non-human serum imposes a lot of limitations in the methods for protein, for enzymes, for substances combined with the proteins in the plasma, and also for methods based on immunochemistry?

Could I have another question? That is for Dr. *Bailly*. I saw your Youden plots, and I understand that you had some special figures, circles or elliptical figures, but as you will remember, every method has its optimal concentration range, as pointed out by Dr. *Richterich* several times in previous Symposia here. Therefore, I don't understand why you try to make such special numerical figures in your Youden plots. If you were to be more accurate, then perhaps logarithmic scales would be more illustrative than the Youden plots.

M. Bailly (France): At this time I cannot make a decision as to whether or not the results are adequate. Two results for each control is not sufficient. The Youden plots with ellipses or circles give a certain indication of accuracy, but will give an indication of precision only if the two pool concentrations are quite the same. If the concentrations are far apart, then we must make an interpretation as it applies to reproducibility.

T. Whitehead (U.K.): I want to refer to Dr. *Stamm*'s paper. You showed a Youden plot where the reference value was in the center of the Youden plot and the data of all the participants had a very small deviation. Nevertheless, they were virtually all on the one side of your reference value, in the right upper side. How do you explain this? Is it due to the systematic error of all participants, or is it due to the method you used for your reference value?

D. Stamm (Germany): This variation depends on the standard used by the laboratories.

Richterich Memorial Lecture

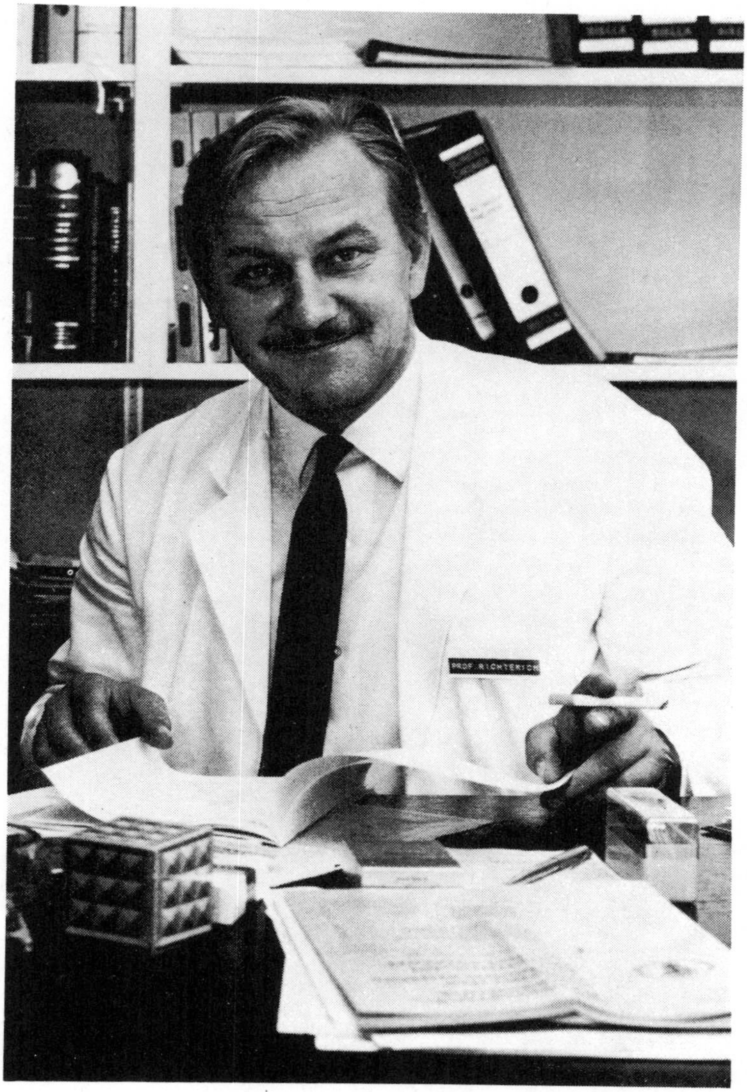

Prof. R. Richterich

Introduction by Prof. H. Aebi

S. Rosalki (U.K.)

As you are all aware, this Symposium has the honour to establish a Memorial Lecture to the memory of the late *Roland Richterich* who was such an active contributor to clinical chemistry and to previous Geneva Symposia.

Prior to his appointment as chief of Clinical Chemistry at the Inselspital, Berne, Professor *Richterich* served as first associate to Professor *Hugo Aebi,* chief of the Institute of Medical Chemistry at the University of Berne, and collaborated with him in many fine research studies. We are delighted to have Professor *Aebi* with us today, to introduce this lecture.

H. Aebi (Switzerland)

Dear Mrs. *Richterich,* or better, Dear Britta, Ladies and Gentlemen,

It is the inevitable fate of man to die; scientists are no exception; however, their lifelong and restless service for progress and the benefit of mankind gives them a fortunate position. The scientist's life continues in a modified manner and in various ways. This is also true for my scholar, later my colleague and friend Professor *Roland Richterich,* who was the victim of a deadly heart attack on Christmas day 1973.

I just said that he is still with us; yes, but in what ways?

1. He stays on in our memory: Many of you certainly remember well how he personally presented and explained with much enthusiasm and devotion the first prototype of his analyzer. This was at the exhibition of the International Congress of Clinical Chemistry held in Geneva in 1969. It is probably more than pure coincidence that the first Memorial Lecture is held at exactly the same place where the Richterich-Greiner Machine was publicly demonstrated for the first time.
2. He is still with us in his publications. This is particularly true for the 3rd Edition and the many translations of his textbook on Clinical Chemistry, a wise and competent companion always ready on the shelf of most clinical chemists, as well as biochemists, to give us his clearcut and frank advice.
3. *Roland Richterich* continues to be around at the place where he worked and where he accomplished most of his achievements. The Chemical Central Laboratory at the 'Inselspital', the University Hospital of Berne is directed now by our common scholar *Jean-Pierre Colombo.* When nominated as successor he also accepted the challenging task of continuing all those professional duties Dr. *Richterich* could not perform due to his untimely death.

The process of fading away is almost as quick as the present pace of progress in science and technology. Therefore, I wish to express my sincere thanks to the organizers and in particular to Mrs. *Divernois,* Secretary of this Congress for having established this *Roland Richterich* Memorial Lecture. It corresponds exactly to the attitude of the scientist, to whom you are reminded by this lecture, that this – and hopefully further sessions – will be devoted entirely to progress in clinical chemistry, and notably to one of the main concerns of *Richterich,* that is 'quality control'.

On behalf of the many friends of Dr. *Richterich* I wish to thank Dr. *Rosalki,* Chairman of this Symposium, for having accepted to be the first speaker to commemorate his fellow colleague. Everybody will agree that Dr. *Rosalki*'s lecture will be an excellent and promising start in 'Seeking the Way'.

Richterich Memorial Lecture

Seeking the Way

S.B.Rosalki, London (U.K.)

Quality control of laboratory practice covers those processes which ensure that the correct result is returned to the right patient.

The road which leads to quality is travelled by controlling the pathways of patient status, sample, determination method, reagents, controls, standards, instruments, and data. Each of these pathways has been sign-posted by the late Roland Richterich, in published work and in contributions to previous Geneva symposia.

In this Memorial Lecture, I shall discuss only determination methods, and shall describe experiences with these which illustrate the need for critical method control. My examples are drawn from clinical enzymology, a discipline to which Professor Richterich's contributions were outstanding.

I shall start by considering creatine kinase isoenzyme demonstration.

By 1962 Prof.*Richterich* and colleagues had shown that serum creatine kinase determination was the most sensitive of all enzyme tests for the diagnosis of myocardial infarction, but that the enzyme could be spuriously elevated as a result of exercise (*Baumann, Escher* and *Richterich,* 1962; *Colombo, Richterich* and *Rossi,* 1962). By 1964 it was known that intramuscular injections could also result in false elevation (*Hess* et al., 1964). In consequence, a 15% incidence of false-positive elevation of *total* creatine kinase activity is found in suspected infarction (*Wagner* et al., 1973). Recently, it has been shown, however, that creatine kinase *isoenzyme* separation can differentiate infarction from these false elevations (*Klein, Shell* and *Sobel,* 1973).

As illustrated in figure 1 and as described by Prof.*Richterich* and colleagues in 1964 (*Burger, Richterich* and *Aebi,* 1964), three isoenzymes of creatine kinase may be separated electrophoretically; a fast-moving form, prominent in brain tissue, and known as the BB isoenzyme; a slow-moving form, prominent in muscle and known as the MM isoenzyme; and a hybrid form of intermediate mobility known as the MB isoenzyme.

Whereas with most demonstration techniques normal sera and post-exercise or post-injection sera show only the MM isoenzyme (*Klein, Shell* and *Sobel,* 1973), the MB isoenzyme appears in post-infarct sera (*Sjövall* and *Voigt,* 1964; *Van der Veen* and *Willebrands,* 1966). Demonstration of the MB iosenzyme is therefore valuable in cardiac diagnosis (*Konttinen* and *Somer,* 1972; *Roe* et al., 1972; *Smith,* 1972).

Almost all electrophoretic techniques for creatine kinase isoenzyme demonstration use

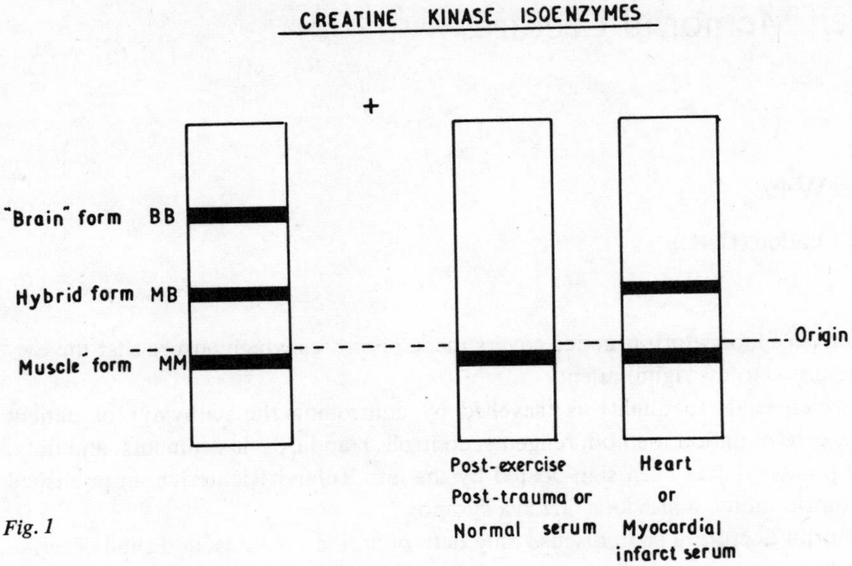

Fig. 1

staining or fluorescence methods similar to that which I described in 1965 for isoenzyme staining following separation on cellulose acetate (*Rosalki,* 1965).

In this procedure (fig. 2) the enzyme acts on creatine phosphate and adenosine diphosphate (ADP), and the adenosine triphosphate (ATP) liberated is coupled to glucose, hexokinase, glucose-6-phosphate dehydrogenase and nicotinamide-adenine dinucleotide phosphate (NADP). The reduced NADP (NADPH) formed, fluoresces strongly in ultraviolet (UV) light, or can be used to reduce a tetrazolium salt to produce coloured staining bands at the sites of isoenzyme activity.

$$\text{Creatine phosphate} + \text{ADP} \xrightarrow{\text{CPK}} \text{creatine} + \text{ATP} \quad (1)$$

$$\text{ATP} + \text{glucose} \xrightarrow{\text{hexokinase}} \text{glucose-6-phosphate} + \text{ADP} \quad (2)$$

$$\text{Glucose-6-phosphate} + \text{NADP} \xrightarrow[\text{dehydrogenase}]{\text{glucose-6-phosphate}} \text{6-phosphogluconate} + \text{NADPH} \quad (3)$$

Fig. 2. Determination of creatine kinase (CPK).

Quality control and standardization of isoenzyme procedures has, in general, been notoriously neglected (*Rosalki,* 1974). Published procedures used to demonstrate the MB isoenzyme, have failed to provide evidence that the conditions chosen were optimal for the demonstration of this particular fraction. This despite the fact that each isoenzyme is known to differ in its kinetic properties (*Dawson* and *Fine,* 1967).

As shown in table 1, for MB isoenzyme demonstration different workers have used creatine phosphate substrate concentrations varying between 2 and 28 mmol/l. Sometimes the *same* workers have used different concentrations in different studies.

Table 1. Creatine phosphate concentrations used for MB isoenzyme demonstration.

Reference	Creatine phosphate mmol/l
Somer and Konttinen, 1972 a	2
Somer and Konttinen, 1972 b	6
Smith, 1972	15
Roe et al., 1972	28
Goto, 1974	2
Anido et al., 1973	7
Anido et al., 1974	10

To determine optimal conditions for the MB form, I have isolated this isoenzyme from human heart using a chromatographic technique similar to that utilized by Prof. *Richterich* in 1963 for lactate dehydrogenase isoenzyme separation (*Richterich, Schafroth* and *Aebi,* 1963).

Figure 3 shows the MB isoenzyme in nearly pure form, demonstrated by fluorescence, in a chromatographically separated heart fraction (Fraction C 9). A post-infarct serum containing this isoenzyme is also shown.

Fraction | *Activity U/l 37 °C*

C9 | 6800
Neat serum
D6
5
4
S6
5
4

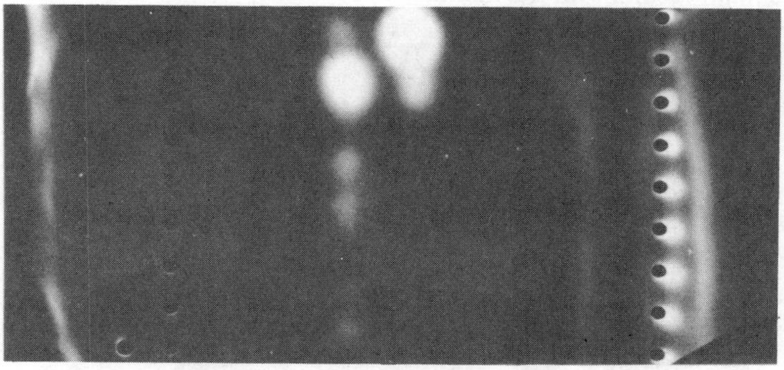

MM MB Anode

Fig. 3
Creatine kinase isoenzymes of DEAE-Sephadex separated fractions of human infarct serum or heart homogenate

With purified MB isoenzyme, I have examined the effect of variation of creatine phosphate concentration on enzyme activity. As shown in figure 4, at 37 °C, the temperature usual in staining and fluorescence methods, creatine phosphate concentrations above 20 mmol/l are required for near-optimal activity. Values below 10 mmol/l are clearly sub-optimal.

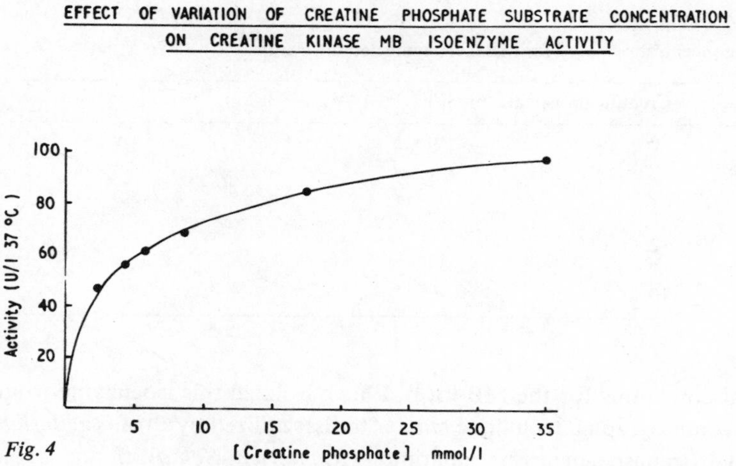

Fig. 4

The need for high creatine phosphate concentrations in the fluorescence technique is clearly shown in figure 5. All three creatine kinase isoenzymes are shown. Fluorescence is very obviously diminished at the lowest creatine phosphate concentration (4.5 mmol/l). These results were obtained with a Dade isoenzyme marker of animal origin (DADE Division, American Hospital Supply Corporation, Miami, Florida 33152, U.S.A.), but I have confirmed similar results with the human isoenzymes.

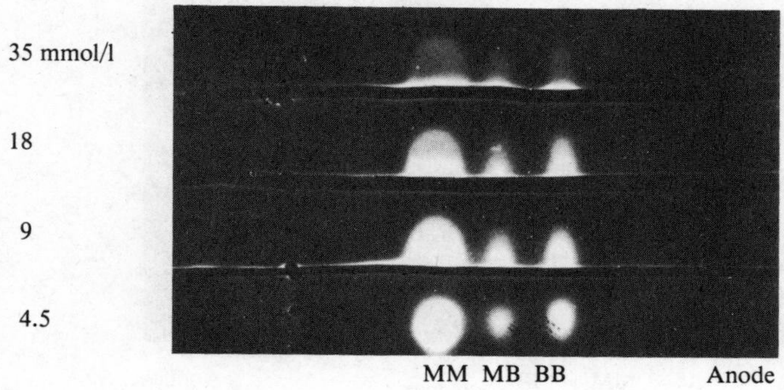

Fig. 5 Effect of variation of creatine phosphate concentration on creatine kinase isoenzyme fluorescence

From the purified MB isoenzyme I have prepared stable liquid and lyophilised control materials for standardization of the isoenzyme method:

Figure 6 shows their use to demonstrate the sensitivity of the staining procedure. On the photograph, the MB isoenzyme is seen to be stained at an activity level of 20 units per litre (U/l) at 37 °C, on the original it is clearly visible even at an activity level of 10 U/l at 37 °C, corresponding to less than 10% of the upper limit of normal for *total* creatine kinase in serum with the determination method used. The upper limit of normal for this being 140 in females and 200 in males.

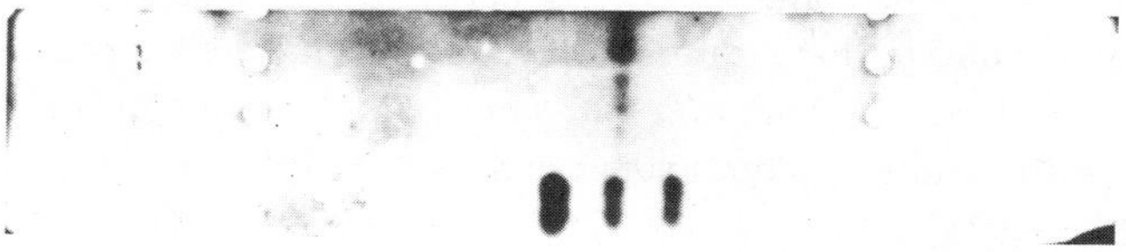

Fig. 6 Standardisation of creatine kinase isoenzyme staining

My studies of creatine kinase isoenzymes have also revealed new *clinical* information, an objective in all method studies. An increase in the MB isoenzyme in serum in the absence of overt muscle disease has generally been considered diagnostic of myocardial injury (*Roe* et al., 1972; *Konttinen* and *Somer,* 1973), though its occasional unexplained presence has been seen in apparently normal subjects (*Smith,* 1972).

Figure 7 shows that it may appear in serum not only in overt myopathy – (Patients 1 and 2) – but also in clinically normal female carriers of Duchenne muscular dystrophy (Carriers 1, 2, and 3).

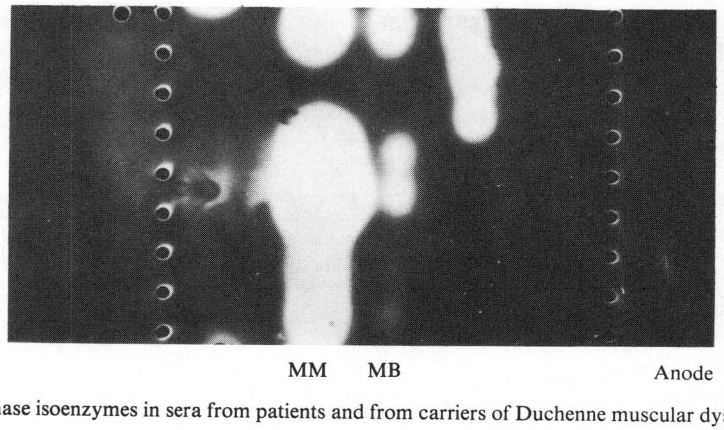

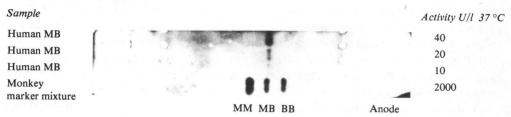

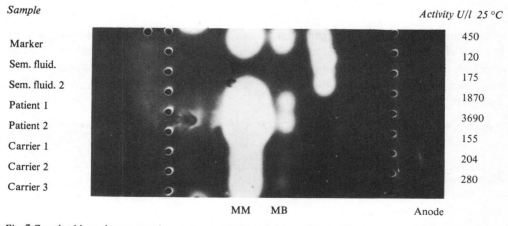

Fig. 7 Creatine kinase isoenzymes in sera from patients and from carriers of Duchenne muscular dystrophy

We should remember that Professor *Aebi*, Professor *Richterich* and colleagues were amongst the first to convincingly demonstrate the value of *total* serum creatine kinase levels in the *detection* of such carriers (*Aebi, Richterich, Colombo* and *Rossi* 1961/1962, *Richterich, Rosin, Aebi* and *Rossi*, 1963).

I now wish to discuss some problems with *total* creatine kinase methodology.

The procedure which I described in 1966 (*Oliver*, 1955; *Rosalki*, 1966; 1967) has now been almost universally adopted for creatine kinase determination.

I would draw your attention to three aspects of the reaction (fig. 2). Firstly, the number of organic phosphates present, both as substrate (creatine phosphate and ATP), as product (glucose-6-phosphate) and as coenzyme (NADP). Secondly, that the measured product is NADPH. Thirdly, that a thiol is added for enzyme activation.

With this reaction, sera with high *alkaline phosphatase* levels may show spuriously low *creatine kinase* values, and it has been suggested that phosphatases may interfere with the method (*Mueller* et al., 1975).

As shown in table 2, however, neither alkaline phosphatase itself nor 5'nucleotidase appear responsible, for addition of purified alkaline phosphatase or 5'nucleotidase to infarct serum creatine kinase is without effect, and liver serum alkaline phosphatase is not inhibitory. Also, β-glycerophosphate addition to serum, which would nullify alkaline phosphatase effects (*Belfield* and *Goldberg*, 1968), does not increase the *creatine kinase* activity of high alkaline phosphatase serum.

Table 2. Effect of phosphatases on creatine kinase determination.

1. Calf intestine, alkaline phosphatase (1000 U/l 37 °C)	No effect
2. Snake venom, 5'nucleotidase (150 U/l 37 °C)	No effect
3. Serum alkaline phosphatase (liver) (280 U/l 37 °C)	No effect

Note: 1. Phosphatase or water mixed 50 : 50 with infarct serum (CPK 170 U/l 25 °C)
2. β-glycerophosphate 20 mmol/l had no effect on CPK activity (9 U/l 25 °C) of high phosphatase serum.

My studies show that low creatine kinase activities with high phosphatase sera, are most marked when *glutathione* is used as thiol activator. This is shown in table 3, in which a low phosphatase serum had identical activities with either glutathione or cysteine as thiol, whereas a high phosphatase serum shows creatine kinase activity with cysteine but none with glutathione.

Table 3. Effect of reagent thiol on CPK activity (U/l 25 °C) of high and low alkaline phosphatase sera.

	Glutathione 20 mmol/l	Cysteine 20 mmol/l
High phosphatase (315 U/l 37 °C)	0	8
Low phosphatase (42 U/l 37 °C)	30	30

Glutathione reductase (fig. 8) in sera may, in part, be responsible. Sera with high alkaline phosphatase levels may be from patients with liver disease or malignancy, in which glutathione reductase activity may also be increased. Reduced glutathione in the reagent system may oxidise on storage, and may oxidise the NADPH formed in the creatine kinase reaction, resulting in falsely low creatine kinase activity (*Weidemann,* 1973).

oxidised glutathione + NADPH → reduced glutathione + NADP

Fig. 8. Action of glutathione reductase

Glutathione reductase, however, only partially accounts for the spuriously low creatine kinase of high phosphatase sera, since this has been observed with reagents using NAD – rather than NADP – dependent glucose-6-phosphate dehydrogenase, also, similar, though reduced effects are observed with other thiols, and I have shown that the low creatine kinase levels may be raised by *further* thiol addition. Table 4 shows higher creatine kinase levels with dithiothreitol (DTT) than with reduced glutathione (GSH), in a high liver phosphatase serum, but *both* values increase and become identical with mercaptoethanol addition.

Table 4. Effect of reagent thiol concentration on CPK activity of high phosphatase serum.

	CPK activity (U/l 37 °C)
1. GSH 20 mmol/l	30
GSH 20 mmol/l + mercaptoethanol 50 mmol/l	42
2. DTT 3.5 mmol/l	36
DTT 3.5 mmol/l + mercaptoethanol 50 mmol/l	43
(Liver serum; alkaline phosphatase 350 U/l 37 °C)	

In my creatine kinase reagent system, I recommended cysteine in preference to glutathione, since *higher* enzyme activities were obtained with this (*Rosalki,* 1967). Thiols may be potent phosphatase inhibitors, and Prof. *Richterich* has confirmed this for cysteine (*Wiesmann, Colombo, Adam* and *Richterich,* 1966).

Table 5 shows an example of alkaline phosphatase inhibition by thiols. The enzyme is almost completely inhibited by cysteine and mercaptoethanol, whereas glutathione is a poor inhibitor.

Though I have shown that non-specific alkaline phosphatase has no effect on creatine kinase measurement, *other* phosphatases such as adenosine triphosphatase (ATP'ase) might cause slight interference. Indeed in 1963, Prof. *Richterich* criticised methods measuring ATP formation because of the theoretical possibility of ATP'ase interference (*Richterich, Rosin, Aebi* and *Rossi,* 1963). It is likely, however, that thiols inhibit not only

Table 5. Thiol inhibition of alkaline phosphatase.

Thiol, mmol/l	Percent inhibition
Cysteine	
10	97
20	97
Reduced glutathione (GSH)	
10	50
20	60
Mercaptoethanol	
10	87
20	91

(Liver serum; activity 230 U/l 37 °C, 15 minute incubation with thiol in assay)

non-specific phosphatase but *specific* phosphatases. Since glutathione is a poor, and mercaptoethanol a good phosphatase inhibitor, the previously demonstrated enhanced creatine kinase activity on mercaptoethanol addition is explained.

I believe,that in the creatine kinase reaction, thiols have a dual role. Firstly, enzyme activation, secondly, inhibition of competing side reactions. A thiol appropriate in type and amount for the first function, may be inadequate for the second.

This is demonstrated in table 6. Addition of extra thiol is without effect on the creatine kinase of low-phosphatase muscle disease serum, whereas, glutathione apart, it increases the activity of a high phosphatase liver serum. Also, whilst activities are near identical with all thiols in the former, they are lowest with glutathione and highest with dithiothreitol in the latter.

Table 6. Effect of doubling thiol concentration on CPK activity (U/l 25 °C), high and low phosphatase sera.

	Thiol × 1	Thiol × 2
High phosphatase		
1. GSH 20 mmol/l	9	10
2. DTT 10	15	19
3. Cysteine 20	12	20
4. Mercaptoethanol 20	12	20
Low phosphatase		
1. GSH 20 mmol/l	118	122
2. DTT 10	120	122
3. Cysteine 20	120	130
4. Mercaptoethanol 20	132	122

High phosphatase (liver serum) 350 U/l 37 °C; low (muscle serum) 40 U/l 37 °C.

It was unfortunate, that in 1970 the German Society of Clinical Chemistry recommendations for creatine kinase determinations (*Bergmeyer* et al., 1970) substituted glutathione for the cysteine I originally recommended. Apart from the inadequacies I have described, Prof. *Richterich* in 1966 had suggested that oxidised glutathione might act as a creatine kinase inhibitor (*Wiesmann, Colombo, Adam* and *Richterich,* 1966). Variable glutathione oxidation on storage might then yield batch-to-batch reagent variation.

Such variation is shown in figure 9. Two batches of reagents from a manufacturer using glutathione as activator are compared with a fluorimetric procedure using mercaptoethanol (*Rokos, Rosalki* and *Tarlow,* 1972). Batch I of the commercial reagent shows creatine kinase activities some 20% lower than Batch 2. Such differences are, of course, quite unacceptable.

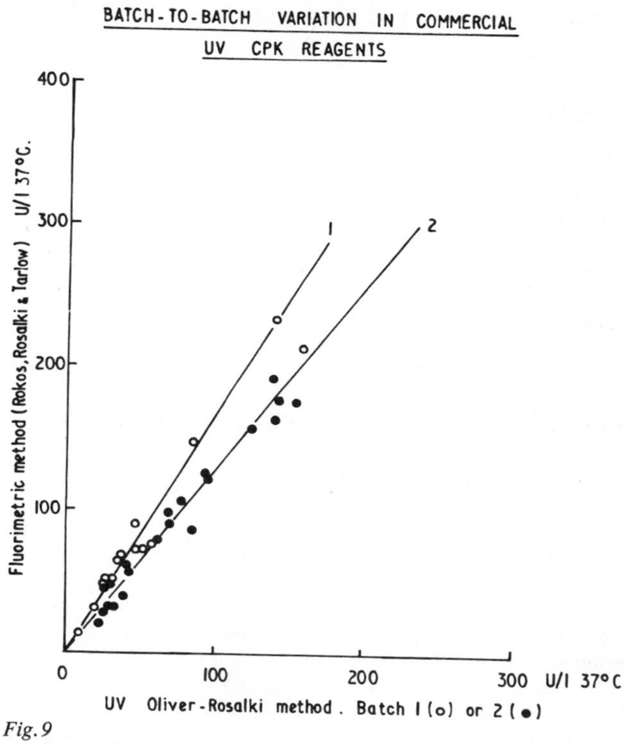

Fig. 9

For all the reasons I have given, it no longer appears proper to use glutathione as activator in the UV creatine kinase method.

I cannot yet make definitive recommendations on the appropriate thiol and its concentration to produce maximal creatine kinase activation combined with maximal inhibition of competing side-reactions, but from the thiols I have studied (glutathione, mercaptoethanol, cysteine, N-acetylcysteine and dithiothreitol), dithiothreitol at a concentration of 20 mmol/l most closely approached this.

Conclusion

The information I have presented has, I hope, emphasised the need for a continual critical approach to our work.

I have considered only methodology and used only examples from clinical enzymology, yet the approach is applicable to all branches of clinical chemistry and to other aspects of quality control.

There are many twists and turns on each pathway on the road to quality, but the way to quality is a way we all must seek. You will have noticed from my many references to the late *Roland Richterich,* how well he sought this way.

I have chosen the title of my lecture 'Seeking the Way' from a poem 'Doctors' by the British poet *Rudyard Kipling,*

> 'Man dies too soon, beside his works half-planned.
> His days are counted and reprieve is vain:
> Who shall entreat with Death to stay his hand,
> Or cloke the shameful nakedness of pain?
>
> Send here the bold, the seekers of the way –
> The passionless, the unshakeable of soul,
> Who serve the inmost mysteries of man's clay,
> And ask no more than leave to make them whole.'

To that great Doctor and Seeker of the Way, *Roland Richterich,* I dedicate this lecture.

References

Aebi, U., Richterich, R., Colombo, J.P., and Rossi, E. (1961/1962): Progressive muscular dystrophy. II. Biochemical identification of the carrier state in the recessive sex-linked juvenile (Duchenne) type by serum creatine phosphokinase determinations. Enzymol. Clin. Biol. *1,* 61–74.

Anido, V., Conn, R.B., Mengoli, H.F., and Anido, G. (1974): Diagnostic efficacy of myocardial creatine phosphokinase using polyacrylamide disk gel electrophoresis. Amer. J. clin. Path. *61,* 599–605.

Anido, G., Fitzgerald, J.C., Soto, A. and Romero, P. (1973): SGOT and CPK isoenzymes in clinical medicine. Quad. Sclavo Diagn. *2,* 137–146.

Baumann, P., Escher, J. and Richterich, R.G. (1962): Das Verhalten von Serum-Enzymen bei Sportlichen Leistungen. Schweiz. Z. Sportmed. *10,* 33–51.

Belfield, A. and Goldberg, D.M. (1965): Inhibition of the nucleotidase effect of alkaline phosphatase by β-glycerophosphate. Nature (Lond.) *219,* 73–75.

Bergmeyer, H.U., Büttner, H., Hillmann, G., Kreutz, F.H., Lang, H., Laue, D., Rick, W., Schmidt, E., Schmidt, F.W., Stamm, D. and Szasz, G. (1970): Recommendations of the German Society for Clinical Chemistry (1970). Z. Klin. Chem. Klin. Biochem. *8,* 659–660.

Burger, A., Richterich, R. and Aebi, H. (1964): Die Heterogenität der Kreatin-Kinase. Biochem. Z. *339,* 305–314.

Colombo, J.P., Richterich, R. and Rossi, E.R. (1962): Serum-Kreatin-Phosphokinase: Bestimmung und Diagnostische Bedeutung. Klin. Wschr. *40*, 37–44.

Dawson, D.M. and Fine, I.H. (1967): Creatine Kinase in Human tissues. Arch. Neurol. *16*, 175–180.

Goto, I. (1974): Serum creatine phosphokinase isozymes in hypothyroidism, convulsion, myocardial infarction and other disease. Clin. Chim. Acta *52*, 27–30.

Hess, J.W., MacDonald, R.P., Frederick, R.J., Jones, R.N., Neely, J. and Gross, D. (1964): Serum creatine phosphokinase (CPK) activity in disorders of heart and skeletal muscle. Ann. intern. Med. *61*, 1015–1028.

Klein, M.S., Shell, W.E. and Sobel, B.E. (1973): Serum creatine phosphokinase (CPK) isoenzymes after intramuscular injections, surgery and myocardial infarction: Experimental and clinical studies. Cardiovasc. Res. *7*, 412–418.

Konttinen, A. and Somer, H. (1972): Determination of serum creatine kinase isoenzymes in myocardial infarction. Amer. J. Cardiol. *29*, 817–820.

Konttinen, A. and Somer, H. (1973): Specificity of serum creatine kinase isoenzymes in diagnosis of acute myocardial infarction. Brit. med. J. *1*, 386–389.

Mueller, R.G., Neville, K., Emerson, D.D., and Lang, G.E. (1975): Depressed apparent creatine kinase activity in sera with abnormally high alkaline phosphatase activity. Clin. Chem. *21*, 268–269.

Oliver, I.T. (1955): A spectrophotometric method for the determination of creatine phosphokinase and myokinase. Biochem. J. *61*, 116–122.

Richterich, R., Schafroth, P. and Aebi, H. (1963): A study of lactic dehydrogenase isoenzyme patterns of human tissues by adsorption-elution on sephadex-DEAE. Clin. Chim. Acta *8*, 178–192.

Richterich, R., Rosin, S., Aebi, U. and Rossi, E. (1963): Progressive muscular dystrophy V. the Identification of the carrier state in the Duchenne type by serum creatine kinase determination. Amer. J. Hum. Genet. *15*, 133–154.

Roe, C.R., Limbird, L.E., Wagner, G.S. and Nerenberg, S.T. (1972): Combined isoenzyme analysis in the diagnosis of myocardial injury: application of electrophoretic methods for the detection and the quantitation of the creatine phosphokinase MB isoenzyme. J. Lab. Clin. Med. *80*, 577–590.

Rokos, J.S., Rosalki, S.B. and Tarlow, D. (1972): Automated fluorimetric procedure for measurement of creatine phosphokinase activity. Clin. Chem. *18*, 193.

Rosalki, S.B. (1965): Creatine phosphokinase isoenzymes. Nature (Lond.) *207*, 414.

Rosalki, S.B. (1966): A capsule test for creatine phosphokinase. Proc. Ass. Clin. Biochem. *4*, 24–25.

Rosalki, S.B. (1967): An improved procedure for serum creatine phosphokinase determination. J. Lab. clin. Med. *69*, 696–705.

Rosalki, S.B. (1974): Standardisation of Isoenzyme Assays, with special reference to lactate dehydrogenase isoenzyme electrophoresis. Clin. Biochem. *7*, 29–40.

Sjövall, K. and Voigt, A. (1964): Creatine-phospho-transferase isozymes. Nature (Lond.) *202*, 701.

Smith, A.F. (1972): Separation of tissue and serum creatine kinase isoenzymes on polyacrylamide gel slabs. Clin. Chim. Acta *39*, 351–359.

Somer, H. and Konttinen, A. (1972a): A method allowing the quantitation of serum creatine kinase isoenzymes. Clin. Chim. Acta *36*, 531–536.

Somer, H. and Konttinen, A. (1972b): Demonstration of serum creatine kinase isoenzymes by fluorescence technique. Clin. Chim. Acta *40*, 133–138.

Van der Veen, K.J. and Willebrands, A.F. (1966): Isoenzymes of creatine phosphokinase in tissue extracts and in normal and pathological sera. Clin. Chim. Acta *13*, 312–316.

Wagner, G.S., Roe, C.R., Limbird, L.E., Rosati, R.A., and Wallace, A.G. (1973): The importance of identification of the myocardial-specific isoenzyme of creatine phosphokinase (MB form) in the diagnosis of acute myocardial infarction. Circulation *47*, 263–269.

Weidemann, G. (1973): Störung der mit GSH aktivierten creatin kinase-Bestimmung im Serum durch Glutathion-Reduktase. Z. Klin. Chem. Klin. Biochem. *11*, 134–135.

Wiesman, U., Colombo, J.P., Adam, A., and Richterich, R. (1966): Determination of cysteine activated creatine kinase in serum. Enzym. biol. clin. *7*, 266–284.

Presentation of Richterich Memorial Medal

H. Aebi (Switzerland)

Dr. *Rosalki,* I wish to thank you so much for this lecture, which brought us all back to the time when *Roland Richterich,* several of my colleagues and myself were studying the isoenzymes of lactate dehydrogenase, creatine phosphokinase and other enzymes. It shows what achievements can be made when the scientist remains faithful to his ultimate goal, and the ultimate goal is to serve; serving for the benefit of mankind.

You have done so, and it is on behalf of the organizers of the Symposium that I present to you this medal commemorating this lecture. It represents the City of Geneva, the place where these Symposia are held. I give you this medal, with many, many thanks.

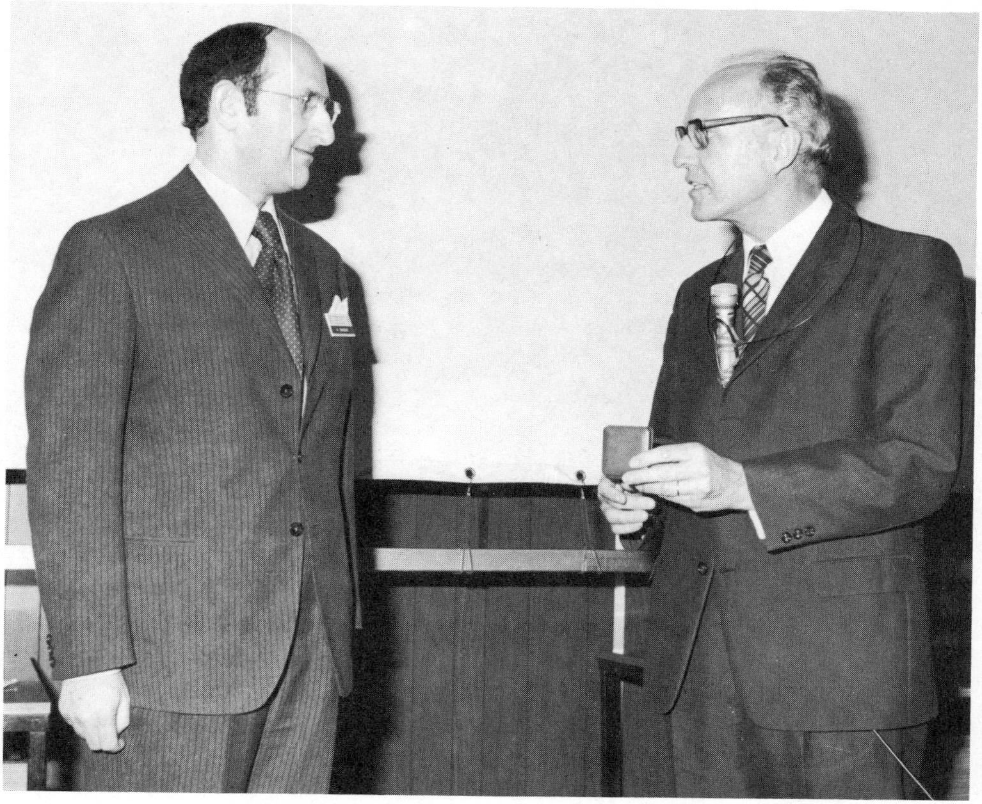

NAD – NADH – NADP – NADPH
Characterization and Purity Assurance

Plenary Lectures

Quality Requirements for β-NADH and β-NAD

W. Gerhardt and *G. Kofoed,* Copenhagen (Denmark)

Key words: 260 and 340 nm absorbance
NAD
NADH
Oxireductase inhibitors
Pyruvate/oxobutyrate reaction rate ratio
Quality requirements
Residual fluorescence

Summary

On the basis of experiments with purified β-NADH, with humidity-induced, and with preformed LDH inhibitors in NADH preparations, an attempt is made to formulate a set of spectrometric and kinetic requirements for quality control of:

a) reference β-NADH.
b) commercially available NADH preparations that will function with the precision required by clinical chemistry.

Reference β-NADH:

1. Relative residual 340 nm absorbance:

$$\frac{\text{solution-residual 340 nm absorbance}}{\text{solution-total 340 nm absorbance}} < 0.01$$

2. Relative residual fluorescence:

$$\frac{\text{solution-residual fluorescence}}{\text{solution-total fluorescence}} < 0.01$$

3. Absorbance fraction:

$$\frac{\text{solution-260 nm absorbance}}{\text{solution-340 nm absorbance}} \leqq 2.27$$

4. Reaction rate ratio:

$$\frac{\text{system-pyruvate}}{\text{system-2-oxobutyrate}} \geqq 1.40$$

It has been known for about 15 years that NADH preparations may contain potent oxidoreductase inhibitors [3, 5, 10, 11, 12, 13, 14][1]. In clinical chemistry and in research, poor quality control of NADH preparations has often been the cause of poor precision in (especially) LDH assays. Still, NADH specifications as shown in table 1 are often encountered in commercial catalogues.

Table 1. Commonly encountered NADH specifications.

NADH, Disodium Salt
High Purity

Table 2 illustrates the variation in reaction rates measured with one preparation of human heart LDH H_4 under S.C.E. conditions [17] and with 13 different NADH preparations. As will be shown, the presence of LDH inhibitors need not necessarily indicate poor quality control at the manufacturing stage, but may be due to such trivia as inadequate packing of the preparation, and subsequent inhibitor formation during storage under unfavourable conditions, especially humidity [1, 5, 6, 7, 13, 14, 18].

Table 2. Relative reaction rates with human LDH H_4 and pyruvate (37 °C, S.C.E. conditions) measured with 13 commercial NADH preparations.

Influence of NADH quality on LDH H_4 reaction rates (S.C.E. Reaction conditions)	
NADH Preparation (nationality)	Relative reaction rate
Dutch	1.00
German	1.00
American	1.00
Danish	1.00
German	0.97
Dutch	0.97
American	0.95
American	0.91
English	0.89
Dutch	0.88
American	0.83
Japanese	0.65
Japanese	0.62

Table 3 shows a more informative set of specifications seen in some catalogues. Assuming that 'per cent' refers to fraction of preparation mass, it may be calculated that for each mole of β-NADH it is necessary to weigh in 830 g of the preparation.

[1] Abbreviations: NADH: Nicotinamide Adenine Dinucleotide (reduced).
LDH: L-lactate: NAD-oxidoreductase (E.C. 1.1.1.27).
S.C.E. Scandinavian Commission on Enzymes.

Table 3. Commercial catalogue NADH specifications. Mass fractions ('per cent of weight') calculated on basis of molar absorption coefficients and enzymatic determination of β-NADH.

Example of current specifications of NADH preparation	
Component	Unspecified kind of quantity
β-NADH (enzym.)	80%
'NADH' $Abs._{340\ nm}$	80%
'NADH' $Abs._{260\ nm}$	81%
Molar mass of preparation: $1.25 \times 665.4 = 830$ g per mole of β-NADH	

Analytical data on the remaining 20% are rarely given. An exception, is one European manufacturing company which accounts for about 96% of preparation mass in their catalogue. However, specifications would be more informative if given in the S.I. system of quantities and units.

In table 4 the author has recalculated a set of analytical data kindly put at his disposal by Boehringer, Tutzing Research department. Column one accounts for a total mass fraction of 0.95 as identified substances. Column two: substance ratio, shows that for each mole of β-NADH the preparation contains e.g. 2.3 moles of sodium and 6 mmoles of β-NAD.

Table 4. Suggested presentation of analytical data on NADH preparations. The original data (mass fractions) kindly put at the authors' disposal by Boehringer Biochemica, research dept. Tutzing. Values have been recalculated on the basis of a total preparation mass of 831.75 g per mole of β-NADH.

Relative residual 340 nm absorbance may include unidentified compounds as α-NADH, 'tail' of NAD absorbance, and LDH inhibitors.

Relative residual 260 nm absorbance is defined as 260 nm absorbance fraction not accounted for by identified compounds absorbing light at 260 nm. Specification of desired value awaits further investigations. Residual 260 nm absorbance includes adenosine containing compounds, LDH inhibitors and others.

Component	Method	Mass fraction	Mole fraction: $\frac{\text{Amount of substance}}{\text{Amount of substance of β-NADH}}$
β-NADH	Enz. LDH $\Delta A_{340\ nm}$	0.80 ±	1.000
Na	Flame photom.	0.065 ±	2.35 ±
H_2O	K. Fischer	0.05 ±	2.31 ±
Alcohol	Gas chrom.	0.03 ±	0.54 ±
A-5'MP	Enzym. AK	0.002 ±	0.005 ±
β-NAD	Enzym. ADH	0.005 ±	0.006 ±
Sum of mass fractions		0.952 ±:	831.75 g per mole of β-NADH

Unidentified substances

Relative residual $ABS_{340\ nm}$:

$$\frac{\text{Total } ABS_{340\ nm} - ABS_{340\ nm}\ \beta\text{-NADH Enz.}}{\text{Total } ABS_{340\ nm}} = 0.015 \pm (98.5\%\ \beta\text{-NADH})$$

Relative residual $ABS_{260\ nm}$:

$$\frac{\text{Total } ABS_{260\ nm} - ABS_{260\ nm}\ (\beta\text{-NADH} + \beta\text{-NAD} + \text{other identified})}{\text{Total } ABS_{260\ nm}} = \text{specif.}$$

Unidentified substances constitute, in the example, about 5 per cent of the preparation mass. Relative residual 340 nm absorbance is then determined: The fraction of initial, total 340 nm absorbance remaining after enzymatic oxidation of NADH with LDH and pyruvate has reached equilibrium [3, 6, 11, 12]. This value expresses the 340 nm absorbance fraction that is *not* due to β-NADH, and is often in the range 0.01–0.05 [3, 6, 11, 12]. It may be as high as 0.15 [6]. It may be due to compounds such as α-NADH and the 'tail' of NAD absorbance [11], and LDH inhibitors.

Similarly, residual 260 nm absorbance in table 4 is defined as: that part of total 260 nm absorbance not accounted for by the calculated sum of identified, measured components as e.g. β-NADH + β-NAD + A-5'MP, adenosine-diphosphate-ribose, nicotinamide, and others.

Relative residual absorbance at 260 nm:

$$\frac{\text{Residual absorbance at 260 nm}}{\text{Total absorbance at 260 nm}}$$

UV absorbance spectra yield a good deal of information on NADH purity. However, they must be interpreted with caution.

Figure 1 shows a spectrum of NADH with superimposed spectra of some commonly occuring contaminants. The 260 nm absorbance peak of a NADH preparation may be the sum of 260 nm absorbances of α + β-NADH, NAD, nicotinamide, AMP, adenosine-diphosphoribose and LDH inhibitors (fig. 1). The 340 nm absorbance peak may be due to α + β-NADH, LDH inhibitor, and 'tail' of NAD absorbance [11].

Figure 1 illustrates the rationale for the use of the 260 nm/340 nm absorbance ratio as a criterion of NADH purity: the fewer contaminants with a 260 nm/340 nm absorbance ratio higher than that of β-NADH, the lower the ratio measured in the preparation. This point is discussed in detail below.

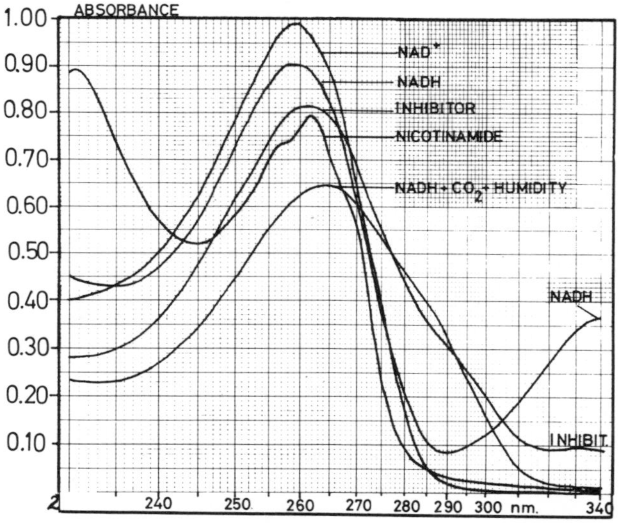

Figure 1. Superimposed UV spectra of β-NADH, NAD⁺, isolated LDH inhibitor, NADH exposed to a carbon dioxide atmosphere at 50 per cent relative humidity at 37 °C for 15 hours and nicotinamide.

The figure illustrates the additive effect of contaminants on both the 260 nm and the 340 nm absorbance peaks measured in actual NADH preparations (from ref. 6).

On the basis of fluorescence measurements a 260 nm/340 nm absorbance ratio of 2.25–2.27 has previously been predicted for a pure NADH preparation with zero residual fluorescence [6]. Preparations with a 260 nm/340 nm ratio of 2.27 have in fact been isolated [9, 11].

However, the 260 nm/340 nm absorbance ratio as a sole criterium of NADH purity is not sufficient.

Figure 2 illustrates this point. The presence of contaminants with 260 nm/340 nm absorbance ratios > 2.27 (fig. 2 [2]) will increase the ratio measured in the preparation compared to that of a pure NADH. In contrast, contaminating compounds with a 260 nm/340 nm absorbance ratio < 2.27 will lower it (fig. 2 [3]); and a combination of the two groups of contaminants in an NADH preparation could conceivably result in a ratio close to 2.27 (fig. 2 [4]). In all three cases, however, the relative residual 340 nm absorbance will be increased (fig. 2 [3, 6]).

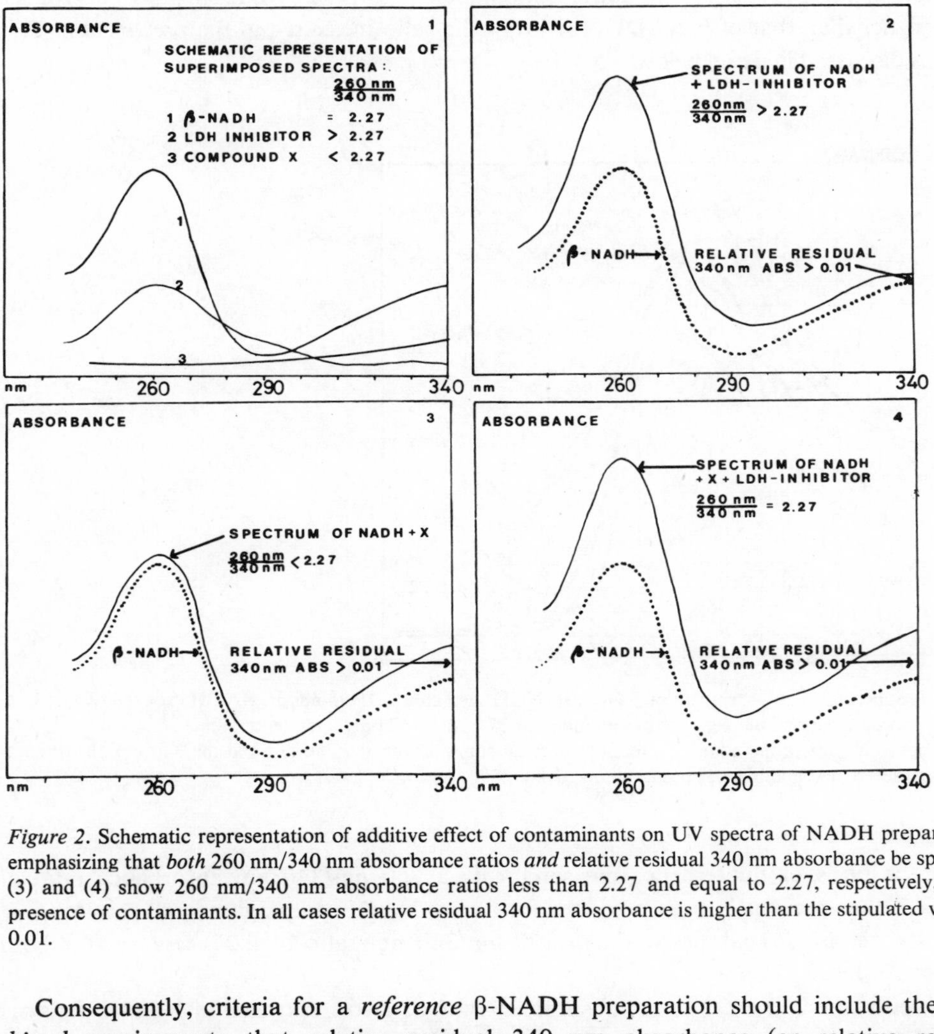

Figure 2. Schematic representation of additive effect of contaminants on UV spectra of NADH preparations, emphasizing that *both* 260 nm/340 nm absorbance ratios *and* relative residual 340 nm absorbance be specified. (3) and (4) show 260 nm/340 nm absorbance ratios less than 2.27 and equal to 2.27, respectively, in the presence of contaminants. In all cases relative residual 340 nm absorbance is higher than the stipulated value of 0.01.

Consequently, criteria for a *reference* β-NADH preparation should include the *combined* requirements that relative residual 340 nm absorbance (or relative residual fluorescence [6, 11, 12]) be less than 0.01, together with a measured 260 nm/340 nm absorbance ratio 2.27 [6, 8, 10].

The molar (linear) absorption coefficients at 340 nm and 260 nm may be other criteria of purity. Recent data by *Bücher* [2] show a value for $\varepsilon_{340\,nm}^{\beta\text{-}NADH} = 621\ m^2 \cdot mol^{-1}$ (38 °C). On the basis of chromatographically purified NADH preparations showing a 260 nm/340 nm ratio of 2.265. *Haid* [9] has calculated $\varepsilon_{260\,nm}^{\beta\text{-}NADH} = 14.1$ (25 °C).

The ratio between the molar absorption coefficients at 260 nm and 340 nm is close to the value of 2.27.

Under unfavourable storage conditions, inhibitors may form in solid samples of NADH. We therefore devised a set-up for storage experiments with NADH under controlled conditions of constant temperature and humidity.

NADH preparations were placed in the center well of Conway units. Constant humidity potassium acetate solutions were placed in the outer annular chamber. The Conway units were sealed by a glass lid with two tubes attached, so that air in the unit might be substituted with oxygen, carbon dioxide or nitrogen. The Conway units were placed at 37 °C for 15 hours in a dark place. After that time, the NADH preparation was dissolved in TRIS-EDTA-HCl buffer, 50 mmol/l, pH 7.7 (25 °C, S.C.E. 3) and adjusted to a concentration of 180 μmol/l [6].

Kinetic properties of thus treated NADH were then investigated with LDH H_4 under S.C.E. reaction conditions [17].

For measurement of catalytic activity, NADH quality should be specified in terms of reaction rate. No primary stable reference enzyme exists. Generally, relative measurements are used as shown in table 2. However, it is possible to measure reaction rates with a constant amount of inhibitor-sensitive LDH under two sets of reaction conditions that differ in their response to LDH inhibitor. *Glenn* [7] and *Rosalki* [16] observed that in the presence of inhibitor in NADH, LDH reaction rate with 2-oxobutyrate was less inhibited than when pyruvate was the substrate. Results could be expressed as a pyruvate/2-oxobutyrate reaction ratio which was independent of LDH total catalytic activity. The value of this ratio will decrease in the presence of LDH inhibitor, depending on the type of LDH used [6, 7, 16].

Figure 3 illustrates the effect of humidity-induced inhibitor produced in the Conway-unit storage experiments. Reaction rates with human LDH H_4 and both substrates decrease as a function of increasing relative humidity, more with pyruvate than with 2-oxobutyrate. The corresponding pyruvate/2-oxobutyrate reaction rate ratios (stippled line, and right ordinate) decrease from the initial value measured without inhibitor. As LDH reaction rates with pyruvate decrease with time after start of the reaction, catalytic activity must be determined from a specified time interval after start. Consequently, the time interval after start, selected as basis for the calculations of catalytic activities must be strictly defined. If early reaction rates e.g. the 15–30 sec. interval after start is used, equipment must be in perfect conditions with respect to mixing. Used as a kinetic NADH quality control parameter at the manufacturing stage, each series should include a minimum of 20 determinations for statistically valid results. Mean and analytical error expressed as e.g. the coefficient of variation should be given. Two examples of poor, respectively strict, control of time intervals used for calculations are shown here:

pyruvate/2-oxobutyrate reaction rate ratio [6]:
n = 16; range 1.38–1.45; mean: 1.41; CV: 1.56%
n = 16; range 1.39–1.43; mean: 1.41; CV: 1.06%

A value of 1.40 has been defined from the 15–30 sec. interval on the basis of numerous experiments [6].

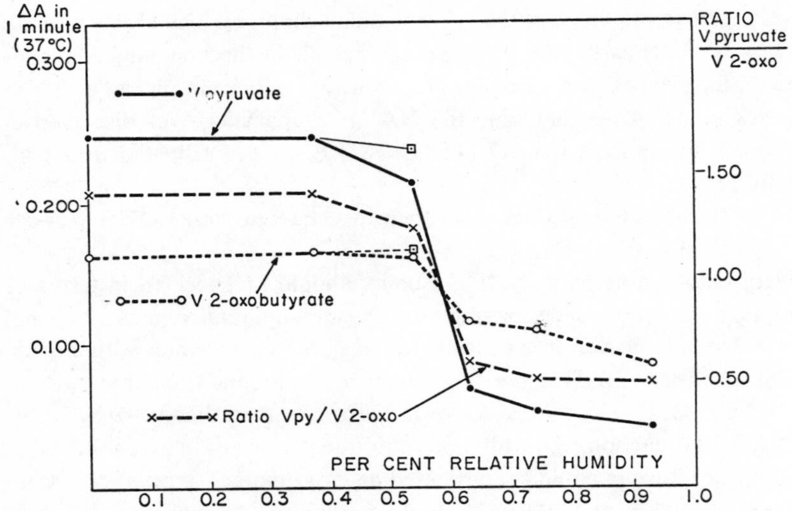

Figure 3. Formation of humidity induced LDH inhibitor under controlled conditions of humidity and temperature in Conway units. Measurements of LDH H_4 reaction rates were made at a constant concentration of enzyme with both pyruvate and 2-oxobutyrate as the substrates. The resulting pyruvate/2-oxobutyrate reaction rate ratio decreases as a function of LDH inhibitor due to the fact that at the same inhibitor concentration the reaction is more inhibited with pyruvate than with 2-oxobutyrate as the substrate.

The numerical value of the resulting ratio depends on the time interval of the reaction selected for calculation of catalytic activity (see text).

⊡——⊡ protective effect of nitrogen substituted for air in the Conway units.

Reaction conditions described in detail in ref. 6.

Table 5 shows the change of the described parameters: 260 nm/340 nm absorbance ratio, relative residual 340 nm absorbance, LDH relative reaction rate with pyruvate, and pyruvate/2-oxobutyrate reaction ratios as function of increasing relative humidity.

Table 5. Change of measured properties of solid samples of NADH preparations exposed to increasing relative humidity for 15 hours at 37 °C in Conway units. For details see text.

Relative humidity (per Cent)	$NADH_2$ appearance	260 nm / 340 nm	Relative Residual 340 nm A (per Cent)	Relative Reaction Rate with Pyruvate (per Cent)	V Pyruvate / V 2-Oxobutyrate
0	white	2.54	2	100	1.41
37	white	2.57	3	99	1.41
53	white	2.62	4	85	1.30
62	yellow	2.80	6	28	0.62
74	yellow	3.34	7	24	0.66
93	yellow, fluid	3.22	8	18	0.50

Table 6 shows the effect on NADH in the storage experiments of the gas acting at the water-solid interface.

In the absence of humidity (laboratory air + silicagel in the Conway unit) NADH tolerates storage at 37 °C for 15 hours well. With laboratory air alone, relative residual 340 nm absorbance was doubled and reaction rate with LDH H_4 and pyruvate decreased by 5 per cent. At 50 per cent relative humidity with laboratory air in the unit, relative residual 340 nm absorbance was increased by a factor 7 and reaction rate decreased by 18 per cent. In an oxygen atmosphere, a higher increase of 260 nm absorbance was observed, probably due to formation of NAD by H_2O_2 [4, 10]. In CO_2, at 50 per cent relative humidity, NADH was destroyed probably due to H_2CO_3 formation in the gas-water interface. In contrast, storage in nitrogen protects NADH against destruction by humidity [4, 6, 10]. Consequently, NADH should be stored under nitrogen in tight containers.

Table 6. Influence of gases on NADH preparations stored under conditions of controlled humidity, temperature and time. Data indicate that NADH preparations be kept under nitrogen.

Effect of Gas on NADH stored in Conway Jars for 15 Hours, 37 °C			
Storage conditions	260 nm / 340 nm	Relative residual $ABS_{340\ nm}$	Relative reaction rate LDH H_4
Dry lab air (Silicagel)	2.53	0.02	1.00
Lab air	2.54	0.04	0.95
50% rel. humidity:			
Lab air	2.64	0.15	0.82
Oxygen	2.83	0.04	0.89
CO_2	54.		
Nitrogen	2.58	0.03	0.94

Table 7 shows that the pyruvate/2-oxobutyrate reaction rate ratios measured in the 13 commercial preparation could actually be used as an estimate of performed LDH inhibitor. hibitor.

Table 7. Pyruvate/2-oxobutyrate reaction rate ratio utilized as quality control of 13 commercial NADH preparations.

Influence of NADH Quality on LDH H_4 Reaction Rates (S.C.E. Reaction Conditions)		
NADH preparation (nationality)	Relative reaction rate	Pyruvate / 2-oxobutyrate rate ratio
Dutch	1.00	1.41
German	1.00	1.40
American	1.00	1.41
Danish	1.00	1.41
German	0.97	1.40
Dutch	0.97	1.40
American	0.95	1.36
American	0.91	1.32
English	0.89	1.32
Dutch	0.88	1.28
American	0.83	1.28
Japanese	0.65	1.29
Japanese	0.62	1.21

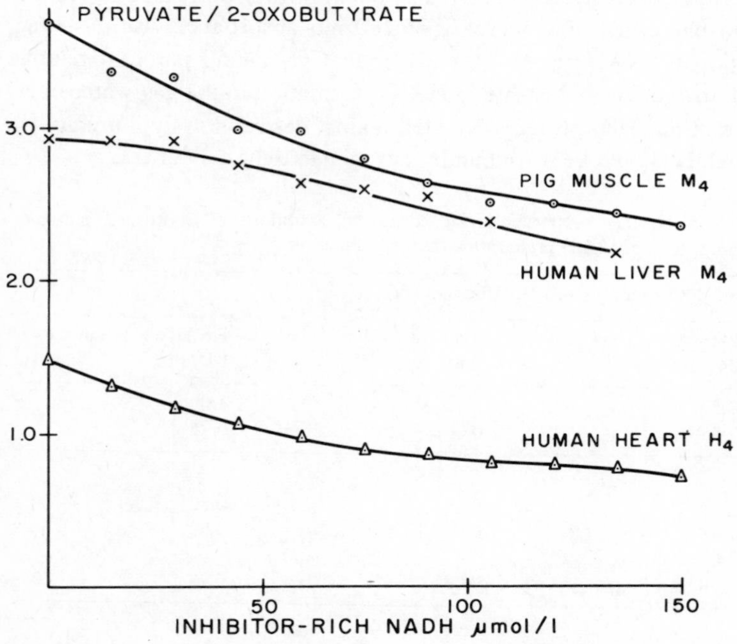

Figure 4. Pyruvate/2-oxobutyrate reaction rate ratios of 3 different LDH controls shown as function of humidity-induced LDH-inhibitor in NADH. The figure illustrates the variation in LDH-inhibitor sensitivity of different species of LDH. Quality control LDH should be at least as inhibitor sensitive as human LDH H_4.

Figure 4 shows that different LDH preparations show different sensitivities to inhibitors in NADH. For quality control in clinical chemistry and elsewhere the species of LDH used, e.g. a human or pig heart LDH H_4 enzyme should be at least as sensitive to inhibitor as are patient sera. Otherwise, values measured with the inhibitor-insensitive control enzyme may well be within tolerances, while LDH in patient sera may be inhibited.

Summing up, the quality criteria for reference β-NADH preparation discussed here are shown in table 8.

Table 8. Summary of suggested spectrometric and kinetic properties of a reference β-NADH.

Characterization of Reference β-NADH Spectrometric and Kinetic Properties	
Parameter	Desired value
260 nm/340 nm absorbance ratio	≦2.27
Relative residual 340 nm absorbance	≦0.01
Relative residual fluorescence	≦0.01
Pyruvate/2-oxobutyrate reaction rate ratio	≧1.40

For β-NADH preparations used in reagents, a secondary set of specifications is required.

As has been shown, a 260 nm/340 nm ratio > 2.27 may be due to non-inhibiting compounds as e.g. β-NAD or nicotinamide. Also on storage of a pure β-NADH, the ratio will increase. Therefore, for routine use, requirements are formulated as follows: NADH should perform kinetically so that reaction rates with human LDH H_4 or pig heart LDH H_4 are within 5% of those measured under identical conditions with a *reference* β-NADH. Pyruvate/2-oxobutyrate ratio should ≧ 1.40 under the conditions specified [6].

Finally it should be mentioned that the inhibitor problem, unfortunately, is not restricted to NADH but encompasses β-NAD as well. Table 9 shows relative reaction rates with LDH H_4, L-lactate, and different samples of β-NAD.

Table 9. Effect of inhibitor in NAD preparations on LDH H_4 reaction rate.

Relative reaction rate (37 °C) NAD^+ preparations		
C	M	B
1.00	0.82	0.60

Reaction Conditions:

Pyrophosphate Buffer	50 mmol/l pH 8.8 (37 °C)
NAD^+	5 mmol/l
D-L lactate	63 mmol/l
Human LDH H_4 (Vol. Fraction 0.083)	

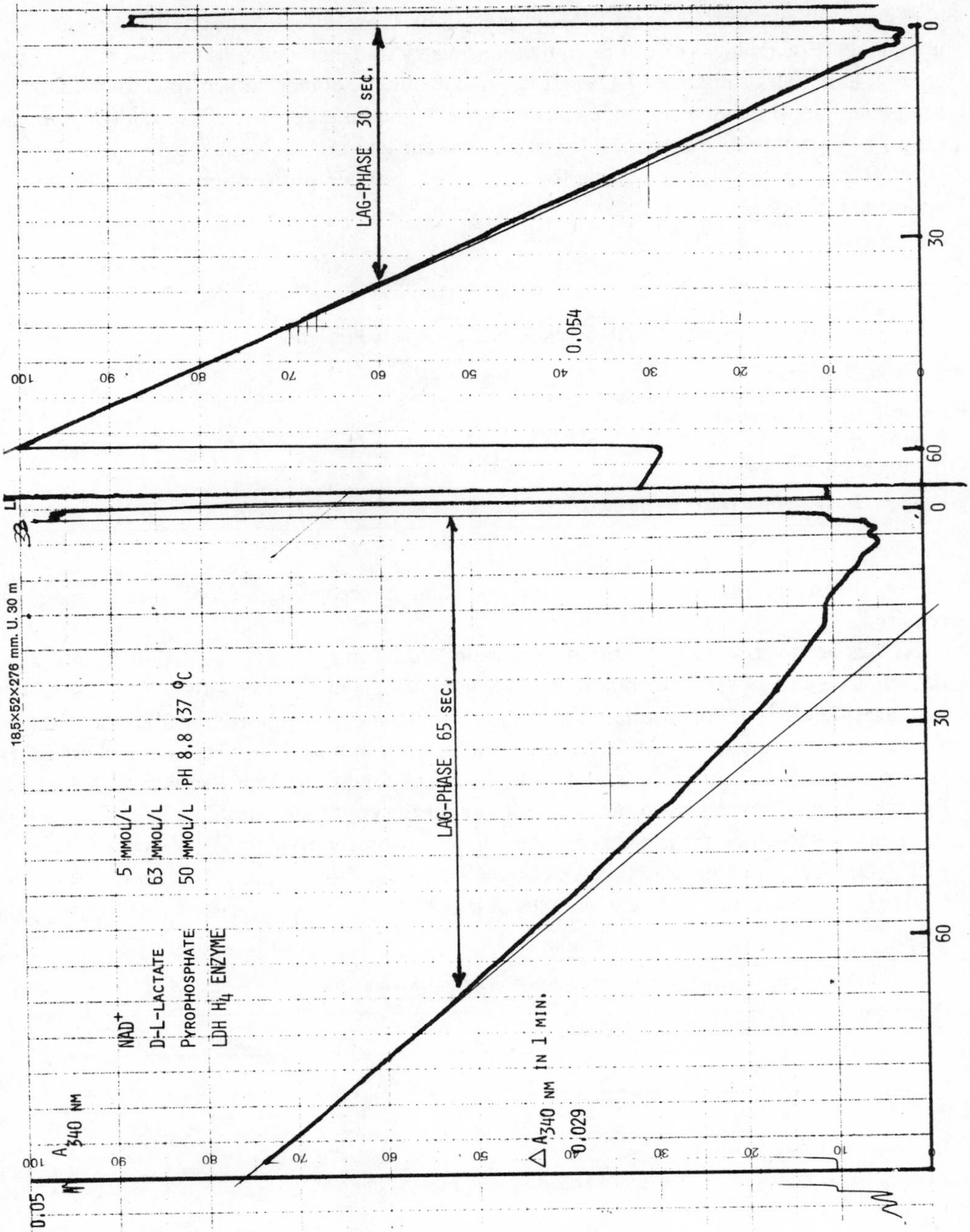

Figure 5. Effect of inhibitor in NAD on LDH H_4 reaction kinetics:
a) Approximately 50 per cent decrease of reaction rate. b) Increase of lag-phase up to more than one minute.

Figure 5 shows that a lag-phase of up to 1 minute is observed in the presence of inhibitor in NAD.

A series of LDH inhibitors in NAD have been described [15] including adenosine, adenosine-5'-monophosphate, adenosine-5'-diphosphate, adenosine-diphosphoribose.

On the basis of enzymatic determination of β-NAD, e.g. with alcohol dehydrogenase, criteria for residual 260 nm absorbance may be specified. With LDH H_4 and L-lactate no lag-phase should be present.

Hopefully, valid quality specifications for NAD will appear in the near future.

References

[1] *Berry, A.J., Lott, J.A. & Grannis, G.F.:* NADH Preparation as They Affect Reliability of Serum Lactate Dehydrogenase Determinations. Clin. Chem. *19,* 1255, 1973.

[2] *Bücher, Th., Krell, H., Lusch, G., Grassl, M., Ziegenhorn, J. & Bermeyer, H.U.:* Molar Extinction Coefficients of NADH and NADPH at Hg Spectral Lines. Z. Klin. Chem. Klin. Biochem. *12,* 239–240, 1974.

[3] *Dalziel, K.:* Some Observations on the Preparation and Properties of Dihydronicotinamide-Adenine Dinucleotide. Biochem. J. *84,* 240, 1962.

[4] *Dolin, M.I.:* Effect of near-ultraviolet irradiation on the peroxide content of solutions of oxidized or reduced diphospho pyridine nucleotide. Biochim. Biophys. Acta *63,* 219, 1962.

[5] *Fawcett, C.P., Ciotti, M.M. & Kaplan, N.O.:* Inhibition of Dehydrogenase Reactions by a Substance Formed From Reduced Diphosphopyridine Nucleotide. Biochim. Biophys. Acta *54,* 210, 1961.

[6] *Gerhardt, W., Kofoed, B., Westlund, L. & Pavlu, B.:* Quality Control of NADH. Evaluation of Methods for Detection of Inhibitors and Specifications for NADH Quality. Scand. J. Clin. Lab. Invest. Suppl. 139, 1974.

[7] *Glenn, J.H.:* Study of an Enzyme Inhibitor Formed From Reduced Nicotinamide Adenine Dinucleotide and its Effect on the Assay of Lactate Dehydrogenase. M. Sc. Thesis, University of Surrey, 1972.

[8] *Grassl, M., Haid, E., Nelböck, M. & Weimann, G.:* On the Quality of Reduced Pyridine Coenzymes. Z. Klin. Chem. Klin. Biochem. *12,* 240, 1974.

[9] *Haid, E., Lehmann, P., & Ziegenhorn, J.:* The Molar Absorptivities of β-NADH and β-NAD at 260 nm. Clin. Chem. (in press).

[10] *Hilvers, A.G.:* Nicotinamide-Adenine-Dinucleotide en zijn Rol in Het Rectiemechanisme van Glyceraldehyde-3-Fosfaat-Dehydrogenase. Hofman-Alkmaar 1964 (Thesis).

[11] *Howell, B.F., Margolis, S. & Schaffer, R.:* Residual Fluorescense as an Index of Purity of Reduced Nicotinamide Adenine Dinucleotide. Clin. Chem. *19,* 1280, 1973.

[12] *James, J., Johnson, B.A. & Schaffer, R.:* Developing NADH as a Standard Reference Material. Proc. Int. Seminar and Workshop on Enzymology. Chicago 1972.

[13] *Lowry, O.H., Passonneau, J.V. & Rock, M.K.:* The Stability of Pyridine Nucleotides. J. biol. Chem. *236,* 2756, 1961.

[14] *McComb, R.B. & Gay, R.J.:* A Comparison of Reduced-NAD Preparations from Four Commercial Sources. Clin. Chem. *14,* 754, 1968.

[15] *McPherson, A.:* Interaction of Lactate Dehydrogenase with its Coenzyme, Nicotinamide-Adenine Dinucleotide. J. Mol. Biol. *51,* 39, 1970.

[16] *Rosalki, S.B.:* Accuracy Assessment from Reference Methods: Isoenzyme Reference Methods with Special Reference to α-Hydroxybutyrate Dehydrogenase Determination. Progress in Quality Control in Clinical Chemistry. Transactions of the 5th Int. Symposium, Geneva 1973. H. Huber Publ., Vienna 1973.

[17] Scandinavian Committee on Enzymes of The Scandinavian Society for Clinical Chemistry and Clinical Physiology: Recommended Methods for the Determination of Four Enzymes in Blood. Scand. J. Clin. Lab. Invest. (in press, 1973).

[18] *Strandjord, P.E. & Clayson, K.J.:* The Control of Inhibitory Impurities in Reduced Nicotinamide Adenine Dinucleotide in Lactate Dehydrogenase Assays. J. Lab. clin. Med. *67,* 144, 1966.

Studies on the Purity and Storage of NADH

M. Härkönen, V. Hänninen, Ö. Wahlroos and *H. Adlercreutz*, Helsinki (Finland)

Key words: Column chromatography
Fluorescence
Gas chromatogram
Infra-red spectrum
Isotachophoresis
LDH inhibitor
Mass spectrum
Storage criteria
UV spectrum

Introduction

Several compounds have been suspected to be the enzyme inhibitors formed in NADH preparations [2, 3, 11, 12]. However, the only ones that exhibit significant dehydrogenase inhibition are adenosine diphosphoribose and some of its analogues. Adenosine diphosphoribose is a frequent contaminant of NADH preparations and acts as a strong inhibitor in frozen alkaline solution [12]. Inhibitors have been isolated from NADH samples exposed to humidity or frozen in alkaline solution [6, 10, 11]. Although their properties in enzyme kinetics, phosphorus and sodium contents, and UV absorption spectra have been studied [5, 6, 10, 11], we know of only one investigation in which the structure of the inhibitor has been investigated by mass or infra-red spectrometry [6].

The usual method recommended for avoiding inhibitor formation is to prepare fresh NADH solutions every time for measurements of enzymes [11]. However, the frequent weighing of small samples of NADH or storage of such samples in pre-weighed bottles under nitrogen [5] is inconvenient; changes may occur in the solid preparation if the same bottle is opened several times, and warming the container to room temperature takes time.

If we knew the structure of the inhibitor or inhibitors, we could better understand the reaction mechanism involved, and could take rational preventive measures, according to the cause. It would also be easier to store NADH as a stock solution, and results would be more reproducible. Therefore, our approach was to study the structure of the isolated inhibitor and to explore the possibility of storing solutions of NADH in a deep-freezer at −75 °C. Deep-freezers of this type are becoming increasingly common, especially in clinical laboratories that use RIA methods, because expensive antisera, especially in dilute form, are more stable at −75 °C than at −20 °C. For comparison, we also tested the effect of storage at + 4 °C and −20 °C. The inhibitors were monitored by the recommended current methods and by new methods (table 1).

Table 1. Criteria for assessing the purity of NADH.

Relative enzymatic activity	=	$\frac{\text{Enzymatic activity with sample NADH}}{\text{Enzymatic activity with reference NADH}}$
Relative NADH content	=	$\frac{\text{Moles of NADH (enzymatic)}}{\text{Moles of NADH (absorption)}}$
260 nm/340 nm absorbance ratio	=	$\frac{A_{260}}{A_{340}}$
Relative residual 340 nm absorbance	=	$\frac{A_{340}\text{ after LDH}}{A_{340}\text{ before LDH}}$
Relative residual fluorescence (365 nm–450 nm)	=	$\frac{\text{F after LDH}}{\text{F before LDH}}$
Relative NAD^+ content	=	$\frac{\text{Moles of NAD}^+\text{ (enzymatic)}}{\text{Moles of NADH (absorption)}}$
Relative strong alkali-induced fluorescence (365 nm–450 nm)	=	$\frac{\text{F acid-treated sample + 6 N NaOH}}{A_{340}}$

Material and Methods

Reagents: The NADH used in the experiments was a pooled sample from Boehringer (Mannheim, Germany), BDH (London, England) and Baker (Deventer, Holland). The reference NADH was purity grade I from Boehringer. The enzymes used were lactate dehydrogenase from pig heart (LDH, E.C. 1.1.1.27) and α-glycerophosphate dehydrogenase from rabbit muscle (α-GDH, E.C. 1.1.1.8) from Boehringer. All other chemical compounds were of analytical grade from Boehringer, the Sigma Chemical Company (St. Louis, U.S.A.) or Merck AG (Darmstadt, Germany). The buffers used were 56 mmol/l Tris-HCl, pH 7.7 (25 °C) (Trismabase, Sigma) and 100 mmol/l sodium carbonate, pH 10.0 (25 °C).

Spectrophotometry and fluorometry: All the UV absorption measurements were made in a Cary 118 C spectrophotometer at 37 °C. LDH activity was measured according to the recommendation of the Scandinavian Society for Clinical Chemistry and Clinical Physiology [13]. α-GDH activity was measured in the same reagent, except that pyruvate was replaced by 0.35 mmol/l dihydroxyacetone phosphate. Fluorometric measurements were performed with a Farrand model A-3 fluorometer and an Aminco Bowman spectrophotofluorometer. Infra-red (IR) spectra from the dried samples (*in vacuo,* P_2O_5) were measured with a Beckman M IR-10 instrument by the macro KBr pellet technique.

Gas chromatography: The instrument used was an F&M model 400 gas chromatograph with a hydrogen flame ionization detector. It was equipped with a 10 m double U-shaped glass column (i.d. 2.5 mm) filled with 1% SE-30 on 80/100 mesh Gas-Chrom Q (Applied Science Laboratories Inc., State College, U.S.A.). The hydrogen flame was supported by oxygen, and nitrogen was used as carrier gas. The samples were injected into the columns in the silylation reagent. The temperature of the column was maintained at 170–180 °C when adenine and nicotinamide were analyzed and at 223 °C when adenosine was analyzed. In the experiments with the inhibitor the column temperature was programmed from 150 to 280 °C.

Gas chromatography-mass spectrometry: Tests were made with an LKB model 9000 gas chromatograph-mass spectrometer, and two different approaches were followed in the studies of the NADH inhibitor. The silylated samples were either chromatographed on a 1% SE-30 column, the temperature programme extending from 150 to 280 °C, or placed in an empty column in the oven, the temperature of which was then increased in the same way. This was done because no direct inlet system was available.

Derivative formation: The compounds were silylated with Tri-sil Z (Pierce Chemical Co., Box 117, Rockford, Illinois, U.S.A.) at +60 °C overnight.

Isotachophoresis: A mixture of the inhibitor, NADH and NAD^+ was analyzed by isotachophoresis, in which the LKB 2127 Tachophor was used, with chloride as the leading electrolyte (5 mmol/l, β-alanine, 0.25% methyl cellulose, pH 3.7) and 5 mmol/l caproic acid as the terminating electrolyte. A 43 cm capillary was used and the current was 80 μA with a starting voltage of 3.0 KV and a final voltage of 24.5 KV. UV-transmittance was measured at 254 nm. A control run was made at 340 nm.

Results and Discussion

Isolation of the inhibitor: Inhibitor-rich NADH was prepared by exposing ca. 50 mg of NADH powder for 3 days in a small open beaker placed inside a larger closed one containing 10 ml of water. The NADH was then dissolved in 500 μl of 5 mmol/l of Tris-HCl buffer, pH 7.4, or in 5 mmol/l ammonium bicarbonate. Column chromatography on DEAE-cellulose or DEAE-Sephadex A-25 (Pharmacia AB, Uppsala, Sweden) was carried out by gradient elution with Tris-HCl or ammonium bicarbonate [11].

A typical chromatogram after elution with Tris-HCl is presented in figure 1. The peaks were identified by the absorption at 260 and 340 nm, and NAD^+ (alcohol dehydrogenase, [10]) and NADH concentrations (LDH, [13]) were determined enzymatically. The fractions between 255 and 300 ml were demonstrated to inhibit LDH significantly. The fractions between the two lines shown in the figure were pooled, lyophilized at −40 °C, dissolved in a small volume of neutralized water, and poured twice through a Sephadex G-10 column to remove the Tris buffer. Elution with neutralized water resulted in a sharp peak of 260 nm absorption in the early part of the curve. The fractions showing 260 nm absorption were pooled, lyophilized and dried over P_2O_5 under a vacuum.

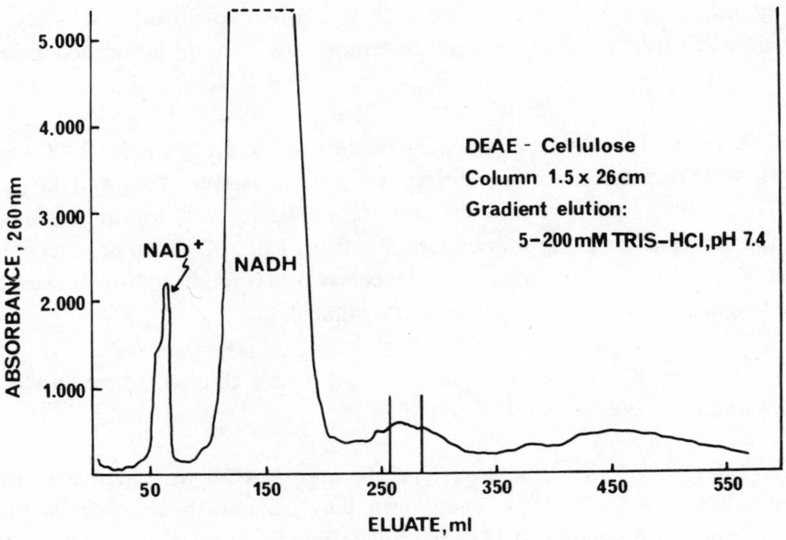

Fig. 1. Separation of NAD^+, NADH and LDH inhibitor on a DEAE-cellulose column. The peaks were identified by 260 nm and 340 nm absorbance and their reactions with lactate dehydrogenase and pyruvate and alcohol dehydrogenase and ethanol. The fractions shown between the two vertical lines were used for further analysis of the inhibitor.

The elution pattern produced by ammonium bicarbonate was similar, except that the broad area of 260 nm absorption after the NADH peak was divided into three subfractions, the middle one showing strong LDH inhibition. When NH_4^+ was removed from this peak by passing the fractions through a Sephadex G-25 (fine) column (2 × 13 cm) the elution pattern was biphasic. Both peaks showed strong LDH inhibition and NH_4^+ was eluted with the latter one. The first fraction, which was devoid of NH_4^+ [9], was used for infra-red spectrometry.

Characterization of the inhibitor: In figure 2 the UV spectra of the isolated inhibitor and some reference compounds are shown. The 260 nm/340 nm absorbance ratio for the inhibitor varied between 9 and 11. The spectrum is like those published earlier [5, 11].

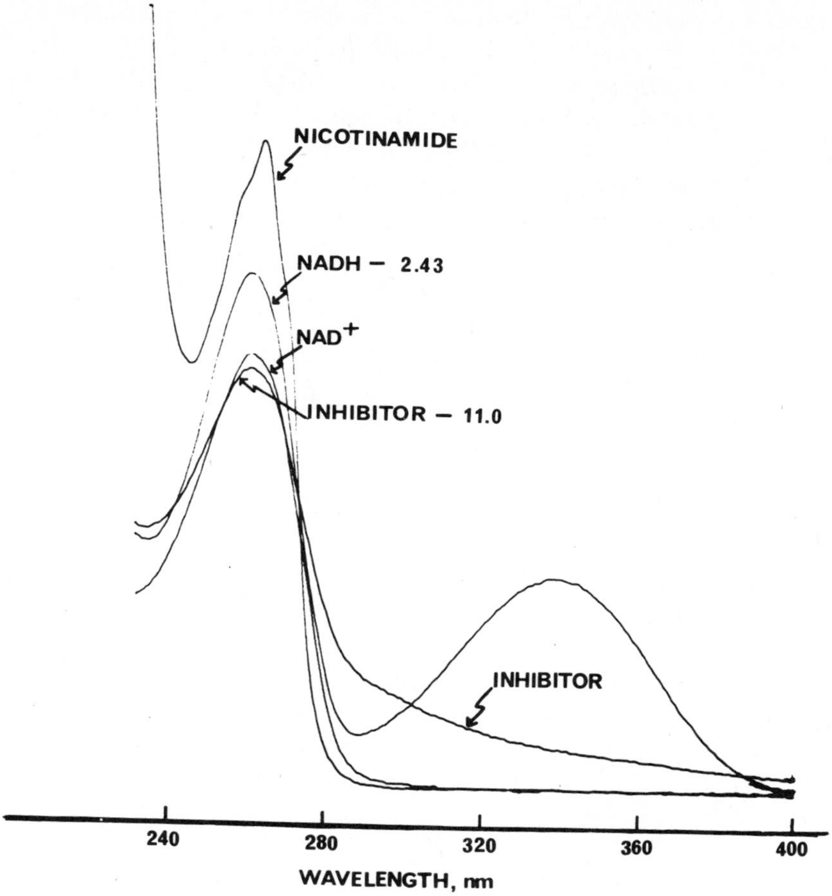

Fig. 2. Absorption spectrum of the LDH inhibitor isolated as described in figure 1. The spectra of some reference compounds are also shown. The numbers indicate the 260 nm/340 nm absorbance ratio.

The spectrophotofluorometric study showed that the inhibitor had a somewhat higher excitation wavelength (350 nm) than NADH (345 nm) (all the wavelengths are uncorrected). Emission maxima of the inhibitor and NADH were located at slightly different wavelengths (460–465 nm). Incubation at 60 °C for 10 min with 6 N NaOH (strong alkali-induced fluorescence, 9) increased the fluorescence ca. 8-fold as compared with the native fluorescence of the inhibitor. The excitation and emission maxima did not differ from those of the similarly treated NAD^+ preparation (365 nm and 465 nm). Treatment with 0.1 N HCl or 0.01 N NaOH (10 min at 60 °C) had no effect on the native or strong alkali-induced fluorescence. In this respect, the inhibitor differs from NADH and NAD^+, which are destroyed by acid and alkali, respectively (compare with the fluorescence characteristics of NADH and NAD^+ in table 2). These observations suggest that the inhibitor is not identical with NAD^+ or NADH, but has some structural slight difference in the pyridine ring. When treated with acid (0.1 N HCl 10 min at 37 °C), however, the compound lost its inhibitory effect although after alkali treatment it was still inhibitory.

The IR spectrum of the inhibitor (fig. 3), was remarkably similar to those of ADP, NMN, NAD^+ (fig. 4) and NADH (fig. 5), except for the 1600–1700 cm^{-1} part of the fundamental region.

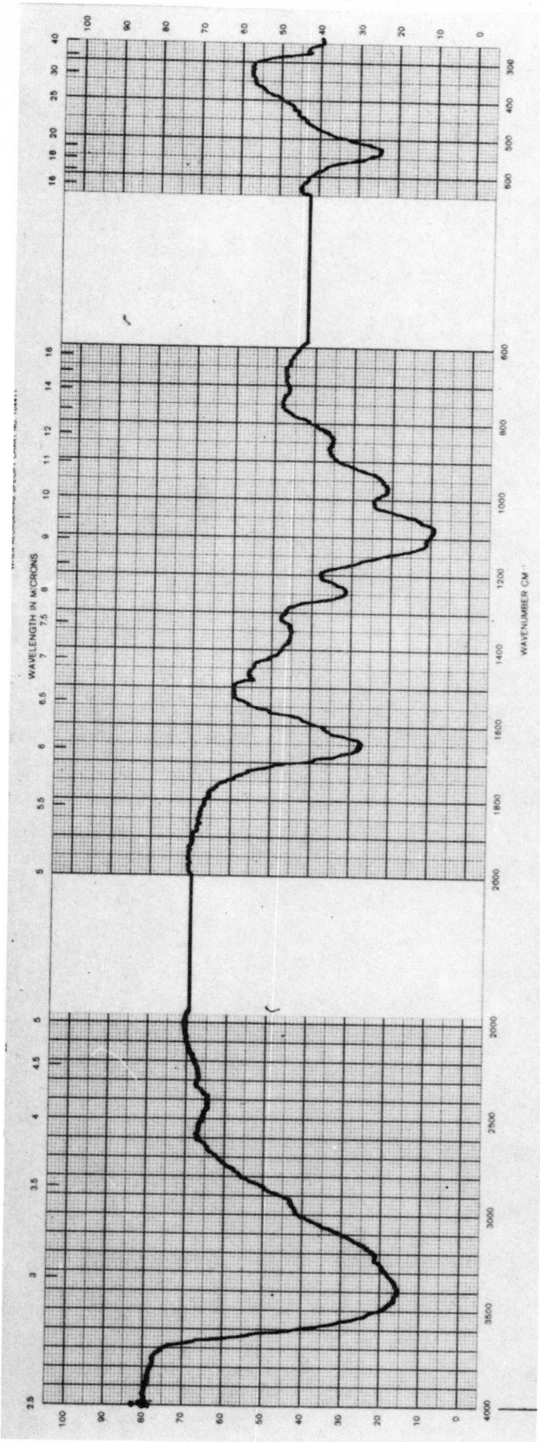

Fig. 3. Infra-red spectrum of the LDH inhibitor isolated on a DEAE-cellulose column by gradient elution with 5 mmol/l – 200 mmol/l ammonium bicarbonate. The fractions showing the strongest LDH inhibition were pooled (50 ml), dried under a vacuum over P_2O_5 and put through a Sephadex G-25 (fine) column (2 × 13 cm). The compound separated into two peaks, the first having the same elution volume as NADH. This peak was completely free from ammonium ion.

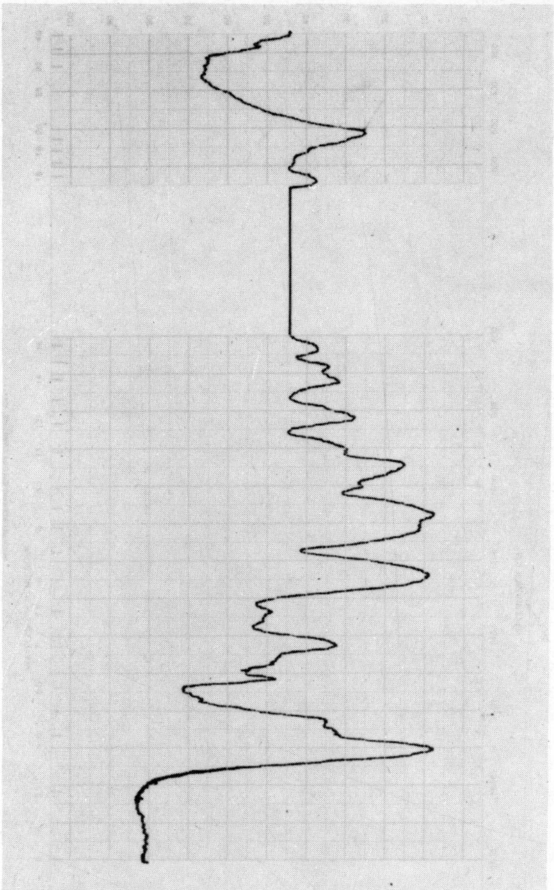

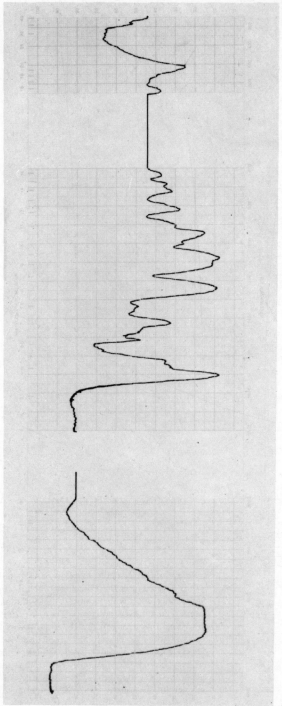

Fig. 4. Infra-red spectrum of the reference NAD^+.

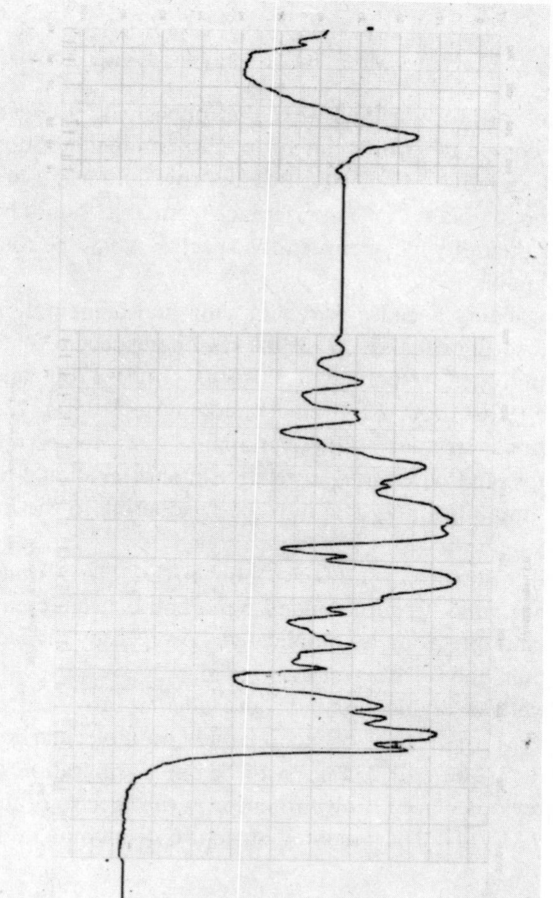

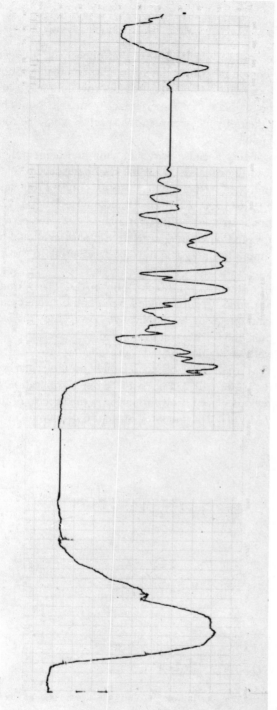

Fig. 5. Infra-red spectrum of the reference NADH.

The inhibitor spectrum was similar to, but not identical with, that published by *Glenn* [6]. It should be observed that *Glenn*'s compound was isolated on a column equilibrated with Tris-HCl buffer, which is difficult to remove completely. Because this author did not describe the subsequent purification of the inhibitor, some interference from Tris cannot be excluded. An alternative explanation for the difference between the spectra, would be that the preparation contains more than one inhibitor.

The IR spectra are rather diffuse, probably because of overlapping and combination bands. The inhibitor spectrum shows absorption bands in all the regions expected for a substance containing heteroaromatic nitrogen structures (500–600, 1400–1700 and 3000–3600 cm^{-1}) as well as phosphate (900–1000, 1250 cm^{-1}) and ribose (1050–1125 cm^{-1}), and does not exclude even an amide structure. The overlapping does not permit further differentiation of functional groups, and differences in relative intensities should be interpreted with caution, because some impurities may still have been adhering to the inhibitor.

The shift of absorption in the carbonyl region (1650–1700 cm^{-1}) for NAD^+, NADH and the inhibitor, suggests a bonded (H-bond) amide group (amide I band bathochromic and amide II bond hypsochromic shift). This interpretation is complicated, however, by the fact that $C = N$ bonds also absorb in this region, and further work is needed.

The mass spectra of the TMS derivatives of nicotinamide and adenine are seen in figures 6 and 7. In the spectrum of the TMS derivative of nicotinamide no molecular ion can be seen and the three ions at m/e 147, 203 and 234 seem to be due to migration of TMS groups. The ion at m/e 147 has previously been shown to occur in the spectra of the TMS derivatives of AMP, ATP and NAD [4]. The assumed structure of nicotinamide TMS is seen in figure 6.

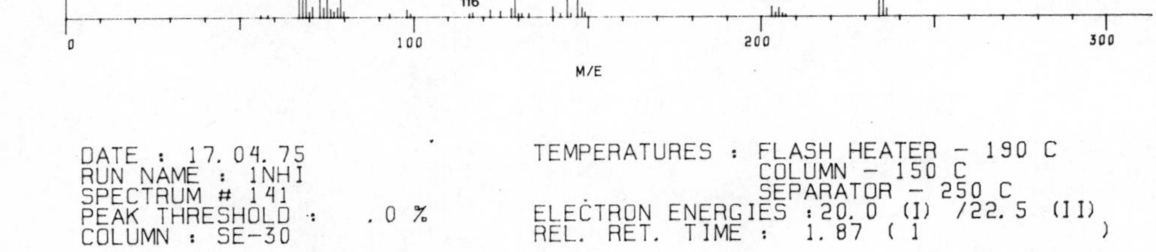

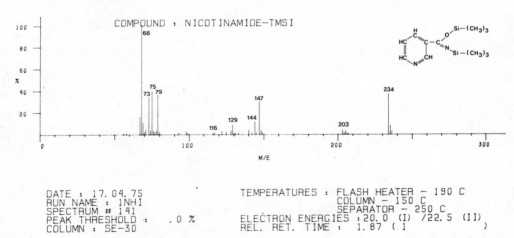

Fig.6. Mass spectrum and supposed structure of the TMS derivative of nicotinamide. The conditions can be seen in the figure. In this case the 'relative retention time' is the absolute time in min.

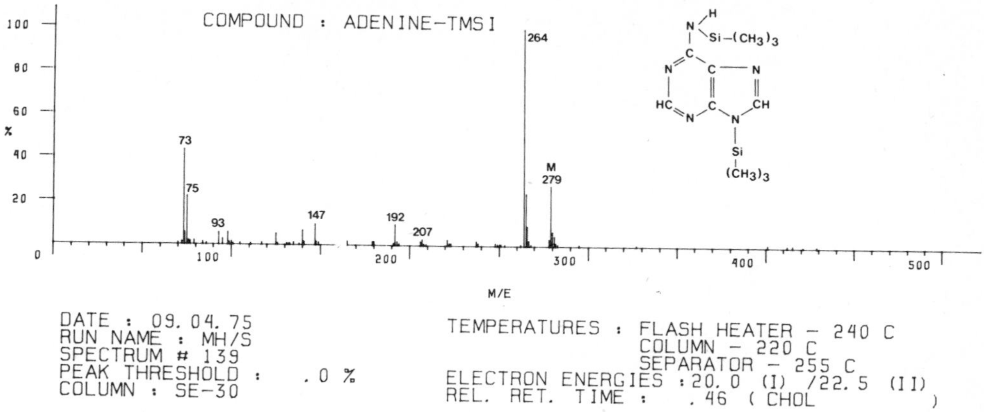

Fig. 7. Mass spectrum and supposed structure of the TMS derivative of adenine. The conditions can be seen in the figure. The retention time is relative to cholestane.

The ions at m/e 67 and 68 are probably the pyridine ring minus one carbon plus one and two hydrogens, respectively, and the ion at m/e 79 is the whole pyridine ring plus one hydrogen. Thus, the interpretation of the spectrum of the TMS derivative of nicotinamide is very difficult. In the spectrum of the TMS derivative of adenine (fig. 7), the molecular ion at m/e 279 and the M-15 ion are prominent. Here, too, the ion at m/e 147 can be seen, but the mechanism of its formation must be different from that described above, because no oxygen is present in the molecule. In addition, typical ions occur at m/e 73 and 75, as in all TMS derivatives of various compounds. The ion at m/e 192 is due to loss of HN-TMS, and the ion at m/e 207 is due to loss of one TMS group. Thus this spectrum is easier to interpret than that of the TMS derivative of nicotinamide.

The two above-mentioned compounds had good gas chromatographic properties and so did the TMS derivative of adenosine, the spectrum of which is shown in figure 8. The spectrum is typical of a TMS derivative. At this point there is no need to go into details of the fragmentation pattern.

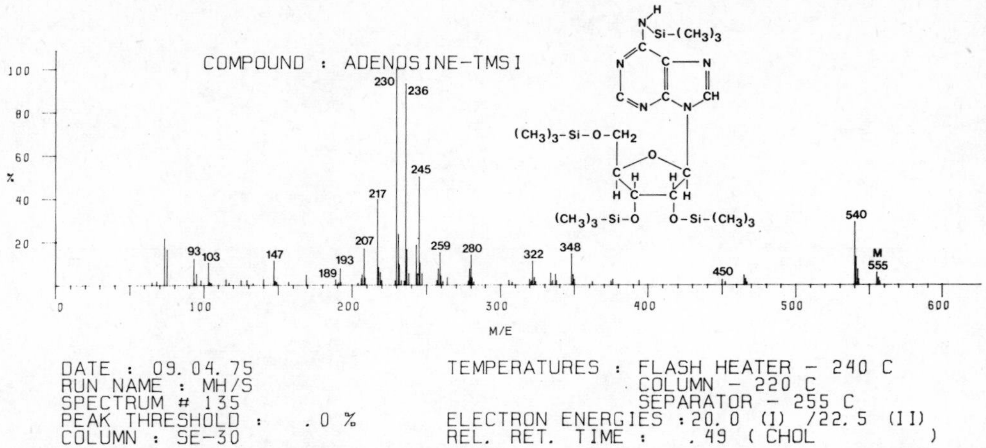

Fig. 8. Mass spectrum and supposed structure of TMS derivative of adenosine. The conditions can be seen in the figure. The retention time is relative to cholestane.

Attempts to chromatograph the silylated derivatives of NADH and the inhibitor were marred by thermal degradation, and, when the inhibitor was chromatographed, the peak formed was irregular and contained at least two compounds. As a result, the mass spectrum varied according to the point at which it was taken. Two spectra of the inhibitor are presented, one obtained by the gas chromatographic technique (fig. 9) and the other by placing the compound in an empty glass column and heating the oven according to a temperature programme (fig. 10). Unfortunately, only the fragments above m/e 100 can be

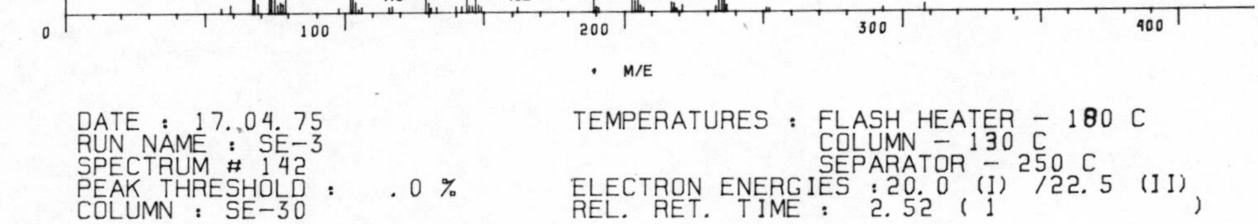

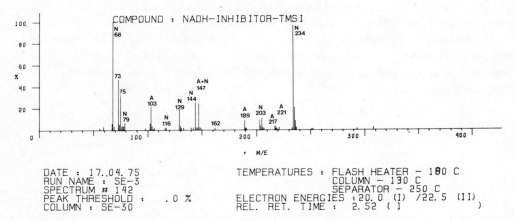

Fig. 9. Mass spectrum of the TMS derivative of the NADH inhibitor. The conditions can be seen in the figure. The spectrum was obtained at the top of the irregular peak obtained. The 'relative retention time' is the absolute time in min. Fragments marked N also occur in the spectrum of nicotinamide TMS. Fragments marked A also occur in the spectrum of adenine TMS.

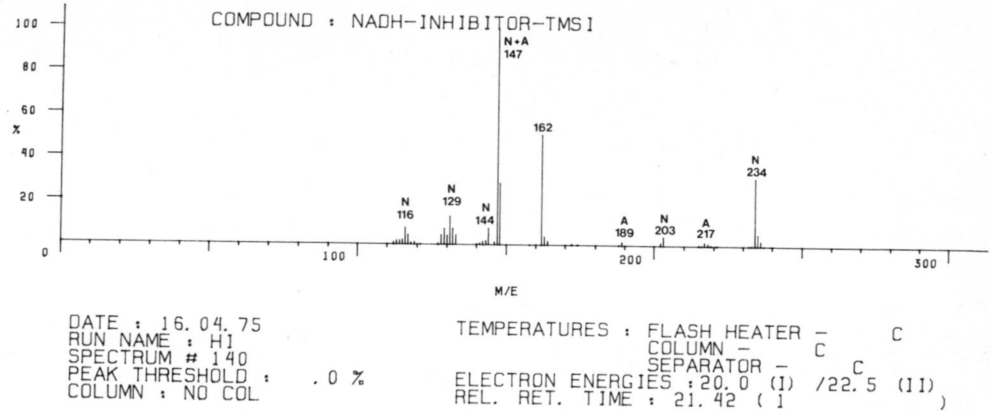

Fig. 10. Mass spectrum of the TMS derivative of the NADH inhibitor. The inhibitor was placed in an empty glass column and the oven heated by a temperature programme starting from 150 °C and increasing at 1 °C/min. The 'relative retention time' is the absolute time in min. Fragments marked N also occur in the spectrum of nicotinamide TMS. Fragments marked A also occur in the spectrum of adenine TMS.

seen in the latter spectrum, because of a mistake in the preprogramming of the computer. However, the spectra are very similar and contain ions from both ends of the NADH molecule, which means that the inhibitor is not very different from the intact NADH molecule. The ions at m/e 147 and 234 are very prominent. In addition to these and the typical nicotinamide ions at m/e 67, 68 and 79, figures 9 and 10 show some other ions (indicated by an N). The structure of these latter ions was not elucidated, but they were also visible in the spectrum of the TMS derivative of nicotinamide (indicated by an N). The ions also seen in the adenine TMS spectrum are indicated by an A.

Thus, although we were not able to obtain a complete spectrum of the molecule, we infer that the inhibitor contains both the nicotinamide and the adenine structures. These findings are not in accord with those obtained by *Glenn* [6], who came to the conclusion that the molecular weight of the inhibitor is only 207. The spectrum obtained by *Glenn* is, in our opinion, an artefact; it is formed mainly by ions which can be found in various derivatives of phthalic acid such as dioctylphthalate (9 ions including m/e 149) and some low-molecular-weight hydrocarbons, oxygen, nitrogen and water. The suggested molecular ion at m/e 207 is a very common background ion, usually derived from column material contaminating the sample or the ion source.

Gel filtration of the isolated inhibitor (Tris-HCl eluted inhibitor) through Sephadex G-10 (2 × 13 cm), G-15 (0.9 × 10 cm) and G-25 (1 × 22 cm), demonstrated that the inhibitor, NAD^+ and NADH have the same elution volume, whereas adenosine and nicotinamide mononucleotide have clearly larger elution volumes (fig. 11). This indicates that we are dealing with a compound which is similar in molecular weight to NADH and NAD^+. The possibility of an NAD-like compound with a dimer structure is not supported by the result of G-25 filtration.

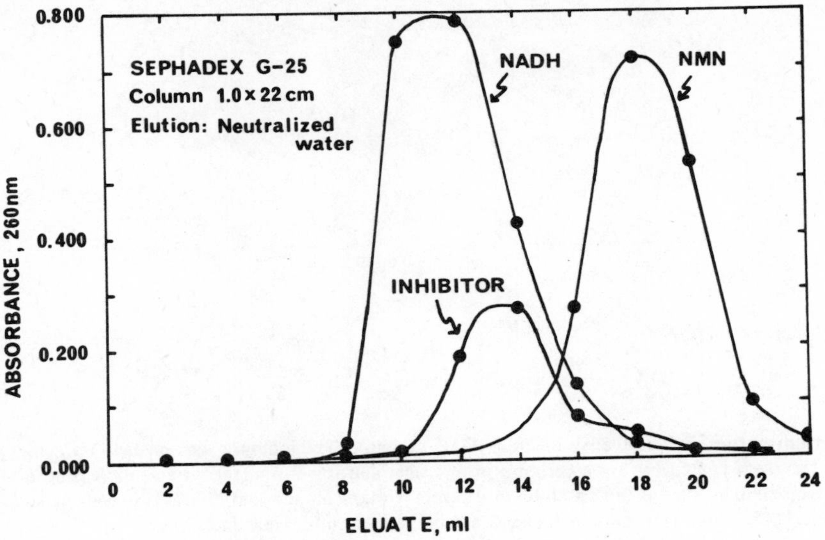

Fig. 11. Gel filtration of the isolated LDH inhibitor on Sephadex G-25. NMN = nicotinamide mononucleotide.

Isotachophoretic separation showed that the inhibitor has a net mobility greater than those of NADH and NAD^+ (fig. 12). The thermal step height of the inhibitor is not very great, indicating that the inhibitor has a high mobility [1]. Thus, analytical isotachophoresis with UV detection should be a valuable aid in the quality control of NADH reagents for enzymatic determinations.

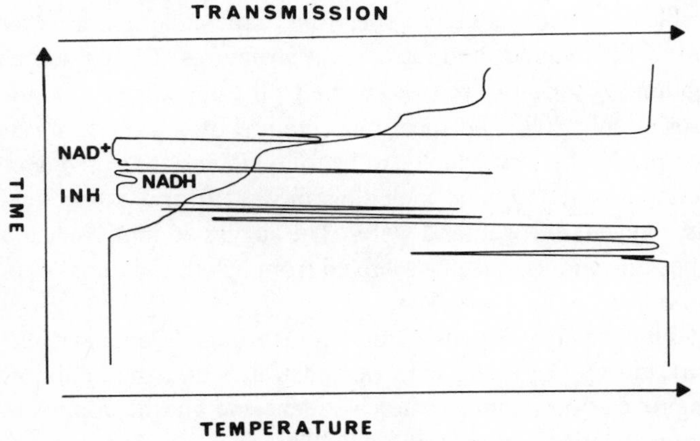

Fig. 12. Isotachophoretic separation of a mixture of the inhibitor, NADH and NAD (the three main components, other bonds are unidentified impurities from the inhibitor preparation). Leading electrolyte is chloride (5 mmol/l HCl, β-alanine, 0.25% methylcellulose, pH 3.7), terminating electrolyte is 5 mmol/l caproic acid. Tension increased from 3.0 to 24.5 KV. Current 80 μA. Run time about 15 min.

Dehydrogenases possess stereospecificity towards pyridine nucleotides. The A-type, e.g. LDH, and the B-type, e.g. α-GPDH, take H^+ from different sides of the nicotinamide ring. Our preliminary results indicate that the inhibitor has less effect on enzymes of the B-type (table 2). A possible speculation would be substitution or addition in the pyridine ring of the inhibitor.

Storage of NADH solutions: For the storage experiments the pooled NADH powder was made up into solutions of 1 mmol/l, 10 mmol/l and 50 mmol/l in ice-cold 56 mmol/l Tris-HCl buffer, pH 7.7 (25 °C), or in 100 mmol/l sodium carbonate buffer, pH 10.0. 1 ml portions of these solutions were transferred to 2 ml Pyrex tubes, which were carefully closed with rubber stoppers and stored at + 4 °C, −20 °C and −75 °C. Freezing was done rapidly in a hexane-dry ice bath. Some of the tubes were also bubbled with nitrogen in an ice bath for 3 min before storage at + 4 °C. Each tube was thawed only once for each experiment. The reference NADH, stored in a tightly closed desiccator over dry silica gel, was carefully weighed every time to make a reference solution in Tris or carbonate buffer.

The criteria for assessing the quality of the NADH preparation are shown in table 1 (for comparison see ref. 5).

Figure 13 shows the formation of inhibitors towards LDH during storage at different temperatures and concentrations. In both buffers, 50 mmol/l NADH at + 4 °C formed inhibitors, so that after storage for 3 weeks there was 20% inhibition. At −20 °C there was also some inhibitor formation at both concentrations, especially in alkaline pH. However, at −75 °C no inhibitors were detectable at any of the concentrations studied in either buffer. Storage under nitrogen, after careful bubbling with it, did not seem to prevent inhibitor formation (fig. 14). Again the high concentration was less stable at + 4 °C. When α-GPDH was used as indicator, the degree of inhibition was similar to that obtained with LDH, but smaller.

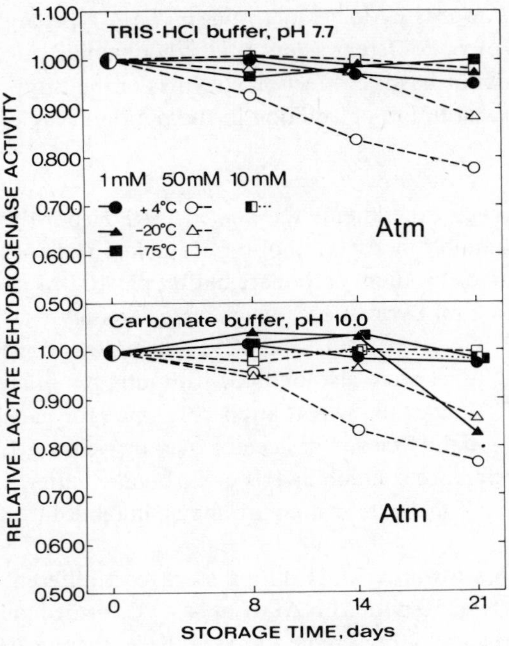

Fig. 13. The effect of storage of NADH solution in various conditions on the relative LDH activity. The buffers were 56 mmol/l Tris-HCl buffer, pH 7.7 (25 °C) and 100 mmol/l carbonate buffer, pH 10.0, NADH concentrations 1 mmol/l and 50 mmol/l, and storage temperatures + 4 °C, – 20 °C and – 75 °C. The relative LDH activity was calculated as explained in table 1. The solutions were under air.

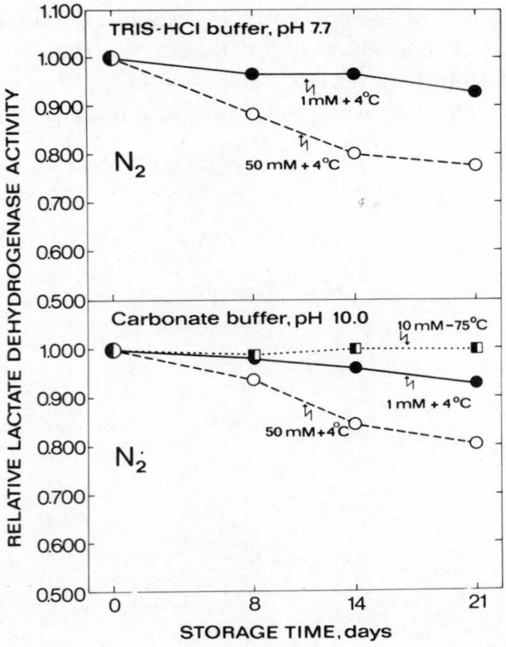

Fig. 14. The effect of storage of NADH solutions under nitrogen on the relative LDH activity. Conditions and concentrations are the same as in figure 13. Note the excellent stability of 10 mmol/l NADH solution in carbonate buffer at – 75 °C.

In Tris buffer the relative NADH content at + 4 °C clearly decreased at both concentrations, whereas in carbonate buffer only the 50 mmol/l solutions did so (fig. 15). At −20 °C some decrease could also be seen, and in carbonate buffer especially the low concentration was more affected. At −75 °C NADH did not change in any of the conditions.

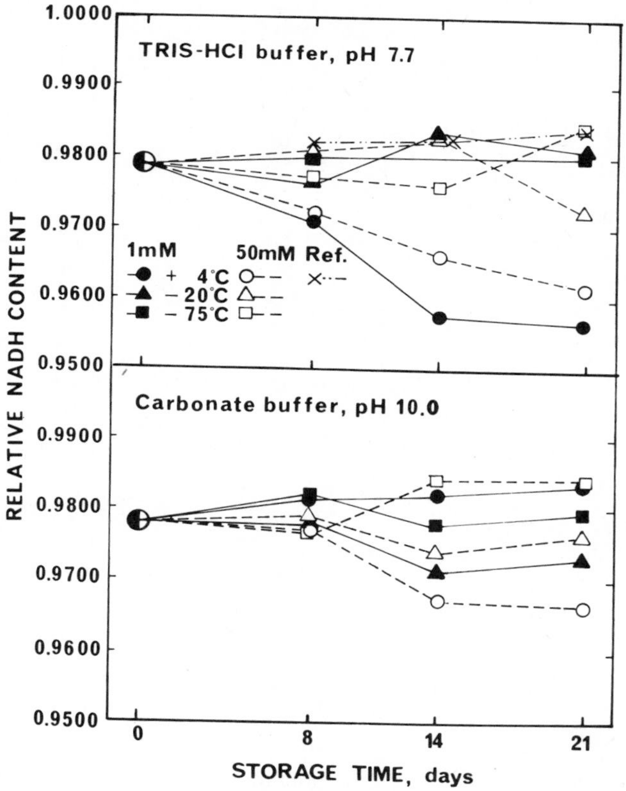

Fig. 15. The effect of storage of NADH solutions on the relative NADH content. The conditions and concentrations are the same as in figure 13. The relative NADH content was calculated as described in table 1.

Figure 16 shows the 260 nm/340 nm absorbance ratios for the same samples. Again, the 50 mmol/l concentrations were less stable at + 4 °C, although in this respect the results seemed somewhat better with the carbonate buffer. At −75 °C there was no change during 3 weeks in any preparations.

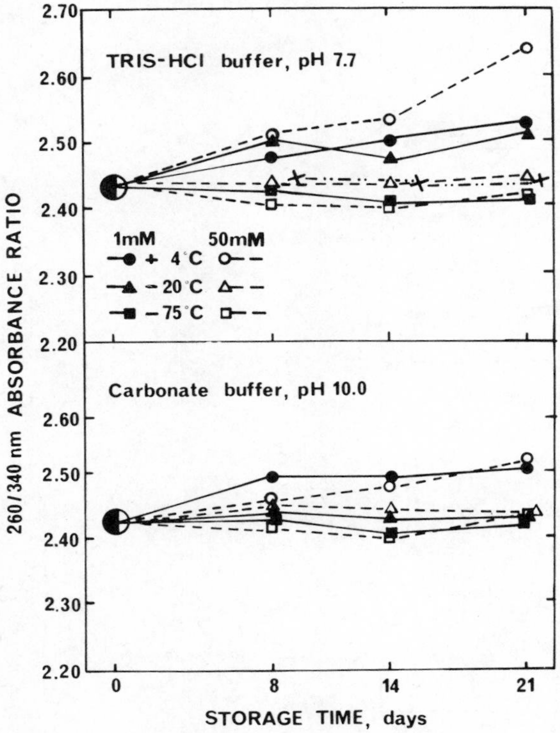

Fig. 16. The effect of storage of NADH solutions on the 260 nm/340 nm absorbance ratio. The conditions and concentrations are the same as in figure 13. The absorbance ratio was calculated as described in table 1. The symbol x shows the absorbance ratio of the reference NADH preparation.

Figure 17 shows the relative residual absorbance at 340 nm. This method is not very good, because measurement of small absorbance differences is not accurate, especially if the photometer is not of high quality. Even with an excellent instrument like the Cary the results were less consistent than in the former test. The samples stored at −75 °C showed less residual absorbance.

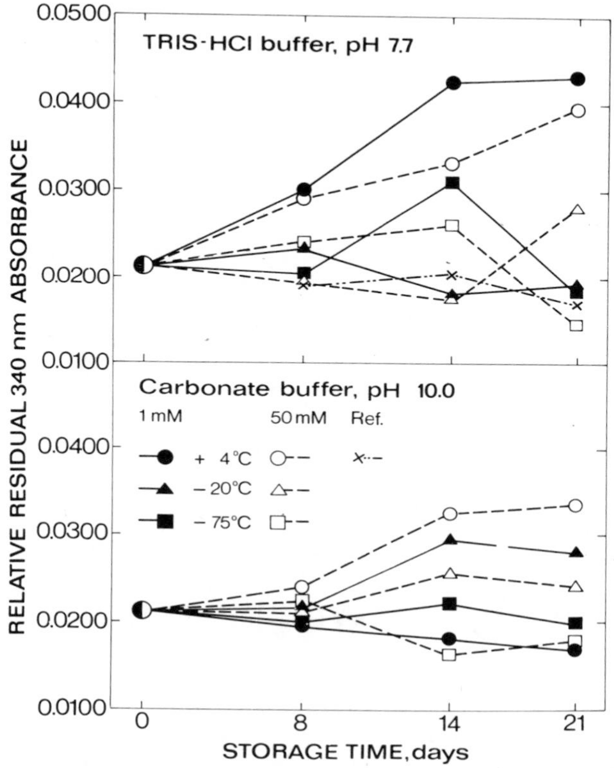

Fig. 17. The effect of storage of NADH solutions on the relative residual 340 nm absorbance. The conditions and concentrations are the same as in figure 13. The relative residual absorbance was calculated as described in table 1. The symbol x shows the relative residual absorbance of the reference NADH preparation weighed at the time of analysis.

Figure 18 shows the effect of storage on the relative residual fluorescence. The result is fully consistent with the previous findings. Note again the stability of NADH at − 75 °C.

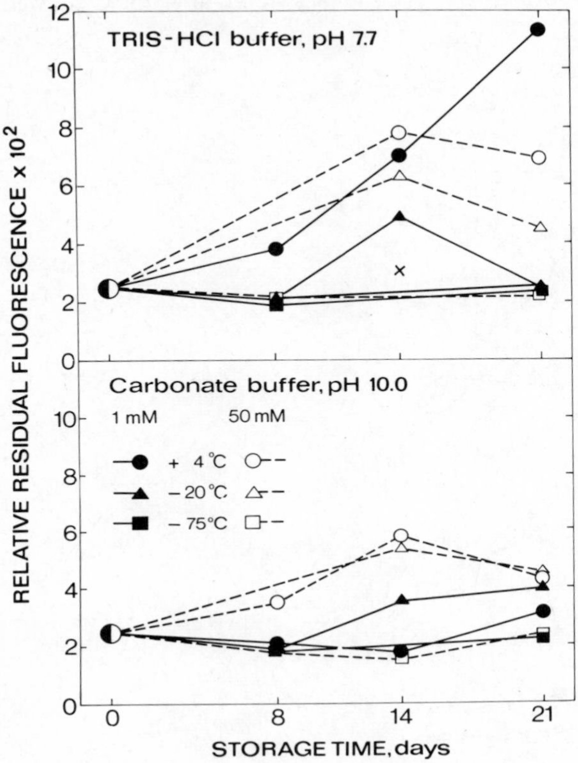

Fig. 18. The effect of storage of NADH solutions on the relative residual fluorescence. The conditions and concentrations are the same as in figure 13. The relative residual fluorescence was calculated as described in table 1. The symbol x shows the relative residual fluorescence of the reference NADH weighed at the time of analysis.

Since the changes seemed to be most pronounced at + 4 °C in 50 mmol/l solution, we studied both buffers to test whether any NAD^+ would be formed at this concentration and if so whether nitrogen would affect the rate of formation (fig. 19). Oxidation of NADH to NAD^+ was much more rapid in Tris than in carbonate buffer, but nitrogen had no preventive effect.

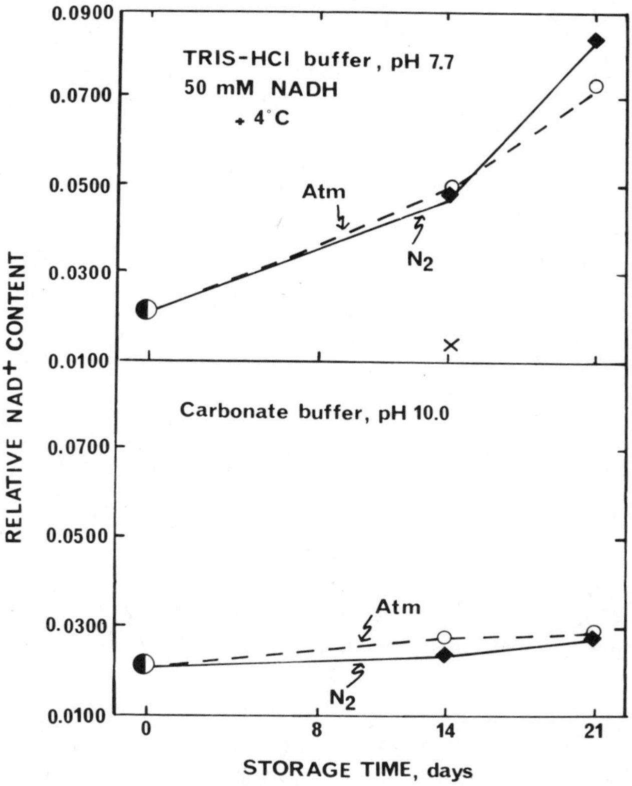

Fig. 19. The effect of storage of NADH solutions under air and nitrogen on the relative NAD^+ content. The storage temperature was + 4 °C. The relative NAD^+ content was calculated as described in table 1. The symbol x refers to the relative NAD^+ content of the reference NADH preparation weighed at the time of analysis.

The same samples were also used to study the strong alkali-induced fluorescence (fig. 20). The curves looked exactly the same as in figure 19, and this test, which is very simple, may be the method of choice for quality control of NADH. However, it mainly measures the amount of NAD^+.

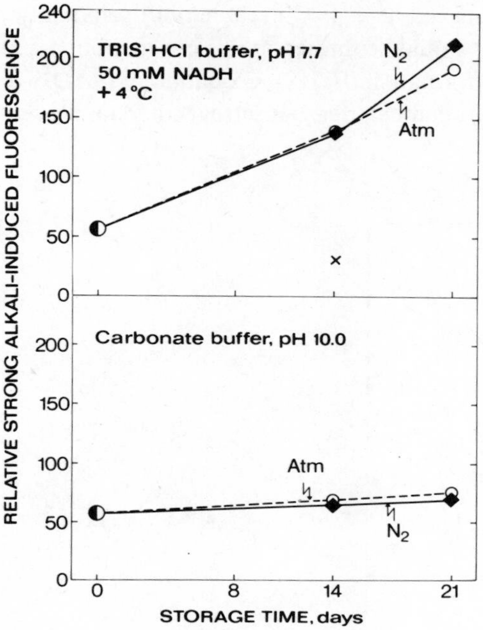

Fig. 20. The effect of storage of NADH solutions under air and nitrogen on the relatively strong alkali-induced fluorescence. The conditions are the same as in figure 19.

Our results on the stability of high and low concentrations of NADH at + 4 °C and −20 °C agree well with the data of *Lowry* and *Passonneau* [9], who found that at + 4 °C dilute solutions are more stable than concentrated solutions, but at −20 °C they break down rapidly.

Our data clearly show that −75 °C is superior to + 4 °C and −20 °C if storage is necessary for more than one week. The difference in the effect of nitrogen on the stability of solid NADH [5] and in solution is not surprising, since in powder form the oxidizable surface of NADH is very large, whereas in solutions only a small number of molecules come in contact with oxygen. Therefore, if NADH is stored in solution there is no need to use nitrogen.

We therefore make the following suggestion for the use of NADH in routine clinical enzymology. Make up, for example, a 17 mmol/l NADH solution in 56 mmol/l Tris-EDTA-HCl buffer, pH 7.7 (25 °C), and store it at −75 °C in aliquots of 5 ml or less according to how many LDH measurements you perform daily in your laboratory. At −75 °C these solutions are stable for at least one month. For LDH measurement the solution is diluted to 1 in 100 with the same buffer; in practice this means that this 5 ml bottle is made up to 0.5 l with the buffer. This is enough for 150–300 LDH measurements.

Conclusions

In table 2 we have summarized the properties of the humidity-induced inhibitor and put forward a suggestion about its structure. It is obvious that the inhibitor we have been talking about is not a single compound, but at least three different compounds. The data presented in the present paper refer to the fraction which has the strongest inhibition towards LDH and has the same elution on Sephadex G-25 as NADH. The inhibitor in question is not a split product of NADH. It seems to differ from NADH and NAD^+ in the pyridine ring, possibly by substitution or addition. In a paper presented in abstract form, *Grassl* et al. [7] came to a similar conclusion.

Table 2. Summary of the properties of the humidity-induced LDH inhibitor and implications for the possible structure.

Properties of the humidity-induced inhibitor	Implications for the possible structure of the inhibitor
UV spectrum: $\frac{A_{260}}{A_{340}} = 9.6–11.0$	Resembles NAD^+ more closely than NADH, but is not identical
IR spectrum: Comparison with NAD^+, NADH, nicotinamide, adenosine, adenine	Similar, but shift in carbonyl region; bonded amide?
Fluorescence: NADH: 345 nm–465 nm INH: 350 nm–460 nm NAD^+ + 6 N NaOH: 365 nm–465 nm (ca. 10^3 ×) INH + 6 N NaOH: 365 nm–465 nm (8 ×)	Resembles NAD^+ more closely than NADH, but is not identical
Acid treatment: Native fluorescence +, (NADH–) H_2O_2 + 6 N NaOH fluorescence +, (NADH–)	
Alkali treatment: Native fluorescence + 6 N NaOH fluorescence +, (NAD^+–)	
Mass spectrometry: Several fragments identical with adenosine and nicotinamide	Contains nicotinamide- and adenosine-like structures
Gel filtration: Elution pattern identical with NADH	M.W. similar to that of NADH and NAD^+
Isotachophoresis: Net mobility: inhibitor > NADH > NAD^+	Assuming the same M.W. as NADH, the difference in charge and/or solvation and/or dissociation constant
Enzyme Inhibition: Different degree of inhibition between the A and B stereospecific dehydrogenases, e.g. LDH (A) α-GPDH (B) 34% 2% 68% 15%	Speculative

However, our results are still incomplete and should be regarded as tentative. More work must be done with several model compounds and enzymes which split the inhibitor into smaller fragments. After isolation,they are easier to handle by the GLC-MS technique and IR-spectrometry.

When the NADH preparation has been tested for its quality in enzyme assays, it can be stored for at least 3 weeks (probably for several months) in 17 mmol/l solution (e.g. 56 mmol/l Tris-EDTA-HCl buffer, pH 7.7) at −75 °C in a deep-freezer. For LDH assay the solution is then diluted 100-fold with the same buffer.

Acknowledgements

The isotachophoretic runs were performed at the Application Laboratory of LKB-Produkter AB, Bromma, Sweden by Miss *Ulla Moberg*, M.A., to whom we wish to express our sincere gratitude. This work was supported by grants from the Medical Research Council in the Academy of Finland and the Ford Foundation, New York.

References

[1] *Beckers, J.L., and Everaerts, F.M.:* The Separation of Nucleotides by Isotachophoresis. J. Chromatogr. *71*, 380–385 (1972).

[2] *Dalziel, K.:* An Inhibitor of Liver Alcohol Dehydrogenase in Preparations of Reduced Diphosphopyridine Nucleotide. Nature *191*, 1098–1099 (1961).

[3] *Dalziel, K.:* The Purification of Nicotinamide Adenine Dinucleotide and the Kinetic Effects of Nucleotide Impurities. J. Biol. Chem. *238*, 1538–1543 (1963).

[4] *Elliott, W.H., and Waller, G.R.:* Vitamins and Cofactors. In Waller, G.R.: Biochemical Applications of Mass Spectrometry. Wiley-Interscience, New York, London, Sydney, Toronto, 499–536 (1972).

[5] *Gerhardt, W., Kofoed, B., Westlund. L.. and Pavlu, B.:* Quality Control of NADH. Evaluation of Methods for Detection of Inhibitors and Specifications for NADH Quality. Scand. J. Clin. Lab. Invest. *33*, Suppl. 139, 1–51 (1974).

[6] *Glenn, J.H.:* Study of Enzyme Inhibitor formed from Reduced Nicotinamide Adenine Dinucleotide and its Effect on the Assay of Lactate Dehydrogenase. M. Sc. Thesis, University of Surrey (1972).

[7] *Grassl, M., Haid, E., Nelböck, M., and Weimann, G.:* Über die Qualität von reduzierten Pyridin-Coenzymen. Abstracts Biochemische Analytik 74 combined with the 1st European Congress of Clinical Chemistry, München 22.–26.4.1974. In Z. Klin. Chem. Klin. Biochem. *12*, 240 (1974).

[8] *Härkönen, M., Suvanto, O., and Kormano, M.:* Glutamate in Post-Natal Rat Testis. J. Reprod. Fert. *21*, 533–536 (1970).

[9] *Lowry, O.H., and Passonneau, J.V.:* Pyridine Nucleotides. In Lowry, O.H., and Passonneau, J.V.: A Flexible System of Enzymatic Analysis. Academic Press, New York, London, p. 8–17 (1972).

[10] *McComb, R.B., and Gay, R.J.:* A Comparison of Reduced-NAD Preparations from Four Commercial Sources. Clin. Chem. *14*, 754–763 (1968).

[11] *Strandjord, P.E., and Clayson, K.J.:* The Control of Inhibitory Impurities in Reduced Nicotinamide Adenine Dinucleotide in Lactate Dehydrogenase Assays. J. Lab. Clin. Med. *67*, 144–153 (1966).

[12] *Strandjord, P.E., Clayson, K.J., and Foley, J.F.:* The Formation of Analogs of Adenosine Diphosphoribose and Their Action as Dehydrogenase Inhibitors. Fed. Proc. *22*, 636 (1963).

[13] The Committee on Enzymes of the Scandinavian Society for Clinical Chemistry and Clinical Physiology: Recommended Methods for the Determination of Four Enzymes in Blood. Scand. J. Clin. Lab. Invest. *33*, 291–306 (1974).

NAD – NADH – NADP – NADPH
Characterization and Purity Assurance

Free Communications

The Molar Absorption Coefficient (ε) of Reduced NAD (NADH)

G. N. Bowers, Jr., *R. B. McComb, L. W. Bond, R. C. Keech* and *R. W. Burnett,* Hartford/Connecticut (U. S. A.)

Key words: Buffer effects
Concentration effects
Glucose-6-phosphate dehydrogenase
Hexokinase
Molar absorption coefficient
NADH
pH effects
Temperature effects

Enzyme reactions utilizing the cofactor nicotinamide-adenine dinucleotide (NAD) are of major importance in biochemical analyses. Clinical enzymology has relied heavily upon measurement techniques based upon the absorption maximum of reduced NAD at 340 nm. The most commonly used reference value of 622 litre $\times$ mol^{-1} $\times$ mm^{-1} for the molar absorption coefficient was determined by *Horecker* and *Kornberg* in 1948 [1]; yet, review of their paper shows a relatively wide spread of values. Improvements in spectrophotometric instrumentation and standardization techniques, as well as the availability of high-purity substrates, coenzymes, and enzymes, suggested that this important biochemical constant might be established with greater certainty. Therefore, we have been attempting to redetermine the molar (linear) absorption coefficient (ε) of reduced NAD at 340 nm over the past few years [2].

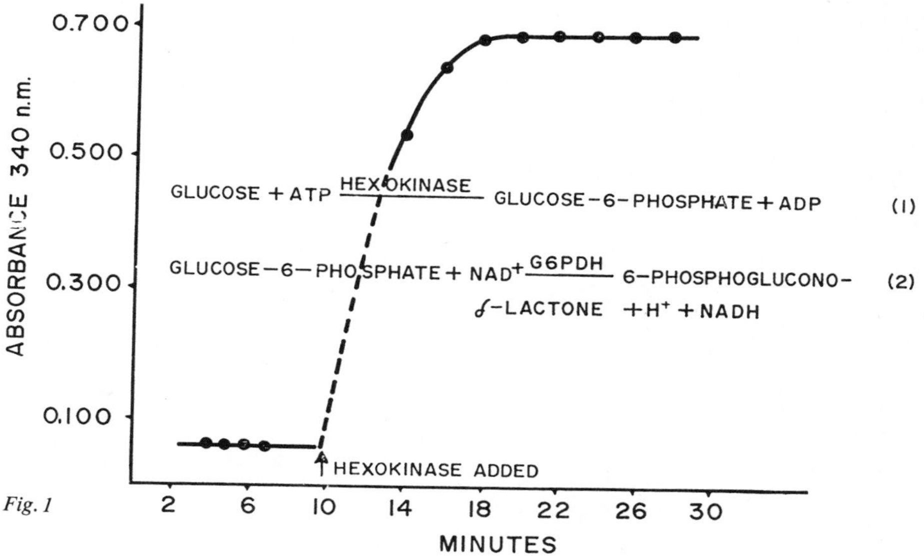

Fig. 1

Figure 1 shows the approach we have used. The increase in absorbance at 340 nm at 25.0 ± 0.2 °C in a 0.1 mol/litre Tris-HCl buffer, pH 7.8 was measured during the stoichiometric conversion of an accurately-weighed amount of pure D-glucose to 6-phosphogluconate according to the reaction given on this figure. The glucose purity of SRM #917 is certified by NBS to be 99.9%. The starting NAD^+ and ATP are available in relatively high degrees of purity, as has been shown by concurrent high pressure liquid chromatography. G 6 PD and hexokinase were likewise high-quality reagents. The G 6 PD was from the bacteria *Leuconostoc mesenteroides* and reacts with either NAD^+ or $NADP^+$.

A weighed amount of NBS glucose was accurately diluted at 25.0 ± 0.5 °C to the desired concentrations with Tris-HCl buffer containing Mg^{2+}, NAD^+, and ATP. A 4 ml portion was placed into a quartz cuvet along with 1 µl of glucose-6-phosphate dehydrogenase. After allowing the sample to equilibrate at 25 °C, the initial stable absorbance vs. air was determined in a Cary 16 spectrophotometer for a 5 to 10 minute period. At this point 2 µl of hexokinase was added, and the reaction time course was followed for approximately 20 minutes with repeated absorbance measurements of the whole system zeroed against air. The reaction was assumed to be complete when the absorbance values remained constant over a 5 to 10 minute period. Based upon the observed delta A, the initial glucose concentration, and the considerations listed in tables 1–3, a corrected value for each determination of $\varepsilon^{340\,nm}_{NADH}$, was calculated.

Table 1. Reagent and reaction considerations.

1. Glucose Purity (99.9% – NBS/SRM#917)
2. Weight of Glucose used
3. Volumetric/Absorbance Changes due to Added Hexokinase + G–6–PD
4. Absorbance Change on Loss of NAD
5. Incomplete or Side Reactions
6. Absorbance Changes in Other Reagents or in Products (6-Phospho-Gluconate, ATP/ADP, and Enzyme-Coenzyme Complexing)

Table 2. Spectral considerations.

1. Wavelength Error
2. Stray Light Error
3. Photometric Error
4. Slit Width Effect
5. Beam Convergence
6. Cell Pathlength
7. Reflectance Errors

Table 3. Other considerations.

1. Volumetric Glassware Recalibrated at 25 °C
2. Balance Accuracy checked (Class S Weights)
3. Air Buoyancy (by calculation)
4. Temperature of 25.0 ± 0.2 °C (vs NBS/SRM#934)

In order to verify the stoichiometry of these reactions, an experiment was carried out substituting ^{14}C-labelled glucose for the NBS glucose. Duplicate experiments using triplicate analyses revealed that less than 0.3% of the original glucose remained in the incubation mixture as either glucose or the intermediate glucose-6-phosphate. Likewise, a ten-fold increase in concentration of either of the enzyme reagents gave no evidence of further changes in either NAD or NADH.

Figure 2 shows the frequency distribution for the 85 corrected $\varepsilon^{340\,nm}_{NADH}$ values which were accepted as being 'within control' subsequent to calibrating all glassware at 25 °C and reconditioning of the spectrophotometer and balances. Statistical treatment of the results gave an aggregate total mean of 631.0 litre × mol^{-1} × mm^{-1} with a standard deviation of 2.8 and a relative standard deviation of 0.44%.

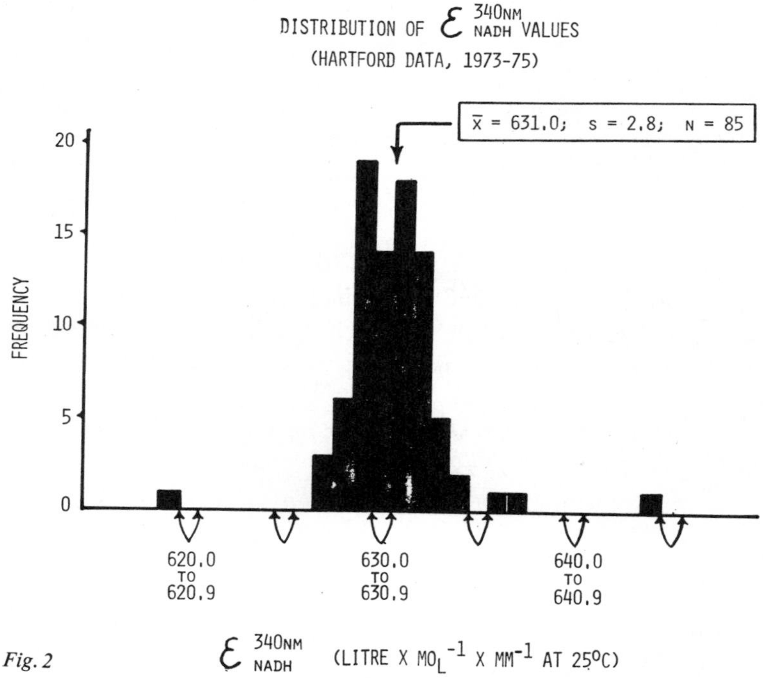

Fig. 2

In order to determine the effect of other parameters on the absorptivity of NADH, experiments were carried out varying the pH and temperature of the buffer, utilizing a simple NADH solution made up in buffer identical to that used in experiments in which NADH was generated enzymatically. There is a significant linear shift in the 340 nm absorptivity of NADH at temperatures ranging from 20 to 35 °C. This change must be taken into consideration in assigning a molar absorption coefficient to a particular system. There is also an effect of pH on the absorptivity of NADH at 340 nm in *Tris-HCl buffer*. A shift of approximately 0.4% change in the molar absorption coefficient occurs per pH unit. NADH is stable for at least 2 hours at 25 °C at pH 7.8 in Tris-HCl buffer[1].

In table 4 the data previously lumped together in figure 2 is grouped at each starting glucose concentration to show the molar absorption coefficient obtained at four different NADH concentrations. These data suggest higher $\varepsilon_{\text{NADH}}^{340\text{ nm}}$ values at the lower NADH concentrations; but after specially-designed experimentation, we can neither prove nor disprove this hypothesis.

Table 4. Molar absorptivity of reduced NAD at 340 nm.

Initial Conc. Glucose mmol/l	X*	S.D.	N	R.S.D.
0.0250	632.3	2.0	10	0.32%
0.0500	632.3	3.5	20	0.55%
0.1000	630.4	2.4	39	0.38%
0.2000	630.1	1.8	16	0.29%
All values	631.0	2.8	85	0.44%

* ε_{340} = litre × mol^{-1} × mm^{-1} at 25 °C in 0.1 mol/l Tris-HCl, pH 7.8.

Summary

1. We question the continued use of one value for the molar absorption coefficient of NADH. It is clear that a single value cannot be used as if it were a universal constant applicable to all systems in clinical enzymology no matter what the chemical buffer, pH and temperature.

2. Our best estimate at this time for the molar absorption coefficient of NADH in 0.1 mol/l Tris-HCl buffer pH 7.8 at 25 °C is 631.0 ± 2.8 litre × mol^{-1} × mm^{-1}.

References

[1] *Horecker and Kornberg:* J. Biol. Chem. *175,* 385, 1948.
[2] *McComb et al.:* Clin. Chem. *20,* 882, 1974.

[1] When comparisons of molar absorptivity in phosphate and tris buffers were attempted, it was found that a measureable decomposition of NADH takes place in the presence of 0.1 molar phosphate ions – even at the slightly alkaline pH of 7.8. The instability of NADH in phosphate buffer, although well documented in the literature, is often ignored in many methods involving the use of NAD^+ in coupled enzyme systems.

The Molar Absorption Coefficients of β-Nicotinamide-Adenine Dinucleotide

E. Haid, P. Lehmann and *J. Ziegenhorn,* Tutzing (Germany)

Key words: Glutamate dehydrogenase
Glycerol-3-phosphate dehydrogenase
Lactate dehydrogenase
Molar absorption coefficient
NAD
NADH

Introduction

At present, for the molar absorption coefficients of the pyridine nucleotides at Hg 334 nm, 340 nm or Hg 365 nm the values 6.0×10^3, 6.22×10^3 or 3.3×10^3 liter·mol^{-1}·cm^{-1} are widely accepted. Recent results from different laboratories along with incongruous data in the literature (table 1) cast doubts on the accuracy of these values.

Table 1. List of previous studies on the molar absorption coefficients of β-NADH

Wavelength nm	Molar absorption coefficient liter · mol^{-1} · cm^{-1}	Reference
Hg 334	6.0×10^3	(3)
334	6.09×10^3 (25 °C)	(6)
340	6.22×10^3	(1)
340	6.3×10^3	(3)
340	6.25×10^3	(4)
340	6.29×10^3 (25 °C)	(5)
340	6.29×10^3 (25 °C)	(6)
Hg 365	3.4×10^3	(2)
Hg 365	3.4×10^3	(3)
Hg 365	3.30×10^3 (25 °C)	(5)
365	3.48×10^3 (25 °C)	(6)
366	3.30×10^3 (25 °C)	(6)

When determining glucose with the hexokinase/glucose-6-phosphate dehydrogenase method, *Haeckel* et al. [7] and *Da Fonseca-Wollheim* [8] obtained results, corresponding to more than 100% of the theory when measured at Hg 365 nm and calculated with the

Enzymes: lactate dehydrogenase (EC 1.1.1.27); glutamate dehydrogenase (EC 1.4.1.3); glycerol-3-phosphate dehydrogenase (EC 1.1.1.8).

above mentioned ε-value. These data coincided fairly well with observations in our own laboratories. Using NADH- or NADPH-dependent reactions for the quality control of highly purified products, at Hg 365 nm, we likewise determined a content of more than 100% with the ε-value of 3.3×10^3. This, together with other information prompted us to revise the molar absorption coefficients of the pyridine nucleotides [9–11]. We describe here our work on the reduced and the oxidized form of β-nicotinamide-adenine dinucleotide.

Hg 334 nm and Hg 365 nm

For the determination of the molar absorption coefficients of β-NADH at the mercury spectral lines of 334 nm and 365 nm, the lactate dehydrogenase or glutamate dehydrogenase assay was performed with carefully purified pyruvic acid or 2-oxoglutaric acid in the presence of excess β-NADH (fig. 1). These analytical systems were chosen because of the favourable equilibrium constants of the reactions [12, 13] and of the low absorbance of the enzymes at the wavelengths studied [11]. Furthermore, the enzyme coenzyme complexes formed did not alter the absorbance of the coenzyme at these wavelengths [11]. Finally, the substrates pyruvic acid and 2-oxoglutaric acid could be obtained with high purity [11]. The purity of the substrates was checked through potentiometric titration, differential scanning calorimetry, moisture analysis, NMR-spectroscopy, gas-liquid chromatography and mass spectrometry [11].

1. $\text{L-lactate} + \text{NAD}^+ \xrightleftharpoons{\text{lactate dehydrogenase}} \text{pyruvate} + \text{NADH} + \text{H}^+$

$$\frac{[\text{pyruvate}] \cdot [\text{NADH}] \cdot [\text{H}^+]}{[\text{L-lactate}] \cdot [\text{NAD}^+]} = 2.76 \times 10^{-12}\ \text{mol} \cdot \text{liter}^{-1}\ \ (\text{pH } 7.0;\ 25\ ^\circ\text{C})$$

2. $\text{L-glutamate} + \text{NAD}^+ + H_2O \xrightleftharpoons{\text{glutamate dehydrogenase}} \text{2-oxoglutarate} + \text{NADH} + \text{NH}^+{}_4$

$$\frac{[\text{2-oxoglutarate}] \cdot [\text{NADH}] \cdot [\text{NH}^+{}_4]}{[\text{L-glutamate}] \cdot [\text{NAD}^+]} = 4.5 \times 10^{-14}\ \text{mol} \cdot \text{liter}^{-1}\ \ (\text{pH } 8.0;\ 25\ ^\circ\text{C})$$

3. $\text{L-glycerol-3-phosphate} + \text{NAD}^+ \xrightleftharpoons{\text{glycerol-3-phosphate dehydrogenase}} \text{dihydroxyacetone phosphate} + \text{NADH} + \text{H}^+$

$$\frac{[\text{dihydroxyacetone phosphate}] \cdot [\text{NADH}] \cdot [\text{H}^+]}{[\text{L-glycerol-3-phosphate}] \cdot [\text{NAD}^+]} = 1.0 \times 10^{-12}\ \text{mol} \cdot \text{liter}^{-1}\ \ (\text{pH } 8.0;\ 25\ ^\circ\text{C})$$

Fig. 1. Assay systems. Equilibrium constants (12–14).

The molar absorption coefficients of β-NADH were calculated according to Bouguer-Lambert-Beer's law from the weighed molar quantities of substrate dissolved per liter of test solution, the light path of the cuvette and the observed change of absorbance after the conversion of the reactants. The measured values were corrected for the proportion of impurities present in the substrates, the buoyancy of the air on weighing of these substances, the change of volume in the course of the test procedure, the beam convergence of the photometer, the multiple reflections in the cell [15], and the self absorbances of all constituents of the analytical systems, which were established by means of separate experiments. The gravimetric determinations were carried out on different precision balances, the optical measuerements on different Eppendorf spectrum line photometers. All instruments were carefully calibrated. Further experimental details are described elsewhere [11].

Following the procedure characterized above, we obtained for β-NADH at Hg 334 nm and Hg 365 nm, respectively, the molar absorption coefficients summarized in table 2. The data observed are in good agreement with recent results of *Bücher* [16].

Table 2. Molar absorption coefficients of β-NADH at 25 °C (11)

Method	Wavelength nm	No. tests	Mean (liter · mol^{-1} · cm^{-1})	Range (liter · mol^{-1} · cm^{-1})
Lactate dehydrogenase assay	Hg 334	56	6.146×10^3	$\pm 0.019 \times 10^3$
	Hg 365	58	3.428×10^3	$\pm 0.011 \times 10^3$
Glutamate dehydrogenase assay	Hg 334	30	6.146×10^3	$\pm 0.009 \times 10^3$
	Hg 365	28	3.432×10^3	$\pm 0.005 \times 10^3$
Total	Hg 334	86	6.146×10^3	$\pm 0.016 \times 10^3$
	Hg 365	86	3.429×10^3	$\pm 0.009 \times 10^3$

260 nm

At 260 nm, the molar absorption coefficients published so far vary from 14.4×10^3 to 16.0×10^3 liter·mol^{-1}·cm^{-1} for β-NADH and from 17.8×10^3 to 18.0×10^3 liter·mol^{-1}·cm^{-1} for NAD [17–21]. Exact knowledge of these values, however, is important to the characterization of the purity of the coenzyme [22].

To examine these data, we carefully purified the reduced form of the coenzyme by repeated chromatography on QAE-Sephadex. Several impurities could be separated from the coenzyme through this procedure. By comparison with the authentic substances on paper electrophoresis, the main constituents were established to be nicotinamide mononucleotide, β-NAD, adenosine-5'-monophosphate, adenosine-5'-diphospho-ribose, and inhibitors of lactate dehydrogenase [10].

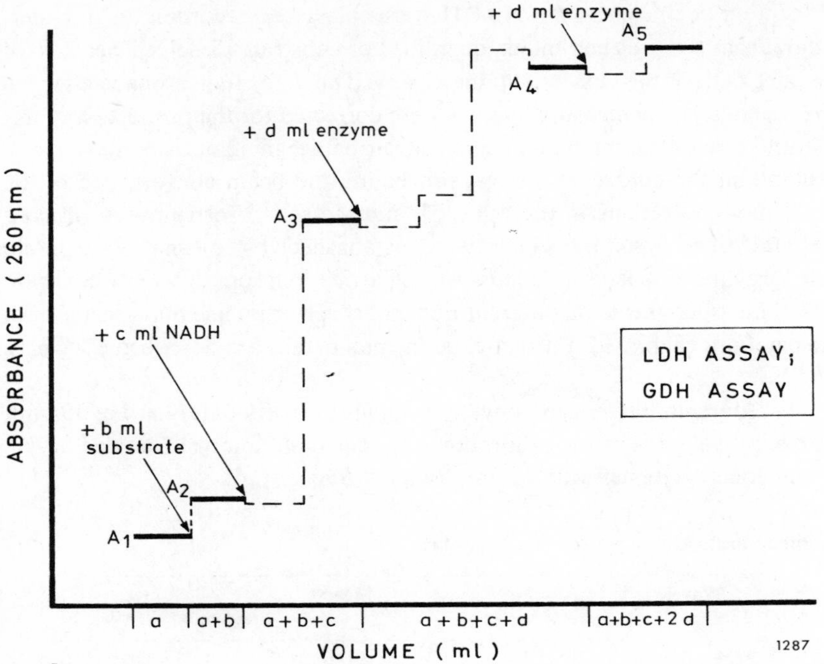

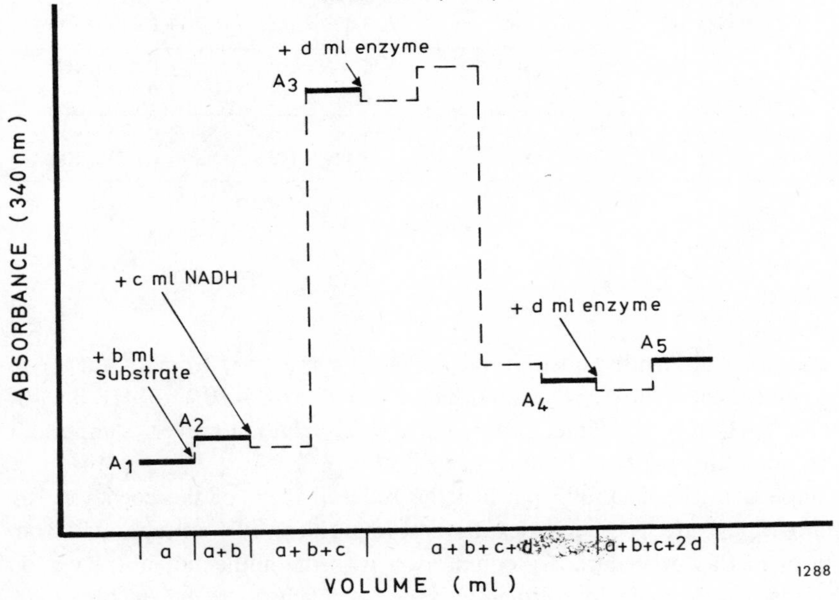

Fig. 2. Outline of the test procedure for the determination of the molar absorption coefficient of β-NAD at 260 nm.

The NADH preparation obtained, which was presumed to be pure, revealed a 260 nm/340 nm absorbance ratio of 2.265. From this quotient, a molar absorption coefficient of 14.2×10^3 liter·mol^{-1}·cm^{-1} resulted for β-NADH at 260 nm and 25 °C (n=205; $\bar{x}=14.17 \times 10^3$ liter·mol^{-1}·cm^{-1}; CV=0.53%). The coefficient was calculated by use of an ε-value of 6.26×10^3 liter·mol^{-1}·cm^{-1} for β-NADH at 340 nm and 25 °C which followed from the absorption spectrum of β-NADH [16] and the results given above for β-NADH at Hg 334 nm. In this case, the optical measurements were conducted on accurately calibrated Zeiss PMQ 2 or PMQ 3 spectrophotometers. For more experimental details see *Haid* et al. [10].

To review the molar absorption coefficients of β-NAD at 260 nm, the lactate dehydrogenase assay and the glycerol-3-phosphate dehydrogenase assay (fig. 1), respectively, were carried out with the pure β-NADH [10]. As outlined in figures 2 and 3, the measured values were corrected for the changes of the volume during the assay and for the self absorbance of all components of the test system.

$$\varepsilon^{260}_{\beta\text{-NAD}} = \frac{2(a+b+c+d)A_4^{260} - (a+b+c)A_3^{260} - (a+b+c+2d)A_5^{260}}{(a+b+c)A_3^{340} - 2(a+b+c+d)A_4^{340} + (a+b+c+2d)A_5^{340}} \times$$

$$\left(\varepsilon^{340}_{\text{substrate}} - \varepsilon^{340}_{\text{product}} + \varepsilon^{340}_{\beta\text{-NADH}} - \varepsilon^{340}_{\beta\text{-NAD}}\right)$$

$$+ \varepsilon^{260}_{\text{substrate}} - \varepsilon^{260}_{\text{product}} + \varepsilon^{260}_{\beta\text{-NADH}}$$

1282

Fig. 3. Formula for the calculation of the molar absorption coefficient of β-NAD at 260 nm.

Referring to the ε-values 14.2×10^3 or 6.26×10^3 liter·mol^{-1}·cm^{-1} for β-NADH at 260 nm or 340 nm, the molar absorption coefficients of β-NAD at 260 nm and 25 °C was established to be 17.5×10^3 liter·mol^{-1}·cm^{-1} (n=85; $\bar{x}=17.47 \times 10^3$ liter·mol^{-1}·cm^{-1}; CV=0.55%).

Concluding remarks

The molar absorption coefficients of the reduced and the oxidized form of β-nicotinamide-adenine dinucleotide observed at 260 nm in our laboratory are lower than any other data reported so far, which suggests that the previously examined coenzyme preparations still contained relatively large amounts of impurities.

By way of contrast, the molar absorption coefficients obtained at Hg 334 nm and Hg 365 nm for the reduced form of the coenzyme are higher than the values published up to the present. Among other things, this might reflect that with the advanced analytical methods applied in the recent experiments the quality of the reference material used could be better characterized than in the previous investigations, most of which date back to more than 15 years.

References

[1] *Horecker, B.L., and Kornberg, A.:* J. Biol. Chem. 175, 385 (1948).
[2] *Beisenherz, G., Boltze, H.J., Bücher, Th., Czok, R., Garbade, K.-H., Meyer-Arendt, E., and Pfleiderer, G.:* Z. Naturforsch. 8b, 555 (1953).
[3] *Beisenherz, G., Bücher, Th., and Garbade, K.-H.:* Methods Enzymol. 1, 391 (1955).
[4] *Wallenfels, K., and Christian, W.:* Methods Enzymol. 3, 882 (1957).
[5] *Hohorst, H.J.:* Biochem. Z. 328, 509 (1957).
[6] *Bücher, Th., Luh, W., and Pette, D.:* In Hoppe-Seyler/Thierfelder, Handbuch der Physiologisch- und Pathologisch Chemischen Analyse VI/A, K. Lang and E. Lehnartz, Eds. Springer Verlag, Berlin, Göttingen, Heidelberg, New York 1964, p. 292–339.
[7] *Haeckel, R., and Haeckel, H.:* In Fortschritte der Klinischen Chemie: Enzyme und Hormone. E. Kaiser, Ed. Verlag der Wiener Medizinischen Akademie, Wien 1972, p. 115–119.
[8] *Da Fonseca-Wollheim, F.:* Z. Klin. Chem. Klin. Biochem. 9, 497 (1971).
[9] *Bücher, Th., Krell, H., Lusch, G., Grassl, M., Ziegenhorn, J., and Bergmeyer, H.U.:* Z. Klin. Chem. Klin. Biochem. 12, 239 (1974).
[10] *Haid, E., Lehmann, P., and Ziegenhorn, J.:* Clin. Chem. 21, 884 (1975).
[11] *Ziegenhorn, J., Bücher, Th., Lehmann, P., Liede, V., Senn, M., and Steingross, W.:* Manuscript in preparation (1975).
[12] *Bergmeyer, H.U., Gawehn, K., and Grassl, M.:* In Methoden der enzymatischen Analyse I, H. U. Bergmeyer, Ed. Verlag Chemie, Weinheim/Bergstr. 1974, p. 512–513.
[13] *Bergmeyer, H.U., Gawehn, K., and Grassl, M.:* Ibid., p. 490–491.
[14] *Bergmeyer, H.U., Gawehn, K., and Grassl, M.:* Ibid., p. 497.
[15] *Burnett, R.W.:* Anal. Chem. 45, 383 (1973).
[16] *Bücher, Th.:* In Quality Control in Clinical Chemistry. G. Anido et al., Eds. de Gruyter Publishers, Berlin 1975.
[17] *Kornberg, A., and Pricer, W.E.,* Jr.: In Biochemical Preparations 3, E. E. Snell, Ed. John Wiley & Sons, New York, London 1953, p. 20–24.
[18] *Rafter, G.W., and Colowick, S.P.:* Methods Enzymol. 3, 887 (1957).
[19] *Siegel, J.M., Montgomery, G.A., and Bock, R.M.:* Arch. Biochem. Biophys. 82, 288 (1959).
[20] *Winer, A.D.:* J. Biol. Chem. 239, 3598 (1964).
[21] *Pfleiderer, G., Woenckhaus, C., and Nelböck-Hochstetter, M.:* Justus Liebigs Ann. Chem. 690, 170 (1965).
[22] *Howell, B.F., Margolis, S., and Schaffer, R.:* Clin. Chem. 19, 1280 (1973).

Stability of NADH-containing Reagent for the Determination of Transaminases on the Greiner Selective Analyzer GSA II

H. Küffer and *P. Degiampietro*, Langenthal (Switzerland)

Key words: Double assay procedure
NADH absorbance ratio 260/340 nm
NADH stability
Transaminase determination

In the determination of the aspartate aminotransferase (AST) and the alanine aminotransferase (ALT) on the GSA II, a blank assay is performed. The assay of the unknown contains L-alanine or L-aspartate, the blank assay contains the same reaction mixture except for L-alanine and L-aspartate. Since side reactions such as unspecific activity of Lactate dehydrogenase (LDH), glutamate dehydrogenase activity in the presence of NH_3, or the reaction of endogenous pyruvate or oxaloacetate, are also measured in the blank assay, the specificity of the determination of ALT and AST is increased.

The double assay procedure on the GSA II permits the start of the reaction with a reagent containing NADH and oxoglutarate. The stability of the reagent could be increased by adding a bicarbonate buffer. The concentration of the buffer was 100 mmol/l, the pH was 10.0. The stability of NADH was observed by spectrophotometric measurement at 260 nm. The value of the 260 nm/340 nm absorbance ratio measured in the reaction mixture at pH 7.4 was maintained at 2.6 for 1 month. Transaminases measured in quality control samples showed no significant deviation over 1 month.

For each determination on the Greiner Selective Analyzer (GSA II), two assays are always performed. This permits a kinetic double assay procedure for enzyme determinations. Several possibilities for a double assay measurement of enzymes have been reported by *Trayser* and *Seligson* [1] and *Küffer* and *Richterich* [2]: In double assays the reaction is started at two different times before reading. However, the Trayser-Seligson procedure is dangerous for routine work where a very large range of enzyme concentration is possible and the approximate enzyme concentration is unknown. This is especially so, if the measurable range is relatively small, as in the UV assay of ALT or AST. It is then difficult to observe whether in one or even both assays the oxidation of NADH is complete.

In the procedure proposed by *Küffer* and *Richterich* [2], the main reaction in the blank assay will not occur, since the specific substrate is omitted. Since with high enzyme concentrations the difference in absorbance reaches a maximum and does not approach zero, as in the Trayser-Seligson procedure, a limit is given which indicates that the analysis has to be repeated with diluted specimen.

Unfortunately, the commercial reagent kits available do not allow one to perform the Richterich procedure for ALT and AST. In the preparation of a new reagent composition, suitable for the GSA II, attention was given to simple handling and long-term stability of reagents.

Materials and Methods

Apparatus

Spectral analyses of NADH-oxoglutarate solutions were monitored with a Zeiss DMR 10 spectrograph. Measurement of enzyme concentrations were done on a GSA II (Greiner Electronic Ltd., Langenthal/Switzerland).

Reagents

All chemicals were purchased from Fluka, Buchs, Switzerland, except the enzymes and NADH which were obtained from Boehringer, Mannheim, BRD. All control sera were obtained from Merz + Dade, Berne, Switzerland.

Stock Solutions

Buffer Solution (EDTA 8.06 mmol/l), TRIS-HCl 124 mmol/l, pH 7.5).

Dissolve 15 g TRIS and 3 g EDTA in about 900 ml distilled water. Adjust the pH to 7.5 with concentrated hydrochloric acid and make up to 1 litre with distilled water. This buffer is stable for at least 6 months at 4 °C.

ALT Substrate Solution (L-alanine 449 mmol/l, EDTA 8.06 mmol/l, TRIS-HCl 124 mmol/l, pH 7.5).

Dissolve 40 g L-alanine by stirring in approximately 900 ml buffer solution. Adjust pH to 7.5 and make up to 1 litre with Buffer Solution. Stable for at least 6 months at 4 °C.

AST Substrate Solution (L-aspartate 225 mmol/l, EDTA 8.06 mmol/l, TRIS-HCl 124 mmol/l, pH 7.5).

Dissolve 30 g L-aspartic acid by stirring and adding by drops 10 molar sodium hydroxide solution in approximately 900 ml buffer solution. Adjust pH to 7.5 and make up to 1 litre with Buffer Solution. Stable for at least 6 months at 4 °C.

Base Solution (sodium hydrogen carbonate 50 mmol/l, sodium carbonate 50 mmol/l, pH 10.0).

Dissolve 4.2 g sodium hydrogen carbonate and 5.3 g sodium carbonate in distilled water made up to 1 litre. Stable for at least 6 months at 4 °C.

Instructions for use

ALT Substrate Reagent (L-alanine 449 mmol/l, EDTA 8.06 mmol/l, TRIS-HCl 124 mmol/l, LDH 12 500 U/l, pH 7.5).

Make up 0.5 ml LDH to 200 ml with ALT substrate solution. In GSA II stable at least one week.

ALT Blank Solution (EDTA 8.06 mmol/l, TRIS-HCl 124 mmol/l, LDH 12 500 U/l, pH 7.5).

Make up 0.5 ml LDH to 200 ml with buffer solution. In GSA II stable at least one week.

AST Substrate Solution (L-aspartate 225 mmol/l, EDTA 8.06 mmol/l, TRIS-HCl 124 mmol/l, LDH 5000 U/l, MDH 11 000 U/l, pH 7.5).

Make up 0.2 ml MDH and 0.2 ml LDH to 200 ml with AST Substrate Solution. In GSA II stable at least one week.

AST Blank Solution (EDTA 8.06 mmol/l, TRIS-HCl 124 mmol/l, LDH 5000 U/l, MDH 11 000 U/l, pH 7.5).

Make up 0.2 ml MDH and 0.2 ml LDH to 200 ml with Buffer Solution. In GSA II stable at least one week.

Cosubstrate Reagent (NADH 0.705 mmol/l, sodium hydrogen carbonate 94.6 mmol/l, sodium carbonate 5.4 mmol/l, 2-oxoglutarate 44.6 mmol/l, pH 8.9).

Dissolve 1.5 g 2-oxoglutarate in approximately 190 ml Base Solution. Add 100 mg NADH and make up to 200 ml with base solution. In GSA II stable at least one week.

Procedure

In the GSA II two times 20 µl are dissolved with 100 µl of bidist. water and distributed into two process tubes. 200 µl of Blank Reagent are added to the process tube leading the blank assay, 200 µl of Substrate Reagent are added to the process tube leading the measuring reaction assay. 6.7 min before reading, the reactions are started in both assays by adding 200 µl of Cosubstrate Reagent. Measurement is made at 366 nm. The difference in absorbance is multiplied by a constant to produce a result in international units at 37 °C *(fig. 1, 2)*. The spectral analysis of the cosubstrate reagent is monitored on a Zeiss DMR 10 against freshly prepared Cosubstrate Reagent where NADH is omitted.

	REAGENT	TIME min x 10	VOLUME I	VOLUME II	ASSAY
	S + DF (X + 100)	100	120	120	
R-1	ALT Substrate Reagent	91	200	–	
R-2	ALT Blank Reagent	77	–	200	
R-3	Cosubstrate Reagent	67	200	200	
	READING	0	520	520	λ = 366 nm

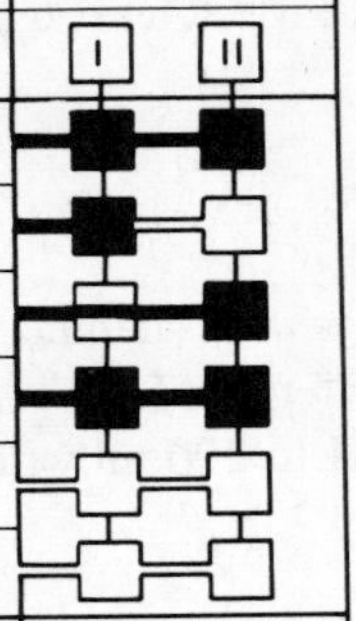

Fig. 1. Method for the determination of ALT on the GSA II.

	REAGENT	TIME min x 10	VOLUME I	VOLUME II	ASSAY
	S + DF (X + 100)	100	120	120	
R-1	AST Substrate Reagent	89	200	–	
R-2	AST Blank Reagent	73	–	200	
R-3	Cosubstrate Reagent	67	200	200	
	READING	0	520	520	λ = 366 nm

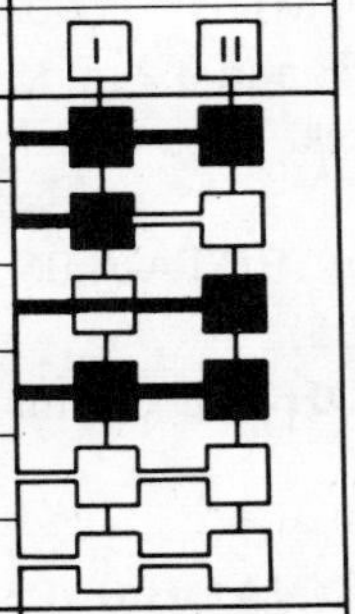

Fig. 2. Method for the determination of AST on the GSA II.

Calculations

Constants: ε (NADH 366 nm) = 3300 litre mol^{-1} cm^{-1}
Sample volume (SV) = 20 µl
Final volume (FV) = 520 µl
Reaction time = 6.7 min

$$c = dA \times \frac{1}{\varepsilon} \times \frac{FV}{SV} \times \frac{1}{t} \times 10^6\ \mu\text{mol min}^{-1}\ \text{litre}^{-1}$$

$$c = dA \times 1176\ \text{U/l}$$

Results and discussion

The daily spectrographic analysis of the Cosubstrate Reagent shows high stability of the reagent. Two solutions observed at the same time show identical results. The absorbance of the Cosubstrate Reagent at 340 nm remains stable over one month. The absorbance at 260 nm slightly increases, probably because of a slow decomposition of 2-oxoglutarate. The measurement of the ratio 260 nm/340 nm, which might be disturbed by the instability of 2-oxoglutarate, follows the increase of the absorbance at 260 nm *(fig.3)*. During the same time and with the same reagents, Monitrol I and II have been measured for ALT and AST in the GSA II. No significant deviation has been observed during the measuring period of over one month.

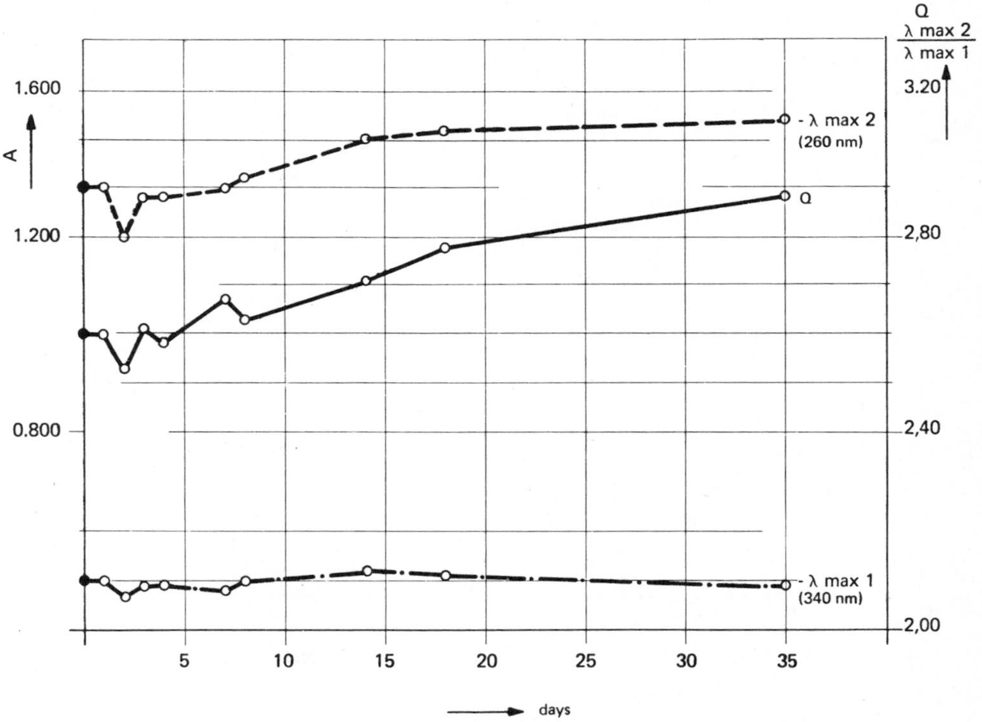

Fig.3. Absorbance of the Cosubstrate Reagent at 260 nm and 340 nm and the quotient 260/340 nm over a period of 30 days.

Over a period of two weeks, the transaminases have been measured in bidist. water, Monitrol XI and Monitrol XII. The measurements were made twice in the morning and twice in the afternoon from Monday till Friday *(tables 1, 2)*. During the whole period, the values for ALT or AST showed no significant decrease nor increase. The day-to-day preci-

Table 1. Evaluation of the stability of the reagents for ALT.

	Zero Solution				Monitrol I X				Monitrol II X			
Day	X_{12}	X_{34}	ΔX_{12}	ΔX_{34}	X_{12}	X_{34}	ΔX_{12}	ΔX_{34}	X_{12}	X_{34}	ΔX_{12}	ΔX_{34}
1	−1	−3	0	−1	19	18	0	0	59	53	2	−1
	−1	−2			19	18			57	54		
2	−1	−4	0	0	17	16	0	2	57	55	−1	2
	−1	−4			17	14			58	53		
3	−3	2	0	2	17	16	1	1	54	52	4	1
	−3	0			16	15			50	51		
4	1	2	−1	−1	12	14	−3	−3	52	54	−2	−2
	2	3			15	17			54	56		
5	−1	3	−1	−1	10	16	−6	2	51	50	0	−3
	0	4			16	14			51	53		
6	4	2	1	−1	16	12	1	2	51	52	−4	1
	3	3			15	10			55	51		
7	6	−3	1	−5	17	16	3	−2	56	53	0	4
	5	2			14	18			56	49		
8	5	5	2	0	15	14	−1	1	53	56	−6	4
	3	5			16	13			59	52		
9	2	2	5	−1	14	15	−2	−3	58	52	4	−2
	−3	3			16	18			54	54		
10	3	2	−1	−4	15	12	0	−5	55	54	−2	1
	4	6			15	17			57	53		
$\bar{X}$					15.55	15.15			54.85	52.85		
S					2.089	2.277			2.834	1.814		
CV					13	15			5	3		
$\bar{X}$		1.300		−0.300		15.35		−0.600		53.85		0.000
S		2.928		1.449		2.167		1.746		2.557		1.962
CV						14				5		

sion of the method calculated with the results of the double determinations [3] was always better than the precision of the daily reconstituted control sera.

We conclude that using a double assay procedure, as in the GSA II, accurate results are produced with a starting reagent containing NADH and 2-oxoglutarate. The stability of the reagents readily permits transaminase determination over at least one week.

Table 2. Evaluation of the stability of the reagents for AST.

	Zero Solution				Monitrol I X				Monitrol II X			
Day	X_{12}	X_{34}	ΔX_{12}	ΔX_{34}	X_{12}	X_{34}	ΔX_{12}	ΔX_{34}	X_{12}	X_{34}	ΔX_{12}	ΔX_{34}
1	2	3	2	3	12	13	−2	−1	45	46	−1	−1
	0	0			14	14			46	47		
2	0	1	−2	−3	9	12	−4	3	42	41	−1	−1
	2	4			13	9			43	42		
3	0	5	1	1	10	14	−4	0	44	45	3	−3
	−1	4			14	14			41	48		
4	3	3	−2	3	14	12	0	−1	47	46	−1	3
	5	0			14	13			44	43		
5	5	5	−2	1	13	13	−3	0	47	48	2	1
	7	4			16	13			45	47		
6	2	2	−1	−2	13	11	−6	1	52	43	−2	3
	3	4			19	10			54	40		
7	4	6	2	−1	13	11	1	−4	48	51	−1	0
	2	7			12	15			49	51		
8	3	5	2	0	12	13	−1	−2	47	48	−1	−1
	1	5			13	15			48	49		
9	5	3	0	−1	13	14	−3	−3	46	47	−1	−1
	5	4			16	17			47	48		
10	2	−1	−2	4	17	14	3	0	47	53	−3	−6
	4	3			14	13			50	59		
$\bar{X}$					13.55	12.95			46.70	47.00		
S					2.259	1.820			3.114	4.449		
CV					17	14			7	9		
$\bar{X}$		3.025		0.1500		13.25		−1.300		46.85		−0.600
S		2.094		2.050		2.048		2.386		3.793		2.210
CV						15				8		

Acknowledgements

We gratefully acknowledge the gift of control sera from Merz + Dade, Berne, the technical assistance of Miss R. Studer and Miss R. Takkinen.

References

[1] *Trayser, K.A. and Seligson, D.:* A New 'Kinetic' Method for Enzyme Analysis Suitable for Automation. Clin. Chem. *15*, 452–459 (1969).

[2] *Küffer, H. and Richterich, R.:* Methodology for Enzyme Determinations on the 'GSA II'. Quad. Sclavo Diagn. *9*, 61–68 (1973).

[3] *Doerr, R. and Stamm, D.:* Methodenvergleich der Gesamteiweissbestimmung im Serum. Z. Klin. Chem. Klin. Biochem. *6*, 304–309 (1968).

The Contribution of Spectrophotometric Instrument Month to Month Variability to the Precision of Molar Concentration Measurements using the Molar Absorptivity Constant for NADH

Two Years of Spectrophotometric Precision Monitoring using United States National Bureau of Standards Absorbance Standards at 3 Absorbance Levels

B.E. Copeland, C.A. Hirsch, D.W. Grisley, A. Doherty and *A. Gough*, Boston (U.S.A.)

Key words: Molar absorption coefficient
NADH
Spectrophotometric variability

The purpose of this paper is to estimate the effect of the use of the NADH molar absorptivity constant upon concentration measurements made using methods which use the NADH indicator system.

The total error due to the NADH spectrophotometer combination will include (1) the day-to-day variability of the spectrophotometer used, (2) the possible systematic errors in the establishment of the molar absorptivity constant itself, and (3) the systematic errors introduced by different spectrophotometers.

There has been a disagreement among experts as to the 'true' value for the molar absorptivity constant. Current proposals by *McComb* et al. [1] and *Bücher* et al. [2] are approximately 1.5% apart.

$$\frac{6.22^{1} \text{ to } 6.31^{2} \times 10^{3} \text{ absorbance units}}{1 \text{ mol/l} \cdot 1 \text{ cm}} = \begin{array}{l}\text{Molar Absorptivity}\\ \text{Constant NADH 340 nm}\end{array}$$

The availability of stable absorbance glass filter standards (NBS) [3] for use in checking the accuracy and day to day reproducibility of spectrophotometer absorbance measurements makes it possible to measure the systematic bias and the expected precision over an extended period.

The use of these NBS spectrophotometric absorbance standards after a two year period will be reported for our spectrophotometers.

Method and Equipment

1. Research level spectrophotometers
   Three DU Beckman Spectrophotometers
   One DBG Beckman Recording Spectrophotometer

2. U.S. National Bureau of Standards [3]
   Glass Spectrophotometer Absorbance Standards
   Standard Reference Material 930
   'Glass Filters for Spectrophotometry'
   Set and Filter Identification Number: 1-88, 2-88, 3-88
   Calibrated for absorbance at 440, 465, 590, and 635 nanometers wavelength
   Office of Standard Reference Materials
   U.S. National Bureau of Standards
   Gaithersburg, Maryland U.S.A.
   J. Paul Cali, Chief

In accordance with the requirements of the College of American Pathologists Inspection and Accreditation Program [4], each spectrophotometer was checked once a month with the series of three spectrophotometer standards at four wavelengths in the visible range. At the same time, a wavelength check was done using a mercury emission source or the helium emission peak. Any significant deviation from standard absorbance values or from wavelength calibration (± 2 nanometers) resulted in corrective repair or maintenance action.

Results

Table 1 shows the results of eighteen to twenty-three sets of absorbance standard readings. The difference in each spectrophotometer total number of readings and the total possible number of readings; i.e., twenty-four, represents down time for that instrument. The spectrophotometers were in daily use in a busy hospital laboratory.

The standard deviation of the average difference between the NBS value and the observed average value is the square root of the sum of the variances. It can be shown that the variance of the NBS value does not contribute to the SD of the average difference.

The precision estimates show a relative standard deviation (coefficient of variation) under actual working circumstances over a 2 year period of 0.77–1.4% at the 0.48 absorbance level; 0.83–1.05% at the 0.68 absorbance level; and 0.78–0.98% at the 0.92 absorbance level. These measurements were made at 440 nm.

The accuracy of absorbance observations on three glass standards by the four spectrophotometers showed respectively (as above) maximum differences of $\pm 0.84\%$, 0.44%,

Table 1. Summary of monthly absorbance standard readings at 440 nanometers wavelength

Filter number:	1–88			2–88			3–88			
Instrument	Mean	SD	RSD	Mean	SD	RSD	Mean	SD	RSD	N
DU # 1	.475	.007	1.40	.680	.006	.83	.934	.007	.78	23
DU # 2	.478	.004	.77	.678	.006	.83	.931	.007	.79	18
DU # 3	.472	.005	.97	.674	.006	.87	.926	.008	.83	21
DGBT	.478	.005	1.01	.678	.007	1.05	.924	.009	.98	18
NBS standard	.476[3]	–	–	.677	–	–	.929	–	–	–
Accuracy range:										
Absorbance:	±.004			±.003			±.005			
Percent:	±.84%			±.44%			±.54%			

$$RSD = \frac{SD}{\text{average}} \times 100 = \text{Relative standard deviation}$$

and 0.54% of nominal value. The United States National Bureau of Standards 'relative uncertainty' estimate [6] for the glass standards is ±0.5% of nominal value (systematic bias 0.4% and precision 0.1%).

Discussion

At each absorbance level the four spectrophotometers had comparable precision values, with one borderline exception. The month to month precision for all instruments averaged 0.92%. The total range was 0.77 to 1.40, with 11 to 12 values between 0.77 and 1.05. These values are larger than those reported [5] for the NBS Carbon Yellow Filter and Chance ON 10 Standard Absorbance Filters in the College of American Pathologists Standards Laboratory – 0.002 and 0.0008 1 SD, respectively.

The 440 nanometer readings were the closest calibration point to the absorbance maximum of NADH at 340 nm. It would be ideal to have a glass absorbance calibration standard closer to the NADH maximum. At present, only liquid standards are available. Until these calibration materials are available from NBS, the 440 nm estimates are used to estimate variability and precision.

When the molar absorptivity of NADH is being determined, the spectrophotometer used should be under strict maintenance and standardization programs which approximate the requirements of the College of American Pathologists spectrophotometer; i.e., monthly wavelength and absorbance calibration.

United States National Bureau of Standards estimates the uncertainty of its absorbance standards as a total of 0.5% absolute. 0.1% represents 2 SD precision estimate and 0.4% represents systematic bias.

The companies producing spectrophotometers do not provide guidelines for precision and accuracy monitoring. No company has as yet given specific criteria for day to day precision or for accuracy relative to the NBS absorbance standards.

Since it is usually practical for regular clinical laboratory procedures to be done as single analyses, the month to month precision estimates would apply. For studies of molecular constants where it is necessary to collect many replicate observations, the precision of the average measurement will be SD average $= \frac{\text{SD individual}}{\sqrt{\#\ \text{observation}}}$

Conclusions

1. The spectrophotometers tested closely approach the 'relative uncertainty' value for the United States National Bureau of Standards. The accuracy of observed values is close to optimum within the present state of the art.

2. Proposed molar absorptivity values for NADH which differ by ±0.8% (i.e., 6.22[1] to 6.31[2])[1] may be due to absolute differences between spectrophotometers. With the present state of the art, a correspondence within ±0.5% would seem to represent the optimum attainable.

3. Of the total day to day inherent variability of methods using the NADH indicator system, an average of 0.92% Relative Standard Deviation (RSD) can be attributed to spectrophotometric variability.

4. A range from ±0.44 to ±0.84% absolute concentration can be assigned to systematic bias between instruments.

[1] $\frac{6.22^1 \text{ to } 6.31^2 \times 10^3 \text{ absorbance units}}{1\ \text{mol/l} \cdot 1\ \text{cm}}$

References

[1] *McComb, R.B., Bond, L.W., Keach, R., Burnet, R.W., Bowers, G.N.:* A Redetermination of the Molar Absorptivity of Reduced NAD. Clin. Chem. 20, 882 (1974).

[2] *Bücher, T., Krell, H., Lusch, G., Grassl, M., Ziegenhorn, J., Bergmeyer, H.U.:* Molar Extinction Coefficients of NADH and NADPH at Hg-lines, Munich, 1st European Congress of Clinical Chemistry, 1974.

[3] *Mavrodineanu, R.:* Solid Materials to Check the Photometric Scale of Spectrophotometers. NBS Tech. Note 544, Menis, O. and Shultz, J.I., ed., p. 6–17, U.S. Government Printing Office, Washington, D.C., 20402 (Sept. 1970). *Ibid.* NBS Tech. Note 584, 1971.

[4] Standards for Accreditation of Medical Laboratories (Revised September 1974). College of American Pathologists, 7400 North Skokie Blvd., Skokie, Illinois 60076, U.S.A., Commission on Laboratory Inspection and Accreditation.

[5] *Copeland, B.E., King, J., Willis, C.:* The National Bureau of Standards' Carbon Yellow Filter as a Monitor for Spectrophotometric Performance. Amer. Journal of Clin. Path. 49, 459 (1967).

[6] Calibration Certificate and Instruction Sheet, Standard Reference Material 930, Glass Filters for Spectrophotometry. U.S. National Bureau of Standards, Office of Standard Reference Materials, Gaithersburg, Maryland, U.S.A.

NAD Quality Control

Standardization of methods for the selection of an NAD coenzyme

S. Schwartz Riera, C. Pascual Mostaza, E. Canadell Anguera, M.R. Segura Cardona, A. Tirado Canals, A. Casals Torrella, Barcelona (Spain)

Key words: Alcohol dehydrogenase
Chromatography
Enzyme inhibitor
Kinetic data
NAD
Spectrophotometry
UV absorbancy

Introduction and Statement of Problem

Several authors have considered the problem of convenient quality control of their analytic results.

This problem becomes of particular importance in enzymatic assays, especially in the measurement of the activity of enzymes which require coenzymes [1, 2, 3, 5, 6, 7, 8].

In this report, we have approached the problem from two classic points of view: assay of β-NAD content and its ratio to other compounds present in the raw product, and assay of the activity of combined enzyme/coenzyme-substrate. We have combined the use of conventional analytic systems with another system to allow quick and easy clarification of quality control.

For these, we use cationic exchange resins that allow separation of different compounds with absorbancy at 260 nm and a single point screening system that demonstrates the enzyme/coenzyme-substrate combination.

The main scope of our work is the standardization of an analytic system that permits the selection of an NAD coenzyme from available sources.

Material

NAD Preparations

The following NAD preparations were investigated:
- NAD SERVA 30311 tetrasodium salt. Purity: 80%–85% total weight.
- NAD SERVA 30311. Purity: not specified.
- NAD BOEHRINGER 15300. Grade II. Control No. 7174246. Purity: 89% total weight.

- NAD GENERAL DIAGNOSTICS. Lot 0918120 from LDH assay kit. Purity: not specified.
- NAD SIGMA. Grade III. Nº D-5755. Lot 101 C-7390. Purity: Approx. 98%.
- NAD SIGMA. Grade V. Nº D-8007. Purity: 99%.

Buffers and Substrates

NAD determination:
- Tetra-sodium-diphosphate-10 hydrate (Merck No. 6591) 75 mmol/l.
- Semicarbazide hydrochloride (Merck No. 7722) 75 mmol/l.
- Glycine (Merck No. 4201) 22,6 mmol/l.
- Ethanol (Merck No. 983) 17 mmol/l.
  General Conditions: pH = 8.7 at 25 °C.

Enzyme

NAD determination:
- ADH from yeast. Alcohol: NAD oxidoreductase EC 1.1.1.1. No. 15418. Boehringer. Control No. 7015418. Crystalline suspension in 2,4 mmol/l ammonium sulphate solution.
  200 U/mg Dilution for kinetic measurements 1200 U/l.

Methods

Spectrophotometric Measurements

Measurements were carried out at room temperature in 3 ml quartz Suprasil cells, 10 mm light path, on a DB-GT spectrophotometer equipped with a Deuterium light source.

1. *Enzymatic measurements of* β-*NAD*
   We prepared aqueous solutions of NAD from the various sources, at a concentration of 1 mg/ml, enzymatically assaying the β-NAD concentration by the following technics.

a) β-NAD
- Buffer: Tetra-sodium-diphosphate/Semicarbazide/Glycine
  Substrate: Ethanol .... 2.90 ml
  Mix and read E_1
- Solution of NAD .... 0.10 ml
  Mix and read E_2
- ADH suspension .... 0.005 ml
  Mix, monitor reaction and read E_3

– Add again ADH .... 0.005 ml

Mix and read E_4

Calculation $\Delta E = (E_3 - E_2) - (E_4 - E_3)$

E_1 = non specific absorbance of product

Calculation of concentration

$$C = \frac{3.05}{\varepsilon \cdot 1 \cdot 0.10} \Delta E \text{ (micromol/ml, sample)}$$

$$C = \frac{3.05 \cdot 0.663}{\varepsilon \cdot 1 \cdot 0.10} \Delta E \text{ (mg/ml sample)}$$

$\varepsilon 340 = 6.22$

2. We prepared the various NAD solutions at a concentration of 100 micromol/l in Sørensen buffers with pH ranging between 2 and 10, and of constant ionic strength at 0.5 mol/l.
   Ultraviolet absorbance spectra between 190 nm and 360 nm were measured in quartz cuvets of 10 mm light path in a spectrophotometer Beckman Acta III, Series Century. Spectra were read against convenient buffer in the sample cuvets. Absorbancy was measured at 209 nm and 260 nm and the ratio 209 nm/260 nm calculated.
3. We similarly measured the spectra, keeping pH at 7 and changing the ionic strength at 0.5 mol/l to 3.5 mol/l.

Cationic Exchange Chromatography

To study the purity of the different preparations of NAD we used an *Unichrome Aminoacid Analyzer,* with analytic conditions as shown in table 1, and assayed elution peaks at 260 nm as well as the area ratio between them.

Table 1. Cationic Exchange Chromatography

Unichrom amino acid analyzer	
Column size	69 × 0.9 cm
Resin	M – 72 (Beckman)
Hight of resin column	48.5 cm
Column flow rate	64.86 ml/h
Column back pressure	12 Kp/cm
Buffer	Sodium citrate (0.2 N)
Run control	70 min
Sample size	0.06 ml (0.25 n mol)
Spectrophotometer	Mod. D B–G T (Double beam operation Beckman)
Cuvette pathlength	10 nm
Wavelength	260 nm
Recorder ranger	100 mv
V. Recorder	0.6 nm/min

Kinetic Measurements

We used the same analytic system as described for the enzymatic assay of β-NAD, but with enzyme concentrations of 1200 U/l for ADH, β-NAD, a Beckman DB-GT spectrophotometer, equipped with a Beckman 10″ recorder, reading at 340 nm, temperature 25 °C and with continuous recording.

Coenzyme concentrations for NAD were 1480 micromol/l, and 50%, 25%, 20% and 10% dilutions of this.

For that solution and each dilution we calculated the rate of absorbance increase Δ E/minute.

Results are illustrated by Lineweaver-Burk plots.

Single-Point Screening System to study Enzyme/Coenzyme-Substrate Combination

For comparison of the effects of different NAD preparations on enzyme/coenzyme-substrate combination, we tested a single point, screening system based on the differences of extinctions obtained in a single period of time for the same concentrations of β-NAD.

Results

All samples of NAD were identically analyzed under the conditions referred to in the previous section. We carried out a minimum of 10 assays for each tested product.

Study of NAD

1. *Enzymatic Measurements of β-NAD*

When making the enzymatic measurements of β-NAD content, we obtained the results, shown in table 2.

Table 2. Enzymatic measurements of β-NAD

NAD	Initial absorbancy (340 nm)	Concentration β-NAD
NAD 1	0.010	75%
NAD 2	0.012	73%
NAD 3	0.0097	83%
NAD 4	0.0060	89%

2. *Deflection of 209 nm Absorbance Peak at 209*

In table 3 we can see that the influence of pH variations using Sørensen buffers, with ionic strength steady at 0.5 mol/l, on the recorded U.V. spectra of NAD from the different commercial sources.

We notice the presence of two peaks, one at 260 nm and the other around 209 nm (fig. 1). The point of maximum absorbancy of the latter may deflect from 209 nm, the deflection ranging from 204 nm up to 234 nm. We studied the deflection of the 209 nm peak of the different types of NAD, classified according to their β-NAD content. We did not find any significant difference (table 4).

Table 3. Deflection of Absorbance Peak at 209 nm

pH	NAD 1 (β-NAD 75%)	NAD 2 (β-NAD 73%)	NAD 3 (β-NAD 83%)	NAD 4 (β-NAD 89%)	NAD 5 (β-NAD 85%)	NAD 6 (β-NAD 100%)
2	213	213	212	214	212	212
3	230	236	230	230	230	234
4	230	230	230	230	230	230
5	216	216	216	218	215	213
6	208	208	209	207	205	206
7	210	210	210	210	205	210
8	213	213	213	213	215	213
9	223	222	221	222	220	221
10	223	224	221	222	222	220

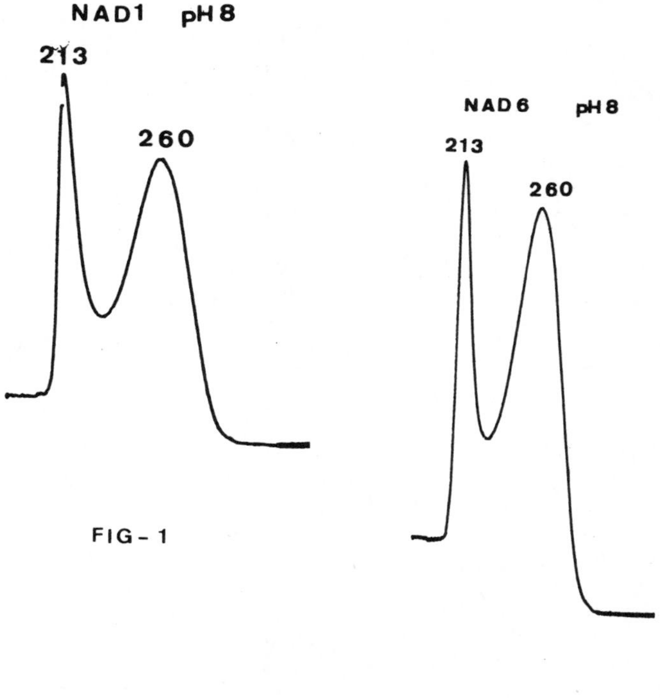

FIG-1

Table 4. Deflection of Absorbance Peak at 209 nm

Correlation		
	NAD 1 (75%) r = 0.9822	With NAD 2 (72%) tg = 1.126
	NAD 3 (83%) r = 0.9886	With NAD 4 (89%) tg = 1.012
	NAD 5 (85%) r = 0.9625	With NAD 6 (100%) tg = 0.974
	NAD 1 – NAD 2 r = 0.9825	With NAD 3 – NAD 4 tg = 0.893
	NAD 1 – NAD 2 r = 0.9817	With NAD 5 – NAD 6 tg = 1.022
	NAD 3 – NAD 4 r = 0.9738	With NAD 5 – NAD 6 tg = 0.8475

3. Maximum Absorbance of the Deflection Peak/260 nm Ratio

In tables 5 and 6 we give the ratio between maximum absorbance of the deflection (209 nm) peak and the absorbance at 260 nm. We did not find any significant difference between the various groups. When studying the influence of ionic strength variation, keeping pH steady (table 7), we also did not find any significant difference between products with different β-NAD concentrations.

Table 5. Ratio between Deflection Maximum Absorbance/260 nm

pH	NAD 1 (β-NAD 75%)	NAD 2 (β-NAD 73%)	NAD 3 (β-NAD 83%)	NAD 4 (β-NAD 89%)	NAD 5 (β-NAD 85%)	NAD 6 (β-NAD 100%)
2	1.191	1.082	1.108	1.143	1.226	1.105
3	0.480	0.500	0.500	0.530	0.500	0.450
4	0.525	0.439	0.500	0.480	0.500	0.370
5	0.822	0.750	0.863	0.931	0.898	0.844
6	1.631	1.438	1.622	1.586	1.575	1.541
7	1.624	1.299	1.404	1.447	1.489	1.476
8	1.179	1.039	1.157	1.020	1.206	1.113
9	0.546	0.398	0.460	0.576	0.598	0.541
10	0.494	0.430	0.448	0.475	0.520	0.411

Table 6. Ratio between Deflection Maximum Absorbance / 260 nm

Correlation	NAD 1 (75%) r = 0.9893	With NAD 2 (73%) tg = 0.8394
	NAD 3 (83%) r = 0.9885	With NAD 4 (89%) tg = 0.9359
	NAD 5 (85%) r = 0.9962	With NAD 6 (100%) tg = 1.0393
	NAD 1 - NAD 2 r = 0.9764	With NAD 3 - NAD 4 tg = 0.9448
	NAD 1 - NAD 2 r = 0.9873	With NAD 5 - NAD 6 tg = 1.0163
	NAD 3 - NAD 4 r = 0.9871	With NAD 5 - NAD 6 tg = 0.9279

Table 7. Influence of Ionic Strength in UV Spectra Keeping pH Steady at 7

Ionic Strength	NAD 1 (75%)		NAD 2 (73%)		NAD 3 (83%)		NAD 4 (89%)		NAD 5 (85%)		NAD 6 (100%)	
	Deflec	Ratio	Deflec	Ratio	Deflec	Ratio	Deflec	Ratio	Deflec	Ratio	Deflec	Ratio
0.5	208	1.754	208	1.581	208	1.527	208	1.555	208	1.562	209	1.611
1.25	208	1.559	208	1.459	208	1.430	208	1.545	208	1.656	209	1.648
3.50	208	1.548	208	1.433	208	1.430	208	1.461	208	1.565	209	1.509

4. *Relationship between Absorbance of Compounds at 260 nm/NAD*

Through cationic exchange chromatography we separated two major fractions, which we shall call A and B. Fraction A is systematically present in smaller proportion and is featured by an elution volume of 12.5 $\pm$ 0.5 ml. Fraction B, shows an elution volume of 45 ml $\pm$ 1 ml. In some chromatograms (figs. 2, 3, 4, 5) other less important peaks can be noticed, and these appear in an inconstant manner.

Comparing the areas under peaks A and B (fig. 2) we see that there is a relationship with the product content of β-NAD (table 8).

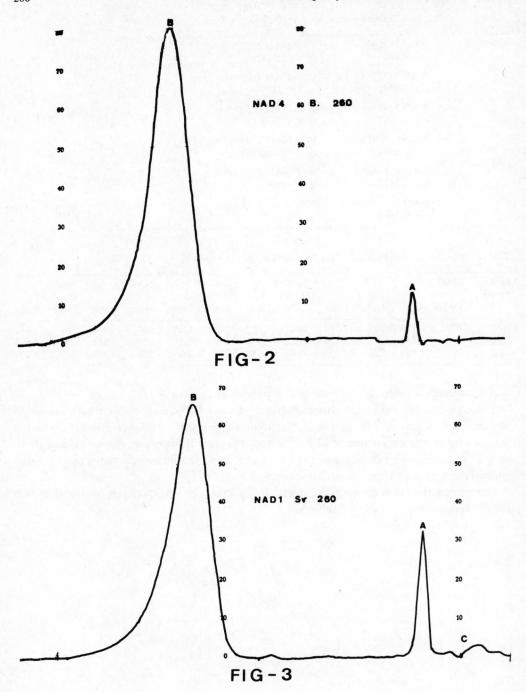

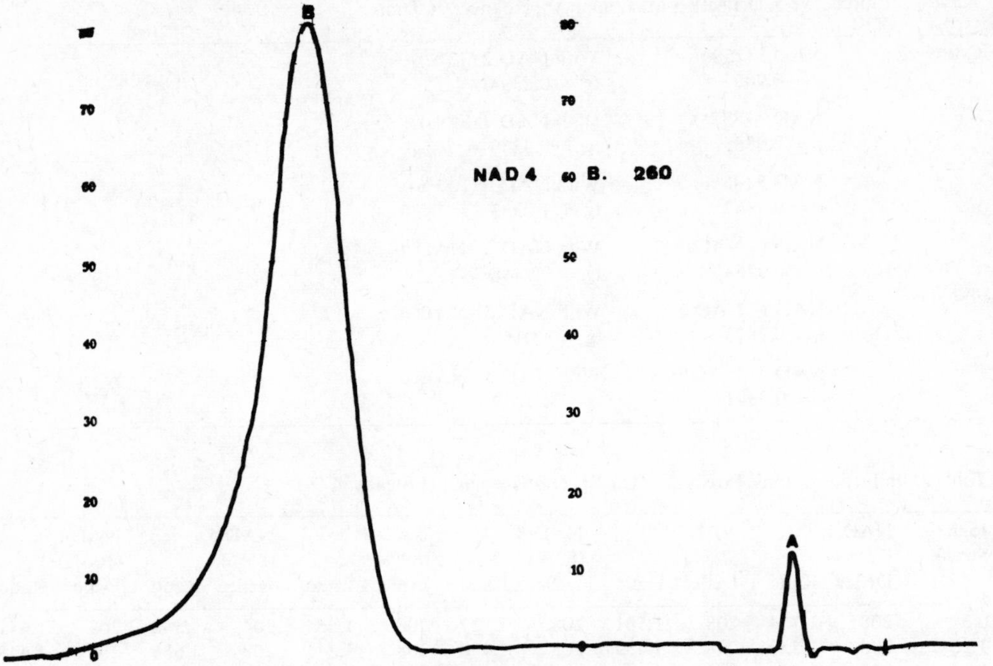
B
NAD 4 B. 260
A
70
60
50
40
30
20
10
0

FIG-2

B
NAD1 Sv 260
A
C
70
60
50
40
30
20
10
0

FIG-3

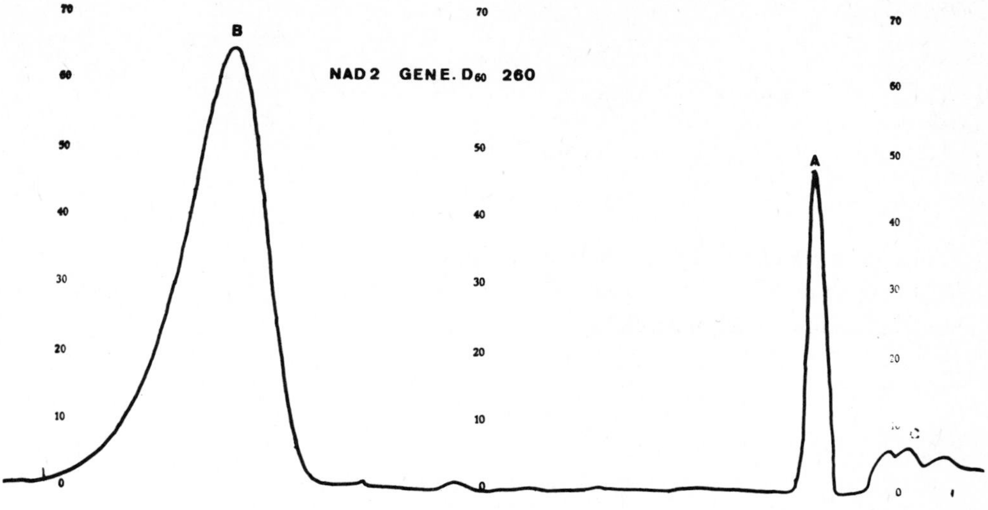
NAD 2 GENE. D60 260
B
A
70
60
50
40
30
20
10
0

FIG-4

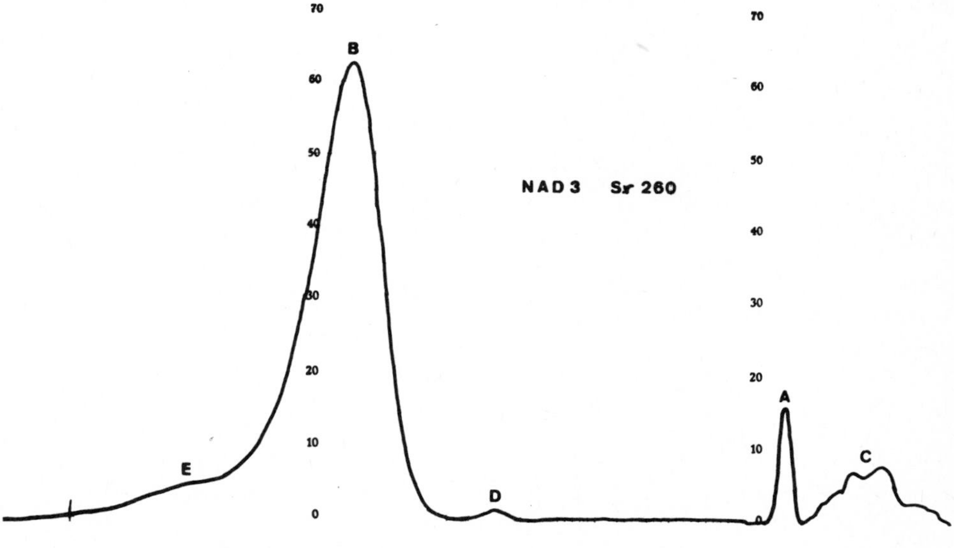
NAD 3 Sr 260
B
A
C
D
E
70
60
50
40
30
20
10
0

FIG-5

Table 8. Ratio Peak A/B

Product	Purity	Ratio
NAD 4	88.9%	0.037
NAD 3	83%	0.058
NAD 1	75%	0.100
NAD 2	73.3%	0.160

5. *Comparison Kinetic Study of Inhibitor Presence*

We obtained the results displayed in figure 6. This shows the presence of competitive inhibitors in the different commercial grade products.

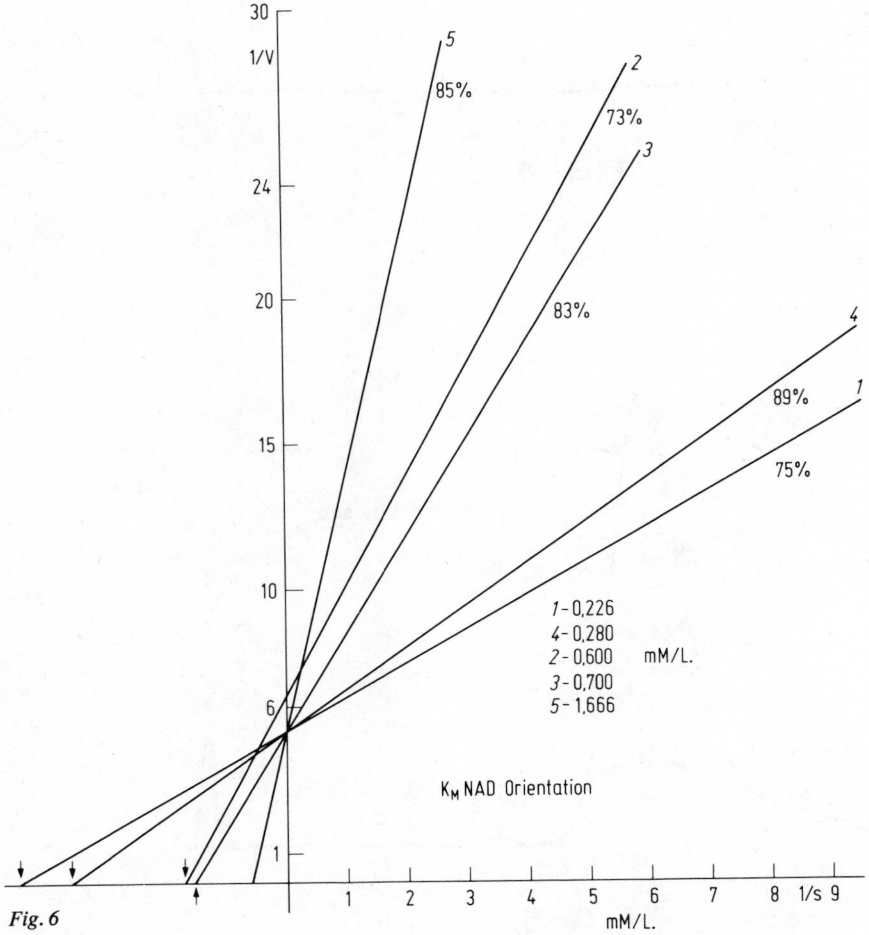

Fig. 6

6. *Single Point Spectrophotometric Characterization of Enzyme/Coenzyme/Substrate Binding*

By placing on the ordinate axis the δ E/m of the reference product, which we consider to be the one containing the least inhibitors and on the abscissa axis the problem product, we obtained a straight line, which specifies:

a) that if the tangent is equal to 1, there is equality of enzyme/coenzyme/substrate linkage

b) that, in comparison to the reference material, binding will be lower the lower the tangent.

Results are displayed in figure 7.

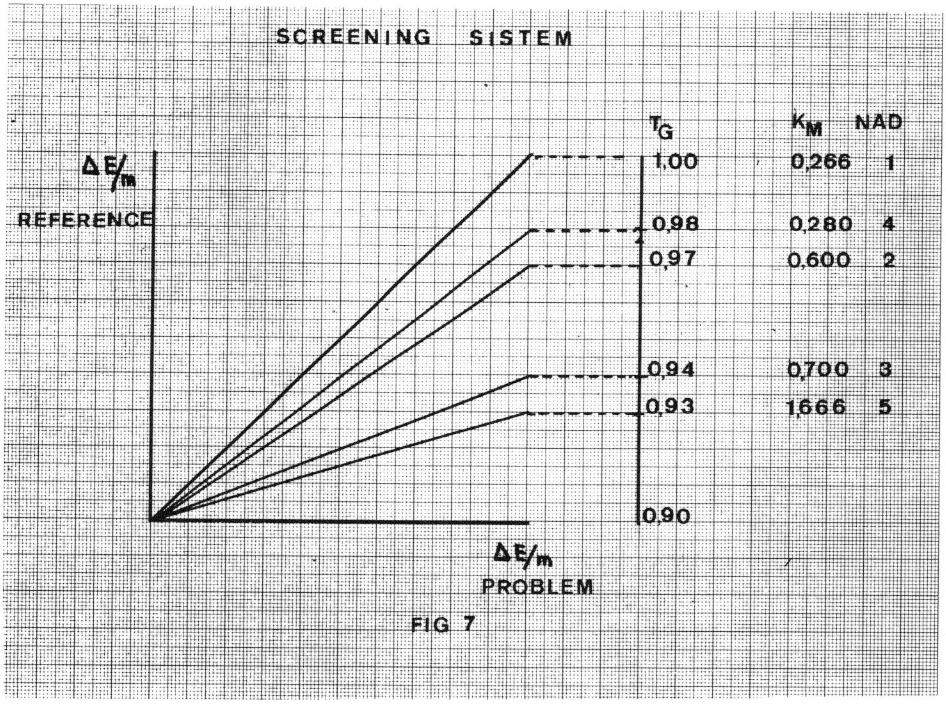

FIG 7

Discussion and Conclusions

We have approached the problem of NAD quality control by combining the use of classic analytical systems with others which allow quick and easy enzyme control.

The work is in two parts. One the study relating to the β-NAD concentration and purity, and the other to the study of the affinity of NAD coenzyme from different sources for a single enzyme/substrate system.

We studied the β-NAD concentration by classic enzymatic analysis, in every case with a perfect agreement of our data with that provided by the commercial firm.

We studied the product's purity by U.V. scanning between 190 nm and 360 nm changing the pH (*Sørensen*'s buffers), keeping the ionic strength constant at 0.5 mol/l, and changing the ionic strength from 0.5 mol/l to 3.26 mol/l, keeping the pH steady at 7.

The results did not furnish any data useful for assaying purity.

Contaminating substances result in absorbancy peaks at 260 nm, as found by *Gerhardt, W.* and *Coll* [6] when studying NADH quality control. These we have been able to remove by cation exchange chromatography.

Comparative study of the chromatograms from different NAD preparations allows us to state that all products show two major peaks. U.V. spectroscopy between 200 nm to 360 nm wavelengths shows that these are symmetrical and homogenous in their composition.

There can also be seen in the chromatograms other peaks of lesser significance and irregularly present.

The enzymatic study of both peaks has shown that the B peak has coenzyme activity.

However, comparison of the areas of the A and B peaks showed that this was related to the product's purity. Moreover, product kept in bad storage conditions showed the biggest number of accessory peaks (fig. 5) and biggest Km.

We studied the relationship of the different NAD coenzymes to a single enzyme/substrate system, estimating the Km's from the Line-weaver-Burk plots.

To simplify the study of the inhibitor we have developed a screening system which compares a coenzyme of known affinity with that of the unknown. With this, placing activity with the reference coenzyme on the ordinate axis and activity with the unknown coenzymes on the abscissa axis, the coenzyme showing the highest tangent will be that having the least inhibitor content.

Since the ΔE required for this plot could be obtained by enzymatic testing of the β-NAD (working with the enzyme properly diluted), a single analytic process can be used to test both product purity and for the presence inhibitors.

References

[1] *Babson, A.L. and Arndt, E.G.:* Lactic dehydrogenase inhibitors in NAD. Clin. Chem. *16,* 254 (1970).

[2] *Bergmeyer, H.V.:* Methods of Enzymatic Analysis. Academic Press. New York N.Y. (1965).

[3] *Bergmeyer, H.V.:* Standardization of Enzyme assays. Clin. Chem. *18,* 1305 (1972).

[4] *Boehringer,* Mannheim: Biochemical information (1973).

[5] *Chilson, O.P., Costello, L.A., Kaplan, N.O.:* Effects of freezing on enzymes. Fed. Proc. *24,* 55 (1965).

[6] *Gerhardt, W., Kofoed, B., Westlund, L., Paklu, B.:* Quality control of NADH. Evaluation of methods for detection of inhibitors and Specification for NAD quality. Scand. J. Clin. Lab. Invest. Vol. *33,* Suppl. 139 (1974).

[7] *Guilbault, G.G.:* Enzymatic methods of analysis. Ed. R. Belcher and H. Freiser. Pergamon Press, Oxford (1970).

[8] Scandinavian Committee on Enzymes of the Scandinavian Society for Clinical Chemistry and Clinical physiology. Recommended methods for the determination of enzymes in Blood. Scand. J. Clin. Lab. Invest. 33, 291 (1974).

[9] Sigma Technical Bulletin n° 106 B March (1972).

A Convenient Enzyme System for the Evaluation of NADH Preparations

J. L. Giegel, J. MacQueen and *G. Anido,* Miami/Florida (U. S. A.)

Key words: Enzyme inhibitors
Hydroxybutyrate dehydrogenase
Inhibitor test system
Lactate dehydrogenase
NADH

Introduction

A great deal of information has been gathered in recent years on the determination of inhibitors in NADH preparations. Much of this work is being presented at this Symposium and it is obvious that one can determine inhibitor levels with a high degree of reliability. There are many approaches to this, but most are beyond the scope of smaller laboratories. During the course of many years of studying the acceptability of NADH we have utilized numerous analytical techniques to determine NADH purity. The most satisfactory method, however, has been the evaluation of NADH by enzymatic techniques. It was our intention in this study to develop a simple system which any laboratory doing kinetic determinations of enzymes could utilize to determine the acceptability of NADH preparations.

We examined two enzymatic systems, LDH and HBD, for sensitivity to inhibitor. As a source of enzyme either pooled normal serum or human erythrocyte LDH was used. In addition, a collaborative study was conducted to evaluate the effect of inhibitor on clinical results.

Materials and Methods

I. Reference NADH Preparations

Commercially available NADH was selected for the study because of its uniformity. Three sizes (1.0, 5.5 and 10 mg/vial) of NADH, lyophilized and stored under vacuum (DADE) were used. Each vial was reconstitued with sufficient volume (i. e. 0.4, 2.5, or 4.0 ml) of distilled water to yield a final NADH concentration of 0.11 mmol/liter in the assay system. This material was found to be identical to a sample of NADH labeled 98% pure (Sigma).

II. Inhibitor-enriched NADH Preparations

Vials of the reference NADH preparation were opened and the contents were exposed to ambient temperature (ca. 22 °C) and humidity (ca. 70%) for 24 hours. One ml of distilled water was added to each vial; the contents were frozen and lyophilized to prevent further degradation. Lyophilization preserves the inhibitor at a constant level.

III. Enzyme Assay Systems

a) *LDH Assay System:* The method of Gay, Bowers and McComb, Clin. Chem. *14,* 740, 1968 was used. The reagent consists of
Buffer: 0.1 mol/liter tris, pH 7.44 (25 °C)
Substrate: 0.75 mmol/liter sodium pyruvate

b) *HBD Assay System:* The method of Rosalki and Wilkinson, Nature 188, 1110, 1960 was used. The reagent contains
Buffer: 60 mmol/liter potassium phosphate pH 7.4
Substrate: 4 mmol/liter sodium α-oxobutyrate

c) *Enzyme Sources:*
1. Pooled normal human sera
2. Purified human erythrocytic extract (see Section IV for preparation).

NADH Assay System

To obtain maximum reproducibility, assay systems were developed for LDH and HBD which contained all reactants except NADH. The reaction was started by the addition of either the reference NADH preparation or inhibitor-enriched NADH as a concentrated solution. In this way, small errors in the volume of NADH added have little effect on the observed activity.

LDH and HBD assay systems were prepared using both the normal serum source and the erythrocyte LDH source. Pilot designations were:

SLC: serum LDH
RLC: red cell LDH
SHC: serum HBD
RHC: red cell HBD

Three ml aliquots of each liquid reagent preparation were dispensed into 9 ml amber vials and were lyophilized. These were stored at 4 °C until used. Pilots prepared with the serum source showed a slight decrease in observed activity following lyophilization due to LD_5 lability.

IV. Preparation of Red Cell LDH

Separation of enzyme protein from hemoglobin was done according to a modification of the Method of *Hennessey* et al., J. Clin. Invest. 41, 1257, 1962. Human blood was hemolyzed and treated with DEAE cellulose at pH 7.0, such that the protein is adsorbed. The protein was desorbed with 0.5 mol/liter KCl, and precipitated with a 50% saturated solution of ammonium sulfate. The precipitate was dissolved in phosphate buffer pH 6.8; excess salt was removed by dialysis against phosphate buffer pH 6.8 (24 hours, 4 °C). Isoenzyme fractionation of the solution indicated that it was mainly LD_1 and LD_2.

Results

The reference and inhibitor-enriched preparations were examined in each of four assay systems. Figure 1 is the LDH assay system using normal serum as a source of LDH and is typical of the results obtained with the other three systems. Several experiments are shown in this figure. To determine the type of inhibition, the amount of inhibitor was kept constant and increasing amounts of reference preparation were added. The results shown in figure 1 are compatible with a competitive inhibitor. Also shown in figure 1 is the effect of adding increasing concentrations of inhibitor-enriched NADH, illustrating the dramatic level of inhibition achieved. Small amounts of inhibitor-enriched material were also added to a fixed, optimal amount of pure NADH. The inhibition observed is quite dramatic, indicating the sensitivity of the LDH system to inhibitor. Similar studies were conducted with different levels of inhibitor in the preparation, and each inhibitor preparation was characterized by physical methods.

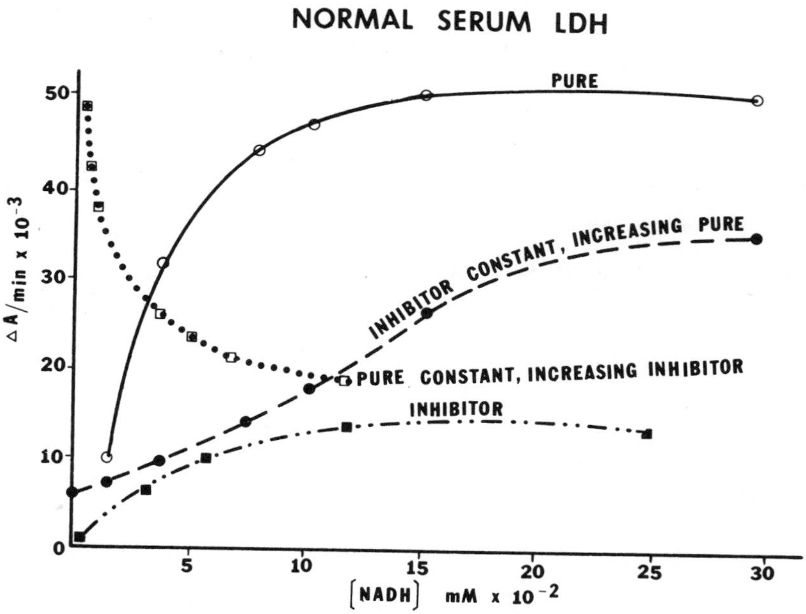

Fig. 1. The effect of Reference and Inhibitor-Enriched NADH on Normal Serum LDH activity. Assays performed at 37 °C.

Figure 2 is an example of the type of correlation obtained between physical measurements and enzymatic activity. Two inhibitor preparations with different levels of inhibitor were compared by their absorbance at 340 and LDH activity. The absorbance and activity of the reference preparation was assigned a value of 100%. One can see that the correlation with 340 absorbance is quite good. As indicated by extrapolation of the graph; it is possible to have some 340 nm absorbing material with no enzymatic activity. Similar studies using the 260/340 ratios gave similar sensitivities. On this basis, it appears that the enzymatic approach should be more sensitive to detecting low levels in inhibitor than would be the determination of physical characteristics.

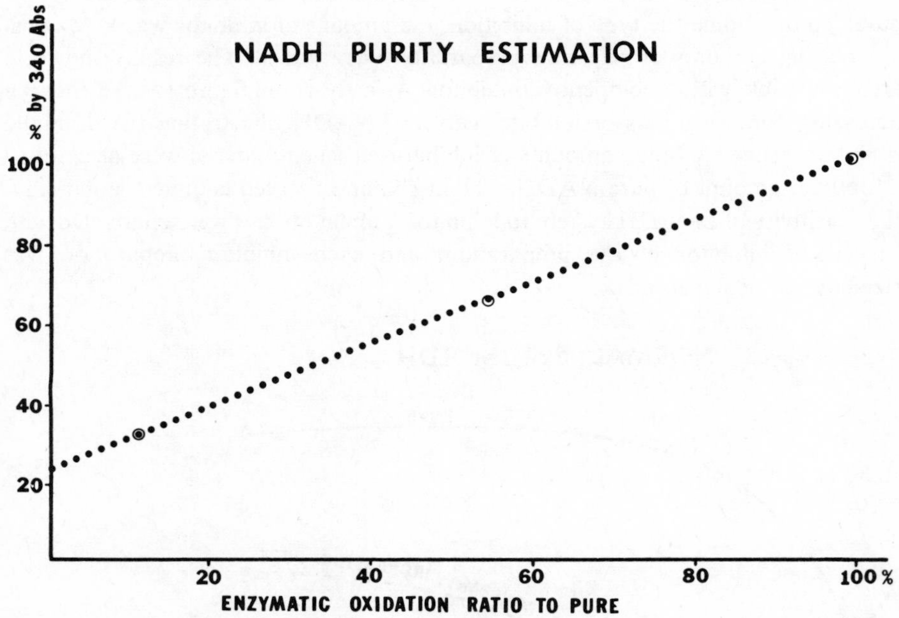

Fig. 2. Correlation between 340 nm Absorbance and observed LDH activity using Reference and Inhibitor-Enriched NADH.

Figure 3 is an example of the spectral characteristics of the NADH preparations used in figure 2. One can see that the 340 nm absorption decreases dramatically while the 260 absorbance increases. Although the 260/340 ratio is more sensitive than the absolute absorbance at 340 nm the extrapolation of this ratio vs. enzymatic activity is still greater than zero, again indicating the inherent sensitivity of the enzymatic measurement of inhibitor.

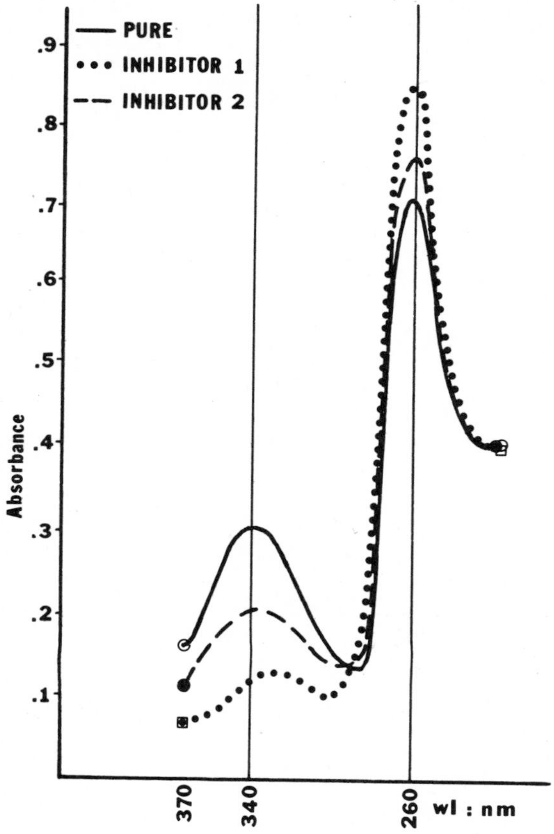

Fig. 3. Spectral characteristics of Reference and Inhibitor-Enriched NADH.

In figure 4 the results with the erythrocyte LDH assay system using the reference and inhibitor-enriched preparations are shown. There is a slight inhibition of activity at high levels of both the reference and inhibitor preparations, however, the percent activity remaining (the comparison of the reference and inhibitor activities at a given concentration) remains fairly constant over a considerable concentration range. Thus small errors in the amount of NADH added have very little effect on the measured activity.

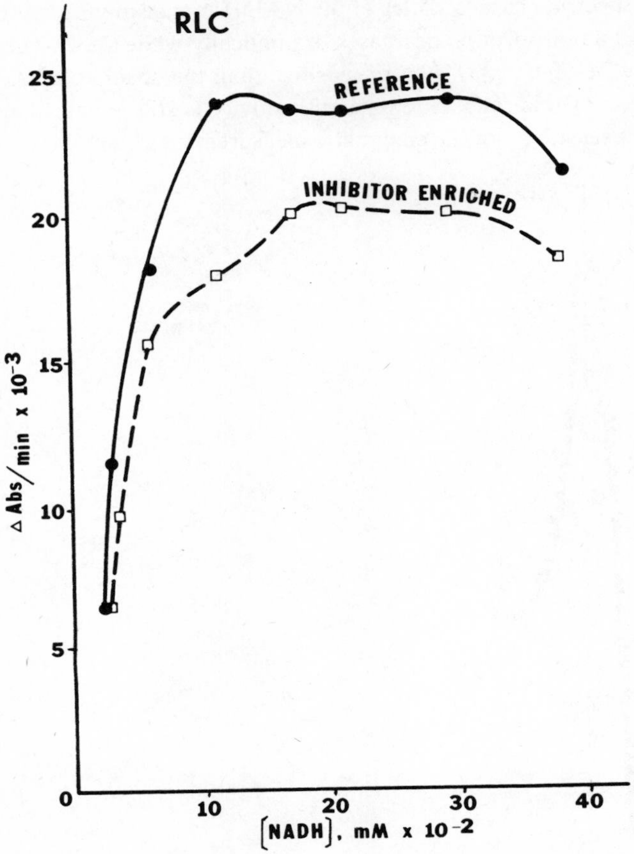

Fig. 4. Effect of concentration of Reference and Inhibitor-Enriched NADH on LDH assay system using Erythrocyte LDH.

Figure 5 is a similar graph using the HBD assay system with normal serum as a source of HBD. Again, the percent activity remaining between the inhibitor-enriched and reference material is fairly constant over a wide concentration range. These observations, shown in figure 4 and 5 were the basis of starting the reaction by adding NADH to minimize pipetting errors in handling the small volume of material. In this way, a pooled assay system can be prepared which contains the LDH source, and large volumes of this can be pipetted quite easily. This approach minimizes the random error in comparing two lots of NADH.

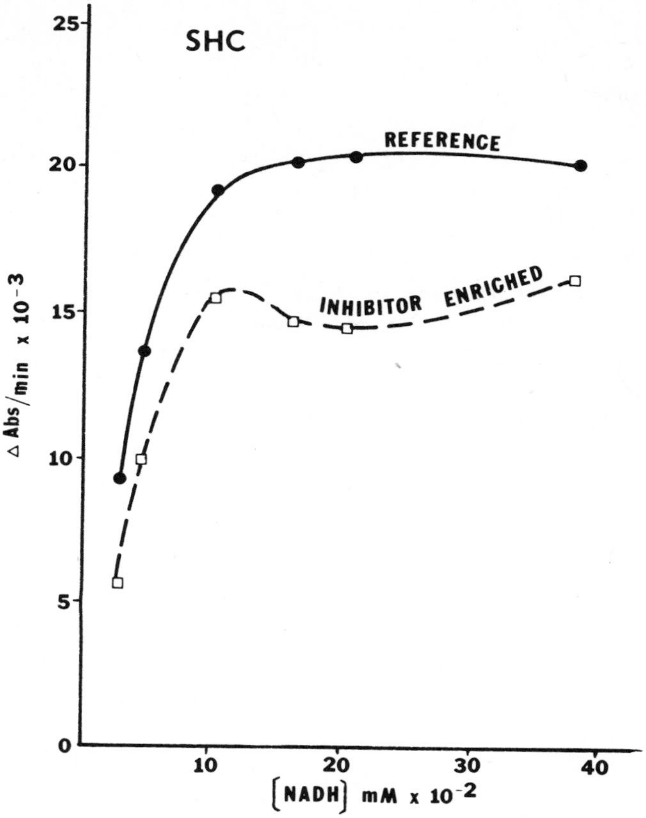

Fig. 5. Effect of concentration of Reference and Inhibitor-Enriched NADH on HBD assay system using normal serum as source of HBD activity.

Collaborative Study

The materials for the NADH assay system along with reagents for the determination of LDH and HBD activity were sent to Drs. Henry and Rappoport for a clinical evaluation using patient specimens under routine laboratory conditions. The goals of this study were first, to determine whether the NADH assay systems provided sufficient sensitivity to detect inhibitor without resort to physical characterization and second, to determine the effect of inhibitor-enriched preparations on LDH and HBD results using conventional assay systems. The results of this study are presented separately by Dr. Henry and Dr. Rappoport at the Symposium.

Summary and Conclusions

Since it is well known that lyophilized preparations of NADH stored under vacuum retain their stability for many years, it is possible for a laboratory to select a reference NADH preparation to compare future lots of NADH for acceptability. This can be done by preparing an LDH assay system using normal serum as a source of LDH and starting the reaction by the addition of a concentrated solution of both the reference NADH preparation and the investigational lot of NADH. Since pipetting errors are minimized in this way, one can determine whether the lot under investigation is different from the reference material with a high degree of reliability. This simple test, coupled with a comparative determination of 340 nm absorbance of both the reference and investigational lot, appears to be adequate for detecting small levels of inhibitor. In the absence of a reference preparation, one must resort to careful spectral investigation of each lot, coupled with a determination of the LDH/HBD ratios.

Clinical Studies of a System for the Evaluation of NADH Purity: Part 1

A. E. Rappoport and *W. D. Gennaro*, Youngstown, Ohio (USA)

Key words: Hydroxybutyrate dehydrogenase
Inhibitor test system
Lactate dehydrogenase
NADH

Clinical scientists have long been concerned with accuracy and precision in their measurements of enzyme activities utilizing beta-nicotinamide adenine dinucleotide (NAD) and its reduced form (NADH). These coenzymes often contain inhibitors, caused by improper purification methods or unsuitable storage conditions, and thus exert a significant effect on reaction kinetics [1].

As part of a project by Dade to develop a system suitable to evaluate the presence of inhibitors in NADH preparations, a clinical evaluation of the inhibitor problem was undertaken at The Youngstown Hospital Association Department of Laboratories.

Pure (reference) and deteriorated NADH preparations and test system samples containing pyruvate and 2-oxobutyrate substrates were furnished a month apart by Dade in two separate shipments. The clinical evaluation included human plasma and red cell LDH samples sent as part of the Dade test system and plasma from selected cases of malignancy, cardiac, liver and miscellaneous syndromes from our hospital population.

Rate reaction studies were carried out on each sample using reference NADH and inhibitor-containing NADH. Studies were performed for both pyruvate and 2-oxobutyrate substrate systems using a Perkin-Elmer ratio-recording spectrophotometer – Model 124-D, employing a thermostatted cell compartment maintained at 37 °C (± 0.5).

Dade Test System Samples

Reaction rate studies were performed on a total of 10 normal human plasma test samples by both pyruvate and 2-oxobutyrate substrate systems. In addition, 10 test samples of human red cell material were studied for enzyme activity in both systems. Reference and inhibitor-containing NADH were used in both systems and for all samples. Per cent activity and inhibition of the reaction caused by deteriorated coenzyme were measured.

Figures 1 and 2 demonstrate the relationship of the two substrate systems employing reference and inhibitor-containing NADH for normal human plasma samples.

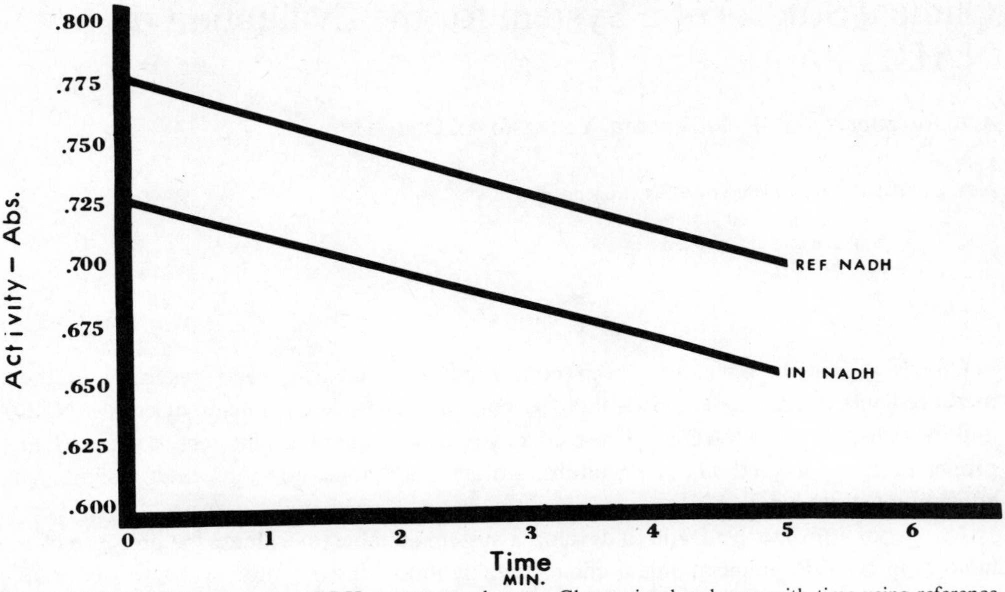

Fig. 1. SLC-101-B human serum LDH, pyruvate substrate. Change in absorbance with time using reference (REF) and inhibited (IN) NADH. Note similar slopes.

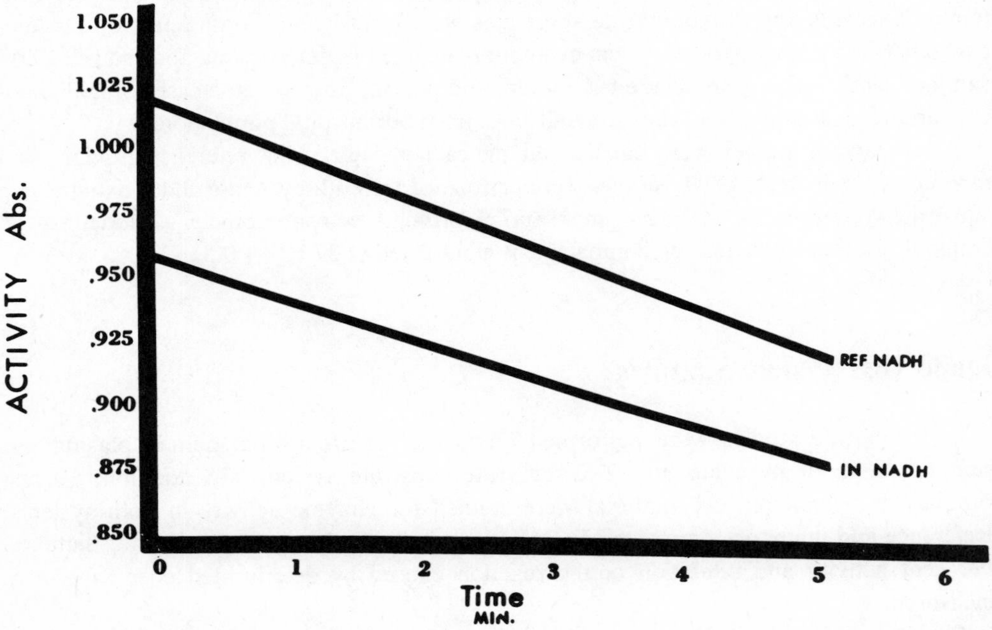

Fig. 2. SHC-201-B human serum HBD, 2-oxobutyrate substrate. Change in absorbance with time using reference (REF) and inhibited (IN) NADH. Note similar slopes.

It can be seen that 'zero' order kinetics are maintained by both NADH preparations. Figure 3 shows the per cent activity remaining with the inhibited NADH for each system and type of sample employed. This clearly shows the slower reaction-rate effect caused by the inhibitor-containing enzyme.

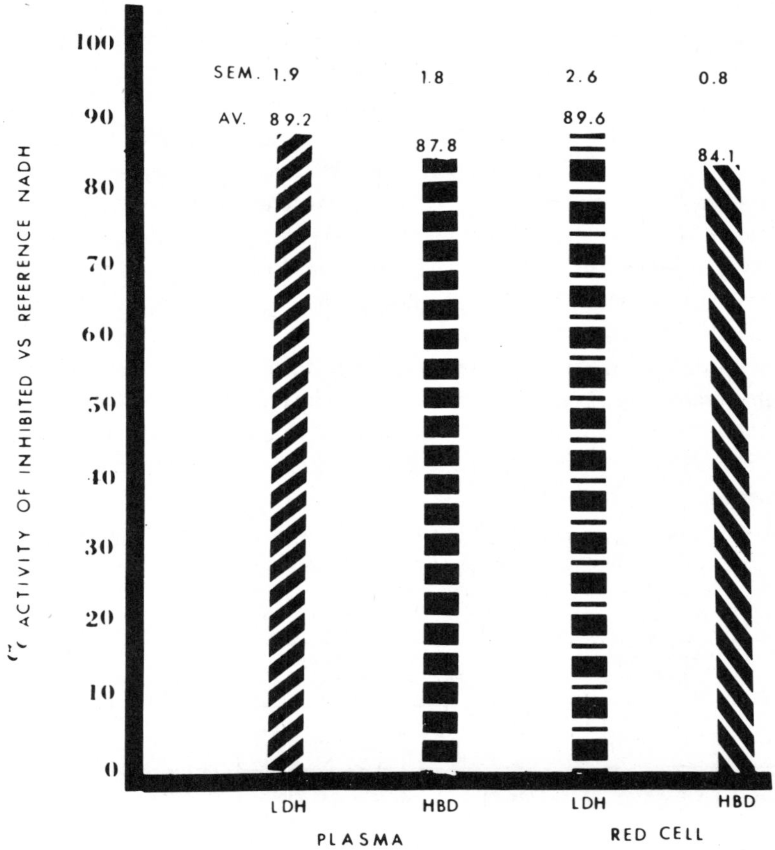

Fig.3. Comparison of LDH and HBD activity in the test system samples plasma and human erythrocytes.

It should be noted that this system which employs test vials containing lyophilized substrate, buffer and enzyme, provides a convenient and simple method to evaluate newly prepared batches of NADH and to maintain quality control for those lots of currently used coenzymes. The system is independent of errors due to pipetting of sample since the reaction is initiated by addition of NADH.

Patient Data and Discussion

Employing the same test format to determine per cent activity remaining when using inhibited NADH, plasma samples were obtained from selected patients and the average change in absorbance/min. was determined in both the pyruvate and 2-oxobutyrate systems. In addition, isoenzyme patterns were performed on all samples using cellulose acetate separation, and quantitation by means of a Beckman Densitometer.

The patients were grouped into four clinical categories where total LDH might be expected to be elevated and where the isoenzyme patterns could be altered. Complete profiles of approximately 30 tests as routinely performed by our automated laboratory were obtained. All data were reduced through a T&T-LDM dedicated laboratory computer connected on-line to an IBM 370/135. Patient order entry and laboratory result transmission was achieved through *Divots* [2, 3]. The clinical information was provided by the attending physicians to substantiate the diagnoses. Where indicated, pathologic anatomic examinations were performed.

Table 1 shows the data derived from a total of 40 patient samples assayed by both the pyruvate and 2-oxobutyrate test systems employing both reference and inhibitor-containing NADH obtained in the 3rd shipment. The average change in absorbance/min. is expressed as per cent activity of the inhibitor-containing NADH compared to the reference NADH reactions.

Table 1. Statistical analysis of % activity and % inhibition of deteriorated NADH – compared with reference NADH in LDH and HBD test systems of normal, DADE, and hospitalized patient's samples.

	LDH		HBD	
	Patient Samples	DADE Test Samples	Patient Samples	DADE HBD Test Samples
NO. OF SAMPLES	40	20	40	20
MEAN % ACTIVITY OF INHIBITED NADH	86.2	89.4	86.4	85.9
MEAN % INHIBITION	13.8	10.6	13.6	14.1
RANGE % INHIBITED ACTIVITY	72-110	72-100	73-105	78-100
SD	11.0	7.1	5.0	4.7
COV. (%)	12.8	7.9	5.8	5.5
SEM.	1.67	1.59	0.8	1.05

The range of per cent activity, SD, CV and SEM are included in table 1. It can be seen that the mean per cent activity with the inhibited NADH is very close for patient and Dade test samples in both assay systems. Whereas the mean per cent activity in the LDH patient system is smaller, the spread of results around the mean is considerably wider and thus shows a larger SD and CV. Since the data in table 1 are in terms of per cent activity of the inhibited NADH reaction compared to the reference coenzyme reaction, one would expect patient LDH system results to resemble those observed in the Dade samples. This correlation is present in the HBD system. One possible explanation for the discrepancy seen in the patient pyruvate system may be found in the fact that these seriously ill people exhibited wide variations and considerably elevated total LDH values. Such differences in LDH activity were not encountered in the Dade samples which were derived from normal subjects.

Shifts in isoenzyme subunits observed in our patient population also may have contributed to the wide spread of per cent activity around the mean value in the LDH assay system.

Consistent patterns of more or less per cent activity were not demonstrated in our patient samples where total LDH was significantly elevated, compared with patients possessing normal total LDH.

Table 2. % activity and inhibition caused by deteriorated NADH compared with reference NADH in LDH and HBD determinations in various clinical conditions.

PATIENT DATA-SECOND STUDY		CANCER-LEUKEMIA	CARDIAC	LIVER	MISCELLANEOUS
	NO. OF PATIENTS	5	3	8	3
L	MEAN % ACTIVITY OF INHIBITED NADH	74.2	78.3	78.6	73.3
D	MEAN % INHIBITION	25.8	21.7	21.4	26.7
H	SD.	6.1	1.5	3.7	0.6
	COV.(%)	8.3	1.9	4.7	0.8
PATIENT DATA-THIRD STUDY					
	NO. OF PATIENTS	10	10	4	11
L	MEAN % ACTIVITY OF INHIBITED NADH	93.4	81.0	86.3	85.7
D	MEAN % INHIBITION	6.6	19	13.7	14.3
H	SD.	19.6	5.1	5.3	7.8
	COV.(%)	20.9	6.3	6.1	9.1
H	MEAN % ACTIVITY OF INHIBITED NADH	86.1	85.8	84.1	88.1
B	MEAN % INHIBITION	13.9	14.2	15.9	11.9
D	SD	6.9	1.7	1.8	6.8
	COV.(%)	8.0	2.0	2.1	7.7

A correlation was made of our derived patient data for both pyruvate and 2-oxobutyrate test systems in terms of four clinical categories as shown in table 2. Two separate groups of patient studies are shown since the NADH preparations, furnished to us at different times, appeared to yield different activities. The second study indicates that the mean per cent inhibition of the reaction for the LDH system is consistent in all four clinical groups. The third study data show rather consistent per cent inhibition of the LDH reaction except in the Cancer-Leukemia group whose ten patients display a rather marked diminution in per cent inhibition. This decrease in per cent inhibition was not observed in the HBD system for the same patients.

Isoenzyme patterns with subunit elevations were correlated to the disease syndromes. Typical isoenzyme patterns of the disease were not observed in all cases, although it is admitted that we may have missed the characteristic patterns usually seen at optimal times. However, adequate correlation existed to allow analysis of per cent activity of inhibited NADH in the LDH and HBD test systems in terms of isoenzyme subunit changes, as depicted in figure 4.

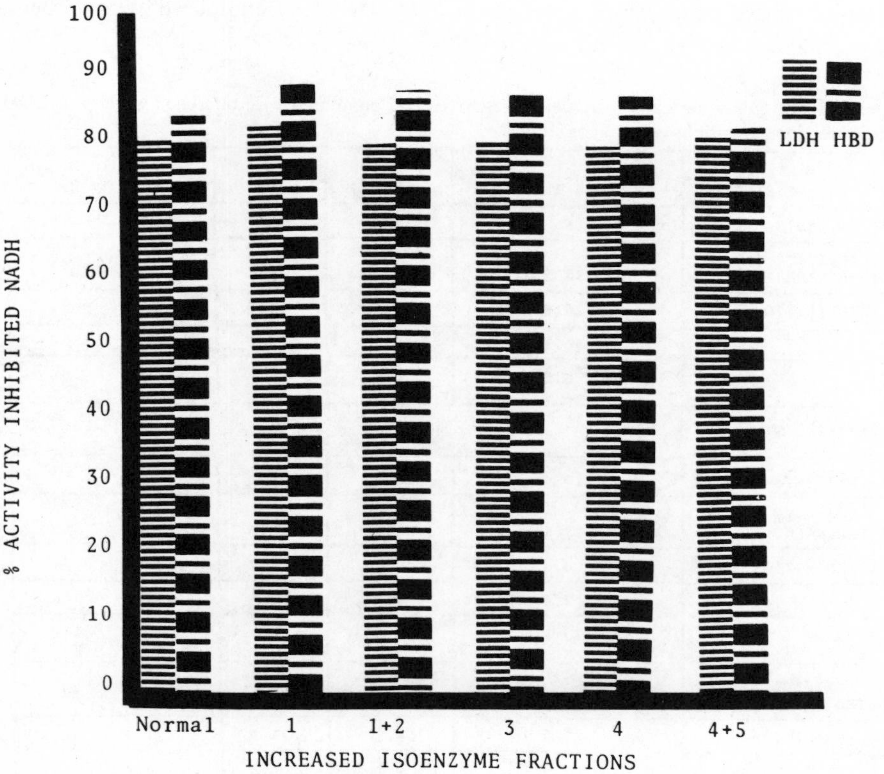

Fig. 4. Comparative data showing % activity of inhibited NADH vs. Reference NADH in LDH and HBD test systems of patient samples correlated with isoenzyme patterns.

This clearly shows that greater per cent activity is displayed by inhibited NADH in the 2-oxobutyrate system than in the pyruvate system. This is in agreement with *Rosalki* [4] and with *Glenn* [5], who found that the humidity induced, inhibitor in NADH preparations regularly inhibits the reaction rate with pyruvate substrate to a greater degree than with 2-oxobutyrate.

Our patient sample data fail to disclose any significant increase or decrease in per cent activity of inhibited NADH as compared to reference NADH when increases in subunits LD_1, LD_2, LD_3, LD_4, and LD_5 were observed. Small differences in mean values were encountered, but these variations are well within the standard error of the methods employed.

Summary

Evaluation of the Dade system for testing inhibitor-containing NADH preparations, demonstrates no consistent evidence that factors other than purity of NADH contributed to the rate of the reaction, assuming that all procedural and environmental factors such as pH, temperature, etc. are standardized.

Our data, with few exceptions, substantiate previous observations that the presence of inhibitors in NADH preparations cause significant decreases in activity for both pyruvate and 2-oxobutyrate substrate systems. These are technically significant since such systematic errors could yield apparent good precision data but poor accuracy, and thus lead to erroneous clinical interpretations.

Acknowledgement

This project was supported by *Grant* No. HS 00060-05 from the PHS Health Resources Administration and Division of Health Systems Design and Development.

References

[1] *Gerhardt, W., Kofoed, B., Westlund, L., and Pavlu, B.:* Quality Control of NADH. Supplement of Scand. J. Clin. Chem. 1974.

[2] *Rappoport, A.E.:* 2001 Today: Computer That Talks Tells Doctors Laboratory Findings. Modern Healthcare, p. 16m–16p, February 1975.

[3] *Rappoport, A.E.:* An On-Line Centralized Computer-Coupled Automated Laboratory Information System Using Touch-Tone Card Dealer Telephone and Audio-Response Technology for Test Order Entry and Result Retrieval. National Computer Conference, Anaheim, California, May 21, 1975.

[4] *Rosalki, S.B.:* Accuracy Assessment from Reference Methods: Isoenzyme Reference Methods with Special Reference to Hydroxybutyrate Dehydrogenase Determination. Progress in Quality Control in Clinical Chemistry. Transactions of the 5th International Symposium, Geneva 1973. Hans Huber Publ., Vienna 1973.

[5] *Glenn, J.H.:* Study of an Enzyme Inhibitor formed from reduced Nicotinamide-Adenine Dinucleotide and its effects on the Assay of Lactate Dehydrogenase. M. Sc. Thesis, University of Surrey 1972.

Clinical Studies of a System for the Evaluation of NADH Purity: Part 2

J. B. Henry and *G. W. Sage*, New York (USA)

Key words: Hydroxybutyrate dehydrogenase
Inhibitor test system
Lactate dehydrogenase
NADH

Much concern has been expressed recently about the formation of inhibitors in reduced nicotinamide adenine dinucleotide (β-NADH or simply NADH) by exposure to atmospheric gases, water vapor, low pH, etc. and the effect of such NADH with inhibitor on enzymatic assays employing this coenzyme [1, 2, 3, 4, 5]. Various investigators have sought methods of determining and specifying NADH quality, preserving it from degradation and developing a standard reference material [1, 4, 5].

Results which show that human liver LDH M 4 is less sensitive to small inhibitor concentrations than human heart H 4 [1, 5] raise the possibility that there may be some clinical use for inhibited NADH. The percent inhibition compared with a reference NADH (i.e., NADH without apparent inhibitor) might bear a relationship to certain diseases states or isoenzyme distributions. The ratio of pyruvate to 2-oxobutyrate activity, which is also a function of inhibitor concentration and 2-oxobutyrate concentration [1, 5], might be another such indicator.

In view of these considerations, the objectives of this study were to:

1. Evaluate a reference system to assay NADH in terms of inhibition.
2. Identify the effect of inhibited NADH versus a reference form of the coenzyme in clinical enzyme assays of lactate dehydrogenase[1] (LDH) with pyruvate and 2-oxobutyrate as substrate. The latter will be referred to as hydroxybutyrate dehydrogenase (HBD).
3. Quantify the effect of inhibited NADH versus a pure (reference) form in clinical enzyme assays of LDH and HBD.
4. Delineate the effect of LDH isoenzymes using inhibited versus reference NADH.

Dade[2] prepared reference systems discussed in a previous paper by Dr. *Giegel* and his associates, with which to assess the pure and inhibited NADH preparations. These

[1] L-Lactate: NAD oxidoreductase EC 1.1.1.27

[2] Dade, Division of American Hospital Supply Corp., Miami, Florida 33152

reference systems contained lyophilized human serum or erythrocyte LDH, buffer and pyruvate or 2-oxobutyrate substrate and are referred to as SLC, RLC, SHC and RHC respectively. The reference systems were reconstituted with distilled water. Since they contained the enzyme, buffer and substrate, pipetting errors were minimized. Pure or inhibited NADH was then added, the rates measured, and the activity with inhibited and pure NADH determined prior to expression as percent (%) of inhibited over pure NADH activity.

LDH and HBD activity were then measured using the reference system with pure and inhibited NADH for 32 patient specimens covering a wide range of diseases, lysed normal human erythrocytes and tissue extracts from heart, liver and skeletal muscle obtained post mortem. Again the percent activity with inhibited NADH was determined.

Experimental procedure

The reference systems, SLC, SHC, RLC, and RHC were reconstituted with 3 milliliters of distilled water and incubated at 37 °C. One hundred µl of NADH was added, the sample mixed by inverting it several times and rapidly transferred to a preheated cuvette in a Gilford[3] 2000 spectrometer. The initial change of absorbance per minute at 340 nm was measured. The cell compartment was maintained at 37 °C (±0.5 °C). Typical curves for these systems are displayed in figures 1 and 2. The curves are linear, i.e., the systems obey zero order kinetics, for five or more minutes. All reagents as well as the pure and inhibited NADH were supplied by Dade.

[3] Gilford Instruments Laboratories, Inc., Oberlin, Ohio 44074

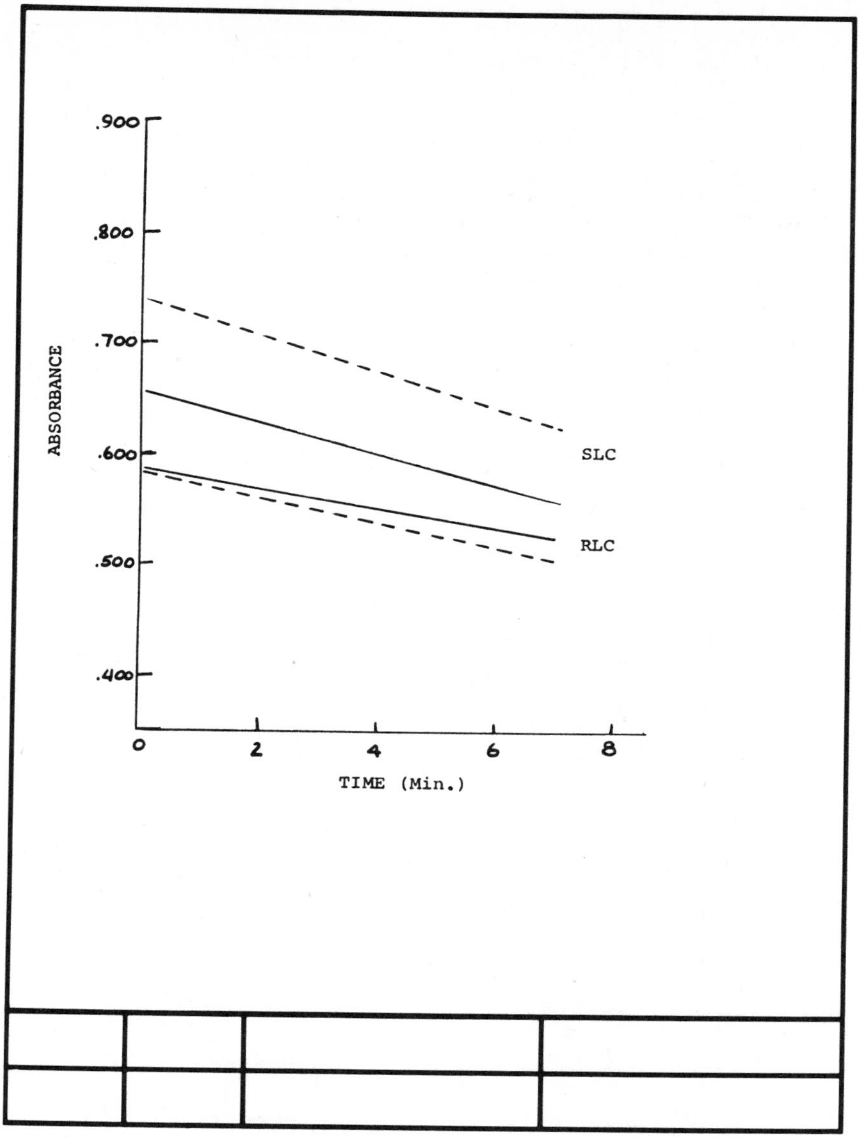

Fig. 1. Absorbance vs. time for SLC-101 B (Human serum) and RLC-302 B (Red cell) – Pyruvate substrate reference systems.
Solid lines: Inhibited NADH
Dashed lines: Reference NADH

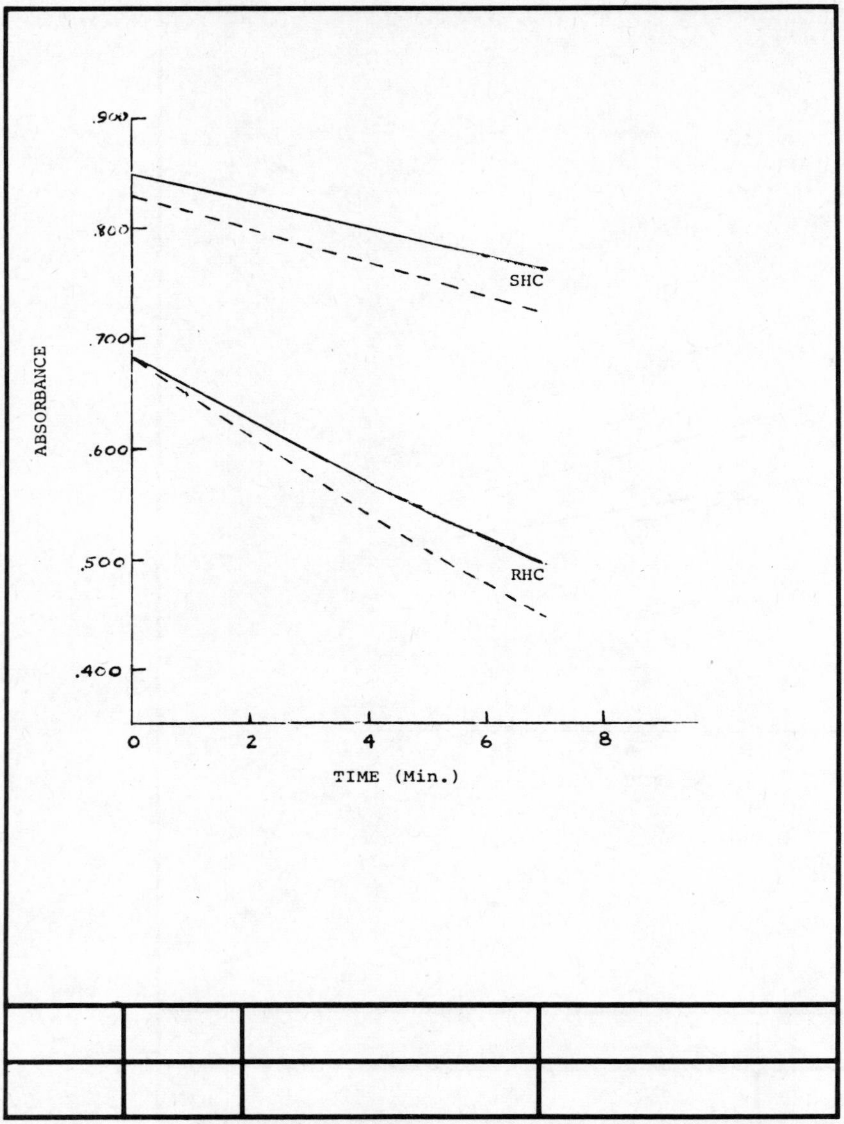

Fig. 2. Absorbance vs. time for SHC-201 B (Human serum) and RHC-402 B (Red cell) – HBD substrate reference systems.
Solid lines: Inhibited NADH
Dashed lines: Reference NADH

Patient specimens were measured by incubating 3 milliliters of pyruvate or 2-oxybutyrate substrate at 37 °C adding 50 microliters of specimen and proceeding as for the reference systems. Once the patient specimen was added, the solution was incubated for less than one minute prior to assay. Although our procedure departed from the usual Dade LDH and HBD procedure, it permitted patient specimens and reference systems to be handled in an analogous fashion using the same vials of reference and inhibited NADH.

Results

The activity of the reference systems using pure and inhibited coenzyme is shown in table 1. The day-to-day precision obtained with inhibited NADH did not compare favourably with the pure material. This shows, as one would expect, that it is more difficult to preserve a deteriorated product than a pure one. The average percent decrease in activity of the reference systems was 18.5%.

Table 1. Results with reference systems.

System	$NADH_2$	#	Mean (A/Min.)	S.D. (A/Min.)	C.V.	$\frac{\text{Inhibited}}{\text{reference}} \times 100$
SLC	Reference	9	.0171	.0007	4.1%	85%
	Inhibited	9	.0144	.0011	7.6%	
RLC	Reference	9	.0117	.0010	8.9%	81%
	Inhibited	9	.0095	.0015	15.4%	
SHC	Reference	9	.0166	.0010	6.3%	79%
	Inhibited	9	.0131	.0013	9.6%	
RHC	Reference	9	.0332	.0017	5.0%	81%
	Inhibited	9	.0270	.0027	10.0%	

Patient specimens whose activity was measured for LDH and HBD activity also had their LDH isoenzymes determined using Corning[4] ACI electrophoresis system and scanned with quantification employing a Clifford[5] densitometer. Diagnoses were arrived at from an analysis of clinical information and laboratory data.

Although we had hoped to group patients into categories according to disease state or prominent isoenzyme band, most of the patients had complications or multiple conditions which precluded such an allocation. An example of this problem is that of C.P. whose Zymogram is shown in figure 3. Although she had hepatitis and a markedly elevated

[4] Corning Scientific Instruments, Medfield, Massachusetts 02052
[5] Clifford Instruments, Inc., Natick, Massachusetts 01760

bilirubin, slow moving LDH 4 and 5 isoenzymes are not the most prominent isoenzymes. Furthermore, 32 patients did not constitute a sufficiently large sample to generate a sizeable number of patients in any category.

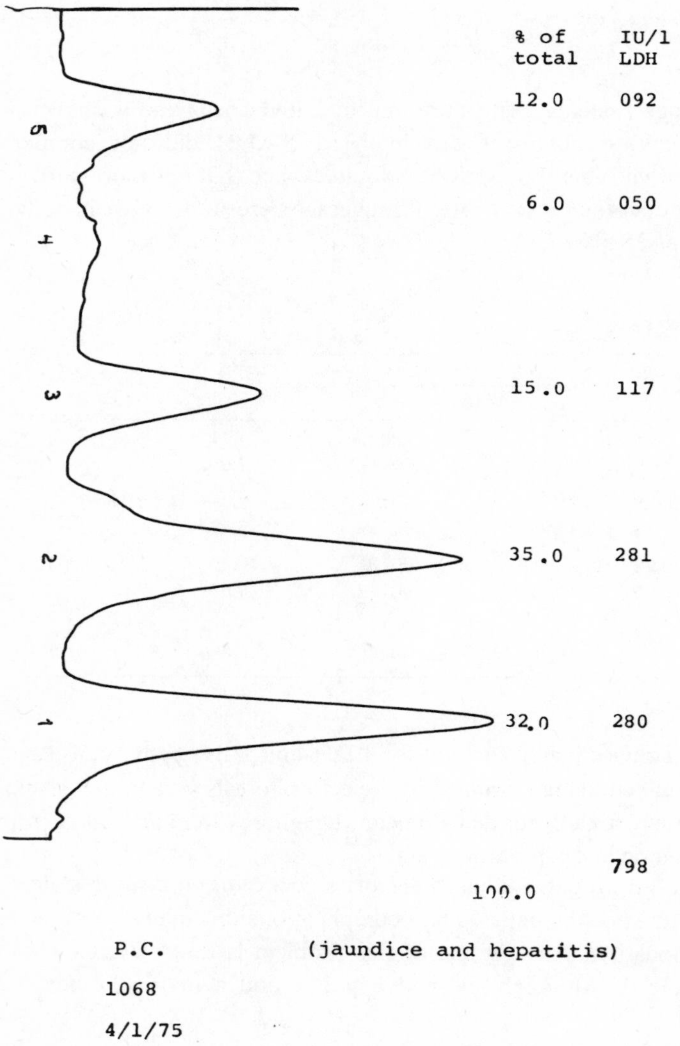

Fig. 3. Zymogram of serum from patient with jaundice and hepatitis.

Figures 4 and 5 show our results of percent activity with inhibited NADH for LDH and HBD. Patients with apparently 'uncomplicated' liver disease or myocardial infarction are so indicated. Results with tissue extracts and reference systems are shown for comparison. The mean percent activity with inhibited NADH for patient specimens were 75 and 80% for LDH and HBD, respectively. Our inhibition of *both* the patients and the reference samples was somewhat greater than that obtained in the preceding paper at the Youngstown Hospital Association which would indicate differences in the NADH which developed in shipping or storage. The extent of inhibition was the same with different specimens obtained from the same patient.

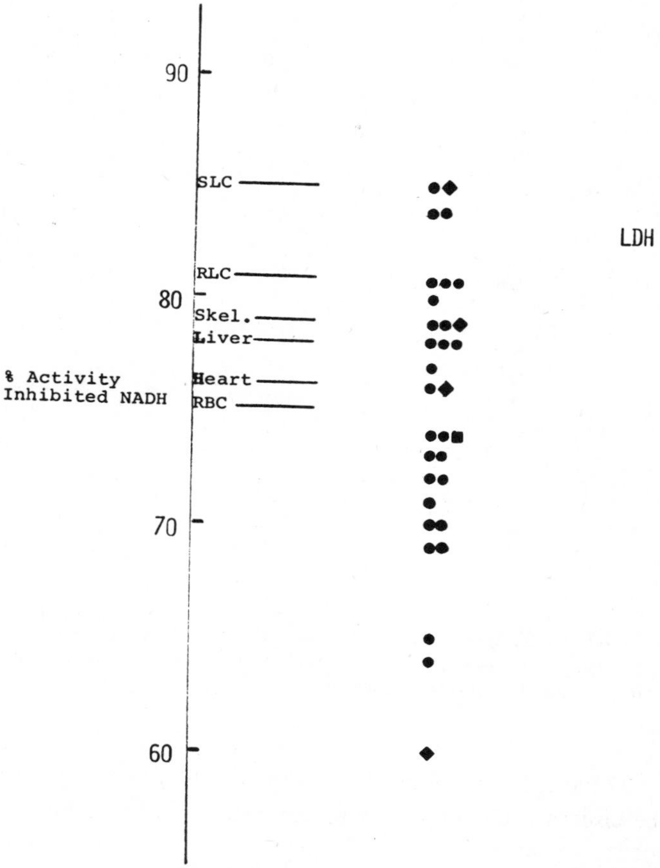

Fig. 4. % activity inhibited NADH for LDH with 32 patient specimens, tissue extracts, and reference systems. Specimens denoted with a diamond or a square are cases where clinical findings and isoenzyme patterns are primarily consistent with a myocardial infarction or liver disease respectively.

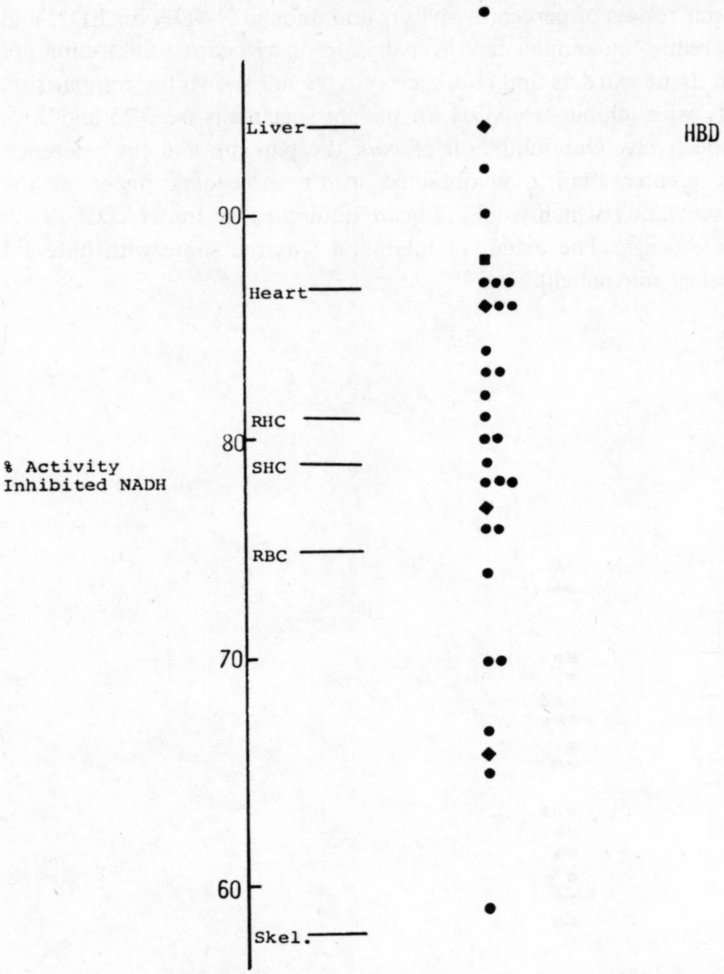

Fig. 5. % activity inhibited NADH for HBD with 32 patient specimens, tissue extracts and reference systems. Specimens denoted with a diamond or a square are cases where clinical findings and isoenzyme pattern are primarily consistent with a myocardial infarction or liver disease respectively.

The percent inhibition for the 32 patients range from 15 to 40% for LDH and 1 to 41% for HBD. No patterns could be discerned by comparing the percent activity of inhibited NADH with disease state or isoenzyme pattern.

Figure 6 shows the percent ratio HBD : LDH (R) of inhibited NADH for the patients studied. The mean value obtained for patients was 1.12. Once again the values of this ratio revealed no correlation with disease states.

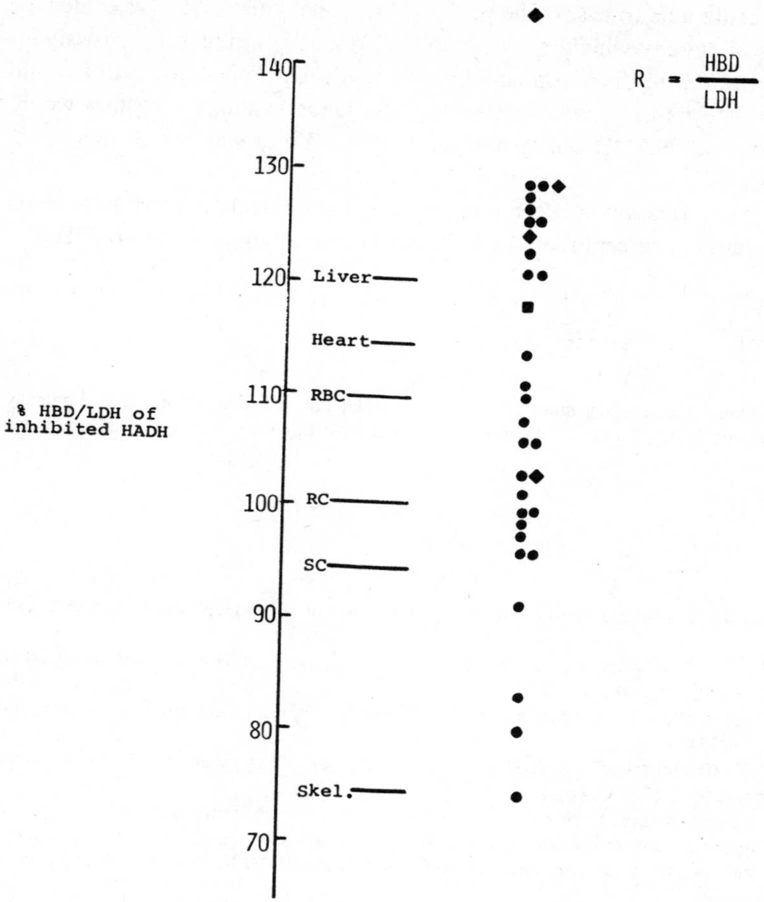

Fig.6. % ratio HBD/LDH for inhibited NADH with 32 patient specimens, tissue extracts, and reference systems. Specimens denoted with a diamond or a square are cases where clinical findings and isoenzyme pattern are primarily consistent with a myocardial infarction or liver disease respectively.

Conclusion

The assay system developed by Dade for the evaluation of NADH purity was evaluated, and we conclude that this is a practical and sensitive system for assessing NADH quality. When the evaluation system was prepared from erythrocytes, RLC and RHC did not seem to offer any advantages over that prepared from serum, SLC and SHC, to justify the additional cost of the product.

The importance of being able to assess the purity of the coenzyme NADH is evidenced by the substantial loss of activity which results from the presence of inhibitors. Grossly inaccurate enzyme values and misdiagnosis could easily result. Of course, a control would ordinarily be used to detect this problem. However, the Dade evaluation system would enable one to check out the NADH purity independently and in a way which minimizes errors due to pipetting.

From our pilot study, no relation between disease state or isoenzyme pattern in patients was manifest by differences in percent reduction of activity of pure to inhibited NADH.

Acknowledgement

We wish to thank the Clinical Chemistry staff at the S.U.N.Y. Upstate Medical Center and especially *Carole Ozark, Joseph Yourno,* M.D., *Lawrence Virgilio,* M.D. and *Rita Carmen* for their assistance in this project.

References

[1] *Gerhardt, W., Kofoed, B., Westlund, L. and Pavlu, B.:* Quality Control of NADH. Supplement to Scand. J. Clin. Chem. 1974.

[2] *James, J., Johnson, B.A. and Schaffer, R.:* Work at N.B.S.: Developing NADH as a standard reference material. Unpublished communication.

[3] *McComb, R.B. and Gay, R.J.:* A comparison of reduced-NAD preparations from four commercial sources. Clin. Chem. *14*, 754, 1968.

[4] *Berry, A.J., Lott, J.A., Grannis, G.F.:* NADH preparations as they affect reliability of serum lactate dehydrogenase determinations. Clin. Chem. *19*, 1255, 1973.

[5] *Rosalki, S.B.:* Accuracy assessment from reference methods: Isoenzyme reference methods with special reference to hydroxybutyrate dehydrogenase determination, in Progress in Quality Control in Clinical Chemistry. Transactions of the 5th International Symposium, Geneva 1973. Hans Huber Publ., Vienna 1973.

Comparison of Mammalian Tissue Extracts and Evaluation of a System for the Detection of Enzyme Inhibitors in NADH Preparations

S.B.Rosalki, London (U.K.)

Key words: Enzyme inhibitors
Hydroxybutyrate dehydrogenase
Inhibitor detection
Inhibitor test system
Lactate dehydrogenase
LD isoenzymes
NADH
Temperature effects

In the 1973 Geneva Symposium (*Rosalki,* 1973), I described experiments on the effect of moisture-induced inhibitors in NADH preparations on the lactate dehydrogenase (LD) and hydroxybutyrate dehydrogenase (HBD) activity of human tissues, and the use of human heart LD_1 and its HBD : LD ratio for inhibitor detection.

I have extended these studies, by examining the sensitivity of LD and HBD from six mammalian species (Cat, Dog, Human, Ox, Pig, and Rat) to inhibitors in moisture-exposed NADH.

For the initial experiments, diluted aqueous homogenates of liver, heart, and heart heated to 65 °C for 30 minutes, from all six species were examined, within-a-day, in triplicate, with the LKB 8600 Reaction-Rate Analyzer using fresh NADH, and NADH from the same batch exposed overnight to a moist atmosphere.

Results and reaction conditions are summarised in tables 1 and 2 and results are illustrated in figure 1. As shown in this figure, LD activity (the total column height) in homogenates of liver (abbreviated as L) heart (abbreviated as H), and heart heated to 65 °C for 30 minutes (abbreviated as HH), is inhibited more than HBD (cross-hatched column height) in all six species. In this experiment up to 80% inhibition of LD was observed compared with inhibition not exceeding 20% for HBD.

For LD, heated-heart preparations from Dog, Man and Ox show the greatest inhibition and heart is more inhibited than liver in all species, though this is minimal in the Ox and Pig. For HBD, the pattern is similar, with heated-heart and heart preparations showing the greatest inhibition, again with anomalous results in the Ox and Pig.

Table 1. Percent inhibition of LD activity with moisture-exposed NADH.

	Liver	Heart	Heated Heart
Cat	39	67	63
Dog	38	64	80
Human	39	64	71
Ox	61	64	74
Pig	52	63	60
Rat	36	63	63

Note:
1. LD inhibited > HBD all tissues.
2. Heated-heart inhibited > heart; dog, human, ox.
3. Heart > Liver, minimal for ox, pig.
4. Reaction conditions: 0.067 mol/l phosphate buffer; 0.15 mmol/l NADH; 0.76 mmol/l pyruvate; 25 °C, pH 7.4.

Table 2. Percent inhibition of HBD activity with moisture-exposed NADH.

	Liver	Heart	Heated Heart
Cat	6	18	—
Dog	9	16	20
Human	6	14	18
Ox	10	13	15
Pig	16	18	18
Rat	8	16	18

Note:
1. Inhibition Heated Heart > Heart (minimal)
2. Inhibition Heart > Liver (minimal ox, pig)
3. Reaction conditions: 0.067 mol/l phosphate buffer; 0.15 mmol/l NADH; 3.3 mmol/l α-oxobutyrate; 25 °C, pH 7.4.

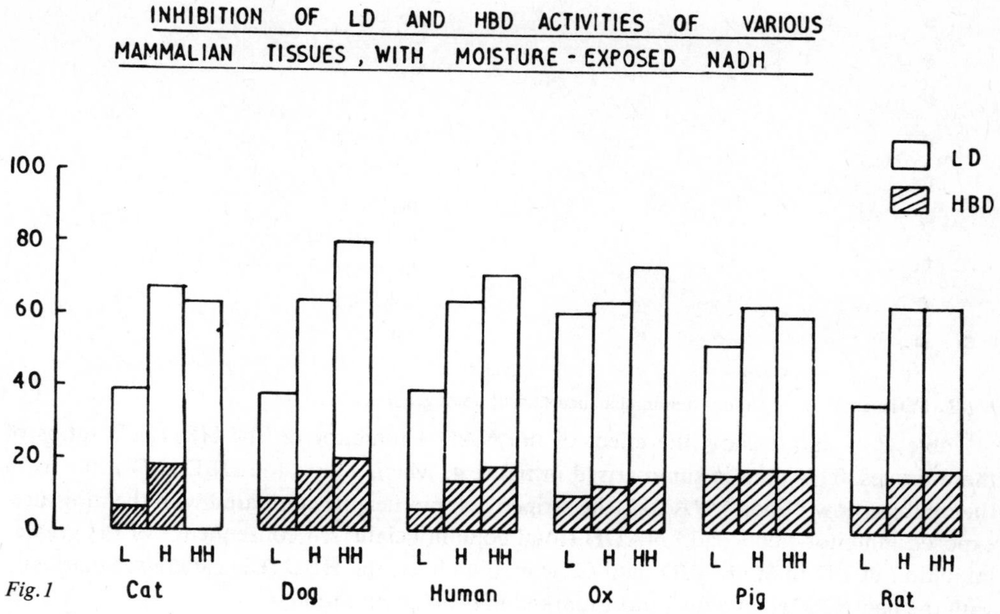

Fig. 1

Figure 2 shows the LD isoenzymes in the *liver* of these species. The pattern in the Ox and Pig differs markedly from that of the other animals, a finding in accord with the anomalous response of their enzymes to inhibitor. As shown in figure 3, the *heart* LD isoenzymes of Ox and Pig also show distinctive patterns.

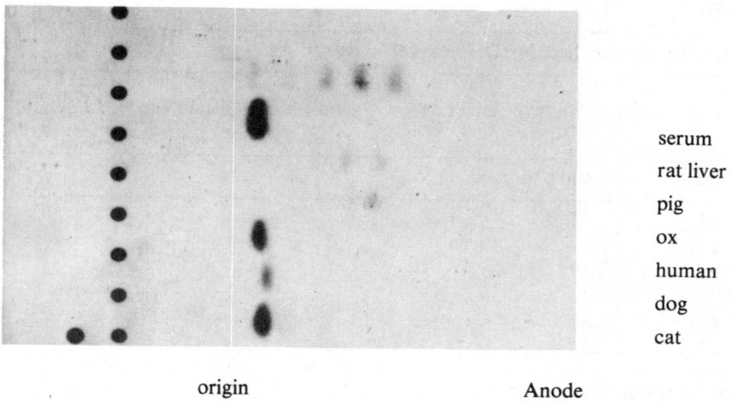

Fig. 2. LD isoenzymes of various mammalian liver tissue homogenates

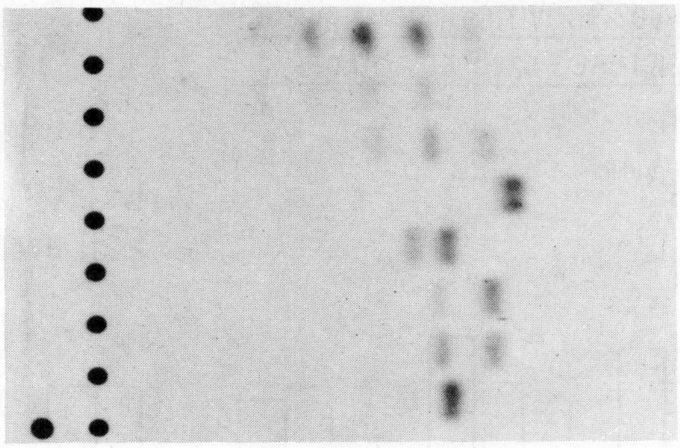

human sera
rat heart
pig heart
ox heart
human heart
dog heart
cat heart

origin Anode

Fig. 3. LD isoenzymes of various mammalian heart tissue homogenates

Tables 3, 4 and 5 show the effect of the NADH inhibitor on the HBD:LD ratios of these tissues. This data is summarised in figure 4, which shows the HBD:LD ratios with the inhibitor-low ('good') NADH (the striped column height) compared with the moisture-exposed inhibitor-rich ('bad') NADH (total column height). In consequence of the greater inhibition of LD than of HBD, and of heart than liver, the HBD:LD ratio *rises* markedly with the bad NADH, an effect most marked in heart preparations.

Table 3. HBD/LD ratios of liver homogenates with inhibitor-low ('good') and moisture-exposed inhibitor-rich ('bad') NADH.

	'Good' NADH	'Bad' NADH	Ratio Bad/Good
Cat	0.17	0.26	1.53
Dog	0.16	0.23	1.44
Human	0.22	0.34	1.55
Ox	0.49	1.12	2.29
Pig	0.56	0.98	1.75
Rat	0.21	0.30	1.43

Note: Increased HBD:LD ratio with 'bad' NADH; marked in ox and pig.

Table 4. HBD/LD ratios of heart homogenates with inhibitor-low ('good') and moisture-exposed inhibitor-rich ('bad') NADH.

	'good'	'bad'	Ratio bad/good
Cat	0.76	1.92	2.53
Dog	0.76	1.75	2.30
Human	0.76	1.85	2.43
Ox	0.56	1.36	2.43
Pig	0.74	1.64	2.22
Rat	0.70	1.59	2.27

Note: 1. Increased HBD:LD ratio with bad NADH.
2. Increase, heart > liver.

Table 5. HBD/LD ratios of heated-heart homogenates with inhibitor-low ('good') and moisture-exposed inhibitor-rich ('bad') NADH.

	'good' NADH	'bad' NADH	Ratio bad/good
Cat	–	–	–
Dog	0.93	3.67	3.95
Human	0.81	2.31	2.85
Ox	0.63	2.02	3.21
Pig	0.69	1.43	2.07
Rat	0.64	1.41	2.20

Note: 1. Increased HBD : LD ratio with bad NADH
2. Least for pig and rat
3. Increase, heated heart > heart (except pig, rat).

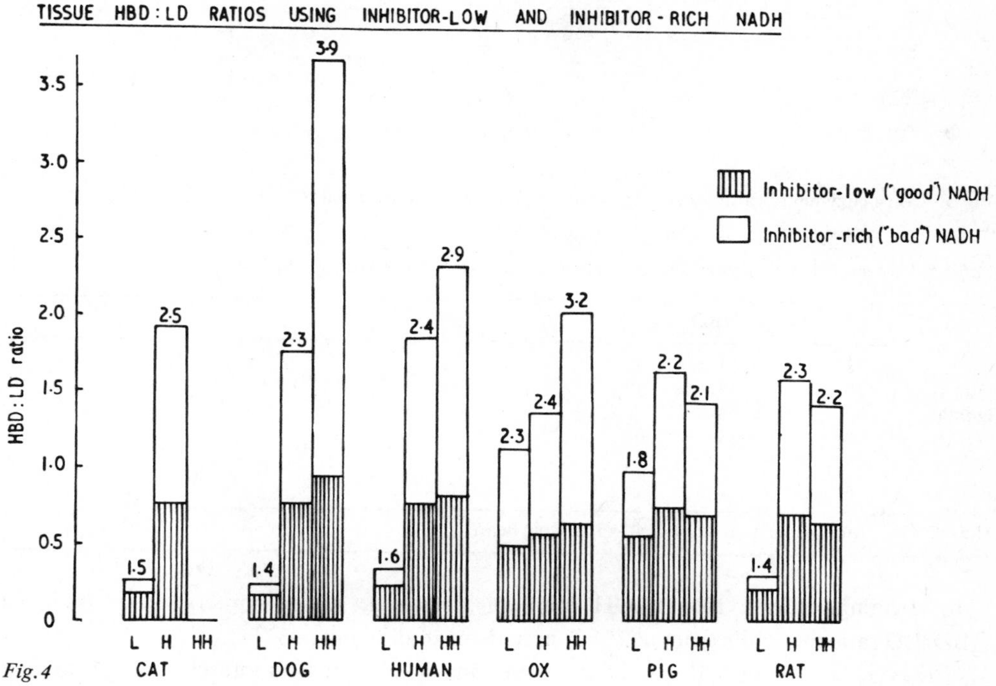

Fig. 4

The numbers at the top of the column in figure 4 compare the HBD : LD ratios obtained with the 'good' and the 'bad' NADH. The higher the number, the more useful is the preparation for 'moisture'-inhibitor detection. This value is highest in heated-heart preparations of Dog, Human and Ox, with the dog preparation showing the highest value.

However, in additional experiments (see, for example, tables 7, 8 and 9) heated dog-heart preparations were only marginally, if at all, superior to the human. Thus, human heated-heart extract, containing almost exclusively LD_1 (figure 5) remains a suitable preparation for inhibitor detection. It may also be noted, that the LD and HBD activity of heart tissue of Dog, Man and Ox was reasonably heat-stable (table 6), whereas that of the other species was heat-labile, the cat heart preparation being so much so that accurate ratios could not be obtained.

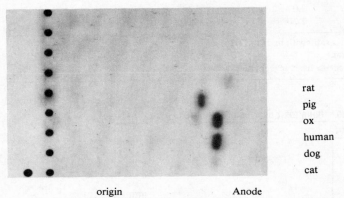

Fig. 5. LD isoenzymes of various mammalian heated heart tissue homogenates

Table 6. Percent residual enzyme activity in heart homogenates heated for 30 minutes at 65 °C.

Animal	LD	HBD
Cat	1	1
Dog	36	44
Human	60	64
Ox	29	33
Pig	15	4
Rat	8	2

Note: Marked heat-lability of cat > rat > pig heart.

In defining criteria for NADH inhibitor detection, some workers have used the HBD/LD ratio determined not at 25 °C, as in these studies, but at 37 °C.

However, in human and dog heart tissue, and in human post-infarct sera, containing mainly LD_1 and LD_2, as shown in the experiments summarised in tables 7, 8 and 10, with the chosen reaction conditions, moisture-exposed NADH produces greater inhibition at 25 °C than at 37 °C and this is more marked for LD. In consequence, both LD and HBD determinations become less sensitive to such inhibitors when performed at 37 °C, but the assay system, and the HBD/LD ratio (tables 9 and 11) then becomes less suitable for inhibitor detection.

Table 7. Effect of assay temperature on percentage inhibition of LD activity with moisture-exposed NADH.

	25 °C	37 °C
Dog		
Heart	53	25
Heated heart	58	25
Human		
Heart	53	23
Heated heart	56	23

Note: Reduction in LD inhibition at 37 °C.

Table 8. Effect of assay temperature on percentage inhibition HBD activity with moisture-exposed NADH.

	25 °C	37 °C
Dog		
Heart	14	13
Heated heart	17	9
Human		
Heart	15	5
Heated heart	15	6

Note: Reduction in LD inhibition at 37 °C.

Table 9. Effect of assay temperature on HBD : LD ratio using 'good' and 'bad' NADH.

	25 °C			37 °C		
	Good NADH	Bad NADH	Ratio Bad/Good	Good NADH	Bad NADH	Ratio Bad/Good
Dog						
Heart	0.73	1.32	1.82	0.48	0.55	1.15
Heated heart	0.82	1.61	1.97	0.52	0.62	1.19
Human						
Heart	0.75	1.36	1.82	0.47	0.58	1.23
Heated heart	0.78	1.53	1.95	0.52	0.63	1.21

Note: 1. Decreased HBD/LD ratio at 37 °C.
2. Impaired differentiation, good – bad NADH at 37 °C.

Table 10. Effect of temperature on percentage inhibition of enzyme activities in post-infarct sera by moisture-exposed NADH.

	HBD	LD
25 °C		
Serum 1	29	72
Serum 2	25	71
37 °C		
Serum 1	18	43
Serum 2	23	42

Note: 1. Inhibition LD > HBD.
2. Inhibition 25 °C > 37 °C.

Table 11. Effect of temperature on HBD:LD ratio of post-infarct sera using 'good' and 'bad' NADH.

	'Good'	'Bad'	Ratio Bad/Good
25 °C			
Serum 1	0.64	1.63	2.55
Serum 2	0.65	1.68	2.58
37 °C			
Serum 1	0.49	0.69	1.41
Serum 2	0.47	0.62	1.32

Note: 1. HBD:LD 'Bad' > 'Good'
2. HBD:LD 25 °C > 37 °C
3. Differentiation (Bad/Good) impaired at 37 °C.

In addition to these studies on tissues extracts, and fresh post-infarct serum, I have examined a system for enzyme inhibitor detection, prepared by DADE (DADE Division American Hospital Supply Corporation, Miami, Florida 33152), in which enzyme and substrate are lyophilised, and the reaction is started by NADH addition. This system avoids sample pipetting error, and permits convenient comparison of NADH preparations. Normally, minor volumetric variation in added NADH has little effect.

Two preparations, designated SLC 101 and SHC 201, were examined. In the former, serum is lyophilised with pyruvate substrate, in the latter serum is lyophilised with 2-oxobutyrate substrate. Both preparations were examined in duplicate, both at 25 °C and at 37 °C using a Vitatron UFD photometer, and were compared with a human heated-heart preparation. The reaction was started by the addition of reconstituted lyophilised NADH preparation, 63 A or reconstituted NADH from the same batch exposed to moisture prior to lyophilisation (NADH 63).

It can be seen from table 12, that at both temperatures the LD preparation shows greater inhibition with the inhibitor-rich moisture-exposed NADH than does HBD. However, at 25 °C, this is lower than that of the comparison heated human-heart LD.

Table 12. Effect of NADH 63 A c.f. – NADH 63 on enzyme activity

	Activity (U/l). NADH 63A	NADH 63	Percent inhibition
25 °C			
SLC 101 (LD)	60	35	42
SHC 201 (HBD)	58	41	30
Human heated-heart LD		–	64
37 °C			
SLC 101 (LD)	105	54	48
SHC 201 (HBD)	87	61	30
Human heated-heart LD		–	39

Unlike the fresh tissue and serum preparations previously examined and the comparison human heated-heart preparation, the lyophilised enzyme failed to show any reduction in inhibitor effects at 37 °C compared with 25 °C. This may be an effect of lyophilisation. However, it should be noted that total activities of the lyophilised preparations were low and, therefore, unsuitable for accurate determination of inhibitor effects.

If the enzyme reaction is to be initiated by coenzyme, it was considered important to ensure that preincubation of enzyme with *substrate* does not exert a protective effect from inhibition. Table 13 shows that both HBD and LD of human heart and heated-heart are identically inhibited by moisture-exposed NADH when the reaction is started by substrate following 15 minutes pre-incubation at 25 °C with NADH, or by NADH following similar pre-incubation with substrate.

Table 13. Effect of preincubation of sample with substrate ('NADH start') of enzyme inhibition by moisture-exposed NADH.

	'Substrate start' % inhibition	'NADH start' % inhibition
HBD		
Human		
heart	15	13
heated heart	15	13
LD		
Human		
heart	53	55
heated heart	56	57

Note: Preincubation with substrate without effect.

Summary

This study has shown:

1. That for each of the six species examined (Cat, Dog, Human, Ox, Pig and Rat), LD was more sensitive to inhibitors in moisture-exposed NADH than HBD, and heart LD was more sensitive than liver.

2. Heated-heart preparations containing mainly LD_1 from the Dog, Man and Ox, were the most inhibitor-sensitive, with human-heart LD_1 providing a suitable preparation for inhibitor detection.

3. Inhibitor effects in tissue extracts and sera were more readily detectable at 25 °C than at 37 °C. Inhibitor *detection* is, therefore, more sensitive at 25 °C, though inhibitor *effects* on clinical specimens would be less in assays carried out at the higher temperature.

4. Lyophilised serum preparations did not show temperature differences in inhibitor effects.

5. The pre-incubation of enzyme with substrate rather than with co-enzyme in the LD and HBD assays exerted no protective effect from inhibitors in NADH preparations.

References

Rosalki, S.B. (1973): Accuracy Assessment from Reference Methods: Isoenzyme Reference Methods with Special Reference to α-Hydroxybutyrate Dehydrogenase Determination. Progress in Quality Control in Clinical Chemistry. Transactions of the Vth International Symposium Geneva 1973. Publisher: Hans Huber, Bern, p. 105–126.

Temperature Dependence of Difference-Absorption Coefficients of NADH Minus NAD$^+$ and NADPH Minus NADP$^+$ in the Near Ultraviolet[1]

Th. Bücher, G. Lusch and *H. Krell,* Munich (Germany)

Key words: Glutamate dehydrogenase
Molar absorption coefficient
NAD
NADH
NADP
NADPH
Temperature effects

Rationale of proceeding

As demonstrated by figure 1 the dihydroband [1] of NADH moves to shorter wavelengths with increasing temperature [2, 3]. The maximum of absorbance is shifted from about 340 nm at 0 °C to about 338.5 nm at 38 °C. The corresponding maxima of NADPH are located at about 0.5 nm longer wavelengths as compared to NADH at these temperatures.

---

[1] A preliminary report on these investigations has been communicated [4].

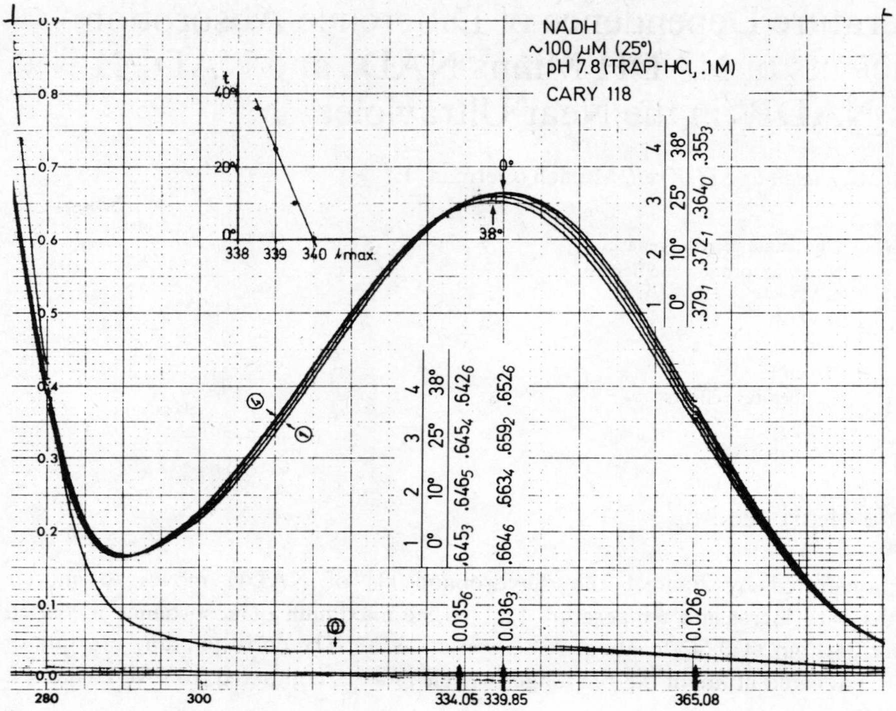

Fig. 1. Sequential recording of absorbance spectra of a solution of NADH at 0 °C, 10 °C, 25 °C and 38 °C. (Pathlength of silica cell 1.000 cm; period, 1 sec; scan speed, 0.2 nm per sec; slit width, 0.15 mm; auto gain.) Buffer solution served as reference. After scanning at 38 °C the sample was readjusted to 25 °C and then β-NADH enzymatically oxidized as shown in fig. 2. Trace O represents the residual absorbance of α-NADH and of impurities. At the wavelengths indicated by arrows at the abscissa, the scan was interrupted and the digitized absorbance values noted as shown by inserted tables. For further details see sections 1.2 and 2 in the text.

In addition to the shift parallel to the wavelengths scale, with increasing temperature, a broadening of the bell shaped dihydrobands of both pyridine nucleotides is observed. The maximal extinction coefficient at 38 °C is about 1.5% lower than that at 0 °C.

As figure 1 also shows, wavelength shift and broadening lead to the effect that the molar extinction coefficients at 334 and 292 nm are essentially independent of temperature and type of pyridine nucleotide in the range investigated. This important observation is further substantiated in the upper section of table 1 for one of these 'quasi isosbestic points'. Fortunately enough, here the sharp and invariant mercury line 334.15 nm is available.

Table 1. Ratios of molar extinction coefficients at 334.15 nm and at 365.1 nm ± SEM

At 334.15 nm:		
NADH, 25 °C/NADPH, 25 °C (n = 9)	$1.000_7 \pm 1‰$	(1)
NADH, 25 °C/NADH, 0 °C (n = 4)	$1.003_2 \pm 1.5‰$	(2)
At 365.1 nm:		
NADH, 25 °C/NADPH, 25 °C (n = 9)	$0.975_1 \pm 3‰$	(1)
NADH, 25 °C/NADH, 0 °C (n = 4)	$0.952_5 \pm 3‰$	(2)
NADPH, 25 °C/NADPH, 0 °C (n = 4)	$0.954_3 \pm 6‰$	(2)

(1) Spectral line Photometer, see sections 1.1 and 4.
(2) Spectrophotometer, see sections 1.2,2 and 3.

Consequently, in order to achieve step by step the desired absolute molar absorption coefficients at distinct temperatures and wavelengths, two types of measurements were performed and their results were combined. It is an essential aim of our presentation to introduce this mode of proceeding.

By means of an accurate spectrophotometer, absorbance spectra of reduced and oxidized pyridine nucleotides were recorded at temperatures between 0 °C and 38 °C. The amounts of pyridine nucleotides and of solvent in the absorption cell were constant in each set of measurements. By division through the solvent densities at the different temperatures the absorbancies were related to a constant molarity. However, the exact value of this molarity was not known; thus ratios of extinction coefficients at relevant wavelengths and temperatures resulted from these measurements, the absorbance at 334.15 nm serving as denominator, as listed in table 2.

Table 2. Temperature dependence of ratios of extinction coefficients (± SEM)

°C	n	$\frac{\Delta\varepsilon_{340.0}}{\Delta\varepsilon_{334.15}}$	$\frac{\Delta\varepsilon_{365.10}}{\Delta\varepsilon_{334.15}}$
NADH:			
0°	5	$1.029_5 \pm .3‰$	$0.579_3 \pm 2.3‰$
10°	3	$1.028_6 \pm 3‰$	$0.567_0 \pm 2.3‰$
25°	4	$1.018_8 \pm .2‰$	$0.551_7 \pm .5‰$
38°	4	$1.014_1 \pm 3‰$	$0.541_2 \pm 1.6‰$
NADPH:			
0°	4	$1.036_3 \pm 1.8‰$	$0.602_3 \pm 4.6‰$
38°	3	$1.018_8 \pm .5‰$	$0.560_4 \pm 2.5‰$

In order to achieve absolute calibration by means of a spectral line photometer, the decrement of extinction of reduced pyridine nucleotide by enzymatic oxidation was measured at Hg 334 at 25 °C. 2-oxoglutaric acid served as titrating hydrogen acceptor for both pyridine nucleotides. These measurements were also performed at Hg 365 as demonstrated by tables 1 and 3.

Experimental

1. Invariance of extinction coefficients at 334.15 nm

1.1 For the comparison of the extinction coefficients of NADH and NADPH at 25 °C the glutamic dehydrogenase system has been chosen. This system:

$$\text{2-oxoglutarate} + NH_4^+ + \text{NADH (NADPH)} + H^+ \overset{\text{Glutamic dehydrogenase}}{\rightleftharpoons} \text{Glutamate} + NAD^+ (NADP^+)$$

has been proposed to us by Dr. *M. Grassl.* It allows the determination of extinction coefficients of both pyridine nucleotides with the same test solution, since glutamic dehydrogenase exhibits the same specific activity with NADH as with NADPH as hydrogen donor.

The test solutions contained 80 μM of 2-oxoglutarate in 0.1 M triethanolamine-HCl buffer pH 7.6, 0.15 M NH_4Cl and NADH or NADPH in a 1.5 to 2 fold stoichiometric excess. The buffer was prepared with distilled triethanolamine. The reaction was started by adding 50 μg beef liver glutamic dehydrogenase. Measurements were performed with an Eppendorf Digital Photometer 6114 at 25 °C.

Table 1, first line, shows the mean of the ratios of extinction coefficients from nine measurements with three separately prepared test solutions together with its standard error. Corrections were applied in these calculations as described in section 4.

The corresponding ratio at Hg 365, resulting from the same set of measurements, is shown in table 1 third line. Here NADPH exhibits a 2.4% higher molar extinction than NADH. The slope of the absorption curve at 365 nm is −5% per nm. With the assumption that the absorption curves of both pyridine nucleotides are equal in shape, the increment in extinction of 2.5% may be divided by the slope of – 5% per nm in order to estimate the wavelength difference of maximum positions of NADH and NADPH. The resulting value of −0.5 nm is in agreement with the readout from the absorption curves.

1.2 The temperature dependence of extinction coefficients of NADH at 334 nm has been evaluated as exemplified by figure 1.

A chromatographically purified preparation of BaNADH was transformed into the sodium salt by addition of Na_2SO_4 and diluted in 0.1 M triethanolamine – HCl buffer, pH 7.8, prepared from distilled triethanolamine.

Special silica windowed thermostating holders[2] for the solvent and the sample cell were fixed into the sample compartment of a Cary Model 118 spectrophotometer. A slow stream of dry nitrogen was led through the sample compartment and through the cell holders in order to avoid condensation of water at lower temperatures.

---

[2] We are indebted to Mr. Josef Grimm for the construction of the special holders.

First the absorption spectra of the NADH solution were recorded at different temperatures. The sequence corresponds to the numbers heading the small tables which are inserted into the figure.

Also, the instruments wavelength drive was arrested during recording at 334.05 nm (and two other relevant wavelengths as seen in the figure) and the digitalized absorbance data noted. By division through the density of water at temperatures of measurement, and multiplication by the density of water at 25 °C, they were corrected for the contraction resp. extension of the solvent.

Secondly, at 25 °C the β-NADPH was oxidized by addition of a small excess of pyruvic acid and of lactic dehydrogenase as demonstrated in figure 2. The remaining absorbance (base line) was recorded (scan 0 in fig. 1). It was corrected by subtracting the small contribution of excess pyruvate (33 μM; absorbance $5 \cdot 10^{-4}$ at 334nm).

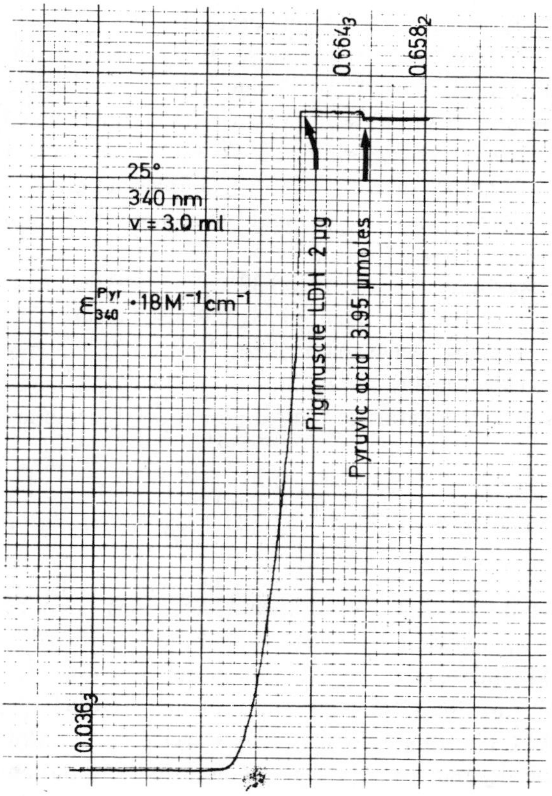

Fig. 2. Oxidation of β-NADH by addition of pyruvic acid and lactic dehydrogenase. The correction of the resulting base line (trace O in fig. 1) for the absorbance of excess pyruvate is explained in section 2 of the text.

The corrected absorbances were subtracted and the ratio calculated as shown in table 1, second line. In the transition from 0 °C to 25 °C the differential absorbance NADH minus NAD^+ exhibits a small but probably significant increase of 3 ‰. No further significant increase was observed between 25 °C and 38 °C. The corresponding ratio of 1.000 has not been included into the table for the following reason: at higher temperatures a slow oxidation of NADH is seen. Its extent can be estimated by a comparison of the absorbance value at 25 °C and 339.5 nm in figure 1 (column 3, fourth line) and the initial absorbance shown in figure 2. The first value was measured before, and the second after the scanning at 38 °C. The time difference was about 40 min., and the decrease of NADH specific absorbance 1.6 ‰.

2. *Ratios of extinction coefficients λ 340/λ 334.15 and λ 365.1/λ 334.15 of NADH between 0 °C and 38 °C*

The experimental setup has been already described in the preceeding section. In the course of scanning, the instruments wavelength drive was stopped at the following indications of the wavelength counter: 334.2 nm, 340 nm, 365.3 nm. (The arrest caused minor disturbances in the scan, especially at 365 nm as seen in figure 1.) When checked with a Mercury pencil arc the exact wavelengths were determined to be 334.05 nm, 339.85 nm and 365.1 nm. The digitalized readout of absorbance was noted. Examples are given in the small tables inserted into figure 1. The slope of the absorption curve at 334 nm is 0.9% per nm. Thus the readout at 334.05 nm was multiplied by a factor of 1.0009 in order to get the absorbance at 334.15 nm. The corresponding correction for 339.85 → 340.00 nm is negligible. The absorbance at 365.1 nm was used as such, since this wavelength corresponds rather closely to the 'weighted average' wavelength of the triplet Hg 365 (see below). Corrections for absorbance of excess pyruvate were $5.3 \cdot 10^{-4}$ at 334 nm, $5.0 \cdot 10^{-4}$ at 340 nm and $1.1 \cdot 10^{-4}$ at 365 nm. The resulting ratios of the extinction coefficients are presented in the upper part of table 2.

3. *Ratios of extinction coefficients λ 340/λ 334.15 and λ 365.1/λ 334.15 of NADPH at 0 °C and 38 °C*

The data are presented in the lower part of table 2. The experimental setup was essentially the same as described in the preceeding section with the following alterations. About 110 μM reagent grade Na_2 $NADP^+$ and 7 mM glucose-6-phosphate sodium salt were dissolved in 0.1 M triethanolamine HCl-buffer pH 7.8. The absorption curve of this solution was recorded at 25 °C. Then 3 μg/ml glucose-6-phosphate dehydrogenase were added. After the completion of transhydrogenation, the desired temperature was adjusted and the absorption spectrum scanned. The whole procedure was repeated for each temperature, since the plateau of reduction was only stable for half an hour. Then, a slow decrease in absorption was observed, especially at higher temperatures.

4. Provisional molar extinction coefficients at Hg 334 and Hg 365 as determined with the glutamic dehydrogenase system

The experimental setup has already been described in section 1.1. An analytical grade sample of 2-oxoglutaric acid provided by Boehringer, Tutzing, served as reference substance. From potentiometric titrations (point of equivalence at pH 8.6) the preparation was estimated to be $99.0 \pm 0.3\%$ pure. This value was used in the calculations of the molarities of the test solutions. Within the limits of experimental error, it is confirmed by further detailed investigations of the sample by the Boehringer staff. Table 3 presents the means of 9 measurements with 3 separately prepared test solutions. Photometry and titration contributed about equally to the error. With each test solution, values for both pyridine nucleotides and both wavelengths were measured. The following corrections were applied in the calculations:

a) Decrement of initial extinction by dilution by the addition of enzyme solution (0.5%).
b) Increment of final extinctions by added enzyme protein (about 0.4% of $-\Delta E$).
c) Contribution of 2-oxoglutarate to the initial extinction.

Corrections for beam divergence, multiple reflection and fluorescence were not applied. They were estimated to be at least one order of magnitude smaller than the experimental standard error.

The molar extinction coefficient of NAD^+ and $NADP^+$ at both wavelengths is about 2–3 $M^{-1}cm^{-1}$ (personal communication of Dr. *Ziegenhorn*). This small value must be added if the absolute molar extinction coefficient of the reduced pyridine nucleotides is desired.

Table 3. Provisional molar extinction coefficients at Hg lines at 25 °C

	334.15	365
NADH	6145	3409
NADPH	6141	3496

Standard error of means are: in the titrations of the reference substance $\pm 3\%$ and in the photometric determinations $\pm 3\%$.

Conclusions

From the data reported here the following considerations appear to be relevant for practical analytical work.

1. At Hg 334 the molar extinction coefficients of NADH and NADPH are practically equal and independent of the temperature of measurement. Since modern spectral line photometers allow measurements at Hg 334 with high accuracy, this line is recommended if precise analytical results are desired.

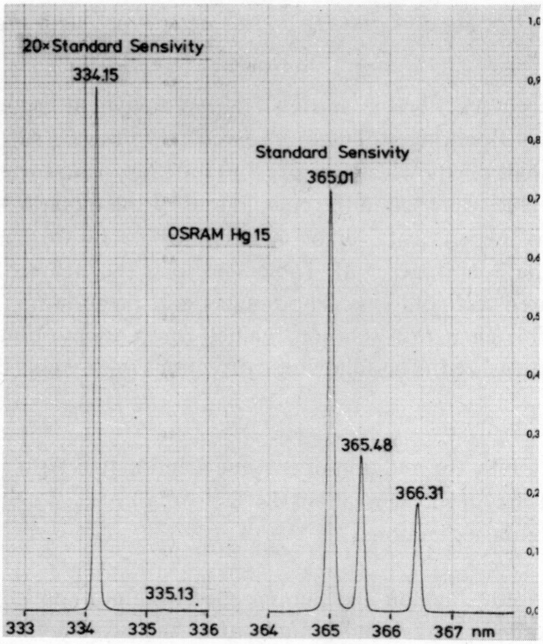

Fig. 3. Relative intensities of the lines constituting Hg 334 and Hg 365 of a mercury arc lamp used in commercial spectral line photometers[1]. Note that the band width of the lines represents partly the slit width of the recording instrument (Cary 118; slit width 0.01 mm corresponding to spectral band widths of 0.09 nm at 365 nm and 0.08 at 334 nm).

It should be mentioned that Hg 334 is a doublet of the lines 334.15 and 335.13 [5]. However, as shown by the scan in figure 3 the relative intensity of line 335.13 is extremely low (0.2% of Hg 334). Hence, the resulting deviation of the weighted average from 334.15 is negligible (0.002 nm).

2. At other wavelengths the extinction coefficients are dependent on temperature and type of nucleotide. A probable explanation of these effects is the existence of reduced pyridine nucleotides in solution in more than one conformation ('open' and 'closed' form). First order reaction kinetics have been found in fluorometric relaxation measurements after temperature jumps with solutions of NADH and NADPH [6]. As a practical consequence, it must be expected that the molar extinction coefficients are also dependent on the ionic strength of the solution and are influenced by the presence of complexing cations (e.g. Mg^{2+}).

3. In a first approximation, the absorbance spectrum of NADPH at a given temperature

[1] We are indebted to Dr. *H. Schwab* for these measurements and to Dr. *D. Bouchain,* Eppendorf Gerätebau *Netheler* & Hinz G.m.b.H., Hamburg, for technical support.

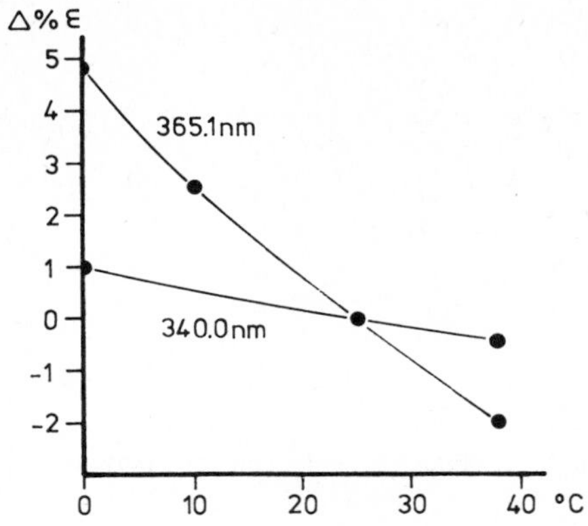

Fig. 4: Temperature dependence of extinction coefficients of NADH at 340 and 365.1 nm referred to 25 °C.

can be regarded as equal to the absorbance spectrum of NADH at a 10 °C lower temperature. This is also in agreement with the kinetic constants measured in [6].

The results of enzymatic metabolite determinations using $NADP^+$ or NADPH as photometric indicator at Hg 365 are 6% too high if the value $3.3 \cdot 10^3$ is used as molar extinction coefficient of NADPH.

4. In figure 4, percental changes of the molar extinction coefficients of NADH at 340 nm and 365.1 nm between 0 °C and 38 °C are plotted. The molar extinction coefficients at 25 °C served as reference values. In the vicinity of 25 °C the changes are −0.4 ‰ at 340 nm and − 1.5 ‰ at 365.1 nm per one °C.

With respect to Hg 365 its triplet structure cannot be neglected (see fig. 3). The weighted average depends on the vapour pressure of the Mercury lamp and the characteristics of the spectral line filter used. The slope of the absorption curve at 365 nm is −5% per nm. Thus the correct molar extinction coefficient of reduced pyridine nucleotides is somewhat dependent on the type of spectral line photometer used. The weighted average of the triplet recorded in figure 3 is 365.32 nm in agreement with [5].

5. The molar extinction coefficients presented in table 3 are considered as provisional, since the preparation of 2-oxoglutaric acid used as reference substance contains, besides water, impurities of unknown composition. We are convinced, however, that the true absolute coefficients fall into the range of our experimental error of ± 0.6% for the following reason: The molar extinction coefficient for NADH of $3.4 \cdot 10^3$ at Hg 365 and 25 °C based on carefully distilled and titrated pyruvic acid which was reported earlier [7] is confirmed by the new measurements with 2-oxoglutaric acid as reference substance.

With the ratio, given in table 2, the provisional molar extinction of NADH at 340 nm and 25 °C is calculated to be 6260 ± 40.

Acknowledgements

This investigation was supported by the Deutsche Forschungsgemeinschaft, Sonderforschungsbereich 51 and the Fonds der Chemischen Industrie. Substantial help and cooperation with many colleagues of the staff of Boehringer Biochemica, Tutzing, are gratefully acknowledged. Most kindly *W. Neupert* has revised the manuscript.

References

[1] *Warburg, O.* (1938): Ergebnisse der Enzymforschung *7*, 210.

[2] *Bücher, Th., Luh, W. and Pette, D.* (1964): In Hoppe-Seyler/Thierfelder, Handbuch der Physiologisch- und Pathologisch-chemischen Analyse, 10. Aufl., Bd. *VI*/A, 292.

[3] *Malcolm, A.D.B.* (1973): Anal. Biochem. *55*, 278.

[4] *Bücher, Th., Krell, H., Lusch, G., Grassl, M., Ziegenhorn, J. and Bergmeyer, H.U.* (1974): Z. Klin. Chem. Klin. Biochem. *12*, 239.

[5] *Netheler, H.* (1970): In Methoden der Enzymatischen Analyse, H.U. Bergmeyer ed., 2. Aufl., Band I, 145.

[6] *Czerlinski, G. and Hommes, F.* (1964): Biochim. Biophys. Acta *79*, 46.

[7] *Beisenherz, G., Boltze, H.J., Bücher, Th., Czok, R., Garbade, K.H., Meyer-Arendt, E. and Pfleiderer, G.* (1953): Z. f. Naturforschung *8*, 555.

NAD-NADH-NADP-NADPH Symposium

Discussion

S. Rosalki (U. K.): Do we know whether the inhibitor in NAD is particularly sensitive to the H 4 isoenzyme as is the inhibitor in NADH?

W. Gerhardt (Denmark): No, I have no data on that, but I would suspect it would be. These reactions really need further investigation.

Unidentified speaker: Dr. *Gerhardt,* I think that in pure NADH preparations the ratio of 260 to 340 nm is quite a good indicator of inhibitor content, but one should state that NADH can be stabilized, for example, by albumin and other substances which have a high absorbancy at 260, so that commercial preparations of NADH might be very suitable for LDH determinations even if they have unsuitable ratios.

W. Gerhardt (Denmark): I agree completely, and that was one of the points I was making. The 260/340 ratio may well be higher than 2.27 and the preparation still be perfectly suitable, but this would be defined by the criteria that I set up to compare it with the reference preparation, and to decide if it performs kinetically as prescribed.

S. Rosalki (U. K.): Could I ask you, Dr. *Ziegenhorn,* why you are recommending molar absorption coefficients at 334 nanometers and at 365 nanometers, which are to two significant figures, but for the 340 values you show three significant figures?

J. Ziegenhorn (Germany): At 365 nm, the absorption curve of NADH has a big slope and is very sensitive to small changes of temperature. Furthermore, the center of the mercury line triplet depends on the vapor pressure in the lamp. Therefore, I should say for routine work the first decimal place is enough at this wavelength.

S. Rosalki (U. K.): Well, wouldn't you say the same would apply at 334 nanometers as at 340 nanometers?

J. Ziegenhorn (Germany): The ε-values of NADH are dependent on various parameters: Wavelength, temperature, ionic strength, etc. For these reasons, one should reflect on the desirability of using in routine work only two significant figures, even at or near the wavelength maximum of the coenzyme.

F. Redondo (Spain): Dr. *Bowers,* you have shown the variation of the molar absorbance coefficient for NADH with different conditions of pH and temperature, and I would like to know if you have checked the absorbancy in these conditions in the immediate vicinity of 340 nanometers, for example at 339.7, 339.8 or 340.2 nanometers.

G. Bowers (U. S. A.): If you are asking which is the maxima, it is actually a little below 340. Although I do not remember the exact figure, I think it is like 339.7, but it is not exactly 340. We stayed with 340 because that was the conventional wavelength that everybody was interested in and in all of our work we used the setting at 340.

F. Redondo (Spain): I wonder if with the change in pH or in another variable there could be a shift in the peak of maximum absorbance?

G. Bowers (U. S. A.): I think this is a good observation and I cannot give you much more on that. Some of the shifts you noticed may be related to the fact we did not sit on the lambda maximum. I would not think from our own observations that we are talking about more than one part, or two parts in a thousand though. It's a very small shift but there is one there.

Th. Bücher (Germany): As you have seen, there are some discrepancies between the molar extinction coefficient of Dr. *Bowers* and what we find.

S. Rosalki (U. K.): At this stage I would like to ask Professor *Bücher*, Dr. *Bowers* and Dr. *Ziegenhorn* to comment on whether this discrepancy might relate to some peculiarity of the different measuring systems, perhaps from the use of a coupled enzyme system, as compared with a direct enzyme system?

G. Bowers (U. S. A.): I am going to play very safe in my answer in stating we have only studied one system intensively. However, about 10 years ago we tried to purify first sodium pyruvate and then potassium pyruvate through a number of crystallizations, and then heating it until we had dehydrated it and actually found loss of weight. In going through an LDH system, we felt at that time that we had a molar absorptivity of about 628, and that is what led me on to believe that the absorbance was higher than what was commonly being quoted. Now that is the only other experience I have, but it does not compare with the type of controls that we have exercised here. I have no doubt that as one moves to other systems you are going to find that the answers are going to be different, but in what order of magnitude and whether it will explain these discrepancies or not I don't know.

S. Rosalki (U. K.): May I ask why the absorptivity coefficient should be different in different systems if one is using a pure reagent?

Th. Bücher (Germany): I think we both have standard means of measurement in the range of one part per thousand, so I think that's clear answer to your question, Dr. *Rosalki*.

J. Frei (Switzerland): I have a question to Dr. *Gerhardt*. It is a useful procedure to compare the activities of two enzymes, in this case LDH and GLDH, I guess, using the latter as a reference enzyme, both requiring beta NADH for activity measurement. We must be absolutely sure that the second enzyme, the reference enzyme, is not influenced by this inhibitor, or not affected by another inhibitor. How can you do this?

W. Gerhardt (Denmark): I am not sure I understood your question. Did you ask whether I used two enzymes to determine the quality of NADH?

J. Frei (Switzerland): Yes, I understood this.

W. Gerhardt (Denmark): I used two substrates and one enzyme. It was the H_4 enzyme of human heart which Dr. *Rosalki* among others has shown as most sensitive to certain types of inhibitors in NADH. The two substrates were oxobutyrate and pyruvate, and it was the reaction ratio obtained with this one preparation of enzyme and the two substrates that was used as a measure of the presence of inhibitor in NADH. I did speak about several enzymes also, but that was in terms of different sensitivities to the presence of an inhibitor.

W. Gruber (Germany): It may be stated that different enzymes are inhibited by different inhibitors in NADH preparations. We have seen preparations which do not inhibit LDH but do inhibit GLDH and vice-versa. But, may I ask a question to Dr. *Bowers*. I remember your paper on the same topic on my visit to Hartford. On both occasions you had a coefficient of extinction at 340 nm of 6.31, but at that time you had not yet introduced correction factors for the residual absorbancy of NAD, for absorbancy changes coming from glucose to glucose-6-phosphate and from ATP to ADP. So is it correct to assume that these corrections must be negligible, as your coefficient of extinction did not change since then, even after you had introduced these corrections?

G. Bowers (U. S. A.): On a slide, we were trying to show you the sign of each of the corrections, and they turn out to pretty much nullify each other. However, the corrections were made, and our paper, which we are preparing now, will be essentially an elaborate discussion of how we tried to standardize each step, so that anyone else might examine that and challenge it. When you start pushing spectroscopy down to a part in a thousand and beyond, one does have to make these corrections and be aware of them. On the other hand, you have to consider such things as the convergence of the light path. The calculations of that is not a simple factor. We went back to the actual engineer at Cary who had supposedly done this originally. After hunting through all of his papers and spending a week, he came back with a figure that agreed with what we thought it might be, reasonably well, at about 1 to 2 parts in a thousand as adding to the path length because of the beam convergence. We have tried to get that type of systematic bias out. Now, if one is looking at another instrument, the question is whether one is going to correct for it or not. I think this will have to be stated about each of the values that people come up with, and that is exactly the format in which we presented this. If it appears that there were no corrections, and there have been a substantial number of them, it is because they cancel each other out.

Th. Bücher (Germany): I would like to make a general comment to the papers by Dr. *Gerhardt* and Dr. *Küffer*. I must apologize as I do not know what the standard method is for testing LDH, but I would like to warn the auditorium against the use of tris buffer with keto acids because tris reacts with keto acids. This is well known and published. The danger of tris has been dramatically apparent in our experiments on measurements of the extinction coefficient of NADH. It is not possible to get a correct answer and value with tris. Neither is phosphate buffer apparently a good system. No disturbances were observed with triethanolamine-HCl buffer, especially, when prepared from distilled triethanolamine and hydrochloric acid.

W. Gerhardt (Denmark): You are perfectly right about tris reacting with keto acids. This is a well-known phenomenon. For instance, if you try to keep a solution of pyruvate, or what is even worse, to freeze a solution of pyruvate in tris, you have quite a loss. I do not know if you were present yesterday when I talked about phosphate buffer accelerating destruction of NADH in solution at both 4 degrees and minus 20. What you are talking about is the equilibrium situation with pyruvate; but what I was aiming at was the reaction rate, which is somewhat different. We have not observed any differences in the reaction rate under standardized conditions in either tris or phosphate buffers of the same ionic strength and pH and with two different species of LDH.

Th. Bücher (Germany): Did you at any time run your experiment using triethanolamine hydrochloride?

W. Gerhardt (Denmark): Yes, we have tried it, but not in many experiments, I regret to say. We did try it at the beginning of our work with the Scandinavian method. At that time we compared several buffers. We only observed the reaction rate and in my opinion, there is no doubt that NADH is more stable at least in the tris than in the phosphate buffer.

R. Sommer (Austria): I would like to ask Dr. *Küffer* about the problem of checking linearity. As we know, it may be affected by the activity of the patient serum and, especially in the LDH-reaction, the linearity of the reaction rate is not given. How did you check this problem? And the second question, why do you measure at 366 nanometers and not at 334 or 340 nm?

H. Küffer (Switzerland): In answer to your first question about linearity, please notice that linearity may be treated as a stoichiometrical problem; or you can follow linearity down to 50% decrease in absorbance of NADH. There the linearity can be measured well. Now this linearity is from 0 to 200 International Units when using 60 microliters of sample, it is about 0 to 400 International Units with 20 microliters, and is 0 to 800 International Units using 10 microliters. We have however, a difficulty, the higher the range of the linearity the lower is the absolute precision of the result.

The second question was about 366 or 334 or 340 nanometers. As you know, we have a decreasing absorbance with time and we cannot have an indefinitely high absorbance to start with. We have to start with an absorbance which is still measurable. Altogether, high linearity is something we do not want to measure at an optimum of absorbance. We prefer to read at 366 because the molar absorptivity is not as high as that of 334. In this way we can use more NADH in our solution. A second reason, is that the intensity of the mercury line at 366 is much higher than at 334. Accordingly, the technical linearity of the photometer is better at 366.

Th. Bücher (Germany): Professor *Härkönen,* did I get right that the inhibitor has no dihydroband? That it does not show the band at 340 which NADH shows?

M. Härkönen (Finland): It did not show the band at 340.

Th. Bücher (Germany): Could it not be that there are changes of substitution just in the pyridine ring. Would you think that the inhibitor really contains an aromatic ring; a ring of pi electrons?

M. Härkönen (Finland): I am sorry, I meant a pyridine ring not a nicotinamide ring. You see, the inhibitor fluoresces. However, since you don't get any enhanced fluorescence with strong alkali with NADH, as you do with NAD^+ and with this inhibitor, it may mean that the ring resembles NAD^+ more closely than NADH. However, it is very difficult to give a conclusive answer.

W. Gruber (Germany): We have studied the same fraction quite extensively and have reported our results at the Analytica Meeting last year in Munich. We can say that we obtained nearly the same results. This fraction mainly appears under conditions where dimerization of NADH is favored, due to concentration, and so our last idea was that this could be a dimeric substance from NADH. Indeed, if you synthesize NADH dimer, it will be eluted just in the same fraction.

The substance is very unstable. It behaves like this fraction which is eluted from NADH. It has the same fluorescence but it does not inhibit LDH; our impression is that this substance is not the inhibitor but a destruction product of it.

S. Rosalki (U.K.): Would you say that the inhibitor is a high molecular weight compound or a low molecular weight compound? And, if so, would you care to speculate on what its molecular weight is?

W. Gruber (Germany): It is very difficult to calculate the molecular weight of the compound no matter what methods are used. If you try to make molecular weight determinations by gel filtration or some other method, it is very difficult, due to the instability of the fraction.

M. Härkönen (Finland): In the Sephadex elution, it appears in the same position as NADH does. Accordingly, the molecular weight should be close to that of NADH and it can not be a dimer.

W. Gruber (Germany): We have done with our inhibitor substance just the same chromatographic experiments, and our substance smears along on the column. So, in this one respect, the substance we have worked with is not the same as yours as we cannot get good peaks in the range of NADH or anywhere.

M. Härkönen (Finland): What happens if you treat your compound with acid; does it still show inhibitory properties; or does it lose the inhibitory properties?

W. Gruber (Germany): I do not have data on that.

E. van Kampen (Holland): I wonder if any elementary analysis has been done on this product.

W. Gruber (Germany): When elementary analysis is performed, there may occur changes in – let's say – the nitrogen contents occurring on dimerization, so that the results are within the limits of accuracy and precision of the determinations.

W. Gruber (Germany): Dr. *Bücher,* as manufacturers of reagents, we think that it is of great importance for us to get new values for the coefficients of extinction which can be published and used nationwide, Europewide or even worldwide. Of course, one could say: 'Well, there is a small uncertainty of plus-minus a small fraction.' However, when we have to print instructions for the user, we need the exact data of what to print. Can we say after hearing your lecture that you recommend for NADH at 25 degrees centigrade and at a wavelength of 334 nanometers a value of 6.12?

Th. Bücher (Germany): I have tried to outline the mentioned value at 334.15 as being practically independent of the temperature in the physiological range or in the practical range. The values you mention at 365 nanometers at 25 degrees centigrade should really be corrected if the measurements are made at other temperatures, say 30 °C or 38 °C. The values at 340 nanometers, in my opinion, have only a historical reason because this value does not correspond to the absorbance maximum. You should not stick to 340 nanometers, which I think is nonsense, because this is the maximum of only one substance at zero degrees centigrade. If you look for a wavelength, then I would ask for the maximum wavelength at different temperatures or at a given temperature. If you ask for the value at 340, I have given you the ratio for the different temperatures including 25 °C. Now, what I would like you to know is that I calculated from the data a value which is about 1% less than the values determined by Dr. *Bowers.* I think we should discuss this discrepancy.

W. Gruber (Germany): May I just state at this point that it would be most useful to have a natural constant for the coefficient of extinction of such an important substance as NADH. It appears that the only wavelength that indeed seems to fit this concept is around the 334 nanometers, whereas at all other wavelengths, it is a natural variable. Is this right?

Th. Bücher (Germany): Yes, that is my opinion, but you know of the immobility of the International Federation of Clinical Chemistry. However, that is not my problem. What I have presented here is only my hobby. I should apologize that my abstract as published in the Conference Manual is so poor because I had only the occasion of the last week to evaluate the wealth of data which was generated.

H. Bergmeyer (Germany): Dr. *Bücher* and Dr. *Bowers,* it is absolutely necessary that we clarify the discrepancies between your results at 339 nanometers. Dr. *Bowers,* I think, agrees that the maximum at 25 °C lies approximately at 339 nanometers. The worldwide use of measuring in clinical chemistry at this wavelength should be promoted. We should really switch over from 340 to 339; but, if we have discrepancies in the absorption coefficient of about 2% or more, then this is not satisfactory and we need a final value for use in routine work in clinical chemistry. Perhaps it might be possible if you both would discuss a little bit more your data as they apply to your systems.

G. Bowers (U. S. A.): I certainly can agree that we need to be measuring at the maximum of 339 and this has been done except that it is very recent. I would say that the only observation that I can make at this point is that, if we were not on the maximum, it would only tend to make the value slightly higher. I do not think this is a major problem.

Th. Bücher (Germany): Dr. *Bergmeyer,* for the practitioner in your field, I think it is not very important if the shift is by 1% or more. I think he has in his laboratory other internal constants. In my opinion, what is more necessary for the practitioner is that he has available a wavelength which is practically as free as possible from error. This – I think – is the main objective of my contribution. Of course, I knew that Dr. *Bower's* results are 1% higher than ours. This forced me to look into my data with special care in order to detect any source of error that may explain the possibility of a shift up of 1%, and so, may I ask you a few questions of you:

- I think you should substantiate the nature of your corrections.
- What is the extinction coefficient of gluconolactone at 340 nanometers?

G. Bowers (U. S. A.): I do not believe we can give you one except that empirically we have looked at the system and find that we are not conscious of a bias related to the products or any of their intermediates. I know that this is inadequate and, in the paper which will be forth-coming, we will direct ourselves to such an observation. We have looked up the extinction contributed by each of the enzymes, the dilution factors, and we do not find other than for the slight change in volume that this has affected the system.

Th. Bücher (Germany): But you see gluconolactone is no enzyme. I would like to come to the contribution of the enzyme proteins later on. The molar extinction of ketoglutaric acid is 20 at 334 nm and that of pyruvic acid is 18 and this has been measured and corrected for. Since the audience considers this matter to be important, we should have all this information in order to make a decision. The next question would be the contribution of the enzyme additions. For instance, what amounts of enzymes did you add, and what was their contribution to the extinction at 340?

G. Bowers (U. S. A.): Correction was made for them at 340. I can not give you an exact extinction for each; but they were corrected for in terms of their extinction as well as for their volume. But I will have to come up with the data. We added one microliter of one of them and two microliters of the other. I will have to go back to my text for confirmation.

Th. Bücher (Germany): Microliters or micrograms?

G. Bowers (U. S. A.): Microliters. For a total of 4000 microliters.

Th. Bücher (Germany): We only added 5 microliters of glutamic dehydrogenase but this really contributed two milliunits to the extinction.

G. Bowers (U. S. A.): The extinction resulting from these were indeed corrected for. I cannot give you the exact extinction but it was corrected for as well as volume correction.

Th. Bücher (Germany): Yes, but you see Dr. *Bowers,* you say it has been corrected but to decide this 1%, we must really know how it has been corrected and by what figures.

G. Bowers (U. S. A.): That would be the data we will discuss in the paper.

Th. Bücher (Germany): That is only a proposition for the publication. For this meeting, we should cover all details. The next point is that, in our measurements, everything was performed in the same laboratory. The preparation of the reference substance, the titration of the reference substance, the dilution and the preparation of the system. You relate to 99.9% purity of glucose but this has not been checked in your laboratory. I would like to know if this is the mono or the dihydrate of glucose?

G. Bowers (U. S. A.): All I can refer you to is that we are starting with a material that is probably as well known as any material available to anyone and it is available to everyone here. If you turn to the IFCC Symposium, you will see on page 382 the type of certification data that has gone behind this starting material. It was not done in our laboratories and it would totally be impossible for us to produce the analytical grade of material this was. This is a standard reference material from the National Bureau of Standards (USA).

Th. Bücher (Germany): Did you dry the preparation in your laboratory?

G. Bowers (U. S. A.): The material specifically said that it should not be dried. The loss of weight on drying is less than 0.01 to 0.02% by weight (see data NBS Certificate of Analysis, Standard Reference Material 917, D-Glucose [Dextrose]).

U. S. Department of Commerce
Frederick B. Dent
Secretary
ional Bureau of Standards
ıard W. Roberts, Director

National Bureau of Standards
Certificate of Analysis
Standard Reference Material 917
D-Glucose (Dextrose)

B. Coxon and R. Schaffer

This standard reference material is certified as a chemical of known purity. It is intended primarily for use in the calibration and standardization of procedures for glucose determinations employed in clinical analysis and for routine critical evaluation of the daily working standards used in these procedures.

Purity	99.9	percent
α-D-Glucopyranose	greater than 99.0	percent
β-D-Glucopyranose	less than 1.0	percent
Moisture	0.06	percent
Ash	0.002	percent
Insoluble Matter	0.001 to 0.006	percent
Nitrogen	less than 0.001	percent

Specific Rotation

$[\alpha]_{D}^{20}$ = +53.2 ° (at equil., *c* 20.1 in water)

$[\alpha]_{546}^{20}$ = +62.8 ° (at equil., *c* 20.1 in water)

$[\alpha]_{D}^{20}$ = +112.6 ° (initial *c* 10.05 in methyl sulfoxide)

The value for the purity has an estimated inaccuracy of ±0.1 percent.

The D-glucose used for this standard reference material was obtained from Pfanstiehl Laboratories, Inc., of Waukegan, Illinois. Analyses were performed by R. F. Brady, Jr., B. Coxon, M. M. Darr, T. E. Gills, E. C. Kuehner, R. A. Paulson, T. C. Rains, T. A. Rush, W. P. Schmidt, J. H. Thomas, and W. L. Zielinski of the Analytical Chemistry Division.

The overall direction and coordination of technical measurements leading to the certification were under the chairmanship of R. Schaffer.

The technical and support aspects concerning the preparation, certification, and issuance of this standard reference material were coordinated through the Office of Standard Reference Materials by T. W. Mears.

Washington, D. C. 20234
November 18, 1970
Revised September 20, 1973

J. Paul Cali, Chief
Office of Standard Reference Materials

The only impurities detected in this standard reference material were moisture and traces of inorganic compounds. Paper, thin-layer, and high-pressure ion-exchange chromatographic techniques revealed no organic impurities.

The proportion of the α-D-glucose anomer was estimated by three methods. The ratio of the β-anomer to the α-anomer was found to be 0.5:100 by gas-liquid chromatography (glc) after per(trimethylsilyl)ation of the solid standard material for 10 min at 0 °C using N-(trimethylsilyl)imidazole in anhydrous pyridine to minimize possible mutarotation. Use of this glc technique on partly melted standard material showed that the proportion of the β-anomer increased markedly during melting. Differential scanning calorimetry of the standard material, contained under nitrogen in unsealed aluminum pans, showed the α-D-glucose content to be 99.4 percent. This value represents only the proportion of anhydrous α-D-glucopyranose present, since the method treats β-D-glucose, or hydrates of α-D-glucose that are stable up to the melting point, as impurities. However, proton magnetic resonance spectroscopy at 90 MHz indicated the ratio of β-anomer to α-anomer to be 0.9:100. This determination was performed 10 min after dissolution of 100 mg of D-glucose in 0.5 ml of methyl sulfoxide-d_6, by integration of the doublets due to the anomeric hydroxyl groups.

Optical rotations were obtained by use of an automatic polarimeter and a high-precision manual polarimeter.

The moisture content reported was determined by the Karl Fischer and near infrared methods. As only 0.01 to 0.02 percent in weight was lost on drying at 70 °C/1-2 torr for 100 hr, the analyses reported herein were performed on the undried standard reference material.

The ash content reported was determined by ignition of 20-g samples at 750 °C; the undissolved residue, on 10-g samples. Turbidimetric assays of solutions of the standard showed the presence of chloride at 2 ppm and sulfate at 3 ppm. Neutron activation indicated chloride at 4 ppm.

Emission spectrometric analysis of the ash from this standard reference material showed calcium to be approximately 5 ppm; magnesium and silicon each less than 0.1 ppm; aluminum, boron and iron each less than 0.05 ppm; and copper, less than 0.01 ppm.

Atomic absorption spectrometry of the standard reference material indicated that it contains less than 0.5 ppm of magnesium. Flame emission spectrometry indicated the content of calcium to be 1 ±0.5 ppm, and sodium to be 2.9 ppm.

This Standard Reference Material is intended for "in vitro" diagnostic use only.

This material is for use as a standard in clinical chemistry. A 1 percent standard solution of glucose may be prepared by weighing 1.000g of SRM 917 into an 100-ml volumetric flask. The flask is then filled nearly to the mark with 0.2 percent benzoic acid solution and agitated until solution is complete. The flask is then filled to the mark with 0.2 percent benzoic acid solution. One ml of this solution contains 0.01g (10mg) of glucose. The benzoic acid solution should be prepared from ACS Reagent grade benzoic acid. Appropriate size samples of this solution are analyzed by the exact procedure used for the submitted specimen of body fluid.

To prepare glucose solution of lower concentration the appropriate aliquot is pipetted into a 100-ml volumetric flask and diluted with 0.2 percent benzoic acid solution.

This Standard Reference Material should be stored in a well-closed container at room temperature (30 °C or less). It should not be subjected to heat or direct sunlight during storage. Refrigerated storage is recommended. Under proper storage, experience at NBS indicates this material to be stable for at least 5 years. If the material purity degrades beyond the limits certified, purchasers will be notified by NBS. It is recommended that material not be used after 5 years from date of purchase.

All constituted solutions of D-Glucose should be clear and without indications of bacterial growth of any kind.

References:

[1] R. D. Henry, Clinical Chemistry, Principles and Practice, pp. 625-656, Hoeber Medical Division, Harper & Row, New York, New York 10016 (1967).

[2] N. W. Tietz, Fundamentals of Clinical Chemistry, pp. 154-163, W. B. Saunders Co., Philadelphia, Pa. 19105 (1970).

This Standard Reference Material has been measured and certified at the Laboratories of the National Bureau of Standards, Gaithersburg, Maryland. All inquiries should be addressed to:

Office of Standard Reference Materials
Room B311, Chemistry Building
National Bureau of Standards
Washington, D. C. 20234

The date of issuance and certification of this Standard Reference Material was November 18, 1970.

Th. Bücher (Germany): How much was the loss on drying?

G. Bowers (U. S. A.): Very small. But the Bureau does not recommend it, and the actual loss is in the data sheet for glucose. We will make sure that this is shown in the paper, but again, as far as I know, the credence of the measurements here have been checked by half a dozen techniques and I personally have no reason to feel that there is anything in my laboratory that I could do to give this greater credence. It is open to everyone's inspection by looking at the NBS criteria, and besides the material is available for everybody to look at.

Th. Bücher (Germany): You see, the philosophy would be that, if the purity is 99.9 and the values obtained in the experiment are higher than that of our group, then we should look again into the purity of the substance, just because our values are lower. On the other hand, if you have the dihydrate and it lost water, then the content might be 101% of what you calculated as the molecular weight. And so, I might suggest that this should be checked out.

G. Bowers (U. S. A.): I think that the credence given these materials in general may not be appreciated here, but they have been under all sorts of attack by our Scientific Community in the United States for years, and very rarely have these been substantially altered. The history of a material like glucose, for instance, probably went through 2 years of intensive analytical work with half a dozen techniques and it is all thoroughly described. So it is a starting material that we give credence to.

S. Rosalki (U. K.): I feel that two distinguished scientists like Dr. *Bowers* and Dr. *Bücher* should be given the opportunity of meeting together to sort out the reasons for their discrepancies. I feel sure, personally, that the reasons will not turn out to be differences of materials or of technique. The differences must be due to differences of systems, and that may well become clear during their more private exchanges. I think Dr. *Bücher* has done us a great service during this Symposium and I would hope that we, as clinical chemists, would not be so resistant to change. I believe that a clinical chemist may very readily accept the 334 nanometers mercury line as a suitable wavelength measuring line for enzymatic determinations. The advantages of the line have been very helpfully put by Dr. *Bücher* and the fact that, at this wavelength, both the coenzymes NADH and NADPH are identical in their molar absorptivity and that they are, at least for NADH, temperature independent constitute important points. I think that these points have been taken note of by the clinical chemists here, and your talk today will have a greater effect on us than you may have thought at the start.

W. Gerhardt (Denmark): I wish to ask a question of Dr. *Härkönen*. Did I understand that you performed some stability studies in which you flushed nitrogen through a solution of NADH in neutralized water – and demonstrated that nitrogen exerted no protective effect?

M. Härkönen (Finland): There were other experiments, but this particular one was carried out at + 4 °C because we found the largest changes at that temperature. We found nitrogen to have no effect in solution.

W. Gerhardt (Denmark): The comment that I want to make is that I do not think this is directly comparable to my study because I used a solid preparation which was exposed to both humidity and carbon dioxide, creating carbonic acid, and found nitrogen to have a protective action. I think you indicated your results were in contrast to my results.

M. Härkönen (Finland): No, I did not say that. What I said was, if people are going to store NADH in solution, they might conclude from your study that nitrogen would have a protective action and this is not so.

W. Gerhardt (Denmark): I am sorry. I have a question. The stability study in tris buffer indicated somewhat poorer stability than the data I showed yesterday. You used a pooled NADH from three commercial sources that had a rather high initial 260 over 340 nanometer absorbance ratio. I do have a feeling that there is something autocatalytic about the process. Perhaps if you were to repeat your experiment with a more pure NADH, like the one I used for the experiments I reported yesterday with an initial ratio of 2.3, then the stability perhaps would come out to be a little better.

M. Härkönen (Finland): You suggest that we should repeat everything because we used three different materials as was shown on the slides. I do not think that it makes too much difference, because you have always the starting point there, and you look for the differences as a function of time. I recommended the use of −75 °C since at other temperatures you have changes.

W. Gerhardt (Denmark): Yes, I think that is quite true. By the way, I want to compliment you on your very thorough study of the subject.

B. Copeland (U. S. A.): I would like to ask a question. In view of the fact that the spectrophotometers that we use in our laboratories show variability in excess of the differences of the molar absorptivity constants about which we are talking, can we not accept the fact that it is very difficult in science ever to get an identical number even from two excellent investigators?

Th. Bücher (Germany): If I might answer. In my opinion, the value of the extinction coefficient is clearly known, both from my personal experience and also from what has been done quite independently in Tutzing (Germany). The Tutzing group did their work using ten different photometers. I personally tested my system only with a Cary, which is a monochrometer instrument, and with the Eppendorf, which is a line photometer. I have the data here. There is no systematic difference. I think we should not give way to these thoughts; they are too dangerous.

Th. Bücher (Germany): I have a question for Dr. *Giegel*. Is there any influence of pyruvate concentration on the inhibitor?

J. Giegel (U. S. A.): We did not examine that in this system.

Th. Bücher (Germany): Is there any competition due to pyruvate? You see, the different isoenzymes are distinguished in their substrate inhibition by pyruvate, and it is known that the substrate inhibition of heart LDH, is much more prominent than of LDH_5, so this might be perhaps what you are seeing. What was the concentration of pyruvate used?

J. Giegel (U. S. A.): It was 0.8 millimolar. Our system was not designed to analyze the effects of pyruvate on the inhibitor, although that is an interesting suggestion.

W. Gruber (Germany): May I ask what was the reason for the study? Was it to check for inhibiting impurities in NADH preparations, or was it to differentiate between different LDH isoenzymes?

J. Henry (U. S. A.): We were looking at both. We were looking for a simple practical system to monitor NADH in terms of its relative impurity and to identify its less than optimal performance. We also wished to see if the use of inhibited, versus normal NADH could show any particular categorization, of either clinical patients or other appropriate specimens, which in turn may reflect LDH isoenzymes.

S. Rosalki (U. K.): At the 1973 Symposium I showed that a human heated-heart preparation was a useful preparation for the detection of the moisture type of inhibitor of NADH preparations; but the specification of a human heated-heart preparation was too crude. What was required was a standard form of preparation to be readily available to the clinical laboratory for this purpose. A partial aim of the study described by Dr. *Giegel*, was to provide such a preparation as a convenient means of moisture-inhibitor detection and see how it would perform with various batches of NADH.

W. Gruber (Germany): As availability of human heart is limited, for a similar reason, we purified isoenzymes from human and pig origin in exactly the same manner. As we described in Munich last year we could show that there are really no differences in any catalytic respect between human and pig LDH isoenzymes, even as far as inhibition by inhibitors in NADH are concerned. So, we think in order to check impurities in biochemicals, the best way would be to take the most pure system possible. But, if you wish to use an impure system, then you can add the purified enzymes to serum of different species in order to carry out the experiments.

S. Rosalki (U. K.): I think that was visible in the slides of different tissues I showed. In fact in those studies there was evidence that dog heart LD-1 was perhaps the most sensitive, even more sensitive than the human. There are, of course, disadvantages in dog heart, and to a certain extent in the pig preparations in that the isoenzyme pattern is very different. Certainly the pig preparation reacts quite distinctly in the HBD reaction as compared to human preparations.

W. Gruber (Germany): You can show large differences in impure preparations, such as extracts and the first steps of purification. But as you continue to purify your enzymes, the differences are lost.

S. Rosalki (U. K.): One of the interesting things that showed up in this study, was the difference in performance of lyophilized material compared to material in the native state.

Hematology Symposium

Plenary Lectures

Quality Control and Hematology I

E.J. van Kampen and *O. W. van Assendelft*, Groningen, The Netherlands

Key words: Counting chamber calibration
Electronic counter calibration
Hemoglobin determination
HiCN standard
Interferometry
Interlaboratory control
Intralaboratory control

In discussing Quality Control in hematology, one is tempted to start with a historical review.

Many fundamental aspects have been recognized by a few at an early stage, namely that quality control should be based on the principles of fundamental analytical calibration and dynamic standardization, aiming at a 'true value'. Dr. *van Assendelft* will later elaborate some details on this point.

Hemoglobin

Some twenty years ago, we started investigating the HiCN-method, which resulted in 1961 in the issue of a HiCN-standard solution, together with a standardized method sheet.

During the first years of this investigation about 20% of clinical chemists decided to introduce this new method in their laboratories (fig. 1). Then in 1961, when the HiCN-standard solution and method sheet were issued, the number increased slowly but steadily, reaching 85% in 1966. Round about 1970 the last of the Mohicans came over to join us. The HiCN-method is now internationally accepted as the first standardized clinical chemical method.

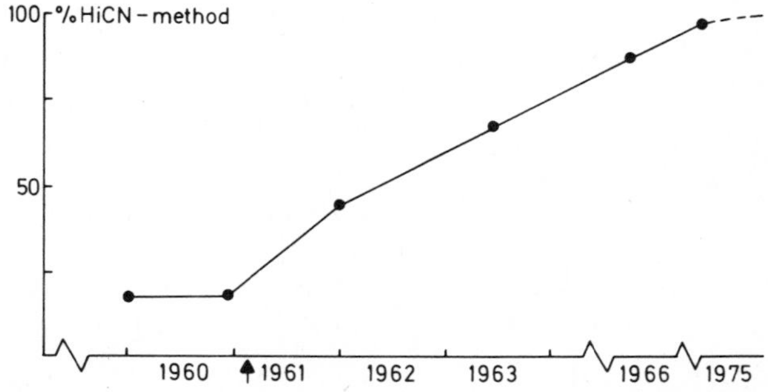

Fig. 1. Increase in the use of the HiCN method from 1960–1975.

The HiCN-standard solution is now used by many laboratories to obtain a calibration point. The concentration of a new standard usually lies at around 60 mg/dl HiCN, corresponding to 15 g/dl ≡ 9.3 mmol/l Hb for a dilution 1:251. Expert panel laboratories from 6 countries determine and check the optical density or extinction (E) of each new standard.

This means, of course, that they do not need to treat the sample, but simply to determine its optical density spectrophotometrically, after wavelength- and optical density calibration. The results of these determinations always revealed a coefficient of variation of Vc ≈ 0.5% (fig. 2).

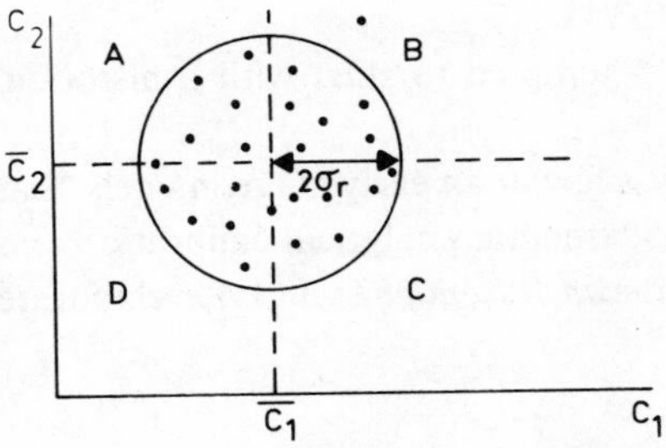

Fig. 2. Youden plot of HiCN standard measurements; Vc ≈ 0.5%.

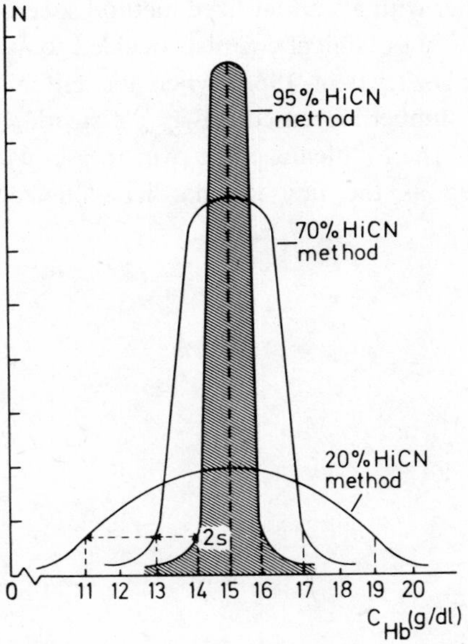

Fig. 3. Decrease of standard deviation of the Hb-determination, using the HiCN method.

In this Youden plot $\bar{c}_1 \approx 50$ mg/dl HiCN and $\bar{c}_2 \approx 60$ mg/dl HiCN; 2 σ, varies from 0.5–0.6 mg/dl, giving a Vc ≈ 0.5%. A perfect circular distribution is shown, caused by a small random error only.

With the standard method sheet and HiCN-reference solutions as weapons of Quality Control, the results of several Hb-trials held in the Netherlands improved considerably. These results, all recalculated to a 15 g/dl Hb-level are shown in figure 3. In parallel with an increasing percentage of HiCN-users the standard deviation of the results became smaller and smaller. The figure shows that 2 σ has decreased from 4 down to 1 g/dl; the coefficient of variation decreasing from 10% to about 3%. This quality control result does give cause for satisfaction, however, one should nevertheless be careful not to rest too soon on one's laurels.

Looking back at figure 2 with Vc ≈ 0.5% and a perfect circular distribution, implying no systematic error, doubt creeps up on us. Do these results give proof that the Hb-determination is performed accurately in each laboratory? In a recent intra-laboratory trial we sent, together with a HiCN-standard, two hemolysates of unknown content. The participants were asked to determine the Hb-concentration in these hemolysates, using the HiCN-method. Behold the results shown in figure 4. The HiCN-standards, represented by crosses, give the well-known circular distribution with a Vc ≈ 0.5%. But sample handling obviously introduced a large combined random and systematic error, resulting in a coefficient of variation of about 5% (dots), a tenfold increase.

One has to come to the conclusion that many clinical chemical laboratories failed in the transition from inter- to intra laboratory control.

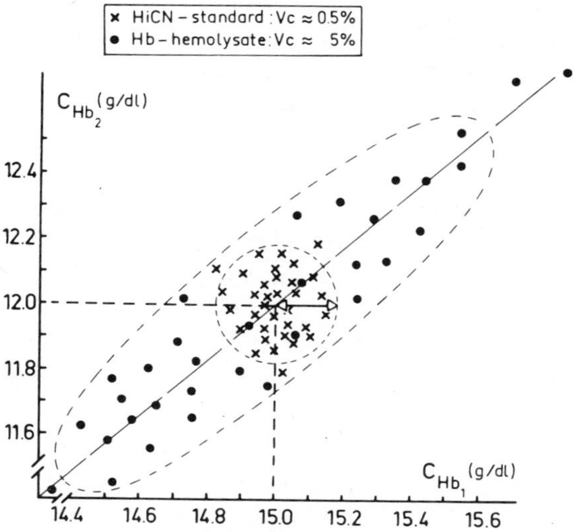

Fig. 4. Youden plot of determinations of:
× HiCN standards, ● Hb content in hemolysates.

Errors made in the trial could be traced back to:

1. dilution errors, automatic dilutors must be calibrated and checked regularly. It is wrong to believe one's supplier!
2. faulty reagents, especially a too low CN^- concentration; this results in too low values. A check on this point can easily be performed.
3. incorrectly calibrated instruments.

A working scheme for reference standards and their general application would seem necessary, Dr. van Assendelft will refer to this in the next paper.

Cell-counting

A second major aspect in hematological quality control is the cell-counting system. Especially because certain parameters derived from C_{Hb} and number of cells play an important part in hematological diagnosis, e.g. the M.C.H. (mean corpuscular hemoglobin).

From investigations made so far it can be concluded:

1. Accurate calibration of automatic cell counting systems, e.g. the Coulter Counter is almost impossible, and certainly not within the scope of an average laboratory.
2. Coincidence in counting, resulting in too low counts, is a special problem.
3. The number of particles counted is dependent on the so called threshold setting, which can be calibrated, but the threshold is strongly dependent on the shape of the particles. This means that adjustment of instruments should be different in cases of spherocytosis (diameter $\ll$ 7 μm) of pernicious anaemia (diameter $\gg$7 μm) or e.g. thallasaemia.
4. Efforts to arrive at some quality control through the use of stabilized erythrocytes or latex particles have failed up till now.

In consequence the (systematic) error can remain quite large, although the reproducibility, i.e. the precision, may be quite good. This in turn leads to a wide normal range for the M.C.H., for instance from $26–38 \cdot 10^{-12}$ g. A range so wide, that it is hardly of any use to the clinician.

How to tackle this problem? The number of cells is given per mm^3 or per l, a volume therefore. What is more obvious then, than to calibrate this volume independently. Several efforts have been made to calibrate a counting chamber as to volume. Measuring the length and the width of the chamber is not the main problem. Measuring the depth, however, is! Filling the chamber ($l \approx 0.1$ mm) with a concentrated dye solution and comparing the measured optical density to the value obtained using a known light pathlength leads to l. This could thus theoretically be a solution. In practice however, this does not work, as we have often experienced. Many errors obviously remain hidden, for instance:

1. The need for vertical positioning of the counting chamber in the spectrophotometer.
2. The clips of the coverglass do not ensure reproducible pressure. The reason for this was discovered later on.
3. The ruled network *in* the chamber, which scatters the light.

The problem of calibrating the depth was solved by Dr. *T. de Boer* and his coworkers[1]. Using both white and monochromatic light in a Michelson interferometer and the interference microscope, they succeeded in measuring the depth of the counting chamber with an error smaller than 1%. In the Michelson-framing the movable mirror of the interferometer has been replaced by that plane of the counting chamber to be investigated. The chamber is arranged in a vertical position, in such a way that both planes of the coverglass and the bottom of the counting chamber are lying in the same vertical position. By moving back the plane of the counting chamber, the number of fringes or interference lines can be counted, each interference line representing a distance equal to ½. This means that the unit of measuring used in determining the depth of the counting chamber is: $\frac{1}{2}\lambda$, e.g. 250 nm $\equiv 250 \times 10^{-6}$ mm, when using light of $\lambda = 500$ nm. Figure 5 clarifies this principle, figure 6 shows the interference lines formed and used for the measurements. When light of e.g. 500 nm is used, about 400 lines have to be counted to bridge a distance of 0.1 mm; $d = 400 \times \frac{1}{2} \times 500 = 10^5$ nm $= 10^{-1}$ mm $= 0.1$ mm.

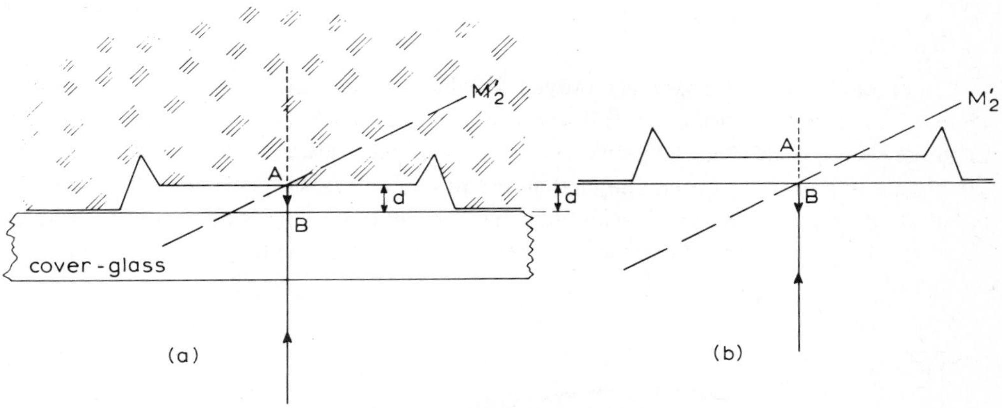

Fig. 5. Principle of the depth-measurement of the counting chamber, using an interference method.

[1] Dept. of Optics, Dr. *Tj. H. de Boer,* Drs. *D. Leijenaar, H. L. Leertouwer*

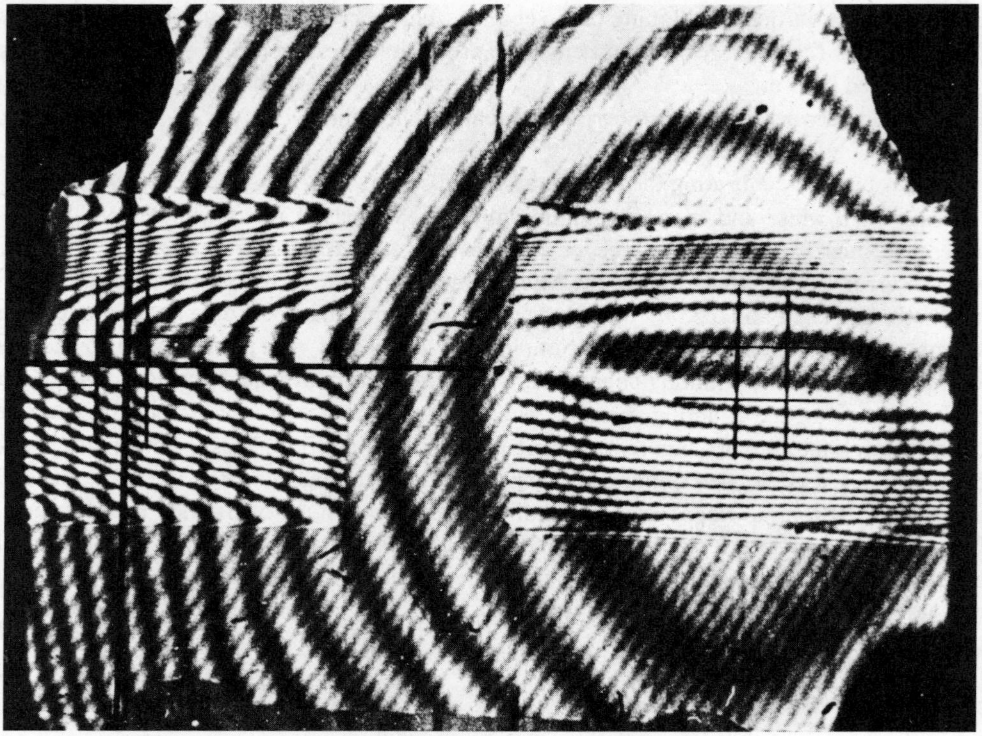

Fig. 6. Interference lines of counting chamber and coverglass.

Before calibration of chambers proved feasible, an erroneous usage of the counting chamber had to be corrected; this error having been made for as long as counting chambers have been used. Clips with layer of cork have always been used to press the coverglass into position. It was shown that, because of cork/glass resistance, the coverglass is forced into a convex shape. Although many believe the coverglass is contained in a perfectly horizontal plane above the chamber, in reality it has a cylindrical shape (fig. 7).

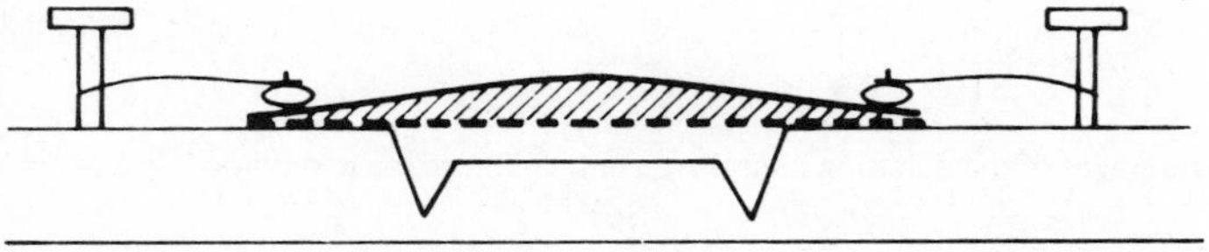

Fig. 7. Coverglass forced into cylindrical shape by clip pressure.

Dependent upon the way of applying and pressing down these clips, a systematic error of up to + 4% is introduced. Replacing the cork layer by two small metal globes, which slide over the coverglass at the same time exerting constant and equal pressure, has solved this problem definitely (fig. 8). Full details are in the process of being published.

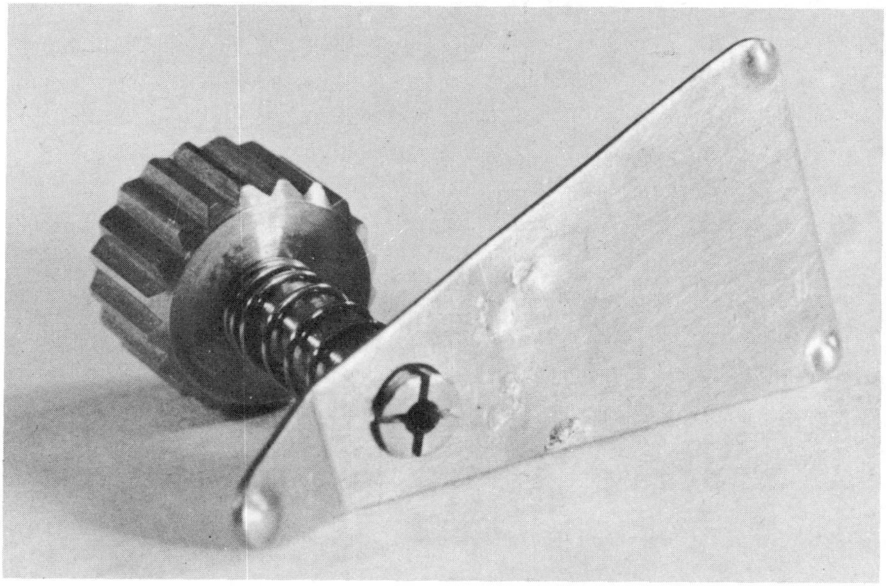

Fig. 8. New coverglass clip.

As an example, the dimension of a counting net ($^1/_{400}$ mm^2) is given. Length = 50.15 ± 0.25 μm, width = 50.00 ± 0.18 μm, depth = 99.8 ± 0.2 μm, content: $25.08 \cdot 10^{-5}$ mm^3; Vc ≈ 0.5%.

Knowing the exact volume of the counting chamber, a completely independent series was set up to count two blood samples containing about 4×10^6 (A) and 2×10^6 (B) erythrocytes per mm^3. Calibrated pipets were used, different medical technicians filled the calibrated counting chambers, after which the filled chambers were photographed (fig. 9), using a Leitz microphoto attachment.

The compartments used for the actual counting were coded, and different medical technicians counted the cells in these compartments from the photographs indicating the compartment coding which they used. As an example the following results are given.

Sample A: $(4.593 \pm 0.114) \cdot 10^6$ erythrocytes per mm^3; Vc = 2.4%; n = 24.

Sample B: $(2.264 \pm 0.072) \cdot 10^6$ erythrocytes per mm^3; Vc = 3.2%; n = 24.

C_{Hb} of these samples were respectively 14.7 ± 0.15 g/dl and 7.0 ± 0.18 g/dl.

Calculation of M.C.H. then yields for sample A $(32.0 \pm 1) \cdot 10^{-12}$ g and for sample B $(31.0 \pm 1) \cdot 10^{-12}$ g.

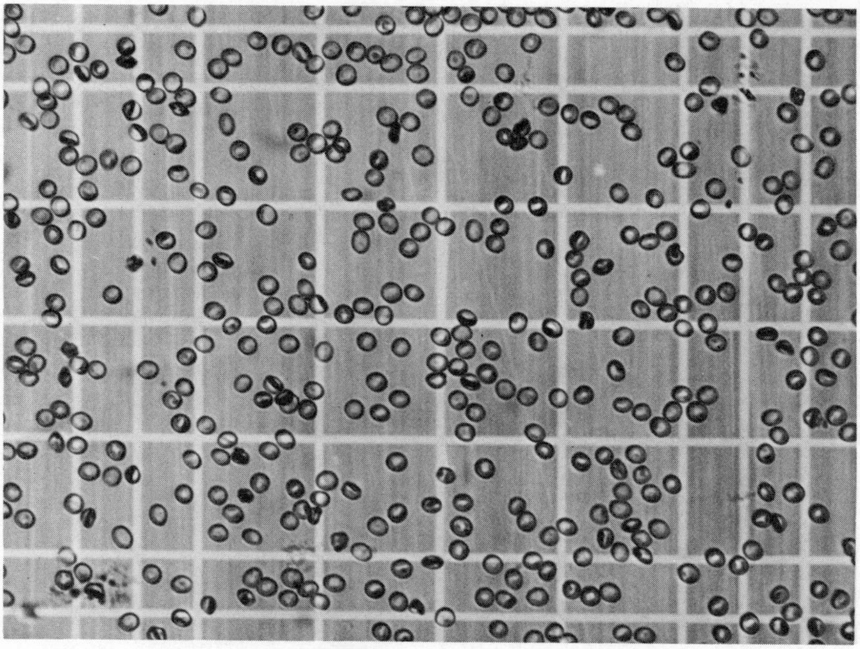

Fig. 9. Photograph of erythrocyte suspension in counting chamber.

At this point we were able to calibrate the automatic cell-counting system and to check its linearity. The samples were counted using a Coulter apparatus. The reproducibility of the electronic counts was within 1%. The values found as well as the values after correction for coincidence counting were compared with the values just mentioned. In our case a correction of −4% proved to be necessary. This correction can be obtained in the instrument by means of varying the threshold setting, but keeping within the plateau-limits. Nevertheless according to our experience, Coulter Counter should explore the possibility of volume adaptation in their instruments.

Summarizing, the following may be concluded:

1. Hemoglobin can be determined with a Vc within 2%, if from interlaboratory control, results are used to take corrective steps as regards the intra-laboratory control programs.
2. Cell counting can be done with a Vc≈2–3%, if one is prepared to calibrate in a fundamental analytical way.

3. Quantities derived from these two, e. g. M. C. H., can be measured, assuming a normal range of 29–35 · 10^{-12} g, with a combined error ($\sigma_{tot} = \sqrt{\sigma^2_{Hb} + \sigma^2_{Er}} \approx 3\%$. This is acceptable, and within e. g. Cotlove's criteria ('Tolerable analytic variation' defined as one half the estimated biological variability; *Cotlove, E., Harris, E.K.* and *Williams, G.Z.,* Clinical Chemistry [1970], *16,* 1028–1032).

Quality Control and Hematology II

O. W. van Assendelft and *E.J. van Kampen*, Groningen (The Netherlands)

Key words: Counting chamber calibration
Cyanide-sensing electrode
Hemoglobin determination
Hemoglobin lysate
HiCN standard
Interferometry
Interlaboratory precision
Intralaboratory precision
Packed cell volume

Both in clinical chemistry and in hematology, we are confronted with an increased demand for greater validity of test results. To meet this demand adequately, every factor in the analytical process leading to a test result must be sufficiently controlled. This includes the training of personnel, instrument performance, the quality of reagents and of reference preparations and the way in which the test is actually performed. The term *quality control* is usually taken to refer to the factor mentioned last, only.

A procedure is said to be under control when both accuracy and precision of the results are within generally accepted, though arbitrary, limits. Accuracy is a measure of the closeness of an estimated value to the true value; precision is a measure of the reproducibility of an estimation. Accuracy is defined by reference to an absolute standard, whenever possible based on international specifications. In practice this is accomplished through secondary (commercial) standards normally used in the laboratory. Precision is assessed by repeated determinations of a (commercial) control preparation.

In quality control, two facts may be discerned. The first is the internal or intralaboratory control. This consists of analysis of control samples selected daily by the laboratory head, and checks both accuracy and precision within the laboratory. The second is the external or interlaboratory control. It consists of the analysis of control samples, usually of unknown content, received periodically from third parties in order to compare accuracy levels of different laboratories. No laboratory can function adequately without a well-defined internal quality control program. The validity of the internal programs must be checked, independently and at regular intervals, through participation in external quality control programs.

The previous paper has already introduced the determination of haemoglobin as an example of an internationally accepted, standardized procedure which can be controlled as to quality, because of the availability of a reference point: international hemiglobincyanide (HiCN) reference solutions of exactly known content.

Table 1. Stability measurements of HiCN reference solutions.

time years	months	40400 D^{540}	D^{540}/D^{504}	60400 D^{540}	D^{540}/D^{504}	70400 D^{540}	D^{540}/D^{504}	80400 D^{540}	D^{540}/D^{504}	90400 D^{540}	D^{540}/D^{504}	00400 D^{540}	D^{540}/D^{504}	10400 D^{540}	D^{540}/D^{504}	20400 D^{540}	D^{540}/D^{504}
0	0	0.391	1.61	0.386	1.61	0.405	1.62	0.383	1.60	0.389	1.61	0.395	1.61	0.413	1.61	0.408	1.61
	3			0.387	1.61			0.381	1.60	0.389	1.61	0.395	1.61	0.413	1.60	0.408	1.61
0	6			0.387	1.61	0.404	1.62	0.386	1.61^{5}	0.388	1.62	0.396	1.61	0.415	1.61^{5}	0.408	1.61
	9			0.387	1.61			0.383	1.61								
1	0	0.389	1.61	0.388	1.61	0.405	1.59^{5}			0.388	1.60	0.400	1.62			0.408	1.62
	3					0.403	1.61							0.414	1.61		
1	6	0.391	1.61			0.407	1.62	0.386	1.61^{5}	0.389	1.62	0.398	1.62	0.414	1.60^{5}		
	9					0.405	1.62	0.385	1.61	0.389	1.61	0.397	1.61	0.415	1.61	0.406	1.61
2	0	0.391	1.61			0.405	1.62							0.413	1.61		
	3					0.406	1.62			0.390	1.61	0.396	1.62				
2	6	0.390	1.61	0.387	1.61	0.404	1.62	0.386	1.61			0.393	1.60	0.412	1.61	0.404	1.61
	9									0.390	1.60^{5}						
3	0	0.391	1.62			0.404	1.61	0.386	1.61			0.393	1.60	0.411	1.61	0.407	1.60
	3																
3	6			0.388	1.61					0.387	1.61	0.393	1.61	0.412	1.61		
	9																
4	0	0.389	1.61	0.387	1.61	0.405	1.61	0.388	1.62	0.387	1.61	0.393	1.61	0.412	1.60		
4	6					0.406	1.60^{5}										
5	0	0.393	1.61	0.386	1.61			0.384	1.61	0.387	1.60	0.393	1.60				
						0.404	1.62										
6	0	0.390	1.62					0.382	1.60	0.386	1.60						
7	0					0.402	1.61	0.383	1.60								
8	0	0.394	1.61			0.405	1.60										
9	0	0.390	1.60														
10	0	0.389	1.60														
11	0	0.390	1.60														

International HiCN reference solutions are prepared yearly by the Dutch Institute of Public Health on behalf of the International Committee for Standardization in Hematology (ICSH). Each new batch is first measured as to content, and controlled as to purity, by ICSH-designated reference laboratories the world over. At present these are laboratories in Germany, Great Britain, Italy, Japan, the Netherlands and the U.S.A. If a new batch is found to conform to the internationally accepted specifications laid down by ICSH, the reference solutions are checked three times at 3-month intervals and then issued for a period of two years. During this period of issue they continue to be checked, now at 6-month intervals. Although any international HiCN reference solution is circulated for only two years, checking as to content and purity has gone on in time in one of the reference laboratories for nearly all solutions prepared since 1964. The results are shown in table 1.

The international HiCN reference solutions are supplied, on request, to National Standardizing Committees and to manufacturers to enable them to compare secondary (commercial) HiCN reference solutions to such a solution guaranteed to meet the requirements laid down by ICSH. To illustrate that these requirements are not always met, an optical density/wavelength (λ/D) curve of a commercial HiCN reference solution recently studied, is shown in figure 1. Purity, as judged from the curve, does not conform to the ICSH requirements. This is apparent from the D^{540}/D^{504} value of 1.34, and from the light absorption maximum around $\lambda = 600–650$ nm. We are possibly confronted in this case by a solution containing a mixture of HiCN and Hi.

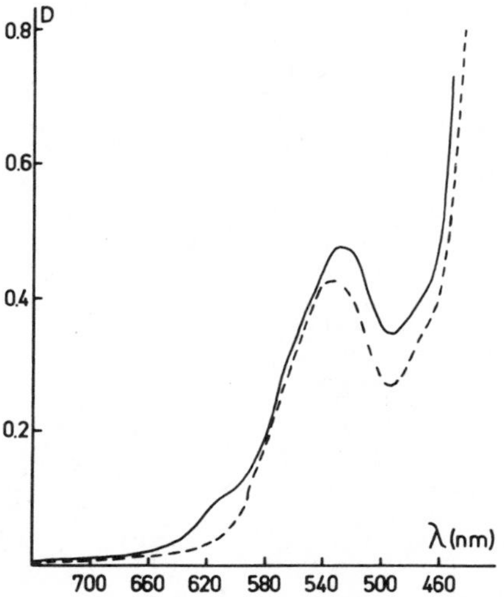

Fig. 1. λ/D curve of (1) a commercial HiCN reference solution (solid line) compared to (2) an international HiCN reference solution (dashed line). D^{540}/D^{504} solution (1) = 1.34, D^{540}/D^{504} solution (2) = 1.61. Optica CF_4 DR grating spectrophotometer, layer thickness 4 cm (1) and 1.00 cm (2), water as blank.

Having available a reference point, a HiCN reference solution of exactly known content, one is able to check the calibration of the measuring instrument used and should thus be able to ensure valid results in the day-to-day determination of haemoglobin. A recent interlaboratory quality control program, however, has already clearly shown this not to be the case. In figure 2 the histogram of the results of haemoglobin determinations on two samples of whole blood (samples 1 and 2) two partly purified haemolyzed blood samples (samples 3 and 4) and a HiCN solution (sample 5), obtained in an interlaboratory trial with 67 *selected* laboratories participating, is given. The histogram shows the instrument calibration to be reasonably well controlled, but rather large errors to have been made in the methods as a whole.

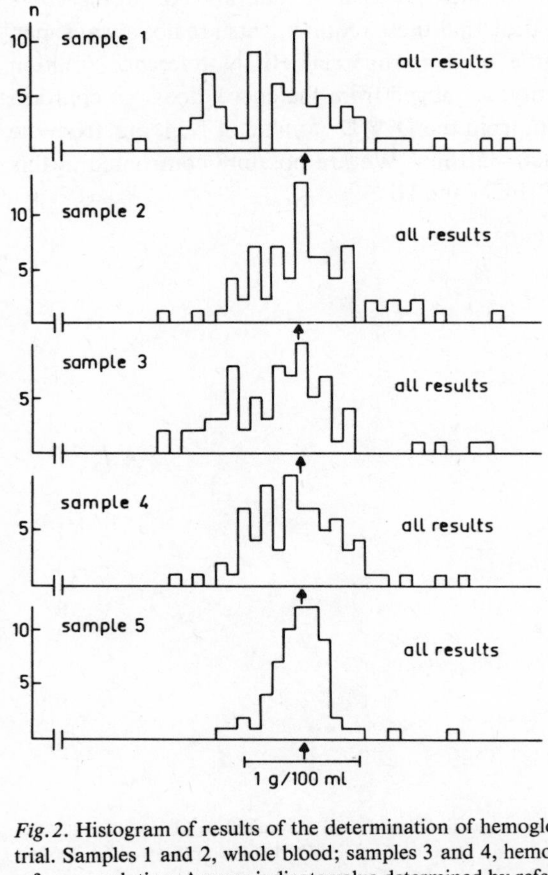

Fig. 2. Histogram of results of the determination of hemoglobin content, by 67 laboratories in an international trial. Samples 1 and 2, whole blood; samples 3 and 4, hemolyzed and partly purified blood; sample 5 a HiCN reference solution. Arrows indicate value determined by reference laboratories.

The different steps in the standardized HiCN method are as follows.

1. Pipette 5.0 ml of reagent into tube,
2. add 0.02 ml blood,
3. mix well and wait 5 min,
4. measure at 540 nm with (spectro)photometer,
5. read or calculate haemoglobin content.

Analysing, the possible errors may be back-tracked as follows.

1. Errors in measurement:
   a) use of non-calibrated instruments,
   b) use of unclean or non-matched cuvettes,
   c) diluted samples turbid.
2. Errors in the conversion to HiCN:
   a) use of aged or faultily prepared reagent,
   b) time lapse to measurement too short.
3. Errors in diluting:
   a) use of non-calibrated pipettes (5.0 ml),
   b) failure to wipe off excess blood,
   c) failure to rinse with reagent,
   d) pipettes insufficiently cleaned.
4. Errors in sampling:
   a) use of non-calibrated pipettes (0.02 ml),
   b) non-free-bleeding capillary puncture.

From the available results it was concluded that measurement errors have been but slight, that errors due to non-conversion or but part conversion were not probable, that errors in diluting were quite probable, that errors in sampling were not to be completely discounted. We are forced to conclude that the availability of a reference solution alone is

Table 2. Stability of partly purified hemoglobin solution.

Time (months)	D^{750}	D^{540}	D^{540}/D^{504}	dilution factor	c_{Hb} (g/dl)
0	.001	$.301^5$	1.59	251	11.1
1	$.001^5$	.302	1.58	251	11.1
2	.001	.300	1.58	251	10.9^5
3	$.001^5$	*.380*	1.59	*200*	11.1
4	.001	*.375*	1.59	*200*	11.0
6	.001	*.375*	1.59	*200*	11.0
12	$.001^5$	.297	1.58	251	10.9

not sufficient for an internal quality control program. The method as a whole must also be checked independently, to which end the availability of a sufficiently stable whole blood or whole blood-like preparation becomes imperative. Such a preparation, a partly purified concentrated haemoglobin solution[1], has been checked as to stability for the past year. The results of checking individual ampoules containing one ml of this haemoglobin solution, stored at 4 °C, are given in table 2.

Also available is a simple method to check the CN^- content of the reagent solution used in the HiCN method. In this method, use is made of a solid state ion-selective electrode with a sensing membrane of AgCN. A diagram of such an electrode is given in figure 3, an example of a calibration line in figure 4. Results of checking concentrated stock solutions of reagent[1] over the past few years are given in table 3.

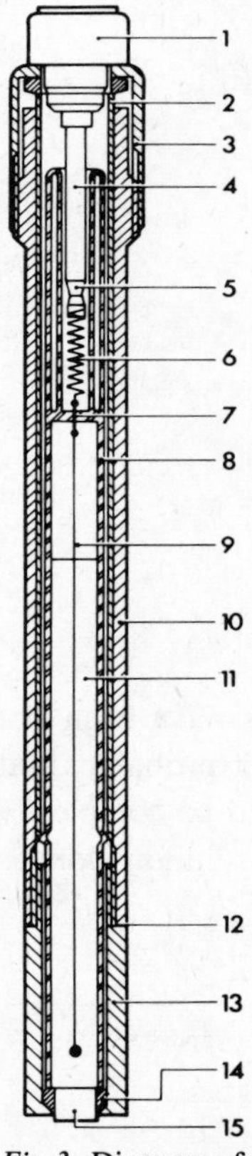

Fig. 3. Diagram of Philips solid state ion-selective electrode IS 550-CN. 1 = plug connector, 2 = screening, 3 = stainless steel cap, 4 = contact pressure pin, 5 = silver contacts, 6 = spring, 7 = platinum wire, 8 = glass housing of internal reference electrode (9), 10 = plastic shaft, 11 = internal solutions, 12 = sealing ring, 13 = membrane housing, 14 = membrane sealing ring, 15 = solid ion-exchanging membrane.

[1] Provided by Merz und Dade A. G., Berne, Switzerland

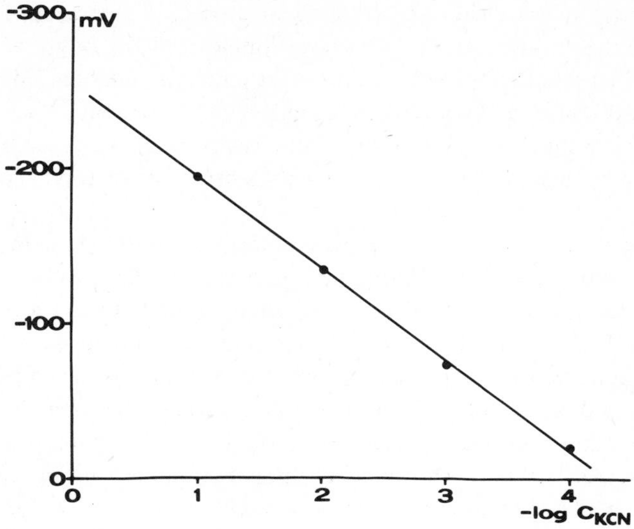

Fig. 4. Calibration line of Philips solid state CN^--sensitive electrode.

Table 3. Results of CN^--content determination of reagent solutions used in the HiCN method.

mV Reagent	Reference*	Reagent	CN^- (mg/l)
1	–230	–217	47.2
2	–217	–202	46.6
3	–242	–243	50
4	–224	–216	48.2
5	–213	–211	49.6
6	–213	–212	49.8
7	–227	–212	46.7
8	–230	–222	48.3
9	–230	–214	46.5
10	–225	–215	47.8

* = freshly prepared reagent containing 50 mg KCN per litre.

With the aid of the tools outlined, HiCN reference solutions to check or calibrate the measuring instrument, a concentrated haemoglobin solution to check the HiCN method as a whole and an ion-selective electrode to check the CN^- content of the reagent solution, it is possible for every haematological laboratory to ensure the clinician of valid results for haemoglobin values of a given patient.

Next to the determination of c_{Hb}, an important part of the haematological laboratory's workload consists of determining the number of cells in a given sample of blood, of giving an indication of cell size and of differentiating the cells within a certain cell population. For many years laboratories have been confronted with a low reliability in cell counting when using a counting chamber and microscope, while major discussion is still taking place as to the value and reliability of the cell volume determined using haematocrit tubes or capillary tubes spun in a centrifuge.

It is thus not surprising, that with the advent of electronic counting apparatus these instruments were enthusiastically introduced into many laboratories. Usually, without previous critical evaluation. Because the reproducibility of the counts thus obtained was shown to be extremely high, many have assumed that the results would also be accurate.

Because, as yet, reference solutions with a proven number of particles sufficiently resembling red cells in whole blood have not become available to allow checking the calibration of such electronic counting systems, we have taken another look at using the much abused counting chamber. As has been shown in the previous paper, the exact dimensions of any commercially available counting chamber can well be measured within but a remarkably small error. Measurement of the interline distances has never been much of a problem, depth measurement has now been proved to be possible with great accuracy. Dr. De Boer and coworkers started an interferometric investigation of counting chambers with the coverglass in position using a modified Michelson interferometer arrangement and an interference microscope for reflected light. Evaluation of the interference images observed, enabled them to obtain very accurate information (precision of measurement up 0.05 µm) about [1] the true shape of the bottom and roof of the counting chamber viz. the ruled area of the recess in the glass slide and the underside of the coverglass when held in position by the clips [2] the shape of the two outer areas of the slide which support the coverglass, [3] the degree of parallelism of the surfaces mentioned above.

They found that the current clips can cause considerable deformation of the coverglass, giving rise to inadmissable errors in the depth of the counting chamber. After having designed and applied a more reliable clip, the coverglass was proved to lie parallel to the chamber bottom. The depth of the counting chamber was next measured with an error of less than 1%.

Table 4. Mean, standard deviation and coefficient of variation of the mean of erythrocyte counts using calibrated pipettes and counting chambers, counting from photographs.

Series*	I		II		III		IV		V	
Chamber*	A		A		B		C		B	
$\bar{x}$ ($\times 10^6$)	4.59	4.59	4.64	4.64	5.00	5.00	4.54	4.54	2.54	2.54
s ($\times 10^6$)	0.114	0.156	0.090	0.154	0.047	0.251	0.040	0.138	0.041	0.093
$cv(\%):\sqrt{n}$	1.01	1.70	0.79	1.65	0.39	2.51	0.36	1.52	0.66	1.84
n	6	4	6	4	6	4	6	4	6	4

* See text.

Using counting chambers and pipettes, both calibrated as to volume, series of measurements were set up in which different technicians using different pipettes filled the counting chamber(s), photographic records of the microscope fields were made and all counting of cells was done from the photographs. A preliminary statistical analysis of the results was performed. A summary of these results is given in table 4.

Using 4 calibrated pipettes, a calibrated counting chamber was filled by one technician (series I, II) or by 4 different technicians (series III, IV, V). Photographs were taken of the two net-rulings (chamber A, B) and counting of cells was done from the photographs by 6 technicians in all series, in series II through V after strict instructions were given. In series IV a second counting chamber (C) was used, the depth of which was determined in the central portion of the net-ruling. A profile of the bottom of this chamber is given in fig. 5; this chamber has been classified a poor specimen. The same sample of blood has been used in the series I through IV, in series V this sample had been diluted 1 : 1 with plasma.

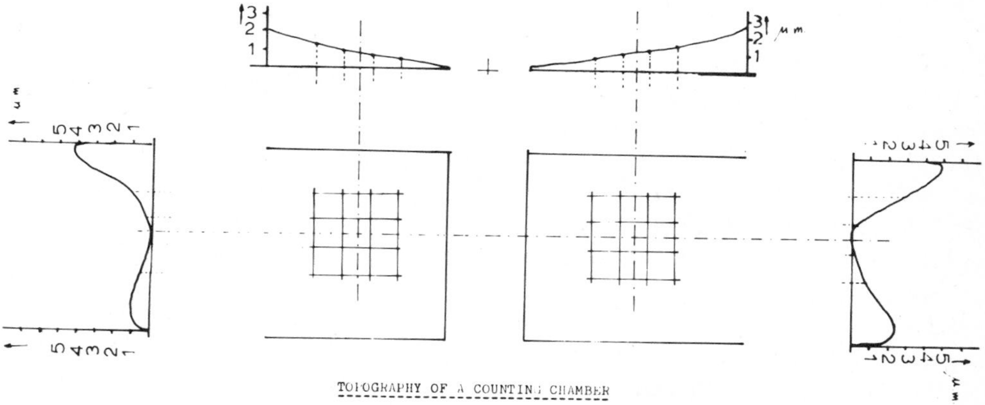

Fig. 5. Profile of the bottom of a counting chamber, as constructed from depth measurements using a modified Michelson interferometer arrangement.

In each series, the mean has been calculated of the results one technician obtained counting the different chamber fillings, as well as the mean the 6 technicians obtained, each counting one and the same chamber filling. From the mean values thus obtained in each of the series, new mean values (given in table 4) have been calculated and, as well, the standard deviations of these mean values together with the coefficient of variation. Because the pipettes had been accurately calibrated, the results give a good indication of the error of filling the counting chamber and of the error made on counting.

The overall mean values, standard deviation and coefficient of variation of the 24 counts in each, have also been calculated and are shown in table 5. It should be emphasized that the standard error of the mean is now obtained by dividing the values for the coefficients of variation given in table 5 by $\sqrt{n}$. This results in the values 0.96, 0.73, 0.95, 0.62 and 0.78 for the series I through V respectively. From these results it may be concluded that independent six-fold counting from photographs of a single chamber filling, using accurately calibrated pipettes, gives an accuracy of the mean lying from 1–2% of the true value.

Table 5. Mean, standard deviation and coefficient variation of all erythrocytes counts, from photographs, by 6 different technicians using calibrated pipettes and counting chambers.

Series* Chamber*	I A	II A	III B	IV C	V B
$\bar{x}$ (× 10^6)	4.59	4.64	5.00	4.54	2.54
s (× 10^6)	0.206	0.167	0.234	0.138	0.097
cv (%)	3.40	3.59	4.68	3.04	3.81
cv (%) : $\sqrt{n}$	0.96	0.73	0.95	0.62	0.78
n	24	24	24	24	24

* See table 4.

One point must be stressed at this time. In this investigation only normal size cells have been used. Problems will inevitably be encountered with electronic counting apparatus when abnormal cells are involved, because accurate results can only be obtained when the threshold setting is such that counting on the plateau is insured. For this reason, no hematological laboratory investigation is complete without visual inspection of cell size and cell shape. When abnormal cells are thus found, cell counting should preferably be done using a counting chamber.

Having a reliable c_{Hb} and cell count at one's disposal, the derived parameter MCH can be calculated to within a more accurate range and thus increases in value for hematological diagnosis. Two other derived parameters are in use for hematological diagnostic purposes: MCV and MCHC. For the calculation of these parameters, knowledge of the relative red cell volume is necessary. The most common and most simple method in use to this end is the determination of packed cell volume or hematocrit value. In this determination, either a large sample is spun for longer periods of time at low speed (macro-method) or a small sample is spun for a short time at high speed (micro-method). Discussion is still in full swing as regards the error made in these two methods, because of the amount of trapped plasma included in the measurement of the red cell column. Both methods, however, show a high reproducibility. Calibration is as yet not possible, due to the lack of blood-like reference preparations containing a known number of particles of known size. For this reason, the ICSH Expert Panel on Packed Cell volume is, at this moment, preparing a document advocating the centrifugation method as the method of choice in daily practice. In that document, the necessity will be stressed of adhering to a strictly standardized procedure. This should result in a range for the MCHC, constant within fairly narrow limits. With more accurate cell counting procedures, it is to be expected that the MCV can now also be determined within narrower and more accurate limits.

In summary, we now find ourselves in a position to accurately determine c_{Hb} and to design an appropriate quality control program; to determine more accurately the number of cells and to design a more appropriate quality control program; to reproducibly determine PCV and to design an appropriate statistical quality control program.

Bibliography

Van Assendelft, O.W.: Spectrophotometry of haemoglobin derivatives. Van Gorcum and Comp., Assen, the Netherlands, 1970.

Van Assendelft, O.W., W.G.Zijlstra and E.J. van Kampen: Haemoglobinometry. Challenges and pitfalls. Proc. kon. nederl. Akad. Wet. C 37, 104, 1970.

Helleman, P.W.: The Coulter Electronic Particle Counter. Aspects and views in counting and sizing of erythrocytes. Academic thesis, Utrecht, the Netherlands, 1972.

Holtz, A.H. and O.W. van Assendelft: Concepts of interlaboratory trials: an international haematological survey. In: Quality Control in Haematology, S.M.Lewis and J.Coster eds., Academic Press, New York/London. In press.

Holtz, A.H.: Some experience with a cyanohaemoglobin solution. Bibl. Haemat. 21, 75, 1965.

International Committee for Standardization in Haematology, Recommendations for haemoglobinometry in human blood. Br. J. Haemat. 13, Suppl., 71, 1967.

Van Kampen, E.J. and W.G.Zijlstra: Standardization of hemoglobinometry. II. The hemoglobincyanide method. Clin. chim. Acta 6, 538, 1961.

Zijlstra, W.G., O.W. van Assendelft, E.J. van Kampen and A.Buursma: The use of an ion-selective electrode for checking the CN content of reagent solutions used in the HiCN method. In: Modern Concepts in Hematology. G.Izak and S.M.Lewis ed., Academic Press, New York/London 1972, p.54.

Hematology Symposium

Discussion

Ph. Mascart (Belgium): Dr. *van Kampen,* this was really a very interesting paper. I would only like to add that once you have calibrated your instruments, the daily mean of truncated results, a system that we have used for several years, is very helpful in distinguishing a trend or any modifications. It is also useful for comparing instruments and stability of instruments. This system is even more useful in the field of hematology, where we do not have available reliable standards or quality control preparations.

E. van Kampen (Holland): I think, Dr. *Mascart,* that we totally agree on this point. The working premise, as you will agree, is that we need a starting point of what is a really acceptable daily mean for the laboratory. Once having that point fixed, then one can proceed, and avoid making a number of systematic errors.

K. von Boroviczény (Germany): I would like to point out that you have a very good possibility for quality control of differential counts if you take smears from surveys where smears are distributed and results are later on sent out to all participating laboratories. The smear then becomes a known sample and you can use it in the normal way, with quality control charts. But there are still two important points lacking in quality control in hematology. First of all, the erythrocyte sedimentation rate. I would like to ask Dr. *van Kampen* if he has some way of controlling this. As you know, in Germany about 97% of all medical doctors, who have a small laboratory in their practice, are performing the erythrocyte sedimentation rate, and I think that it would be very important to have quality control possibilities available to them. The other point where we need something, but have nothing, is on platelet count. Here again, I would be happy to get some good hints.

E. van Kampen (Holland): Dr. *v. Boroviczény,* all the points you bring up must be investigated. During the last two years, the Scientific Committee of the Symposium looked into ways to add hematological quality control to this Symposium. The only project we took on, and we worked on it more than a year, was the calibration of this counting chamber. We wanted to open the discussion on quality control in hematology with this, before considering the erythrocyte sedimentation rate, differentials and their interpretation, and platelet counts, and their quality controls. I hope that, from you, there will be some contributions in these fields.

O. van Assendelft (Holland): Dr. *v. Boroviczény,* as you probably well know, for the erythrocyte sedimentation rate (ESR), one of the expert panels of the International Committee for Standardization in Hematology has prepared a document describing a standardized method. I quite agree with you, that we have no material which we know has a certain sedimentation rate. For the moment, we should wait for the description of the standardized method to be accepted.

A. Klein-Wisenberg (Germany): I should like to ask Dr. *van Kampen* if he could tell us about the availability of counting chambers calibrated by the interferometric way he described? Is it possible to get a limited number of precalibrated chambers and check their performance?

E. van Kampen (Holland): At the moment, we are preparing a description of the calibration procedure, especially for the general physics laboratory. We are prepared to undertake calibration, but I sincerely hope that all of you will not send counting chambers to us to calibrate. If you wait until September or October, when the Transactions of this Symposium will appear, then you will have a very precise description of how to do this calibration. I believe that every general physics laboratory can do the calibration. In the meantime, certainly we are prepared to help you calibrate these chambers. Apart from that, the group that has developed this system promised us, just before we left for this Symposium, that it would be possible to develop a very simple inexpensive calibration instrument. This instrument could then be used by laboratories within a certain geographical area. This will, I hope, be decided by the end of this year.

B. Copeland (U.S.A.): I would like to ask if the laboratories reporting the spread of values that you show for hemoglobin in the survey, were reference level laboratories, using spectrophotometers such as the *Beckman* DU, the Cary and instruments of this caliber?

O. van Assendelft (Holland): The reference laboratories involved in the study all used either a *Beckman* DU or Optica CF or Zeiss Spectrophotometers to determine the reference value. On the other hand, many of the reference laboratories did more than one determination, also using a dilution of 1:251 as in the standardized method. And there, they may well have performed the measurement using a filter photometer.

W. Albath (Germany): Dr. *van Assendelft,* in one of your slides, you mentioned the possibility of error in obtaining capillary blood. All doctors in the laboratory know that during each examination, each test is as good as the materials that are used. So my question is, if there may be any reason why the test can not be performed using venous blood, since the compatibility of the results may be much different from when capillary blood is used.

O. van Assendelft (Holland): I completely agree with you that if we could also perform our sampling for hemoglobin determination by venipuncture, it would be wonderful. But I am afraid, in very many clinics requiring only the hemoglobin content and perhaps the cell count, many technicians are not able to do the venipuncture and/or would still prefer capillary puncture.

G. Cooper (U.S.A.): How satisfied are you with the red blood cell evaluation or reference materials that you are using in your studies?

O. van Assendelft (Holland): I take it that you mean the red blood cells which we ourselves use in the trial, as whole blood. Well, we were very satisfied, because we knew that the samples had reached the user (the participant in the trial), within 7 or 8 days and we had no fear at all of anything happening to the hemoglobin content within that period.

A. Klein-Wisenberg (Germany): You showed quite an abominable spectrum of a so-called cyanmethemoglobin standard, showing a very impressive methemoglobin band at 629 nanometers. Now, this substance exhibits the characteristics of an acid-base indicator, so my question to you is, did you measure the pH on this substance, and can it be inferred that this standard was prepared for a certain procedure or for a certain instrument?

O. van Assendelft (Holland): I hope the pH measurement is being done while I am here in Geneva, because the Friday afternoon before I left I asked my technician to do that. The material you mentioned is put out by a specific company for use with a specific instrument. The label on the bottles says most definitely 'cyanmethemoglobin standard'.

R. Sommer (Austria): In 1974, we performed a hemoglobin survey in Upper-Austria. We used whole blood (CH-35®, DADE) in the normal [1] and abnormal [2] range. I would like to show the slides from that survey and compare them with the data from Dr. *van Assendelft. Slide 1* shows a histogram of the results obtained with specimens 1 and 2. As you see, the results are within a relatively narrow range. *Slide 2:* in the same survey, we also had four different standards: 5, 10, 15 and 20 grams per deciliter. We requested that these standards should be measured as unknown specimens. It was interesting to see that those laboratories which found high values for the standards, also obtained high values for the control-blood. As the speaker mentioned, bad results are due either to poorly calibrated photometers or bad standards. *Slide 3* shows the results after correction by excluding values over ± 3 S.D. The overall CV for specimen 1 is 3.75% and for specimen 2 it is 4.0%. I would like to ask the speaker if the result of a CV of 5% could be due to lack of homogeneity of the material?

Slide 1. 1. Upper Austrian Survey 1974
Hemoglobin Determination

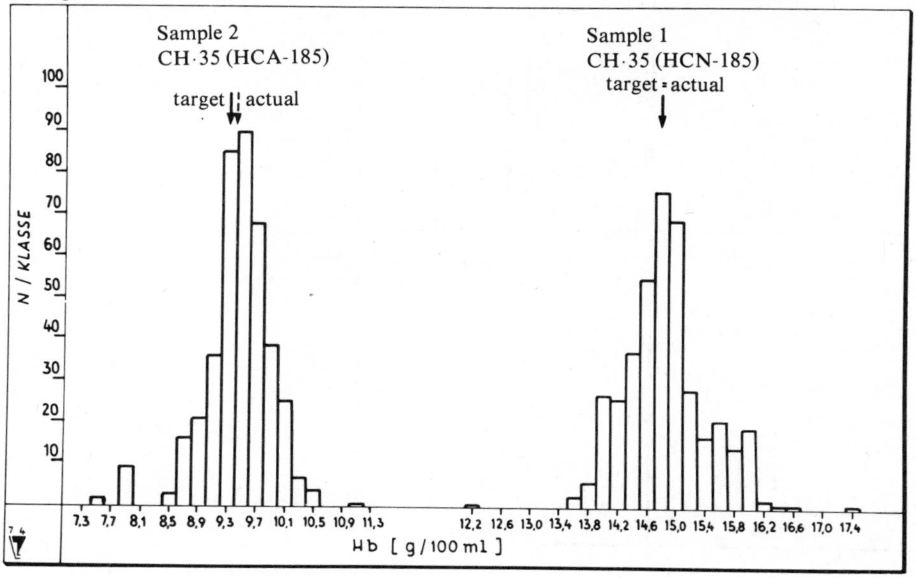

Slide 2. Hemoglobin Standards (diff. Concentrations)

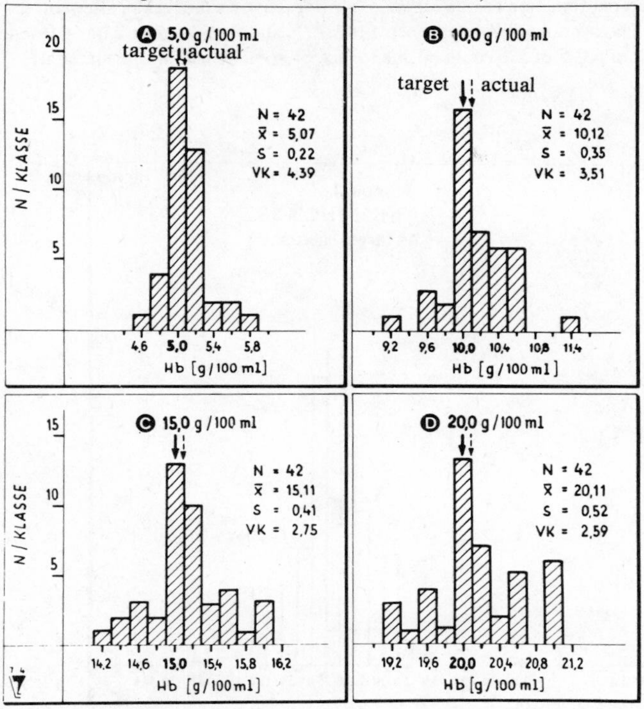

Slide 3. 1. Upper Austrian survey 1974. Hemoglobin determination.

	Sample 1 (CH. 35, HCN-185) Number	Mean value	Dispersion	Coeff. of. var.
Assay value[1]		14.8	(14.2–15.4)	
Result	405	14.81	0.59	4.01%
Corr. (without ± 3s)	402	14.80	0.55	3.75%
	Sample 2 (CH. 35, HCA-185) Number	**Mean value**	**Dispersion**	**Coeff. of var.**
Assay value[1]		9.3	(8.9–9.7)	
Result	405	9.38	0.46	4.88%
Corr. (without ± 3s)	394	9.42	0.38	4.04%
HB – Survey Germany 1970				3.9%
HB – Survey Switzerland 1971				3.5%

[1] Remark: Assay values according to the manufacturer Dade (USA).

E. van Kampen (Holland): From experience in many hemoglobin surveys, one of the first precautions we always take is to be sure of the homogeneity of the sample. Before we dispensed the hemolysate in ampoules, we did a total hemoglobin determination of the bulk preparation; then we proceeded to the dispensing. We did a hemoglobin determination, at the beginning of the dispensing, at the middle and at the end. We sent a few samples for determination to laboratories which we knew had good intra-laboratory control. Once it was established that there was a good homogeneity of the material (and we knew our own measurements were correct, since we correlated with the other laboratories), it was then that the samples were sent around. So, this coefficient of variation of 5% is certainly not due to lack of homogeneity. Apart from this, in the last slide, you showed that there was a coefficient of variation of 4%. So I am not surprised at our results, since the difference between 4 and 5% is not great.

A First Transatlantic, Live Demonstration of a Computerized Audio-Response Communications System of an Automated Clinical Laboratory

A.E. Rappoport, W.D. Gennaro and *R.E. Berquist,* Youngstown, Ohio, U.S.A.

DIVOTS (Direct Input Voice Output Telephone System), is an on-line, audio-response, laboratory communication system (LCS) utilizing a touch-tone telephone for test order entry and result retrieval.

The Youngstown hospital computerized laboratory

A brief description of the functional and structural characteristics of our Data Acquisition System (DAS), Laboratory Information System (LIS) and LCS (DIVOTS) is shown in figure 1.

Every patient's medical data base, accumulated during his entire hospital stay, is stored in the hospital IBM 370/135 computer.

The DAS consists of a dedicated laboratory computer, the T&T, Laboratory Data Manager (LDM). The LDM receives and processes simultaneously, all the analog and digital signals from 15 instruments which have been equipped with appropriate interfaces and sample identification devices which are capable of reading human and machine readable patient specimen information on the samples.

The machine test results are merged with the specimen identification number in the LDM. Manual test results (i.e. Urinalysis) are entered by CRT, Key or Port-A-Punch cards while narrative reports (i.e. Surgical Pathology) are transmitted by the Communicating Magnetic Card Selectric Typewriter (CMC/ST) [12]. The LDM transmits all results by telephone line and to the IBM 370 where they are filed automatically within each patient's master file (PMF).

An Interim Ward Report is printed at 1300 h daily, listing all available test results up to that hour. An updated cumulative Patient Summary Report, listing all results for the past seven [7] days, is printed each evening. This permits chronologic comparison of serial values of the test on a horizontal line, while groups of tests relevant to clinical diseases or substances studied are listed vertically.

DIVOTS' represents an one-line telephone communication loop between Nursing Stations (or physicians' offices) and the laboratory, used to order tests without writing, and to hear completed results as soon as they have been filed in the 370, prior to printing.

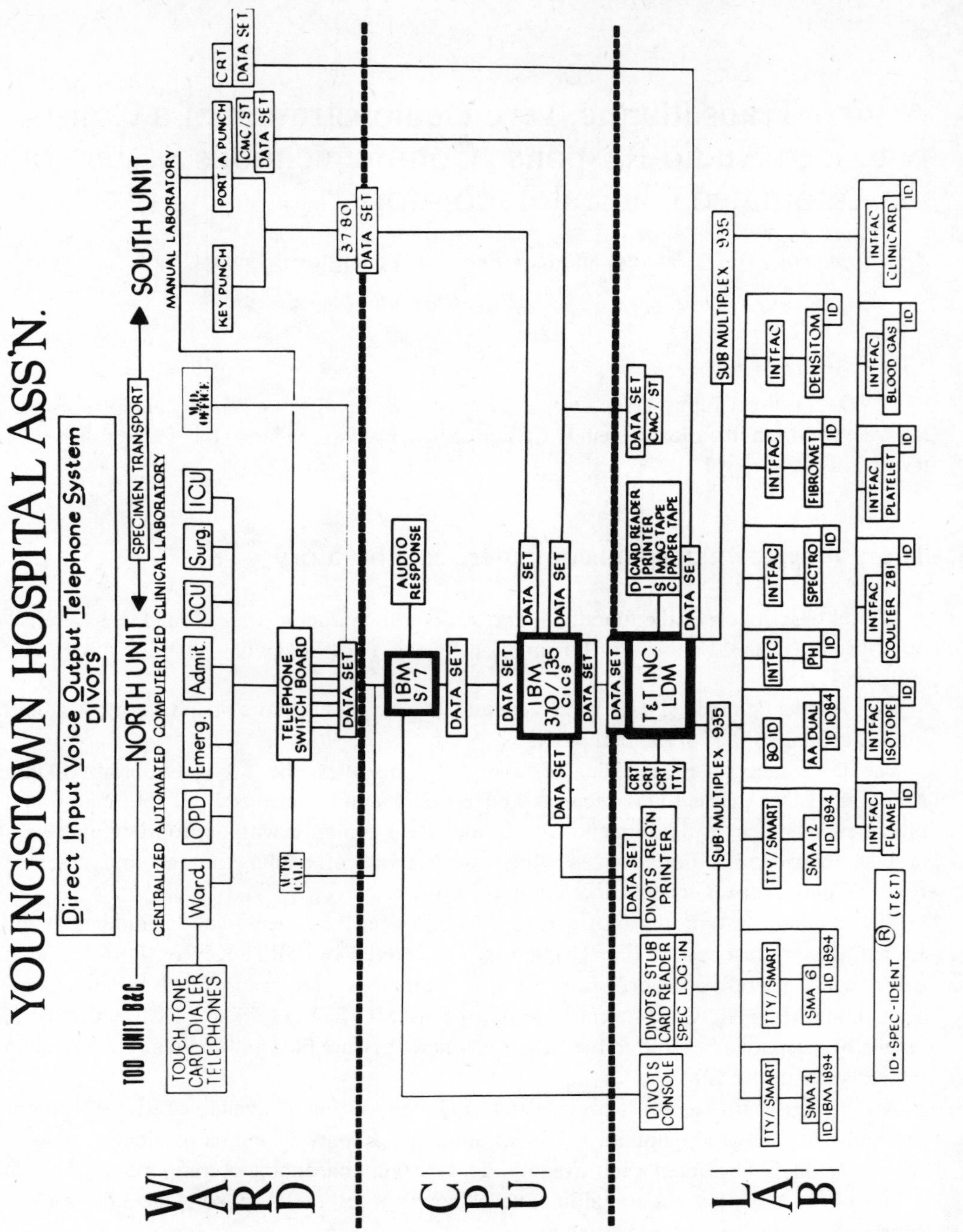

Fig. 1. Flow Chart showing the telephone connections to the System/7 possessing the Autio-Response Unit. This computer communicates with the IBM 370 containing the patient's data base. Note the analytic instruments connected on-line to a laboratory computer (LDM) for data reduction and automatic, on-line transmission to the 370.

DIVOTS consists of an IBM System/7 computer possessing 20 K core, a fixed disk for program storage and a removable disk which possesses a digitized, audio-response, vocabulary of 850 words, appropriate for laboratory medical use. This includes the names of all tests, the letters of the alphabet, numbers, Greek letters and symbols, chemical units, general administrative and technical words, and all descriptive words necessary to report verbally, diagnostic and numeric results, generally by sections of the laboratory performing a wide variety of anatomic pathology and clinical pathology tests.

These words have been dictated previously. The tape has then been processed in the IBM Phonolaboratory where the words were digitized and transferred to the removable S/7 disk.

DIVOTS may be operated from any Touch-Tone (T-T) telephone within the hospital, the attending physician's office or home, or anywhere else in the world. If a T-T phone is not available, small, battery operated accessory 'pads' are available which can be attached to the mouth-pieces of the handset and thus convert a rotary 'phone' to a T-T phone as we shall do tonight.

Three internal automatic hospital switchboard telephone lines and one external, private, commercial line bypassing the switchboard communicate by appropriate Data Sets with the S/7 which also is coupled to the 370 by another Data Set. Programs governing System/7-370 communications and the addresses for the location of all digitized words are located in the 370.

When admitted, the patient's complete demographic data are entered into the 370 computer through a CRT by a clerk in the Admitting Office. The patient is assigned a unique hospital number, and receives an embossed Identification Card and a telephone Dialer-Card with his hospital number punched in it.

The demonstration tonight (carried out with the assistance of Mr. Bernhard and his colleagues of Radio Suisse) will simulate the following process: The patient arrives on the nursing station with physician's orders for tests; the nurse will initiate a telephone call (Extension 461) to the S/7 in Youngstown. The S/7 responds with a high pitched 'beep' and states 'Please enter request'.

Test request is achieved by a code (=1 or =2). In Code 1, the S/7 instructs the clerk in the next step to use DIVOTS, which responds to each successive input with a high-pitched beep indicating to proceed automatically to the next input.

The clerk then inserts the 'Patient Number' by Patient's Dialer Card or enters the number manually by T-T. The S/7 relays it to the 370, which locates the patient's file and spells the name in the S/7, which is verified by the clerk within 2–3 seconds after input, thus verifying the accuracy of the patient's identification. The S/7 checks the patient's ward number and asks for the time of day that the test was requested by the physician.

In the next step, DIVOTS requests the codes of the desired test. This is done by entering an appropriate 4-digit code for each procedure by checking a Test Directory. The test name is verified audibly immediately and thus verifies the correctness of the order. If an error is made, the test may be delected by entering the Asterisk (*) key.

The nine most frequently ordered procedures in our laboratory (i.e. glucose, hemoglobin, SMA) can be ordered by entering a single digit on the T-T pad. Special instructions such as 'Urgent', 'Pre-Operative', 'Next Day', etc. are requested by another single digit, and these instructions are also confirmed audibly. After completion of each patient's order, DIVOTS states 'Order Accepted'. The clerk may now order tests for additional patients or she may terminate the process by 'hanging up'. DIVOTS may talk to, and receive data from the S/7, up to 15 stations simultaneously.

Immediately after entry of the test request, the 370 prints the requisition in the laboratory, complete with the patient's name, age, sex, room and hospital number and the tests desired. These data are entered on human and machine readable punched stub cards which will be attached to the Vacutainer for automatic identification. At the onset of the days transaction, the laboratory clerk transmits to the 370, the 1st pre-printed, human and machine readable requisition (specimen) number which will be merged by the 370 to the printed patient's hospital number. Henceforth, all subsequent, sequentially printed requisitions will be merged automatically with the following patients' hospital numbers.

For non-urgent tests, the 370 will collect all orders for all patients of each ward, collate them by room and bed number and print out sequential patient requisitions every half hour. This simplifies specimen collection for the phlebotomists.

After the DIVOTS order has been processed, the 370 transmits a copy to the LDM to establish a list of anticipated test results. The 370 also bills the patient, counts the test for statistical purposes and reminds the LDM operator if a result is not generated later to satisfy the order.

When the specimen is returned to the laboratory it is 'logged-in' by a special specimen identification device, thus maintaining an 'Audit Trail'. All tests are performed on automated and semi-automated instruments and by manual methods and the results are transmitted to the 370 to be filed in the patients' records.

Retrieval of test results by DIVOTS

Ward clerks and physicians initiate a DIVOTS telephone transaction using Codes #3 for beginners and #4 for experienced clerks to obtain results as early as possible. The patient's name is verified after the hospital number is entered. To guarantee confidentiality, the attending physician must enter his private number to establish his privilege to obtain results. The computer compares that number with his number listed on the patient's record.

One may obtain all abnormal results for that day or any result on any day during the patient's entire period of hospitalization. Single tests or entire profiles are available. The system speaks sufficiently slowly to permit the hearer to write the message, which may be repeated by using the asterisk (*) key.

Auto-call

In the case of urgently required ('stat') results, for seriously ill patients in Intensive Care or Coronary Care Units or for abnormal results of hazard materials (potassium, blood sugar), the 370 will automatically dial the patient's nursing station number as soon as the LDM transmits the test result to the 370. The clerk hears a three-note chime, indicating a DIVOTS 'Auto Call' report. This spells the patient's name(s) and test(s) and states the results. Thus delay between completion of the test and result transmission to the physician is completely eliminated.

Geneva DIVOTS demonstration

Following this description, a successful, live demonstration of DIVOTS was carried out. A telephone call to the U.S.A., A/C 216, 746–7727, was initiated from the Conference Room in the Hotel President, Geneva. Within nine seconds, the S/7 in The Youngstown Hospital laboratory responded audibly and the Test Order Entry routine, as described above, was carried out for 'Patient' Rappoport and was verified immediately.

Results of tests for actual patients *'Wade', 'Walsh',* and *'Jenkins'* were then requested. Within a few seconds, the audience heard these names spelled out, followed by the names of the tests, the dates they were performed, and the results.

Acknowledgement

This project was supported by Grant Number RIS HS 00060 from the National Center for Health Services research, HRA.

The First International Symposium on Quality Control, Tokyo

S.B.Rosalki (Chairman):

Ladies and gentlemen,

In 1974, was held the first International Symposium on Quality Control – Tokyo. We are honoured to have with us Dr. *Kawai,* Chairman of the Scientific and Organizing Committee of that Symposium and it is my pleasure to invite him to say a few words concerning that Symposium and of his plans for the second Tokyo Symposium scheduled for 1976.

T.Kawai, Tokyo (Japan)

First of all, I thank Dr. *Rosalki* and the other scientific committee members of this Symposium for inviting me to the VIth Symposium on Quality Control in Clinical Chemistry.

In Japan, internal quality control programs actually started in some clinical laboratories in 1960. There were several control surveys conducted by various scientific groups. However, from 1967 the Japanese Medical Association with the cooperation of the Japan Society of Clinical Pathology has been conducting nationwide quality control surveys. Although the Japan Society of Clinical Pathology has been in contact with the College of American Pathologists and the World Association of Societies of Anatomic and Clinical Pathology, we have had practically no communication among the Asian countries. Therefore, in June, last year, the first International Symposium on Quality Control, Tokyo, which was similar to this symposium, was held in Japan, covering many countries in the Pacific-Asian zone, sponsored by Dade, Miami, and International Reagents Cooperation in Japan.

I was honored to be the chairman of the Scientific and Organizing Committee, and the Proceedings will be published soon in both Japanese & English. The program was composed of 4 parts. The first part included guest lectures given by Dr. *Büttner* (Germany), Dr. *van Kampen* (Holland), Dr. *Anido* (USA) and Dr. *Saito* (Japan). In the second part, the present status of their quality control programs was reported by many countries, including Australia, New Zealand, Philippines, Hong Kong, Republic of China, and Republic of Korea. In the third part, 5 selected topics were reported by Japanese clinical chemists, including quality control surveys on blood glucose and uric acid determinations, and some problems in Automation.

The last part was one of the most successful. A survey subcommittee was organized to do a careful control survey, especially planned for the first Tokyo Symposium. Two enzyme determinations, alkaline phosphatase and LDH, were selected. Before we sent the samples and reagents to the participating laboratories, a questionnaire on all sorts of determination conditions, was answered by them, so that we might be able to correlate the reported values and the determination conditions. With regards to alkaline phosphatase determination, a total of 6 samples from 3 different sources were sent and were analyzed by the routine methods used in the participating laboratories. With regards to LDH, again, a total of 6 samples from 3 different sources, including M-subunit dominant and H-subunit dominant samples, were analyzed by the routine method, and also with reagents of the same lot, kindly supplied by Dade, Miami. We certainly obtained much interesting information from this survey, but because of the short time available, I will not discuss this further at this time. Full details will be reported in the Proceedings.

Certainly it was a wonderful and successful opportunity for us to meet many colleagues from Asian countries as well as some representatives from this Geneva Symposium. We are planning to have a second Symposium in June, 1976. For this, careful surveys on LDH and plasma prothrombin time determinations will be conducted.

Quality control in the clinical laboratory is a ‘must’ for better patient care, and should not be limited to one laboratory or one nation, but should extend throughout the world. It is our wish to make closer contact with this Geneva Symposium in order to assist our aim of improving laboratory quality.

Thank you.

International Symposium on Quality Control – Tokyo

June 5–6, 1976
Fukiai P.O. Box 24 Kobe, Japan (651)

First Announcement

The Second International Symposium on Quality Control – Tokyo

In this Symposium, several aspects of quality control in the clinical laboratory will be discussed among many participants from the Asian-Pacific Basin and distinguished guests from Europe and America.

Date: June 5 (Sat.) & 6 (Sun.), 1976

Location: Tokyo, Japan

Scientific Program: Guest lectures, free communications, control survey reports

Free Communications: Summaries (400 words) are to be submitted for consideration by the Scientific Committee before December 20, 1975. Only papers on quality control in clinical chemistry and blood coagulation will be accepted.

Official Language: Japanese. Simultaneous translation, English/Japanese will be available.

Membership Fee: Y 10,000 (Japanese currency)
This fee includes lunch during two days, as well as the Reception Party. It also includes the Program, Abstract Volume and the 2nd Volume of the Proceedings.

All Correspondence to:

Masaya Ogawa
Secretariat
2nd I.S.Q.C. – Tokyo
Fukiai P.O. Box 24
Kobe, Japan 651
Tel. (078) 392-1451

Nozomu Kosakai, M.D.
President
2nd I.S.Q.C. – Tokyo

Tadashi Kawai, M.D.
Chairman of Scientific and
Organizing Committee

Chairman's Closing Remarks

Ladies and Gentlemen,

It is now my task to conclude these first two days of the 6th International Symposium on Quality Control sponsored by DADE and by Merz and Dade. Tomorrow the Symposium organisers are pleased to play host to the International Federation of Clinical Chemistry who will present a Symposium on the Clinical Laboratory from an International Viewpoint.

It has become customary at the close of the Geneva Symposium to outline plans for future meetings. The 7th Symposium is planned to take place in Geneva in Spring 1977. It will include plenary lectures, and parallel sessions devoted to both clinical chemistry and haematology, the haematology programme being expanded to include quality control of coagulation, blood grouping, and immunohematological procedures.

In closing, I should like to thank DADE and Merz and Dade for sponsoring this most successful meeting, Mr. *George Darnell,* President of DADE, and our moderator, Dr. *Anido.* A special word of thanks is due to Madame *M. Divernois* for her charming and efficient organisation of the secretarial and social facilities. I also wish to thank all the speakers, and last but by no means least all those who have contributed to the discussions both public and informal which have made this meeting so entertaining and productive.

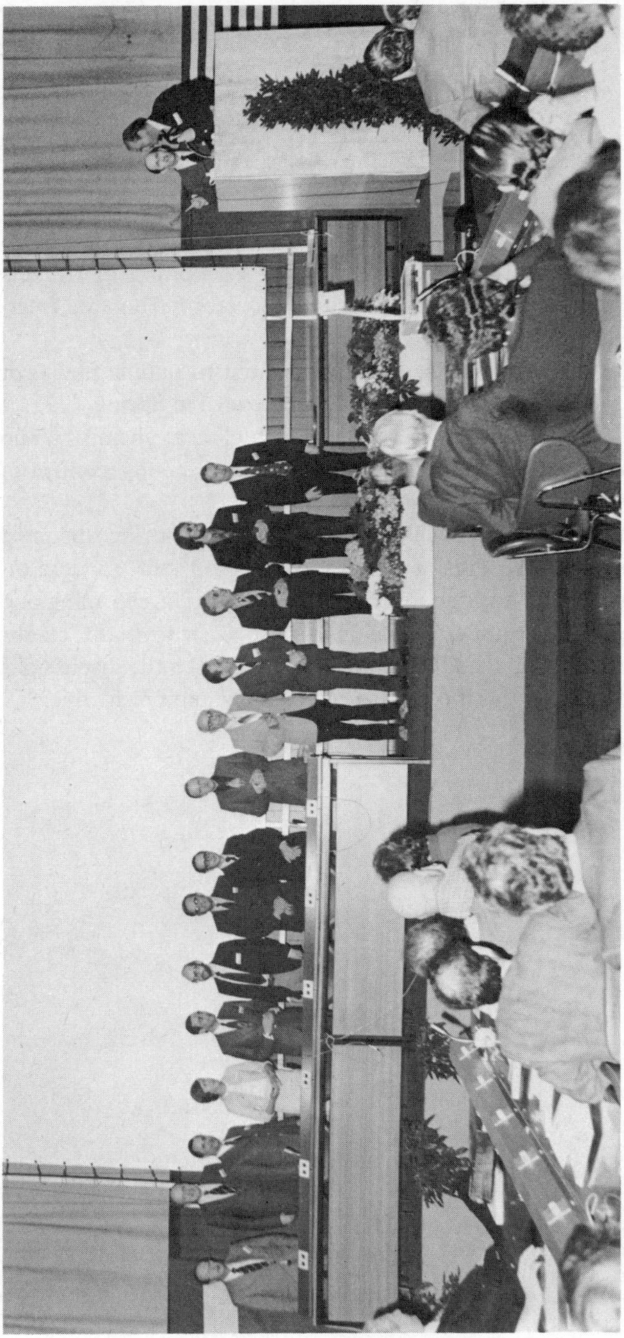

Award Presentations

Award Presentations

Presented by: George M. Darnell[1]

From the initial Geneva Symposium in 1967, it has been our desire to provide a means whereby interested and competent scientists could gather and present data supportive of their efforts in the development of better Quality Control in Clinical Chemistry. We hoped it would also serve as a means of stimulating discussion, relative to differences of approach and analysis.

I feel a great deal has been accomplished in these past nine years – and a base has been established – not only for continued development of Quality Control in Clinical Chemistry – but now for other disciplines, such as just this year's embarkation in Hematology.

In the opening address Dr. *Bürgi* of Switzerland most aptly provided the historical development of the Geneva Symposium and Dr. *Rosalki* of the United Kingdom, our Chairman, has indicated our plans for its continuation and its expansion in other areas of interest. Dr. *Kawai* of Japan has informed you of the development of a similar Symposium in the Pacific Basin with its first meeting last year and their plans for a second meeting to be held in Tokyo in mid-year 1976.

With the recognition of the accomplishments developed in the Quality Control of Clinical Chemistry, the Dade Award Lectures for 1975 were formulated. A sum of $ 1000.00 was provided to the professional society of Clinical Chemistry in each 'interested' European country.

This was to be given to that person they as a society *elected* as a major contributor to the development of Quality Control – to represent that activity in the form of a scientific lecture presentation. I hope this recognition will serve as a stimulus for others to establish goals of contribution and achievement.

The establishment of the *Richterich Memorial Lecture* and its excellent first presentation by Dr. Rosalki will serve as a reminder of this opportunity and responsibility. This latter point of *responsibility* is important and one I feel industry and the professions *share.* Responsibility for continual research, education, and development of improved laboratory medicine.

In closing, I would like to ask each of the Award Lecture winners to come forward as I call their name so that I may on your behalf present to them a medal of recognition of their selection and of their valuable participation in this year's VI International Symposium on Quality Control.

I would be remiss if I did not also recognize the many others that have provided signifi-

[1] President, Dade Division American Hospital Supply Corporation, U.S.A.

cant contributions in the form of presentations, as well as those that participated in the free discussion.

Thank you for your continued involvement, which I hope will remain so that we may have the benefit of your presence at our next European Symposium in 1977. Finally, I hope you all will share with us in recognizing the efforts of Dr. *Rosalki, M. Divernois-Merz,* Dr. *Anido* and the other members of the Scientific and Co-ordinating Committee.

Award Lectures

G. Ceriotti, Italy: Considerations on bilirubin determination
L. Havelec, Austria: Comparisons between determination methods
R. Leclercq, Belgium: Intralaboratory Quality Control using the daily means of patients' results
W. Gerhardt, Denmark: Evaluation of some determination materials used in the Scandinavian Recommended Methods for Determination of Four Enzymes in Blood, and the performance of contrc. .naterials with these methods
A. Hyvarinen, Finland: Control of error and use of standardized reference samples in estimation of the true biological normal range
A. P. Jansen, Holland: Studies on alkaline phosphatases of different origin with an external quality control scheme
A. Martinez, Spain: Evaluation of several commercial controls. Correlation between them
R. Zender, Switzerland: Interlaboratory comparison of both accuracy and precision by a two-sample method
G. R. Cooper, USA: The WHO-CDC lipid standardization program
D. Stamm, West Germany: The determination of assigned values for control specimens: Experimental design and statistical evaluation of the analytical results of reference laboratories
T. Whitehead, U. K.: The role of external quality control schemes in improving the quality of laboratory results
H. E. Solberg, Norway: Computerized techniques for quality control in the clinical chemistry laboratory
C. H. de Verdier, Sweden: Systems analysis of analytical procedures as a means of improving their performance
M. Bailly, France: Discussion of the options followed in processing quality control data

Richterich Memorial Lecture

S. B. Rosalki, U. K.: Seeking the Way

International Federation of Clinical Chemistry

President:	Prof. M. Rubin, Washington, D.C., USA.
Vice-President:	Dr. R. Dybkaer, Copenhagen, Denmark
Treasurer:	Mr. P. M. G. Broughton, Leeds, U.K.
Secretary:	Prof. J. Frei, Lausanne, Switzerland
Associate Secretary:	Prof. G. Siest, Nancy, France

Symposium:

'The Clinical Laboratory from an International Viewpoint'

Session I

Topic: International Criteria for Clinical Laboratory Materials

Session-Chairman: H. Adlercreutz, Finland
Discussion-Leader: J. L. Giegel, USA

International Criteria for Reference Materials

J. P. Cali, Washington, D. C. (USA)

Key Word: Reference materials

1. Introduction

The formal definition of that class of materials called Reference Materials (RM) is now in the process of formulation by several international bodies including the International Federation of Clinical Chemists (IFCC), the World Health Organization (WHO), International Organization for Standardization (ISO), International Organization of Legal Metrology (OIML), and International Union of Pure and Applied Chemistry (IUPAC). That such a large number of prestigious organizations are focusing their energies in this direction gives some indication of the importance of RM's in many diverse measurement systems and areas of standardization. Because international agreement has not yet been achieved on a definition of RM, we will use for purposes of discussion in this paper that of the National Bureau of Standards (NBS), USA:

> 'Certified reference materials (CRM) are *well-characterized* (in terms of end-use and with quality assurance mechanisms specified) and *certified materials* (by international organizations, national governmental laboratories, national standards bodies, or industrial or trade associations), produced in quantity so as to be continually available without regard to national boundaries.' The definition is continued with regard to the uses and purposes for which RM's exist: '(A) to help develop *reference methods* of analysis or test, i.e., methods of demonstrated accuracy; (B) to calibrate a measurement system in order to: [1] facilitate the exchange of goods or services, [2] institute quality control, [3] determine performance characteristics, [4] characterize at scientific frontiers; (C) to assure the longterm adequacy and integrity of the quality control process.'

A shorter, more succinct definition proposed by Professor *M. Puttock* of Australia is: 'RM's are well-characterized materials or devices, generally produced in quantity and generally available, used to calibrate and/or assess a measurement system either in whole or in part. CRM's are reference materials the specific properties of which have been certified by a recognized competent laboratory.'

From these definitions, it may be deduced that RM's play a central, vital role in a wide variety of measurement processes, among them certainly the clinical chemistry measurement system. In fact, as will be shown later, RM's are the vehicle whereby accuracy in measurement is transferred from one part of the measurement network, say, from a national central laboratory, to reference laboratories or manufacturers of reagents, kits or reference sera, to the local hospital or clinical laboratory.

Before setting out the criteria for RM's that should be considered at the international level, it might be well to discuss briefly the role of RM's in the measurement process itself.

2. The Measurement Process

Measurement in science and technology is the process whereby a numerical value is sought and associated with a distinct, specific, and unique property of a material. The magnitude of the number is related to the amount or degree of that property in a particular material or similar class of materials. Here, 'material' is taken in its broadest sense to include all those things that constitute the physical objects of the observable universe.

As pointed out by *Shewart* in 1939 [1], there are two aspects of measurement, one quantitative, the other qualitative. The former aspect concerns number associated with a scale, pointer reading, counter, or the like. RM's belong to this category, because they too have numbers associated with one or more properties in a manner analogous to the numbers on a meter stick, although RM's usually have one number per property rather than a series of incremental values. While a meter stick may have a thousand divisions along its length, each defining one millimeter, a RM of cholesterol will have just one number defining its degree of purity. Thus, the RM represents the quantitative aspect of measurement and is extremely useful where composition is the property being measured.

The qualitative aspects of measurement are included in what is often called the procedure, or the method. Included in this factor are such things as apparatus, reagents, indeed all those things that are used or can affect the course of the measurement. The qualifications of the experimenter or measurer, the sequence of operations, control of the ambient conditions, etc., must be stated in the written method used by the operator to make the actual measurements.

Experience over many centuries has taught man that, if he can agree on one universal set of coherent scales, he can more effectively communicate with his fellow man across time and geographical boundaries. In principle, there is no logical reason why many different sets could not be utilized, as historically they have, but the economic, political, and social benefits of one universal set are so apparent, that most of the world's nations have now agreed to use the set of measurement scales called the International System of Units (Système International d'Unités) and abbreviated as SI. This rational, self-consistent system of units of measurement includes the base units (mass, length, time, electric current, thermodynamic temperature, luminous intensity, and the mole), together with rules for their use [2, 3]. Having defined the units, access to the units is provided through highly developed measurement processes. In some cases one can reconstruct the unit, in others one relies on artifacts such as sets of weights, gauge blocks, and the like whose magnitudes in terms of the unit have been carefully established – especially when the magnitudes met in routine measurement practice are far removed from (i.e., are large multiples or small fractions of) the base unit. The uncertainty in the use of such reference standards is a function of both the method and the process precision. The uncertainty of the assigned value of the reference standards becomes a systematic error of the process in which the artifact is used.

3. Measurement Compatibility

The definition of measurement compatibility flows directly from the most common usage of the word 'compatible' – namely, the ability to get along well together; to agree. If two or more laboratories, each working independently, agree to measure a specific property of a particular lot of stable material, and if each obtains an identical numerical value (within some beforehand agreed on limits of uncertainty), then a compatible measurement network exists. The question, of course, is how does one bring this much sought after result into being? Measurement compatible networks are based on many different modes. In addition to the reference material mode, three of the most widely used are: (a) the calibration of measuring instruments sent to a well-qualified laboratory and returned to the user [4]; (b) the publication of critically evaluated Standard Reference Data, which, if given with detailed preparation and measurement procedures allows the user to use the data directly or to reproduce the original measurements [5]; and, the provision, directly from a central source to the user, e.g., of signals for the measurement of time or frequency[6].

The most appropriate mode in the field of clinical chemistry, where composition is the measurement property most often under consideration, is that embodied in the RM concept. What we must now show is how measurement compatibility is achieved, or at least is capable of achievement, when RM properties are based on accuracy.

3.1 Compatibility Through Accurate Measurement

Every property of a specific, homogeneous, stable material has a number on some scale that is its actual value. This value is often called the 'true value'. In a paper by *Dorsey* and *Eisenhart* [7], and highly recommended for all who are interested in the philosophical bases for absolute measurement experiments, the 'true value' is called the *quaesitum*. Intuitively, most scientists would agree that if all laboratories in a measurement network are proceeding in such a way that each operational step in the process was directly traceable to the 'true value' (for a given property) and that each step was made without error, other than the measured but irreducible random errors always present, then measurement compatibility in that network exists. This logic is based on the assumption that there can exist only *one* 'true value' for the property of the material under examination. Measurements that can be rigorously related to the 'true value' will be called *accurate measurement,* and by definition, or through acceptance of the above philosophy or logic, are compatible. Such measurements must agree.

An accurate measurement system must be free of systematic errors, those errors that would lead one away from the 'true value'. In addition, however, the measurements must also be considerably more precise (reproducible) than the small and usually unknown systematic errors remaining after all is done. Man being imperfect can never with certainty know he has removed every systematic error; he can only be careful and cautious. *Cali* and *Reed* [8] have shown the difficulty of ferreting out systematic errors in an imprecise system.

A full discussion of the nature of systematic error, imprecision and other aspects of measurement are beyond the scope of this paper. The volume on Statistical Concepts and Procedures, edited by *Ku* [9], and the paper by *Eisenhart* [10] on accuracy and precision are highly recommended for readers interested in pursuing these questions further.

From the above discussion, the conclusion may be drawn that if RM properties are founded on accurate measurement, then the RM itself becomes the vehicle whereby accuracy may be transferred throughout the measurement network to help bring about measurement compatibility.

It must be emphasized that RM's *alone* are insufficient to bring about measurement compatibility. Obviously, the methodology whereby the RM is incorporated into the measurement process is of utmost importance. Definitive and reference methods (methods of demonstrated accuracy) are important components of a compatible measurement network. These subjects are discussed by other speakers in this symposium. References to these topics include a monograph by *Cali* et al. [11] on the role of reference materials (called by NBS, Standard Reference Materials) in measurement systems, the paper by *Cali* [12] on problems of standardization in clinical chemistry, and the large number of papers published in a proceedings of a symposium on reference materials and meaningful measurement [13].

4. Criteria for CRM's of Known Accuracy

Although the criteria to be recommended apply in almost all instances to the entire class of reference materials, this discussion will be directed primarily to the sub-class, certified reference materials (CRM). In clinical chemistry where analytical mistakes may have serious consequences in terms of human life, only reference materials of the highest quality and greatest integrity should be used. CRM's whose properties have been measured under the strictest control possible, and whose production, storage and distribution are carried out under close supervision by well-trained, competent specialists are certainly the reference materials of first choice.

The major criteria that should be considered by both producers and users of CRM's are: purity, homogeneity, stability, continuity of both supply and information, availability, and the certification process which may or may not include legal requirements such as labeling. Each of these is discussed in turn.

4.1 Purity

Ideally, every analytical method should have available to it a quantity of the pure material being analyzed (i.e., the analyte). Traditionally, and based on sound scientific principle, standard curves of detector response versus amount of analyte present are first determined using as pure an analyte as can be found. Only when the simplified system (relatively speaking) is clearly understood and under control should the analyst proceed to the usually more complicated aspects associated with the matrix, interferences, questions of specificity and the like.

There are several major factors to be considered in the preparation of a pure CRM.

4.1.1 Moisture

Hydrolysis reactions may occur if significant amounts of water are present. The water may be occluded, absorbed, or present as water of crystallization. When the NBS-CRM urea was certified about 5 years ago, its moisture content was found to be 0.18% by weight – an acceptable level. Recently, upon re-examination, the moisture was found to be at 0.02%. It is most likely that hydrolysis of the urea occurred to form CO_2 and NH_3. In this instance the degradation products, being gaseous, probably escaped with no serious consequences on the urea itself. Moisture content determinations are called for as a matter of routine in all NBS clinical CRM's.

4.1.2 Trace Metals

Depending upon the preparative routes used, and the storage containers utilized, the CRM may contain trace elements as impurities. In many reactions these are totally inconsequential, but if enzymatic reactions are to be used the presence of even parts per million of elements such as copper may cause serious difficulties. At NBS, all clinical CRM's are routinely examined by emission spectroscopy, and where warranted, by more sensitive techniques such as neutron activation analysis, polarography, or atomic absorption spectroscopy (among others).

For example, it is known that copper, even at trace levels, catalyzes the oxidation of cortisol. Therefore, when the NBS cortisol CRM was under measurement for certification, the copper was determined by neutron activation analysis to be 35 ng/g of cortisol, an amount unlikely to produce a significant error in cortisol analytical methods.

4.1.3 Isomeric Interferences

As the organic molecule becomes more complex, the question of the presence of its isomers becomes important. When the NBS bilirubin CRM was first issued this question, although recognized, was largely by-passed because of lack of information available at the time. Since then, two isomers of bilirubin have been found in the natural IX α-bilirubin (the principle constituent of the NBS-CRM). They are III α-bilirubin and XIII α-bilirubin. The extinction coefficients are greatly different: III $\alpha = 65{,}200$; IX $\alpha = 62{,}600$, XIII $\alpha = 52{,}500$. Even a relatively small percentage of either or both of these isomers will introduce a deviation from the accepted absorptivity of the CRM. Additional work is now underway to determine the amount present of the two isomers and to estimate the error in the extinction coefficient of the IX α isomer due to their presence.

4.1.4 Preparative Intermediate Impurities

It is important that the certifying laboratory have full knowledge of the process whereby the candidate CRM was prepared. In many instances the certifying laboratory will have to depend upon commercial sources of supply for the CRM candidate, because these are usually required in kilogram quantities and not amenable to production by most certifying laboratories. At NBS, commercial materials are purchased to NBS specifications, one of which is an agreement to allow NBS scientists to overlook the preparation of the candidate material and to be made knowledgeable concerning all steps in the production process. Thus, when NBS procured its first lot of cholesterol, we were aware that its purification included a bromination step used to produce the cholesterol dibromide, which was then crystallized (for purification purposes) and then dehalogenated to give cholesterol. Determination of the bromine was done using activation analysis. The bromine content of the current lot is 12 µg per g.

4.1.5 Interfering Impurities

The certifying laboratory scientists must be aware of the currently used analytical procedures so that potentially interfering substances in any one given method may be sought and kept below interfering levels. Thus, when NBS procured the lot of calcium carbonate to be used for its calcium CRM, and knowing that strontium was a definite interference in all calcium determinations based on an oxalate reaction, the strontium specification was less than *10* parts per million. The strontium level was then determined very accurately (2.1 μg/g) and constitutes one of the data given on the certificate when this material was issued.

4.2 Homogeneity

Since each issued unit of a CRM carries with it the full certification of the entire lot from which it came, it is clear that the entire batch itself must be homogeneous with respect to all the properties certified. But, to draw by inference that all properties, including those not measured or certified are homogeneously represented is a dangerous assumption and one against which the user should be warned.

With high purity substances, homogeneity with regard to the major constituent is not usually a major problem, and sample sizes for use are not specified. However, with matrix type CRM's (e.g., a proposed electrolytes in serum CRM) the possibility of heterogeneity becomes an important consideration. In such cases, the certificate must specify the minimum amount of the CRM that can be dispensed to ensure the homogeneity of the CRM. In clinical chemistry today this is not a problem, since few, if any, CRM's exist in this category. It will, however, become an important consideration in the years ahead, and especially so with the rapid escalation of micro methods where small samples and small amounts of reagents are used.

The certifying laboratory must again know the full details of the manufacturing process when commercial suppliers are used. Very often the manufacturer can meet the quantity specified only by producing sub-quantities at one time. The various sub-lots are then combined to meet the specified quantity. Unless very careful control is maintained throughout the entire manufacturing process, a heterogeneous product may result. Blending, mixing, and sieving operations may be called for, each of which carries in turn the possibility of error, contamination, etc.

Close quality control and proof of homogeneity requires statistical services and analysis, sometimes of a high degree of sophistication, to minimize cost and use of scarce scientific resources, and to maximize yield of product.

4.3 Stability

Contrary to some statements in the literature, cholesterol, per se, is relatively stable. In over 6 years of testing at NBS, the cholesterol CRM was found to have degraded in purity by less than 0.3%. As a general principle it would seem that stability is associated with purity – the higher the purity, the more stable the material.

Keeping in mind that reaction rates double for every 10 °C increase in temperature, sensitive materials may need to be stored at low temperatures. Both the cholesterol and bilirubin CRM's are stored in freezers at −40 °C. The proposed matrix CRM, electrolytes in serum (now a candidate material) is kept in the frozen state.

Exposure to radiation, especially ultra-violet and to moisture must also be considered. The NBS bilirubin CRM was packaged and then sealed in vials under dry argon gas, wrapped in black paper, and stored in a freezer. Thus reaction with UV and/or moisture is prevented. No appreciable degradation in three years has been noted for this material. VMA is stored in desiccators in the cold to prevent hydrolysis. Users of KCl and NaCl CRM's are warned on the certificate not to expose these to relative humidities greater than 75 and 60 percent, respectively.

As the field moves toward reference materials for proteins and enzymes, stability precautions will be even more severe. Current studies now underway in enzyme chemistry indicate the need for a much greater understanding of basic knowledge than now exists before these very sensitive materials can be produced, certified and stored as reference materials.

4.4 Continuity of Supply and Information

The supplier of CRM's must make a long-term commitment to the field to assure continuity of CRM supply. In the US, where the quality of over 90% of the steel is controlled via a large number of steel CRM's, NBS has been producing, certifying, and supplying these materials uninterruptedly for over 65 years. The same kind of commitment is now being made for the clinical CRM's so that manufacturers and users can count on a continuous supply to help bring about, and then to maintain better, measurement in this field. Obviously, for economic reasons alone, no large measurement network will be based on CRM's unless continuity of supply is assured.

It is also important that continuity of information on CRM's from supplier to user be assured. This will involve the establishment of formal information networks, such as now are being considered by international bodies and agencies, to make new, revised or updated information on CRM's easily and readily available. The supplier of CRM's should take responsibility to make certain that as such information is developed it is fed into the appropriate media networks.

4.5 Availability of CRM's

No international measurement network can or should be based on CRM's that are not freely available across national boundaries, and until such time that truly international CRM's come into being, only CRM's from individual nations that move freely in international trade should be referenced in international standards. Supply of such CRM's should also be adequate to meet international needs.

4.6 Certification

At the present time there is no international agreement on the contents, specifications and format for a CRM certificate in any field. Several international bodies are about to initiate study and to take action on this matter, among them WHO, IFCC, ISO, and OIML. The NBS certificate for the Cortisol SRM 921 (Appendix A) is offered as an example to indicate the kind of information that should be considered in such studies. In the following sub-sections, examples are drawn from the cortisol certificate.

4.6.1 Official or Legal Status

The certifying organization is clearly identified – (NBS), and the official responsible for the certification is identified – *(J. Paul Cali)*. Certificate date and revisions are clearly indicated.

4.6.2 Identification

The certificate applies to a specific lot of material clearly identified by name and number – (Cortisol and SRM # 921). At NBS, when the specific lot of a CRM is exhausted, its renewal is issued with a new certificate and a letter added to the SRM number. Thus, the first renewal lot of cortisol will be numbered SRM # 921*a*.

4.6.3 Statement of Intended Use

The purpose and intended use of the CRM is stated usually in the first paragraph. Here is also placed any warning for the user concerning minimum size of CRM to be taken to avoid heterogeneity.

4.6.4 Certified Values

Whatever properties have been measured and certified should be clearly stated, preferably on the first page. Cortisol has been certified for assay (purity) at 98.9% by weight. Impurities of importance have also been measured and certified. (See appendix for other properties measured.)

4.6.5 Uncertainties

These should be indicated in terms of both inaccuracy and imprecision. Estimated inaccuracy of the cortisol assay is 0.2%. The elemental microanalysis is stated with only an imprecision statement ($\pm$ 2 standard deviations of the mean), while for melting point, the range is given. Ideally, for every property measured there should be shown n, the number of replications, s, the standard deviation of the mean, and $\bar{x}$, the mean. In addition, a statement of the inaccuracy of the certified or recommended final value should also be stated. In the field of organic analytical chemistry, these ideals are just beginning to be met.

4.6.6 Limitations on Use

Cortisol CRM is for 'in-vitro diagnostic use only'. Any other significant limitations, whether technical or legal should be clearly stated.

4.6.7 Directions for Use

As a minimum, one or two references to the use of the CRM should be given. On the cortisol certificate directions for the preparation of standard solutions are given.

4.6.8 Stability Statement and Expiration Date

Stability statements must include conditions for storage – for cortisol this is five years from date of purchase. The expiration date is, in this case, the same.

4.6.9 References

Key references, if available in the open literature, should be given concerning the measurement processes used, material preparation, etc. In this instance, this work has not been published; the references here refer to standard methods for cortisol determination.

4.6.10 Certifying Laboratory(ies)

These should be named and an address given where additional or supplemental information can be obtained.

4.6.11 Date of Issuance

Now a legal requirement in the United States of America.

4.7 Legal Aspects

This topic is covered by other speakers in the symposium. In the United States of America, CRM's are now fully covered in the In-Vitro Diagnostic Products Regulation of the US Food and Drug Administration and cover many of the items and subjects listed above in section 4.7. Obviously, harmonization of the various national legal requirements will be a necessary prerequisite if these and similar materials (reagents, kits, e.g.) are to move freely in international usage.

5. Conclusions and Recommendations

A meaningful, that is, a compatible clinical chemistry measurement system is, in principle, now capable of establishment on an international basis. Such a system based on accurate measurement depends upon the availability of reference materials and reference methods. Unfortunately, both of these, in clinical chemistry, are in short supply, but intensive work is now underway in many nations to improve this situation. What is urgently called for at this time is a coordination of the various national programs now in various stages of development. Such coordination is vital if costly and unnecessary duplication of effort is to be avoided. Resources, especially qualified scientific manpower, are so limited that such waste should not be tolerated. Two international standards efforts in clinical chemistry are now underway. Within the IFCC, an Office on Reference Materials and Methods has been proposed to coordinate these activities, while within WHO, the Office on the Standardization of Diagnostic Materials is now operational. Both organizations should work together to: [1] gather information (worldwide) on the current availability of reference materials and methods; [2] establish and recommend a unified glossary and terminology in the field; [3] recommend priorities for both reference materials and method development; [4] develop a plan whereby qualified national laboratories, or agencies, national or international laboratory networks, national professional societies, national manufacturing associations, or standards groups are assigned various priority items; and [5] sponsor and hold workshops, symposia, and lectures to educate clinical chemists as to the philosophy and methodology of achieving compatible measurement.

Three other international agencies, IUPAC, ISO and OIML are also starting work on other aspects of reference materials, and coordination with these groups is also recommended.

Finally, the criteria given in section 4 for certified reference materials should be given consideration by these groups as appropriate to their goals and purposes.

Acknowledgement

The author is indebted to Mr. *Thomas W. Mears* of the National Bureau of Standards Office of Standard Reference Materials for useful advice and information on the subject matter, especially section 4.

References

[1] *Shewhart, W.A.:* Statistical Method from the Viewpoint of Quality Control, Dept. of Agriculture (Washington, D.C., 1939).
[2] Metric Practice Guide, ASTM designation, E-380-70 (1970), Phila., Pa.
[3] ISO Recommendation R-1000, reprinted by ANSI (New York, New York 1969).
[4] Calibration and Test Services of the NBS, NBS Spec. Publ. 250 (1970).
[5] The National Standard Reference Data System, NBS Tech. Note 747 (1972).
[6] Time and Frequency. NBS Monograph 140 (1973).
[7] *Dorsey, N.E. and Eisenhart, C.:* Absolute Measurement. Sci. Monthly, No. 2, *77,* 103–109 (1953).
[8] *Cali, J.P. and Reed, W.P.:* Symposium on Trace Analysis. NBS-Special Publication (1975) (in press).
[9] *Ku, H.H.* (editor): Precision Measurement and Calibration. Vol. 1, Statistical Concepts and Procedures, NBS Spec. Publ. 300-301 (1969).
[10] *Eisenhart, C.:* Realistic Evaluation of the Precision and Accuracy of Instrument Calibration Systems. J. Res. Nat. Bur. Stand. (US) *67C* (Eng. & Instr.) No. 2, 161–187 (Apr.–June 1963).
[11] *Cali, J.P. et al.:* The Role of Standard Reference Materials in Measurement Systems. NBS Monograph 148 (1975).
[12] *Cali, J.P.:* Problems of Standardization in Clinical Chemistry. Bull. Wld. Hlth. Org. *48,* 721–726 (1973).
[13] *Seward, R.W.* (editor): Proceedings of 6th Materials Research Symposium on SRM's and Meaningful Measurement. NBS Spec. Publ. 419 (1975 – in press).

Appendix A. Standard Reference Materials Currently Available from NBS.

SRM	Type	Purity (%) or Property
911a	Cholesterol	99.4
912	Urea	99.7
913	Uric Acid	99.7
914	Creatinine	99.8
915	Calcium Carbonate	99.9
916	Bilirubin	99.0
917	D-Glucose	99.9
918	Potassium Chloride	99.9
919	Sodium Chloride	99.9
920	D-Mannitol	99.8
921	Cortisol	98.9
922	Tris(hydroxymethyl)aminomethane, pH	99.9
923	Tris(hydroxymethyl)aminomethane, hydrochloride, pH	99.7
924	Lithium Carbonate	100.0
925	VMA (4-hydroxy-3-methoxymandelic acid)	99.4
928	Lead Nitrate	in preparation
929	Magnesium Gluconate	in preparation
930b	Glass Filters for Spectrophotometry	Optical transmittance and absorbance
931a	Liquid Filters for Spectrophotometry	Optical transmittance and absorbance
932	Quartz Cuvette for Spectrophotometry	Optical transmittance
933	Clinical Laboratory Thermometers	0 °C and 25, 30, or 37 °C
934	Clinical Laboratory Thermometer	0, 25, 30 and 37 °C

U. S. Department of Commerce
Frederick B. Dent
Secretary

National Bureau of Standards
Richard W. Roberts, Director

APPENDIX B

National Bureau of Standards
Certificate of Analysis
Standard Reference Material 921

Cortisol (Hydrocortisone)

B. Coxon and R. Schaffer

This Standard Reference Material is certified as a chemical of known purity. It is intended primarily for use in the calibration and standardization of procedures for cortisol determinations employed in clinical analysis and for routine critical evaluation of the daily working standards used in these procedures.

Constituent	Percent
Cortisol	98.9
21-Dehydrocortisol	0.6
21-O-Acetylcortisol	0.2
21-Dehydrocortisone	0.1
Cortisone	0.1
Total Steroids	99.9
Ash	0.002
Insoluble matter	0.001
Loss on drying	0.08

The cortisol assay has an estimated inaccuracy of 0.2 percent.

The cortisol used for this Standard Reference Material was obtained from the Upjohn Company, Kalamazoo, Michigan. Analyses were performed by R. F. Brady, Jr., A. Cohen, B. Coxon, M. Darr, W. D. Dorko, D. P. Enagonio, T. E. Gills, E. E. Hughes, W. P. Schmidt, and S. A. Wicks of the Analytical Chemistry Division.

The technical and support aspects concerning the preparation, certification, and issuance of this Standard Reference Material were coordinated through the Office of Standard Reference Materials by T. W. Mears.

Washington, D. C. 20234
February 15, 1973
Revised December 16, 1973

J. Paul Cali, Chief
Office of Standard Reference Materials

(over)

Identification and quantitation of the four steroid impurities were accomplished by Fourier-transform proton-magnetic-resonance (pmr) spectroscopy and thin-layer chromatography (tlc) performed on fractions from the liquid chromatography of 100 mg of the material in ethanol on a column (91 x 0.8 cm) of poly(vinylpyridine) crosslinked with 8 percent of divinylbenzene. Fractions were eluted with ethanol at a pressure of 4.7 $kg \cdot cm^{-2}$. Tlc of aliquots of the fractions was performed on silica gel GF_{254} using 9:1 (v/v) chloroform-methanol. Equivalent sensitivity of detection was obtained by fluorescence quenching and by spraying with aqueous 20-percent sulfuric acid and heating at 120 °C. All the steroid impurities, except 21-dehydrocortisone, showed similar sensitivity. 4-Androsten-11β-ol-3,17-dione was found in liquid chromatography fractions, but could not be demonstrated directly by tlc of up to 1 mg of the bulk material. Because this compound was readily resolved from mixtures prepared with it and the bulk material and detected in proportion to amounts used for reference, the compound was adjudged an artifact produced during liquid chromatography. On the other hand, the major impurity, 21-dehydrocortisol, did not arise by the known copper-catalyzed oxidation of cortisol, as shown by its unaltered proportion by tlc of the bulk material even after EDTA-treatment of the system to remove copper.

The quantitative proportion of each steroid present in the sample was estimated from the dry weight (W) of the residue of each liquid chromatographic fraction and the measured intensity of the Fourier-transform generated methyl signals characteristic for each steroid, using the expression:

$$m_n M_n = \frac{W h_n M_n}{h_1 M_1 + h_2 M_2 \ldots + h_m M_m}$$

where m_n and M_n are the number of moles present and the molecular weight, respectively of the n_{th} component in a mixture of m components, h_n is the methyl signal intensity of the n_{th} component, and $h_1 \ldots h_m$ are the corresponding intensities of components 1...m, obtained by measurement of the methyl peaks above the methylene envelope of the steroids.

For proof of homogeneity, nine samples were withdrawn from the bulk Standard Reference Material according to a statistical plan. They were analyzed in a commercial carbon-hydrogen-nitrogen microanalyzer and were found to be homogeneous with respect to carbon and hydrogen content within the limits of precision of the method. Solutions of the samples in 95 percent ethanol at 25 °C showed an absorbance maximum at 242 nm with a molar extinction coefficient of 16.1 x 10^3 $liter \cdot cm^{-1} . mol^{-1}$.

Elemental macroanalysis of the material showed carbon 69.49 ± 0.10 percent (2 SD of the mean); and hydrogen 8.39 ± 0.05 percent (2 SD of the mean); the calculated values for cortisol are 69.58 percent and 8.34 percent, respectively.

The Standard Reference Material melted at 219.0-220.5 °C (corrected) when heated in an open capillary tube at 0.5 $°C \cdot min^{-1}$. The resulting pale yellow melt did not solidify on cooling. After sealing in a capillary tube under vacuum, the material melted at 220.5-221.5 °C without yellowing, but did not resolidify.

Thermogravimetric analysis of samples heated under dry nitrogen at 2 $°C \cdot min^{-1}$ showed the initiation of loss of a large proportion of sample weight at 221 °C (uncorrected). However, for samples heated in air, loss of weight began at 204 °C. The attempted application of differential scanning calorimetry to samples heated under nitrogen gave thermograms that were very dependent on the rate and time of heating, and that were not reproducible.

International Criteria for Diagnostic Material

A.L. Louderback, Costa Mesa, California, U.S.A.

Key Words: Control materials
Diagnostic Kits
Fidelity
International standardisation criteria
Reference materials
Standards

The first two days of this Symposium have been devoted to topics relating to 'Quality Control in Clinical Chemistry'. The present discussion is on the subject of 'The Clinical Laboratory from an International Viewpoint'. This paper is on 'International Criteria for Diagnostic Material'.

Table 1 represents the various diagnostic fields of interest. In this table, are seven fields of interest in the clinical laboratory, all of which require some form of quality control. Our present concern is primarily in the area of clinical chemistry with some additional consideration of other topics.

Table 1

1. Immunology
2. Coagulation
3. Hematology
4. Serology
5. Immunohematology
6. Clinical Chemistry
7. New areas:
   a) Toxicology
   b) Radioimmunoassay (RIA)

There are various organizations, such as the World Health Organization (WHO), the International Union of Pure and Applied Chemistry (IUPAC) and the International Federation of Clinical Chemistry (IFCC), which certainly have been considering many of the quality control problems in these different areas. In immunology, standards have been set by the World Health Organization for immunoglobulin A (IgA), immunoglobulin G (IgG) and immunoglobulin M (IgM). As yet these have not been used extensively on an international basis. In the area of coagulation, international standards have been proposed for standardization of prothrombin testing. In therapeutics, an international standard exists for Factors VIII and IX. In coagulation, with its cascading enzyme systems and required cofactors, quality control is difficult due to the use of subjective measurements. In hematology, the efforts of the ICSH have resulted in standardization of hemoglobin analysis by the cyanmethemoglobin procedure and the documentation of the physical characteristics of the reference preparation.

In serology, local governments have cooperated to provide procedures for VDRL testing, but standardization of many serological tests such as for rheumatoid arthritis and lupus erythromatosus are far from complete, despite the availability of WHO serum standards for these serological reactions.

In immunohematology, the recognized serious consequences of error have encouraged worldwide standardization efforts. The WHO provides standards for Anti-A, Anti-B, Anti-D and related factors.

International standardization in toxicology and in radioimmunoassay has barely begun. The advent of gas chromatography as an analytical tool for precise analysis of drugs has made it essential to establish the effect of drugs on clinical laboratory values. An excellent monograph on this topic has been provided by Dr. *D. Young*. The newer field of RIA will require more extensive control in immunology because of the sensitivity of the procedures and the use of radioactive compounds. In addition to testing for hepatitis associated antigen, a wide variety of drugs and enzymes are now determined by RIA procedures. Study of the effects of interfering substances on these sensitive assays has only recently been initiated.

In clinical chemistry, a variety of materials are available for use in clinical laboratories (table 2), these include kits, standards and controls. In the U.S.A. the term 'kit' is used to designate as assemblage of chemicals, possibly including standards, with adequate direction to allow its use as a diagnostic test.

Table 2

1. Kits
2. Standards
3. Controls

Hopefully, the manufacturer would furnish in the direction insert:

1. A list of each of the chemicals and a complete description of contents therein.
2. The exact % or molar basis of the chemicals or constituents.
3. The procedures by which it has been developed along with the pertinent bibliography.
4. Explicit directions for the use of this assemblage, especially including such things as incubation time, temperature and wavelength to be used etc.

In the United States of America at the present time,a report of the College of American Pathology lists 17 different ways for the determination of glucose for diagnostic purposes. The F. D. A. has made a request for descriptions of glucose testing procedures,and has established rigid requirements for the labelling of the so called 'Diagnostic Kits'. It is extremely important for the user to know:

1. 'How a particular kit compares to well accepted procedures:
2. The bias of the procedure
3. The potential interferences with the procedure'

Descriptions of the sensitivity, specificity and interferences pertaining to the use of diagnostic kits will have to be improved if we are to see increased quality of laboratory performance using these materials. The German Clinical Chemistry Society has published standard procedures to be used with each of some 20 commonly used diagnostic procedures. They have gone to great lengths to make recommendations as to what the substrate concentrations are, and temperatures to be used for these procedures, and it is hoped that manufacturers would follow the lead of such organizations as this.

The Scandinavian Society has also taken a lead in this area in defining substrates for enzyme reactions at a particular temperature. The United States of America is now moving in this direction and the Center for Disease Control (CDC) is now actively pursuing this course of action in defining so called well recommended or 'International Reference Procedures' to be used as a basis for comparison of kits.

The second area of interest in diagnostic material is that of standards. If you prepare your own standards, you can perhaps buy the same materials that are being purchased by the commercial manufacturers in the preparation of these standards. The United States National Bureau of Standards is a well known source of such materials and most laboratories would use chemicals either purchased from the Bureau of Standards, or would use chemicals that are standardized by comparison to such materials. In the small clinical laboratory there is a great difficulty in preparing standards, since it requires an excellent analytical balance as well as volumetric equipment. Preparation of adequate standards also requires that 'pure' solvents be used to prepare the solution. These are not always available to the small clinical or hospital laboratory. Likewise time is usually of the essence to complete the duties of the day. For these reasons the preparation of standards has increasingly become the responsibility of commercial sources. This has brought a new problem. At this time, the largest Class A glassware available is the six liter volumetric flask. If the manufacturer makes up six liters only of a standard, and each of the finished products contains 100 ml, this means that only 60 potential units can be made up at one time. The number available for distribution would be decreased by the requirements of production quality control. The manufacture of such small batches is not commercially feasible. What is done in practice in industry is the following.

A large vessel, usually stainless steel, is tared for weight on a kilogram scale. Then 100 or perhaps 200 kilograms of water are added to this vessel. The scales have a resolving power of 200 to 250 grams. Hypothetically, let us suppose that we, as manufacturers, are to prepare 100 liters of a glucose standard solution. A large container is tared, 100 kilograms of water are added to the vessel, and then 100 grams of glucose are added while stirring to complete solution. Also added into this solution is a requisite amount of benzoic acid, used as a preservative. The amount of the specific volume taken up by the benzoic acid and the glucose are negligible compared with the large volume of water, but certainly there is an error in weighing out 100 grams of glucose, plus the error of weighing out 100 liters of water and preparing the solution. In the end result, a practical way of making a large volume of standard solution is obtainable. However, the results are not exactly 100 mg/dl of glucose. The final results may vary somewhere between 97 and 103 mg/dl. Under a general definition of standards, can this material truly be called a standard, or should the manufacturer assay this material against another standard made up with all Class A glassware and microbalances? In this latter case, the standard prepared in large volume would not be a pure standard by definition, but a secondary standard. These are the complications that arise in terms of the manufacture of large volumes of standard solutions. Each of the manufacturers certainly endeavors to do his best in making up competent final products, but these products may not be the same as you would make in your own laboratory under the best conditions.

Concerning point three – control materials, we have the most interesting enigma of all. Control serum is used world wide by laboratories to determine the quality of their work. The criteria of quality need to be established for the normal and the abnormal range. Consequently, control sera are made with the specifications of either all normal or abnormal (abnormal or pathological, can be high or low values).

Besides being used to establish precision of analysis, some laboratories use the same control materials as 'standards'. These control 'standards' are used with manual or automated procedures. For example, some of the clinical laboratories which cannot afford to prepare their own protein standards will use the stated value for total protein, e.g., as listed and defined by the manufacturer. This may be a source of difficulty, since the analytical procedure used by the manufacturer or its consulting or reference laboratory may be an unreported modification of a published method. Thus, the stated value may be the consensus of four or five laboratories each, perhaps, using different standards. In the case of automated procedures the so-called control or reference serum has even more variables. For example, the values assigned for control preparations for the Technicon 12/60 may utilize chemicals made by Company X for several channels, Company Y for others, with the remainder provided by the hospital laboratory. Likewise 'Reference Sera' used to set the instrument response and 'control sera' to monitor precision may be from unrelated sources. The resulting organized chaos may bring about an inexplicable divergence between stated and observed values for various constituents.

This difficult problem is being studied in the U.S.A. by the National Committee for Clinical Laboratory Standards (NCCLS), which has been working some six years now on a final draft of standards for calibration reference and control materials in clinical chemistry. The Food and Drug Administration in the United States of America (FDA) has utilized the white paper prepared by this group of industrial, governmental and laboratory workers, and has published a preliminary call for responses to this proposal.

One of the more important issues examined by the NCCLS is that 'inter-vial differences in concentrations shall not exceed ± 1% of the mean value in more than 5% of the vials'.

This is a reasonable requirement which should be stated on the direction inserts of control serum, assuring that the values for each production lot of a manufacturer meets this statistical norm of the vial to vial fill and contents variation. This would fulfill an important criteria for control materials – namely the amount of variation we can expect for vial to vial variation of control material.

A summary of some of the other NCCLS's positions on these materials is as follows:

1. That calibration materials should contain 'one' well-documented and well tested procedure for each of the major constituents to be examined. The criteria for precision of the assigned values by the NCCLS are comprehensive and well defined. They should allow any clinical laboratory to duplicate the analytical procedure and obtain the stated results. This well documented procedure will be called the 'true value' for each constituent.
2. The number of clinical laboratories to be used by the manufacturer for the assignment of values for reference and control materials is also specified.
3. Additional values as obtained by alternative methods may also be added along with the 'true values'.
4. What then really is the purpose of the reference material? Its main purpose is to enable the clinical laboratory to know how the procedure it is using might compare to the 'true value' for a particular constituent in this serum. Thus the availability of a 'true value' for glucose, for example, can help establish the bias of the procedure in use.

It is hoped, of course, that the manufacturers of instrumentation will be advised by the trends and manufacture instruments capable of the temperature control within the recommended ranges proposed by the International Federation of Clinical Chemistry (IFCC), the International Union of Pure and Applied Chemistry (IUPAC) and other international organizations. The manufacturers of various types of diagnostic kits would then, perhaps, change their procedures to more closely correspond with well referenced international procedures. The establishment of well referenced international procedures, of course, is an international criteria for quality control materials and must be considered as one of the important efforts and goals of the IFCC. In the long run, and this is going to take five to ten years for completion, clinical laboratories will be better standardized and have better quality control than they do today.

I would like to propose that a new term 'Fidelity' be used to describe reference materials. Fidelity in reference serum would mean exactly the same thing as it does in the field of music, namely, the exact reproduction or faithfulness of materials as compared with the original material. For example, in music we have the faithful reproduction of a concerto on tape that sounds exactly the same as if one were present in the auditorium while it was being performed. I propose we use the same term in describing reference serum and the particular reactions of the reference serum with respect to those obtained in the analysis of fresh serum. Doctor Jean Pierre Bretaudiere presented a paper at the Twenty-Sixth

Meeting of the American Association of Clinical Chemists in Las Vegas, Nevada concerning a program on which he has worked for some time. The title was 'Are Quality Control Sera Reliable for Assessment for Laboratory Accuracy in Collaborative Surveys? Consequences for Laboratory Accreditation'. I believe that Doctor Bretaudiere has shown us a new way to examine quality control materials which are being used in our laboratories. His technique assesses how closely the values of control sera compared to fresh serum with respect to bias, and interferences.

Several specifications may be considered for these materials. To do this it would be useful to describe how control sera are prepared. For our products we obtain serum product by double plasmaphoresis, using heparin as an anticoagulant. This heparinized blood is spun down and plasma is removed aseptically from the unit, and the red blood cells are returned to the donor. Then another unit of blood is drawn from this donor, the plasma is collected in the manner previously described, and the red blood cells are returned to the donor. From the two collections of this donor we collect approximately 500 ml of plasma at a time. The donor is usually bled twice a week, so we collect a liter of plasma per week from each donor. The donors, of course, are always checked for VDRL positive serology: for Hepatitis Associated Antigen, type B, both by counter-electrophoresis and RIA and for other parameters indicative of good health. The plasma is later converted into serum in the absence of red blood cells, at our convenience. Thus, the normal coagulation effects take place just as they would naturally in serum, but without hemolysis. The clot is removed from the serum, the serum filtered and stored frozen until ready for use. When a serum pool is required, the material is thawed out and poured into a large container which has been tared so that the final weight of serum can be ascertained. If materials have to be added to the serum to raise the concentration of certain constituents, these can be then added. This large serum bulk is stirred in the cold and passed through several stages of filtration, for clarification and removal of bacteria. After clarification, the material is dipensed into vials which are frozen and placed in the lyophilizer for the freeze-drying. At the termination of the freeze-drying cycle, the chamber where the vials are lyophilized is returned to normal pressure by bleeding in dry nitrogen. The vials are then stoppered in the lyophilizer, removed from the lyophilizer, capped and stored at + 5 °C.

What then are the stages of 'Fidelity' that we can be interested in? One is the clarity of the final solution. As you all know, control sera are more turbid than are normal sera taken from individuals. What then is the reason for this turbidity? The main reason for this turbidity is the change in steric structure of the lipoproteins in the lyophilizer as water is removed. Secondary to this, but adding to it, is the turbidity which is caused by the denaturation of protein in the freezing process. Depending upon how fast the material is frozen, water will tend to freeze first, and thus start concentrating the salts into a small portion of the serum. When the salt concentration rises high enough in the still liquid portion of the serum, it will begin denaturation of some of the proteins. The faster the freezing of the serum before lyophilization, the less turbidity will occur in the final product.

One of the International Criteria for Diagnostic Material then, should be the consideration of clarity as a possible specification for control serum. This is especially significant, since it has been well established that excessive turbidity of serum will cause fluctuation in the results of kinetic assay in the ultraviolet spectral region. This is due to the scattering of light which occurs in a turbid solution. This light scattering increases with decreasing wavelengths.

A secondary specification for 'Fidelity' might be the pH. As we know, the pH of normal serum is in the range of 7.4 ± 0.1. However, this is not true of a control serum. Normally the pH of the control serum, before going into the lyophilizer is adjusted to 6.9 to 7.0. During lyophilization, there is an outgasing of carbon dioxide from the bicarbonate in the serum. After reconstitution of the serum, the pH would seem to rise because of the decreased concentration of the carbonic acid. The pH of most control sera varies usually from 7.6 to 8.6, depending upon the initial pH and the lyophilization cycle in terms of vacuum and temperature maintained during lyophilization. Thus, I am proposing, in terms of 'Fidelity', that a specification be set for pH of the final reconstituted product, since it is well known that pH can effect the stability and activity of enzymes, e.g., acid phosphatase. Should a diluent be included in control serum so that an exact pH can be maintained? If so, some international criteria should be established.

Several years ago a similar problem arose in trying to adjust the pH in control serum without affecting any other values. For example, it is very easy to add sulphuric acid to decrease the pH, since we do not test for sulfate. One cannot use hydrochloric acid because of its effect on the chloride-concentration. The adjustment of the pH towards the alkaline side is far more difficult, since one cannot use sodium hydroxide, potassium hydroxide, calcium hydroxide, etc. The addition of these alkaline compounds would obviously raise the concentrations of sodium, potassium or calcium above the so called normal ranges. The pH of some sera could be adjusted using tris(hydroxymethylaminomethane)(TRIS). This did not affect any of the enzymes, nor any of the reactions in use on the Technicon instrumentation at the time. Only later was it apparent that the amino group in Tris acted as a competitive inhibitor in the Berthelot-urease reaction, giving values approximately one-half of those obtained for urea analysis by the diacetyl monoxime method.

It is evident that the addition of a new component to serum may affect the analysis of others unfavorably. Thus, in this instance, the method used to adjust pH in the control serum turned out to be critical. A third component to be discussed in the 'Fidelity' of control serum is that of additives or preservatives. The philosophy to which we adhere is to try to maintain the composition of the serum as closely as possible to the use situation. For example, in a clinical laboratory, one draws the blood from the patient, and allows it to clot over a one to two hour period and then centrifuges down the red cells. Such a process would be the most faithful reproduction of the actual procedure. However, as described previously, this is not done. Blood is collected in a slightly heparinized solution, neutralized and then allowed to coagulate in the absence of red cells, to avoid the problems associated with hemolysis.

On a production basis in an industrial manufacturing setting, this is the best procedure which can be utilized. Other manufacturers prepare control serum from outdated ACD or CPD blood. They then dialyze the serum to remove all traces of citrate, glucose and phosphate which may be present in the serum, leaving only the protein base. Then all the individual components that were present in the original serum are added as weighed materials.

However, where the difficulty lies, is in not knowing what trace elements may be important in enzyme reactions that one is not putting back into the serum in the correct trace amounts. We certainly know of the importance of magnesium in ATP linked reactions and alkaline phosphatase reactions. We know the importance of zinc, calcium and sodium on other enzyme reactions. However, there is so much that we do not know or understand that I, in my own mind, do not feel that this method is the most faithful reproduction of control serum that can be had at the present time.

Some manufacturers add various types of preservative such as borate, or even antibiotics to their serum to keep down the bacterial flora. We utilize a quick freezing of the serum which has been taken aseptically to keep down the bacterial flora. However, we all know that blood is not sterile and there's always some bacteria that are going to multiply, therefore preservatives are sometimes added. Since the long term effects of preservatives are not known they need to be used cautiously.

In summary then, the term 'Fidelity' or the faithfulness of the product in comparison to the tested serum, would consider the clarity of the material, the pH, and the various additives and/or preservatives used in its preparation. It is necessary to know how closely the control materials approximate human serum. This is especially important for setting automated instrumentation or for use in manual chemistries. Thus, to the greatest extent possible, control material should be human based. However, when used solely for control of precision it should be possible to depend primarily upon animal sources. Control and reference materials in the USA today are prepared – especially for enzymes – from bovine, porcine and equine tissues. Pig heart provides the transaminases, dehydrogenases and kinases. Some investigators have reported that the Michaelis constants of pig enzymes with respect to substrate and cofactor requirements are close to the human. A readily apparent difference is evident however in the use of bromcresol dyes for albumin assay. The dye-binding characteristics of bovine albumin are of a steeper slope than that of human albumin. Therefore, human albumin is the preferred reference material for dye-binding tests for albumin. Nonetheless, the NCCLS and the National Bureau of Standards have advocated the use of bovine albumin as a standard for total protein. Considering the worldwide shortage of human plasma and serum it would seem appropriate to reserve this precious resource for the requirements of blood product fractionation rather than for establishing the precision of clinical laboratory analysis. In addition, with bovine material, for example, there is no extra risk of Hepatitis Associated Antigen Type B in this base material. Bovine material is plentiful, is relatively inexpensive and therefore fulfills many potential international criteria for diagnostic materials.

Another important criterion is in the labelling of the control materials used in the clinical laboratories. Adequate directions must be stated and set forth in the direction insert on exactly how to reconstitute the control serum, how the deionized or distilled water is to be added; or if a buffer is to be utilized, exactly how it is to be added, how long it is to stand to fully solvate the powder before it is mixed. Should this solvation take place at room temperature for an hour period and then be placed at +5 °C or exactly how should this material be put into solution for the best reproducibility? This information is required from the manufacturer. The solvation and solution times of quality control materials from different manufacturers will vary. We're all very familiar with the fact that alkaline phosphatase values will change in control sera depending upon the temperature and time they were placed into solution and the temperature at which they were subsequently maintained. Generally speaking, the values for alkaline phosphatase will rise over the first few hours and then level out. It is an obligation of the manufacturer to present this data in the direction insert as well as the stability of each of the enzymes in his product. Generally speaking, it is my belief that enzyme products should only be used on the day of reconstitution. They should be stored at the temperature recommended by the manufacturer for a particular enzyme, usually around +5 °C. The manufacturer should be able to supply to the user the stability of the enzymes in the lyophilized state with respect to the half-life when stored at +5 °C, +20 °C, +37 °C. This additional information is a most reasonable requirement and it is essential that the clinical laboratory director know the characteristics of the enzyme to be used as a reference standard or control.

It is very difficult, at the present time, for the manufacturer of control materials to compound products for the various types of enzyme determinations with the variety of temperatures which are being used throughout the world; namely, 25 °C, 30 °C, 32 °C, and 37 °C. It would be a tremendous boon to industry were a final and definitive temperature recommended for enzyme analysis. It would also help the manufacturer of equipment used in the clinical laboratory. At the present time, the German Society recommends 25 °C, the Scandinavian Society 37 °C, and in the United States of America both these temperatures and also 30 °C are used. As one who has long been concerned with problems of enzyme stability in control solutions I would urge acceptance of the 30 °C temperature system which has been proposed by the I.F.C.C. Expert Panel on Enzymes and recommended by many societies in the world. This could serve as an 'International Criteria for Enzyme Determination in Diagnostic Materials'. This conclusion is at variance with the suggestion of the German Society for establishing 25 °C as the norm for enzyme and other chemical determinations. Despite their thorough and outstanding studies in support of their recommendation, as well as proposed methodology, it would appear that the higher temperature more closely approaches the technical and political compromise needed to attain international agreement.

While the specification of analytical methodology appears to remove some element of choice for the individual laboratory director, this is not really the situation. It rather requires that his selected method have a known bias in comparison to the recommended and specified procedure. Such agreement would not inhibit the investigation of new procedures and approaches. It would establish mandatory and stringent requirements for those investigators proposing new methods to fully test and document their contribution.

Another area of international interest is that of proficiency testing. Proficiency testing is a mandatory requirement in many countries in order to maintain laboratory licensure. In the United States of America it is a requirement that quality control proficiency testing be done in order to obtain payment from the various health insurance organizations at the Federal or State level. This is also required in several European countries. It can be argued that this external proficiency testing which is required, is not fulfilling the purpose for which it was intended. Because poor performance may result in the loss of a license, many laboratories will take special pains with the proficiency test samples. Multiple replicate analysis by the best staff members and consultation with other laboratories is not an uncommon tactic. To obviate this problem,the proficiency testing program of the State of New York includes hand-delivered and immediate on-site analysis as though the test sample were from a patient. This is an excellent system,but one hardly possible on a national scale.

Another approach for proficiency testing is that of internal testing. At the present time, however, for the control materials utilized by most of the manufacturers, there are generally two different products available. One is normal control serum and the other abnormal control serum. The problem here,very simply,is that all the values in normal serum are essentially normal, and all values in the abnormal serum are essentially abnormal. This is not the way serum specimens come into the laboratory. Usually, only two or three values are abnormal and all the rest are normal. In order to mimic the actual process we prepared a new type of control serum for the clinical laboratory which is to be used in internal proficiency testing. For 21 different constituents, random values are selected by a computer program utilizing the lowest range that is of clinical significance and the highest range. For example,in the case of sodium the low range might be 130 and the high range 165. For potassium the low range might be 3, the high range might be 7. All of the ranges for the lows and highs are then programmed,and random numbers are picked by the computer between the lowest and the highest for each of these separate constituents. Control serum is then made for these separate constituents, with the result that the final values are jumbled up, some low, some high, some intermediate, in the manner that the patients' serum comes to the clinical laboratory. The laboratory director distributes these randomly prepared control samples, for which he has assay results, to the different laboratory workers. From the resulting data he can determine who is doing the best work and who is weak in certain areas. It is then his task to improve the quality control of the laboratory by increasing the skills of a person who is getting poor answers.

With present external proficiency testing procedures the results are the 'best effort of a laboratory' not the 'average effort of the laboratory'. The type of internal proficiency testing which has been described,together with a program of external proficiency in which the samples are brought in fresh and assayed immediately in a routine manner,will provide a real index of quality control.

The International Federation of Clinical Chemistry Expert Panel on Quantities and Units along with the International Union of Pure and Applied Chemistry, has recommended systems for dimensional results of a diagnostic test. This standardization of result reporting is in accord with the metric system for standardization in methodology. This S.I. unit terminology is an excellent method to help in standardization of international clinical chemistry. It is my belief that industrial manufacturers should not only put the results of commonly used diagnostic procedures on the inserts in the older terminology, but should also include extra columns utilizing the IFCC-IUPAC S.I. unit values. After some time, control serum could be labelled only with these units. Of course the units are new and different. In order that a transition be possible we must now begin to teach medical students and future laboratory technologists to use this terminology.

In summary then, the following proposals have been advanced today for International Criteria for Diagnostic Materials.

1. That the calibration serum be prepared with 'Fidelity' or faithfulness to the human serum being analyzed. Such a serum of high Fidelity based on human material would be used as a reference or standard for both automated and manual methods. Control materials for intra laboratory precision could be made from bovine, porcine or equine sources.
2. As rapidly as possible, international agreement must be achieved for such critical subjects as assay temperatures in enzymology and definitive and reference methods.
3. International agreement is required for reagent description and standardization. The pioneering efforts of the German Society provide a useful model for such an effort.
4. The problem of the criteria for diagnostic kits has become acute, due to the variety of products now available, and the sharply increasing use of these convenience products. International agreement is essential on methods of their evaluation and the standards they are to reach.
5. Agreement is needed on the standards for quality control materials, their permissable variability, description, assay, composition, and use.

Acceptability of Quality Control Materials

A.L. Babson, Morris Plains, N.J. (U.S.A.)

Key Word: Control material

The term, 'Quality Control', practically unknown to the clinical laboratory twenty years ago, has its origins in industry. It refers to a system of checks and procedures designed to increase the probability that all units of a product meet the minimum specifications set by the manufacturer. It assumes that the manufacturer knows what the product is supposed to be like. On the other hand, quality control of the products of the clinical laboratory and analysis on unknown patient samples is complicated by the fact that all the samples are different. There is no way of knowing that the numbers reported out of the laboratory are correct. This uncertainty is no doubt responsible for the traditional distrust of laboratory results by clinicians, which prevailed only a few short years ago. Laboratory data were in many cases totally ignored or accepted only if they confirmed an existing diagnosis. The introduction twenty years ago of commercial quality control sera was a major factor in reversing this distrust.

They provided the laboratory and the clinician with an objective criterion to evaluate laboratory performance.

Absolute accuracy is an unattainable ideal. The purpose of a quality control program in a clinical laboratory is to increase the probability that the numbers reported out of the laboratory are sufficiently close to this ideal that they can aid in the determination of the correct diagnosis or prognosis on a patient, rather than hinder this determination. However, quality control materials are only a small part of a quality control program which must also be concerned with sample handling, method selection, reagents, instrumentation and operator technique.

Any particular laboratory analysis will deviate from the true value because of the combined effects of random and systematic errors. Random errors are to a great extent a result of manipulative variations. They affect individual determinations and can be either positive or negative. Systematic errors are always biased one way or the other and can affect a whole series of determinations. Automation has gone a long way to reduce random manipulative errors, but has increased the need for quality controls materials to detect systematic errors, as a machine will grind out wrong answers without moral compunction or the benefit of human judgement. A third type of error arises from interfering substances in occasional samples which can influence, positively or negatively, values obtained with nonspecific analytical methods.

The rationale for using quality control materials is that they can be treated exactly as unknown samples, the presumption being that if the 'correct' assay value is obtained for the control, the entire run of assays is 'in control'. Likewise, if the control value is not recovered, the entire run is questionable. This rationale only addresses itself to the systematic errors in an analytical procedure. By using the same lot of quality control material over a period of time, the laboratory is able to obtain an objective measure of the random error in a procedure as indicated by the observed standard deviation. This value is taken into account in determining if a particular analysis of the quality control material can be considered acceptable.

There are three criteria which should be used to judge the acceptability of quality control materials: 1. they should be similar to the clinical samples being tested, 2. they should have minimal variability within a lot, and 3. the stated value for any particular constituent should be accurate. The last two criteria impose the additional requirement of stability for the quality control material. These three characteristics are not always easy to achieve and are often incompatible. The overall acceptability of any quality control material involves compromises among conflicting desirable properties and balancing what is possible with what is practical. I will examine each of these criteria in turn as they relate to blood serum analyses.

The ideal quality control material for human serum analyses is, of course, human serum itself. However, many of the constituents of serum are not stable. To provide the required stability, the serum is customarily lyophilized. Unfortunately, the process of lyophilization alters the serum in that some of the β-lipoproteins are denatured, resulting in an increase in turbidity. Turbid samples can present problems with some kinetic enzyme procedures and with assays that do not provide for individual blanks. Another problem with human serum that has received a lot of attention lately, is the potential hazard of unnecessary exposure to hepatitis. While screening all raw materials for hepatitis B antigen, as is now done by all manufacturers, minimizes this risk, it doesn't necessarily eliminate it. Possibly more important are as yet unidentified viral diseases that might be transmitted through human serum quality control materials. The use of animal serum as a base for quality control materials would presumably avoid these hazards, but animal serum requires considerable manipulation to approximate the constituent concentrations found in human serum. The point is, what would appear to be the ideal quality control material is not necessarily the most suitable.

Constituents are often added to a serum base to provide abnormally elevated levels for the quality control serum. For most inorganic and organic compounds this presents no problem. For enzymes it is a different story. They are not well characterized and the same enzyme from different tissues or animal species can exhibit markedly diverse behaviour in various assay methods. A few years ago, the National Committee for Clinical Laboratory Standards (NCCLS) in the USA recommended the use of human enzymes in quality control materials. As most human tissues are not readily available for the production of purified enzymes, the availability of the human tissue has often been the sole criterion for selecting which isoenzyme is recommended. Placental alkaline phosphatase, for example, has been recommended because of its availability and stability. However, it is probably the most atypical isoenzyme with respect to kinetic properties. Beef kidney alkaline phosphatase behaves much more like the enzyme in pooled human serum.

If the quality control material is to be used to measure the day-to-day variability of an assay procedure, the material itself should not contribute significantly to that variability. Most quality control materials are lyophilized to ensure long-term stability. Thus two sources of vial-to-vial variability are inherent in this process, variation in fill, which is due to the manufacturer's equipment, and variation in reconstitution volume, which is introduced by the user. The best commercial filling machines available today cannot control volume better than about ± 1%. This approaches the assay precision attainable for some substances such as sodium and chloride. For these assays, a stabilized, liquid control serum would probably be more suitable than lyophilized quality control sera. For the great majority of laboratory procedures, however, the vial-to-vial variability due to fill is not significant.

A potentially more important source of variability can arise from the instability of various constituents before and after reconstitution.

Bilirubin is highly sensitive to light, and, unless precautions are taken to protect the vials and reconstituted samples from light, it can deteriorate significantly. Enzymes are particularly labile, and can deteriorate in the lyophilized vials if they are not properly refrigerated, or are retained after the expiration date. After reconstitution, most enzymes have limited stability. Alkaline phosphatase, on the other hand, characteristically increases in activity for some time after reconstitution of most lyophilized sera. The user must know the stability characteristics of these constituents to obtain uniform analyses.

If the quality control material is to be used only as a daily check on assay precision, it is not even necessary that the actual constituent values be known. However, the value of a quality control material is considerably enhanced if the user knows not only that he is getting the same answer every day, but more importantly, that he is getting the right answer. A great deal of attention is currently being focused on how correct the assigned values should be on quality control materials and how they should be attained. The NCCLS has been working for the past seven years on defining criteria for acceptable standards and control materials. Two considerations must be balanced in any such endeavour: 1. what is the most accurate value attainable within present state-of-the-art techniques, and 2. how accurate must the value be for the quality control material to fulfill its intended function. Unfortunately, groups such as the NCCLS tend to concentrate on the former with little consideration for what is practical. The state-of-the-art at the National Bureau of Standards, with unlimited time, equipment and money, is not the state-of-the-art in an industrial laboratory and bears even less resemblance to that in the average clinical laboratory. There is a real danger that, in their zeal for perfection, regulatory agencies such as the Food and Drug Administration will set unattainable standards for quality control materials that will only result in denying the use of these materials to the laboratories that need them the most.

Another aspect of the NCCLS recommendations that I find totally unrealistic is the identical requirement for accuracy in the labelling of all constituents of a quality control serum. There is no justification for requiring the same degree of accuracy in an amylase value as in a sodium value, for instance. Allowable errors in labelling each constituent in a quality control material should be individually set, based on the clinical significance of variations in the constituent value in patients and a realistic appraisal of the accuracy and precision of the methods generally available to measure that constituent.

There are two ways to arrive at a constituent value in a quality control material. One is by assay and the other is by quantitative addition to a defined matrix. The latter is the most straight-forward and is the way primary standards are prepared. Unfortunately, this fact appears to have been lost sight of in the flurry of excitement and activity by various groups in designing 'optimized' assay procedures and defining reference methods. Accurate reference methods are needed to determine the true concentration of a substance in a complex medium such as serum, because many of the methods in common use are known to be biased or nonspecific. The reference methods are, however, generally too cumbersome for routine use. As long as biased methods are in common use, the true concentration of a constituent in a quality control serum, whether determined by weigh-in or by reference method, may have little meaning for the laboratory using the biased method. For example, consider a quality control serum with an elevated bilirubin being run on an SMA 12/60. Although the true cholesterol level of the control may be known, it will not be the value that the instrument will or *should* reproduce, since it is well known that bilirubin will falsely elevate cholesterol determinations on the SMA 12/60. How then does one go about assigning the 'correct' SMA 12/60 cholesterol value for this control without relying on the instrument itself? This is a real problem.

This problem, however, pales into insignificance compared with the problem of assigning meaningful enzyme values to quality control sera. No matter how pure, enzymes today can only be quantitated in terms of activity. Enzyme activity can be markedly influenced by slight changes in assay conditions or reagents. A great deal of the effort currently being expended on standard reference methods for enzymes is in defining adequate specifications for all the ingredients that go into the reagents. Commercial enzyme kits have often been denigrated, but because of the rigorous quality control procedures many of these kits undergo by the manufacturer, they probably provide less interlaboratory variation in actual use than reference methods would if used in these same laboratories.

If enzymes are on shaky ground in terms of defined values for quality control materials, blood coagulation is a veritable quagmire. Quality control plasmas are merely labelled as normal or abnormal. The experts have been arguing for eight years and can't even agree on whether the plasma or the reagent should be the standard. What, after all, is thromboplastin? But there is no question that we do need standards in blood coagulation and we need quality control materials, however poorly defined. We need standard methods and well defined quality control materials in clinical chemistry. And we need them now. We can't afford to wait seven years to define the ideal method or control material. We need practical methods and controls that represent the real world of today. They can be improved as the technology improves.

Manufacturers of reagent kits, instruments and quality control materials should and will be regulated. But standards of performance should not be unattainable. If they are, these commercial products which have revolutionized laboratory performance will not be available. The loser will be the patient, whose improved care is the rationale for all regulatory activity.

In this brief report, I have touched on some important issues that confront the field of clinical chemistry. These represent my own opinions based on over twenty years experience in the development of quality control materials for the clinical laboratory. The variety and quality of these materials have improved over the years and will continue to do so. Reasonable regulation can spur this improvement. Unreasonable regulation can repress the development of new and improved laboratory standards, reagents and quality control materials.

A System Approach to Calibration and Quality Control Materials

J.L. Giegel, Miami, Florida, U.S.A.

Key Words: Aspartate transaminase
Calibration materials
Control materials
Creatine Kinase
Proficiency test samples

The current practice of clinical chemistry involves the use of control and calibration materials in each analytical series. The use of protein-based calibration materials is becoming widespread and often a single calibration point is used with controls at higher and lower levels. This practice is usually supplemented with analyses of unknown samples from an external source (proficiency testing). Thus, three distinct functions are apparent; however, the materials used for each of these functions at the present time are often similar in composition.

I believe that a great deal of additional information regarding analytical performance can be obtained if these three functions are considered as an integrated system with materials designed specifically for each purpose.

Control Materials

For purposes of this discussion, I will define control materials as serum or protein based materials used for:

1. Quality Control
2. Calibration
3. Proficiency Testing

Each of these functions is separate and distinct. Quality control and calibration are considered internal functions for the laboratory while proficiency testing is usually external.

Quality Control Materials

Currently, quality control procedures are concerned with the evaluation of precision and accuracy of analytical systems. The goal of these programs is to reduce imprecision and inaccuracy. A simple definition of the *function of quality control material is the detection of problems in an analytical procedure before the problems affect patient samples.* This implies that quality control materials are more sensitive to analytical problems than the most sensitive patient sample. This definition may appear incompatible with the goals of reducing imprecision to very low levels. It can be shown, however, that when the analytical system is operating properly, this precision obtained with sensitive materials is equivalent to that obtained with insensitive materials. Based on this simple definition, and in conjunction with suitable calibration materials, a different approach to quality control can be developed.

Calibration Materials

In contrast to quality control materials, *calibration materials should be rather insensitive to minor analytical problems.* The principal advantage of this dual system of a rugged calibrator and sensitive control is that it permits evaluation of analytical problems. In addition, an insensitive calibrator should provide more precise and accurate patient values when the analytical system is functioning properly. If one considers calibration materials in systems which do not include quality control materials, this definition is difficult to justify since very often the calibrator provides some quality control information also.

I have thus far avoided definition of calibration, and will continue to do so. While this discussion is concerned primarily with serum or protein-based calibrators, this systems approach is also appropriate when 'primary standard' calibrators are used. The relative merit of 'primary standards' vs. protein based calibrators is another intriguing area for discussion.

Proficiency Testing Materials

In this system, *proficiency testing is defined as the evaluation of bias between laboratories.* This may involve different laboratories using the same method or different laboratories using different methods for the same constituent. These programs permit the individual laboratory to relate its performance to either a peer group or a reference laboratory. This definition is quite similar to the current concept of proficiency testing. Unfortunately, a great deal of data obtained in current surveys provides little guidance to the individual laboratory in analyzing his problems. The reasons for this are primarily twofold. First, it is difficult (perhaps impossible) to determine the 'true value' of a constituent in a material as complex as serum. Secondly, few methods exist in common use which are free of interferences from some substances found in serum. It is possible, however, to design materials which can clearly identify certain errors in methodology.

Application of the System

The system approach of analytical control is best illustrated by examination of specific methodologies. One important and widely studied clinical determination is the measurement of serum aspartate aminotransferase (AST) activity. One widely used method for the measurement of AST activity is the UV method of Karmen. This reaction is shown in figure 1.

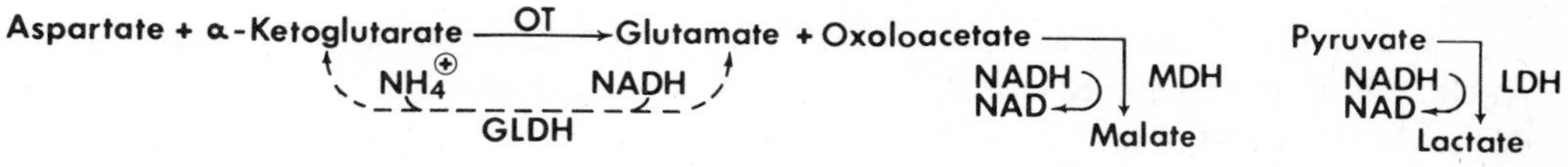

Figure 1. Reactions considered for serum AST determinations.

MDH is used as the linking enzyme to determine AST activity and LDH is often added to consume endogenous keto-acids in the sample. Many serum samples contain GLDH, which can cause problems if reagents contain ammonium ions. In considering a quality control scheme for this method, several parameters need to be considered. Both LDH and MDH may become inactivated in the reagent system; therefore, a sensitive control sample should not contain either LDH or MDH. Moreover, the control should contain significant concentrations of pyruvate or other keto acids to evaluate the effectiveness of the LDH reaction. The presence of GLDH in the control permits the evaluation of ammonium ion contamination in the test method.

Table 1. Sample and reagent constituents of interest in consideration of control materials.

AST reaction contains:	Sample may contain:
1. Aspartate	AST
2. α-ketoglutarate	LDH
3. NADH	MDH
4. MDH	GLDH
5. LDH	NH^+_4
6. Buffers, etc.	Pyruvate

A list of the materials which a sample may contain is shown in table 1 with a list of important materials in the reagent. Many AST methods use protein based calibrators instead of the molar absorbance of NADH for calibration. The properties of an insensitive calibrator are indicated in table 2.

Table 2. Control Materials for AST.

	Calibrator	Quality Control	Proficiency Testing
AST	+	+	+
LDH	+	−	+ or −
MDH	+	−	+ or −
GLDH	−	+	+ or −
NH^{+}_{4}	−	−	−
Pyruvate	−	+	+ or −
Other Interferences			

The composition of an appropriate control and proficiency test sample is also listed in table 2. With the combined use of these materials, one can clearly evaluate problems with either LDH, MDH or ammonium ion contamination in reagents.

Another example of this approach is illustrated in the measurement of creatine kinase (CPK) activity by the method of Rosalki (fig. 2). This method uses a thiol activator to reactivate CPK in the patient sample. An ideal control therefore, should contain inactive CPK to properly evaluate the performance of the thiol compound in the reagent. An insensitive calibrator for this method should contain fully active CPK. In addition, the method of Rosalki contains adenosine monophosphate (AMP) to inhibit myokinase activity. Quality control materials should therefore contain myokinase to evaluate AMP levels.

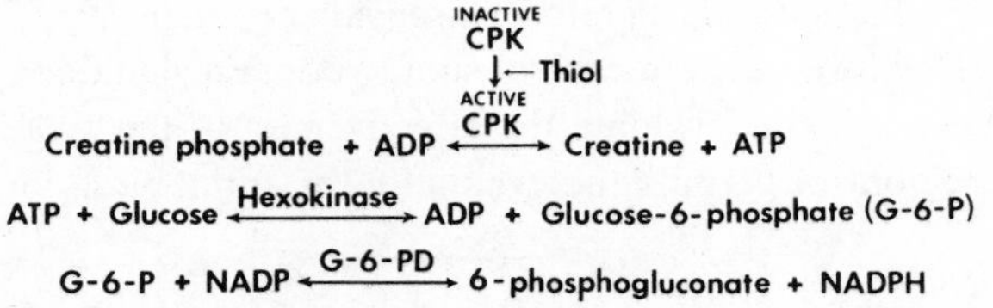

Figure 2. Measurement of CPK activity by the method of Rosalki.

Proficiency testing materials could also evaluate the problems of glutathione reductase when glutathione is used to activate CPK. An outline of control materials for CPK is shown in table 3.

Table 3. Control Materials for CPK.

	Calibrator	Control	Proficiency
Inactive CPK	+	+	+
Activator	+	−	+
Myokinase	−	+	+ or −
Glutathione reductase	−	+ or −	+ or −

This systems approach is not restricted to the measurement of enzyme activities. Many methods are in common use for the determination of triglycerides in serum using enzymatic techniques. Appropriate controls should evaluate the performance of these techniques in relation to known problems, such as glycerol interference, enzyme activity from certain samples, etc. By appropriate analysis of the methodology, one can design optimal materials for quality control, calibration and proficiency testing.

The constituent levels in these materials are basically independent of the composition. Thus, one can use these materials in current quality control schemes to evaluate precision at appropriate constituent levels. These materials thus serve conventional quality control purposes, however, more information concerning analytical problems becomes available.

Comprehensive Control Materials

The goal of most manufacturers of control material has been to add as many constituents as possible to each material. This has been in response to the clinical chemist's request for a single control material for his laboratory. One must recognize that the addition of certain materials may seriously affect the suitability of the control material for some methodologies. It is apparent that the knowledge of the limitations of comprehensive control materials will lead to better direction from the professional community on the future developments of such materials. Obviously, it is not possible to develop control materials for each methodology; however, by consideration of the systems approach described, it appears that more than one control material is required.

International Criteria for Clinical Laboratory Materials

Discussions

W. Gruber (Germany): I should like to underline the paper by Dr. Babson by saying a few words about the influence of precision of methods on confidence limits.

Let us assume different laboratories make determinations on the same sample; then by an analytical procedure it may be established which parts of the variance are of an intra-laboratory nature and which are of an inter-laboratory nature. This is shown in fig. 1.

	$\frac{\text{Variance } \alpha}{\text{Variance } \varepsilon}$ Mean
Protein	0.4
Glucose	
GOD-Perid	0.75
HK/G6P-DH	0.75
GOT/GPT	
Suboptimized and optimized	1.2
Urea	2.3
Creatinine	2.3
CPK	2.7

Fig. 1. Ratio of interlab (α) to intralab (ε) variance

Figure 1 shows that, if one calculates innerlab and interlab increments of variance of laboratory tests, the ratio of both is specific for the different methods (our data were meanwhile confirmed by Dr. Esser, head of the laboratories of the German Landesversicherungsanstalten).

A ratio may be established between the calculated inter-laboratory variance and the intra-laboratory variance. This ratio is quite constant for a given method. In our hands this ratio of inter-laboratory variance to intra-laboratory variance has proved quite convenient to determine which methods are satisfactory. We have established characteristic values for this ratio for different methods. For example, for total protein, the inter-laboratory variance part is lower than the intra-laboratory variance. For glucose the inter-laboratory variance is of the same magnitude as the intra-laboratory part of the total variance. With creatinine the inter-laboratory variance is more than double that of the intra-laboratory variance. It is approximately 1 for the transaminases. For creatine kinase we find a value of 2.7.

These ratios are mean ratios derived from quite a number – 10, 20 – different assays, in which four laboratories took part. But, whether the value exceeds 2 or exceeds 1, it is clear that the confidence limits of assigned values depend on the number of laboratories which take part. If unlimited testing is done, there are other variables besides precision that influence the confidence limits. In practice, always limited numbers of determinations must be done; if altogether 40 determinations are performed, through a complex mathematical function we can correlate these determinations to the confidence limits of the value. If you have two laboratories, you can only reach a certain level of confidence limits for your values, whereas if three laboratories make the same total number of determinations, these confidence limits improve. With five or six laboratories, the range always becomes closer. It is possible to calculate the influence of the inter-laboratory precision of a method on the confidence limits of assigned values (fig. 2).

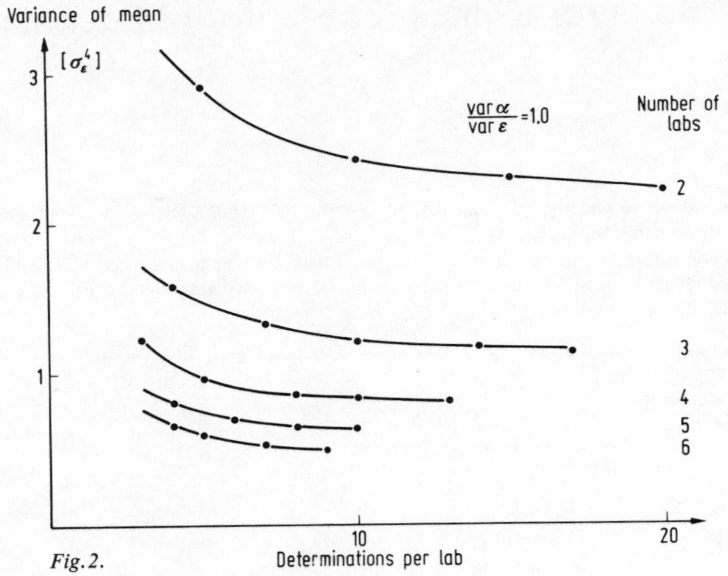

Fig. 2.

Figure 2 shows that, for a given ratio of variance increments and a given total amount of assays the confidence interval which can be reached by consensus analysis of different laboratories, depends on the number of laboratories, which take part.

Figure 3 shows part of what we have calculated. Included are the precision of the methods used and the inter-laboratory precision of the values. The half part of the 95% confidence limits of the values obtained is also shown. For example, if a method has an inter-laboratory coefficient of variation of two, which in most cases is very good, and you want to have confidence limits between 98.5 and 101.5 for an assigned value of 100, then you would need 9 labs. If the state of the art is such that the coefficient of variation of a method is in the range of 4 to 8, between 30 and more than 100, different laboratories are needed to get a value within those confidence limits.

		Interlab variance (CV %)			
	%	1	2	4	8
½	0.5	18	64	248	984
Confidence	1.5	4	9	30	112
Interval	2.5	3	5	13	42
(95% Limits)	5		3	5	12
	10			3	5

Fig. 3. Number of laboratories necessary.

Figure 3 shows that one can calculate the number of laboratories needed for a consensus analysis to reach predesigned confidence limits (in accordance to the NCCLS- and FDA-definitions) for assigned values by methods for which the interlab precision is known as State of the Art.

Just to summarize, the confidence limits of assigned values are influenced by the precision of the method used and the number of laboratories taking part in establishing the assigned values. If you have bad precision and wish to get a very good confidence interval, then you must perform unlimited testing.

U.P.Merten (with *A.v.Klein-Wisenberg* and *V.Schumann*), Germany: The conclusions from the presentation and tables of Dr. Gruber are similar to those reached by the Institute of Standardization (INSTAND), in that several more laboratories are needed for the determination of a target value than previously proposed (e.g. the lecture of Prof. *Stamm:* The determination of assigned values for control specimens). Although Dr. *Gruber* used a different statistical concept in analysing the influence of sample size in confidence intervals, whereas INSTAND calculated the statistical power function for given relevant differences, yet both models showed that a larger number of laboratories are needed. This latter can be seen from the following tables:

Optimal sample size for the one sample problem to lie within a defined percentage deviation of a given target value.

Formula:

$$n = \left(\frac{U\alpha + U\beta}{\alpha/\sigma} \right)^2$$

n = required sample size
u = standardized normal value
α = error I = 5% (twosided)
β = error II =
1–β = power of the test

1. Example: Glucose $\bar{x}$ = 108.0 mg/dl
s = 4.95 (based on 48 single values)
s% = 4.58 (CV)

from former studies with 1800 values
s% = 4.54

95% confidence interval = 4.39–4.59
d = relevant difference to target value

Sample size for power 1–β

$\bar{x}$ = 108.0	d	d%	95%	90%	80%	60%	40%	20%
	0.5	0.46	1274	1030	769	480	285	123
	1.0	0.93	318	257	192	120	71	31
	1.5	1.39	142	114	85	53	32	14
	2.0	1.85	80	64	48	30	18	8
	2.5	2.31	51	41	31	19	11	5
	3.0	2.78	35	29	21	13	8	3
	3.5	3.24	26	21	16	10	6	3
	4.0	3.70	20	16	12	8	4	2
	4.5	4.17	16	13	9	6	4	2
	5.0	4.63	13	10	8	5	3	
	5.5	5.09	11	9	6	4	2	
	6.0	5.56	9	7	5	3	2	
	6.5	6.02	8	6	5	3		
	7.0	6.48	6	5	4			
	7.5	6.94	6	5	3			
	8.0	7.41	5	4	3			

2. Example: Calcium $\bar{x}$ = 7.50 mmol/l
s = 0.3273
s% = 4.24 (based on 1725 values)

95% confidence interval = 4.10–4.39

1–β

$\bar{x}$ = 7.50	d	d%	95%	90%	80%	60%	40%	20%
	0.05	0.67	557	450	336	210	125	54
	0.10	1.33	139	113	84	52	31	13
	0.15	2.00	62	50	37	23	14	6
	0.20	2.67	35	28	21	13	8	3
	0.25	3.33	22	18	13	8	5	2
	0.30	4.00	15	13	9	6	3	
	0.35	4.67	11	9	7	4	3	
	0.40	5.33	9	7	5	3		
	0.45	6.00	7	6	4	3		
	0.50	6.67	6	5	3			
	0.55	7.33	5	4	3			
	0.60	8.00	4	3	2			

When divided by a variance factor of 9, at least 2 mean values, estimated on 2 days, are needed for each laboratory. Thus INSTAND demands about 20 laboratories with mean determinations for at least two days.

B. Copeland (USA): Mr. Chairman, I should like to present on behalf of the Commission on World Standards (COWS) of the World Association of Pathology Societies (WASP) our congratulations to the IFCC on this very useful conference on reference methodology. As Chairman of the COWS of WASP we look forward to continued co-operation between our international societies. As a member of this meeting I should like to speak on two points:

1. the need to separate the current research in reference methodology from day-to-day clinical laboratory practice, and
2. the problem of the lack of quality control with respect to publication of new methods in the world literature.

There is no doubt that it is very important to continue current efforts in reference methodology. In my opinion this will be an effort which will take at least ten years to accomplish. During this time it is important to limit these investigations to university hospital and equivalent workers such as those assembled here today. In my practice, I have seen medical laboratories doing work with excellent precision and of excellent medical usefulness who, nevertheless, are very upset because their average value does not duplicate the labelled average value (let us say an average of urea of 28 mg/dl versus a labelled value of 32 mg/dl).

Necessarily, our efforts in reference methodology will be concentrated on concepts of accuracy, which as you know are extremely difficult concepts and upon which even our leading institutions disagree. We have seen an excellent example of this disagreement with respect to the molar absorptivity of NADH. This is only one of several examples which could be cited. One has only to recall the problem of the accuracy of the molar absorptivity of cyanmethemoglobin which took almost ten years to clarify.

While we are concentrating efforts on reference methodology, we should, in my opinion, continue to encourage the large majority of clinical laboratories to continue their efforts to obtain good within laboratory day-to-day precision. For this purpose, I should like to bring to your attention the concept of large regional day-to-day quality Control Pools as they are currently used in the USA. This idea originated with Dr. *Joseph Preston* of Denver Colorado who organized the first Daily Regional Quality Control Program. The forty hospital laboratories in Colorado combine their purchasing of lyophilized human serum control, thus allowing a considerable saving. The material does not contain any labelled values. On a monthly basis each laboratory submits its daily values and receives in return a composite printout of all average values. Thus, after the first month a reference point for each component is established. With this reference point as guide, all laboratories in the Daily Regional Group can direct their efforts towards the group mean values; thus improving the interchange of patient data between hospitals in the region. The regional average cannot be considered an absolutely accurate value and it may be shown by reference methodology that there is a significant absolute bias with respect to the absolutely accurate value. However, while reference methodology is being developed, the regional average value is a very powerful operational tool which is of great practical relevance.

In the United States there are now approximately sixteen regions. The largest is Illinois with approximately 250 hospitals. Anyone who would wish to obtain material from one of those regions would be welcome. The Massachusetts Society of Pathologists Regional Quality Control Program has already made its material available to a small but vigorous program involving some Eurotransplant group laboratories in the Netherlands.

Again, I should like to emphasize the need to distinguish between the reference method efforts which are essential and which should be carried out by skilled and well-informed workers over the next ten years, and the immediate present need for daily within-laboratory precision and within-region correlation. Both aspects, 'reference level accuracy' and 'within-laboratory daily precision' will eventually be fused. This process must be carefully documented in order to preserve the integrity of the diagnostic medical heretage.

The second area where, at present, there is no quality control is the area of methodology development itself.

Past experience has shown that methodology development is a continuous and dynamic phenomenon. It will continue in parallel with reference methodology development. At the present time there is no effort made to guarantee the validity or the quality of new methods before they are published. Recently, I have had the frustrating experience of trying to set up two newly-published methods which were not workable as published. Often the newly-published methods have a significant bias with respect to previous reference or commonly used methods. Journal editors are most responsible for developing a solution to this problem, but they will not be able to set up quality control of new methods without our help and our stimulation.

Again, I should like to thank the IFCC sponsors of this program for the opportunity to present these opinions.

D. Stamm (Germany): I have only a short remark. Calibration and quality control materials are mentioned in one sentence and everyone may think we use the same material for different purposes, and that the same requirements apply to both. But, the opposite is true. The requirements for calibration materials and calibrated solutions are very different from the requirements for control materials, and we should discuss them under different sections. I did this at the WHO Atlanta Meeting in 1973.

H. Büttner (Germany): I should like to announce that in addition to the paper given by Dr. *Louderback,* the Expert Panel on Nomenclature and Principles of Quality Control of IFCC has in preparation a document on calibration and control materials. The Panel hopes to finish the first draft of this document at the Toronto meeting, so it can be sent out to the Associate Members of the Panel in the near future.

G. R. Cooper (U. S. A.): I agree with Dr. *Babson* that we should be very practical about setting requirements for labeling of serum reference materials. Labeling requirements would probably vary primarily with the attainable accuracy and precision of the reference analytical method and the stability of the reference materials for the particular constituent. With respect the determination of cholesterol, tools are available to label materials within 95% confidence limits of 1% when a large number of analyses are performed with high precision with the manual *Abell* et al. method. It seems practical, therefore, that serum reference materials for the determination of cholesterol should be at least within 95% confidence limits of 2 to 2½% as a general guideline. The CDC Lipids Section offers standardization, through lipid standardization programs, to commercial companies and others who are interested in accurate labeling of serum reference materials.

H. Adlercreutz (Finland): There is an urgent need for reference methods in the field of toxicology and hormone assays, because of the enormous number of radioimmunoassays being developed. I have found out that combined gas chromatography and mass-spectrometry is one good means of controlling radioimmunoassay methods. But there is a need today for deuterated internal standards for use in mass-spectrometry and it is almost impossible to obtain these. I would like to ask the company members here if there is any work going on to synthesize these types of compound for use as internal standards in reference assays.

A. Babson (U.S.A.): I should like to answer Dr. *Cooper's* comment on the accuracy of labeling of these quality control materials. I too would like to see everything labeled to an accuracy within 1%. However, I do not see how this is possible when we have a vial-to-vial variability in fill of 1% on a lyophilized product. As Dr. *Gruber* just pointed out also, unless we have a low enough coefficient of variation within the procedure, it might require an unlimited number of laboratories and analyses to reduce the imprecision down to this level.

G. Vanzetti (Italy): I should like to stress the importance of applying quality control procedures to radioimmunoassays. I can add to Dr. *Adlercreutz'* comments on this subject, that we have made a survey in Italy concerning the reliability of these radioimmunoassays. I must say that there are great differences between laboratories. I believe that this subject would deserve discussion at the next Symposium of Quality Control.

M. Rubin (U. S. A.): I should like to ask the manufacturers of Quality Control materials to what extent it is possible to give full disclosure of the composition of the materials that they are supplying to our colleagues.

J. Giegel (U. S. A.): I think it will be many years before we know the composition of serum. We can disclose what we add to the product and also what is removed, however, we must remember that pooled serum is a very ill-defined raw material consisting of several thousand components. A serious problem that we have to face and learn to live with, is that different pools of material have different levels of interfering materials. We also have to deal with methods which are non-specific. We may eventually achieve methods of greater specificity, however, it is unlikely that we will ever achieve a well-defined control serum as long as we use pooled human serum.

M. Rubin (U.S.A.): I should like to suggest that this is not quite the answer I was hoping to get because we all understand this point. What I am concerned about is the disclosure of the nature of the additives, of the stabilizers, of the distribution of isoenzymes and their tissue sources which has caused us tremendous problems in the use of control materials. I am concerned even about the methods used by a specific manufacturer for assay of the constituents. We all understand that there are necessities of industrial confidence which limit some aspects of the disclosure, but there is a borderline here between the need to know of the scientist and the need of the industry. It is that point I would much enjoy hearing some comments on from our colleagues in industry who are concerned with these problems.

A. Babson (U. S. A.): Yes, of course we are happy to tell everything we know about what we put into our products; in fact I believe we are now legally obligated to do this. In terms of the assay procedures, this becomes crucial, primarily with constituents such as enzymes. Where suitable standard methods do not exist we have developed our own standard methods, which are available on request. Obviously, they are too detailed to include in the package insert of the comprehensive quality control material.

F. L. Mitchell (U.K.): I should like to rise to the defense of the N.B.S. They habe been criticized yesterday. and also today. I think this criticism can be summed up in an accusation that they tend to be 'fiddling while Rome burns'. Many of us are working with the N. B. S. and I would like to say how much we appreciate their work. I think that possibly much of the criticism arises from a misconception of definitive and reference methods. We have had several international meetings involving reference technology recently and on at least one occasion a discussion was a complete waste of time because the people there did not have definitions for definitive and reference methods. These methods have a very important place in Quality Control, but I feel we do not yet have the right conception of their use and it is very important that we do. I think we should remember that it is only necessary for one laboratory in the world to be able to do a definitive method – that is all; and it is only necessary for one laboratory in each country to be able to do a reference method. These are very difficult technics which need only to be done in certain clearly specified laboratories. They should not be criticized just because they are high-powered and cannot be done by everybody.

Session II

Topic: International Criteria for Diagnostic Methods

Session-Chairman: H. Büttner, Germany
Discussion-Leader: G. Anido, USA

Acceptability of Definitive, Reference and Routine Methods

S. S. Brown, Harrow, Middlesex, U.K.

Key words: Definitive methods
Reference methods
Routine methods
Selected methods

Introduction

Working definitions of 'definitive' and 'reference' methods of analysis (table 1) were agreed in a discussion at the 1st European Congress of Clinical Chemistry (Munich, April

Table 1. IFCC-CS, Expert Panel on Nomenclature and Principles of Quality Control – proposal for categorizing analytical methods

Term	Concept	Value obtained for calibration or control material
Definitive method	No known source of inaccuracy (inaccuracy = 0)	Definitive value (best known approximation to 'true' value)
Reference method	After exhaustive testing: inaccuracy = $0 \pm \delta$; (δ negligible as compared to between-laboratories imprecision)	Reference method value (stated or certified)
Method with known bias	Known bias δ as determined	Assigned value (stated or certified)
Method with indetermined bias	Bias not known	

1974), which has since been published (*Z. klin. Chem. Klin. Biochem.*, 1974, *12*, 558). Routine analytical methods may be described as those which are in common, regular, use in clinical laboratories; they may have known or indeterminate bias.

These definitions beg the question of the need to define the analyte. In principle, this may be done fairly easily for the monatomic anions or cations, but it becomes progressively more difficult with polyatomic ions, and with organic compounds – consider for example glucose. With the more complex proteins, including enzymes, a strict chemical definition may not be practicable at all – at least in the sense required by definitive and reference technology. This problem of defining the analyte, is, of course, intimately associated with the need for defining appropriate reference substances and corresponding standards.

The definitions of the three types of method also beg the question of defining the matrix in terms of normality or pathological abnormality; nor do they consider potential interferences from drugs and the like. Such factors are usually investigated before publishing a routine method – should they also be for definitive and reference methods?

It is implicit in the definitions of these methods that only one definitive method and only one reference method for a particular analyte can exist at any one time. It is therefore vitally important that definitive and reference methods command wide acceptability both by clinical scientists and by scientific or governmental bodies which have legitimate interests e.g. pharmacopia commissions, and national or international health organisations. In addition, members of the medical profession must be aware of the importance and long term significance of these concepts – can this be achieved, and can we broaden the narrow view of 'clinical usefulness' by some of our own colleagues?

Definitive Methods

For a definitive method to be acceptable, there are two fundamental requirements. Firstly, the theoretical basis of the method, and the full practical details, should be published and open to scrutiny, so that they can be recognised as sound. Secondly, the method should be carried out in an institution with impeccable credentials, to the highest possible standards of performance. The question must then be asked – should the methods and its findings be accepted as proven, or should the technique be set up and repeated elsewhere? Now since the members of our profession are by nature both conservative and suspicious, it is tempting to maintain that a definitive method should be set up and tested independently of the initiating laboratory. Is this a realistic or an unrealistic attitude, and might the time and effort be better spent in validating reference methods?

In some ways, definitive methods are analogous to the determination of a physical 'constant' such as Avogadro's number, the gas constant, and atomic or molecular weight. Attempts to measure these values are made only rarely, but great credance is attached to the results, even though in historical perspective they may be found to be inaccurate. There is no doubt, however, that once a definitive method is set up, it should be available from time to time in order to check the performance of reference methods derived for the same analyte. This requirement of course places a considerable burden on the initiating laboratory – is there any way around this problem, perhaps involving the use of carefully prepared and stored matrix reference materials (such as analysed sera)?

Reference Methods

A reference method can only be validated, and become acceptable, by strict comparison with the corresponding definitive method. Is it a useful exercise to develop 'candidate reference methods' before the corresponding definitive methods are available? Thus for the clinical reference methods under development (table 2), there are as yet definitive methods only for calcium, electrolytes and lead.

Table 2. Clinical Reference Methods under Development (Source – NBS Newsletter, 1974)

Analyte	Status of method
Calcium in serum	Revision of final protocol being agreed
Electrolytes in serum Lead in blood Uric acid in serum Glucose in serum	Round-robin comparisons in progress
Cholesterol in serum Iron in serum Creatinine in serum	At early planning stage

There should be two tiers of testing reference methods once a preliminary selection of the candidate method has been made. Firstly, there must be the round-robin approach between a network of collaborating laboratories, each engaged in the sequential testing of protocols. At the end of this period of comparison, it is essential that the final method should be written up with great care, and that there should be independent assessment of it, preferably by laboratories in different countries which have not had any detailed involvement in the work so far. Only in this way is it possible to obtain a really objective view of the whole exercise, and uncover obscurities or difficulties which might be experienced e.g. in respect of the general availability of certain reagents, glassware, or instruments. This procedure is vitally necessary if a reference method is to be fully debugged, both to command the respect which it must achieve if it is to be useful, and at the same time to be 'realisable in the real world, by many dozens of qualified laboratories' (*J.P. Cali et al., N.B.S. Special Publication* 260–236, 1972). Just how many laboratories comprise a valid network, both in the round-robin testing and in the independent assessment, is debatable. Certainly, the more elaborate the network, the less chance of carrying the work through to a satisfactory completion; on the other hand, if there are too few critical views, something of importance may be overlooked. All this is time-consuming and expensive, and it may be hard to justify the work in the face of two kinds of criticism: that errors associated with poor sample handling and identification, contamination at the bench etc. make reference technology unimportant for practical purposes; and that the remedying of large imprecision is much more urgent than that of small inaccuracy.

Routine Methods

The criteria for the acceptability of routine methods of analysis are particularly difficult to define since there are so many of them for a given analyte, and because laboratories differ so greatly in their workloads, instrumentation and special skills. It is well to remember that enormously important work has been done in years past using methods which today would not be regarded as acceptable at all. At the same time, there is now good evidence, by way of performance in quality assurance surveys, that methods of doubtful acceptability *may* yield good results in dedicated hands – 'good' here being associated with good precision, but not necessarily good accuracy. In fact, laboratories which achieve good results with doubtful routine methods are those which are least likely to abandon these methods in favour of more acceptable ones. Laboratory directors may become reconciled to performing with a consistent margin of difference in relation to the group mean, and may feel fully justified in doing so. Other directors who find themselves in this position are perhaps less strong-willed, and may utilize a factor in reporting their results to bring them into concordance with the group mean; does this happen more widely than we realise, in respect say of uric acid? The use of correction factors of any kind in routine analysis may be highly undesirable, but protagonists of the view will not be encouraged – let alone persuaded to change their stance unless samples are regularly analysed by a reference method of demonstrably good precision and high accuracy.

In some countries, there are official or unofficial moves to promulgate 'standard' or 'standardized' methods of routine analysis, to be used in conjunction with specimens analysed by referee laboratories. Some see this approach as the quickest and most practicable means of improving laboratory performance – perhaps they are right? But how is the performance of referee laboratories to be monitored and how are the standard methods to be chosen? How relevant is the publication of proposed 'Selected Methods', which are intended for critical scrutiny and assessment by the profession? A very wide variety of such Methods (table 3) has now appeared in the pages of *Clinical Chemistry,* but the mechanism for evaluating reports on them, and hence offering revised and fully tested methods, has not yet been worked out. Is it really possible to achieve this objective in the context of enzyme- or immunoassays? Is a routine method, whether manual or automated, ever going to be acceptable without several years' trial in many laboratories?

The last, but certainly not least, important question is – which body defines the criteria of acceptability of a reference, definitive or routine method, and sets the seal of approval on it? Clearly this could be done at the national level, by one or more societies of clinical chemistry, or perhaps by an organisation such as the British Standards Institute or the U.S. National Committee for Clinical Laboratory Standards. Internationally-agreed criteria and approval would be far better, and the IFCC should take a strong lead in these matters, where necessary offering advice to, or seeking support from, international agencies such as I.S.O. and W.H.O.

Table 3. Proposals for «Selected Methods» published in Clinical Chemistry

Analyte	Author	Reference
α_1-Antitrypsin	A. A. Dietz *et al.*	1974, *20,* 396–399
Trypsin	J. A. Ambrose	1974, *20,* 505–510
Insulin	C. A. Velasco *et al.*	1974, *20,* 700–702
Lecithin: Sphingomyelin	E. H. Coch *et al.*	1974, *20,* 1369–1375
Cortisol (plasma)	A. de la Pean *et al.*	1974, *20,* 1376–1378
Cortisol (urine)	R. E. Juselius *et al.*	1974, *20,* 1470–1476
Prostaglandins, E, F and A	A. F. J. Avletta *et al.*	1974, *20,* 1580–1587
Transketolase	L. G. Warnock	1975, *21,* 432–436
Triglycerides	H. G. Biggs *et al.*	1975, *21,* 437–441

Summary and Conclusions

This paper has set out to pose the kinds of question which usually arise in debates on methodology; indeed, the devil's advocate might say that the paper should have been entitled 'Unacceptability of Definitive, Reference and Routine Methods'.

To stimulate discussion, attention might be focussed initially on just a few questions:

1. Should definitive and reference methods be tested in the context of pathological, or potentially interfering, matrices, as well as normal ones?
2. Should emphasis be placed on preparing and distributing matrix reference materials, rather than on disseminating reference methods?
3. Is it possible to define criteria for the acceptability of routine methods, so as to encourage standardization?

Acceptability of Simplified Methods

D. Kutter, Luxembourg

Key words: Maximal sensitivity
Practical sensitivity
Simplified methods
Specificity
Test strips
Test tablets

Simplified methods (test strips, test tablets) are very widely used, which makes it necessary to establish criteria for their acceptability.

Most of the tests are designed for urine analyses giving qualitative or roughly semiquantitative results. This means that the problem of these tests is not precision, but sensitivity, and – owing to the very variable chemical composition of urine – specificity. These two dimensions determine whether a test gives acceptable results or not.

As all the interesting metabolites are present in very low concentrations even in normal urines, optimal sensitivity is not necessarily the best solution. Values within the normal range should not react! It is impossible to indicate for one reagent a precise value of sensitivity applicable to all urines. This is caused by the variable chemical composition of urine (pH, rH, osmolarity, drug metabolites etc). We, therefore, consider *practical sensitivity,* meaning the lowest metabolite concentration detected by the reagent in 90% of a large number of random specimens. It is determined by testing a large number of urines with a quantitative reference method and by the test strip. Higher concentrations may be adjusted by addition of known quantities of the metabolite. *Maximal sensitivity* is the lowest metabolite concentration reacting positively in 10% of the specimens. Practical sensitivity should be as close as possible to the upper normal limit, without maximum sensitivity falling within the normal range. In that case every positive reaction has pathological significance.

Specificity is a difficult problem in urine analysis. No test may claim to be absolutely specific. False positive reactions may be caused by similar metabolites (urinary mucoproteins reacting as albumin), drug metabolites (sulfa drugs causing false positives with urobilinogen tests based upon Ehrlich reaction) or secondary impurities (oxidising disinfectants simulating glucose). Inhibitors causing false negatives may not be ruled out completely (ascorbic acid inhibiting enzymatic glucose test). I propose to consider as completely unacceptable any reagent yielding more than *10% of unspecific results* in a large series of unselected specimens. A higher proportion of false positives might be tolerated, provided this fact is known and every positive is checked by a more specific method.

I suggest for discussion the folowing criteria for practical sensitivity:

Glucose (enzym.)	50 mg/dl
Protein	20 mg/dl
Ketone bodies	10 mg/dl diacetic acid
Urobilinogen	1 mg/dl
Bilirubin	0.5 mg/dl
Blood	10,000 erythrocytes/ml
Nitrite	0.1 mg/dl
Phenylpyruvic acid	10 mg/dl

Multiple tests strips are considered acceptable only if all the test areas satisfy these criteria.

These criteria should be borne in mind by the producers of quality control urines. Testing strips with such urines gives no guarantee of their practical sensitivity, as the result is obtained only on one specimen. Quality control shows, however, that the test strip is effective and that it is used correctly.

No reagent is indefinitely stable, even in an unopened package. *Reagents which do not bear an expiration date are unacceptable.*

The problem of precision appears for test-strips designed for estimation of blood glucose or blood urea. The more constant composition of blood makes specificity a secondary problem. I propose to consider acceptable such tests which cover the 90% of results within *±30%* of the results obtained by a good reference method. It is preferable that such a tests covers the whole normal and pathological range.

It is now possible to read blood glucose strips in specially designed reflectance meters. As these instruments are rather costly, they should provide definite improvement over the simple visual method. I propose a maximum deviation of *±20%* of the reference method.

Reflectance meters designed for analysis of whole blood can only be checked with whole blood and not with standard plasma. Standard plasma can be used with strips designed for analysis of both whole blood and serum or plasma.

The Development of Simplified Tests

H. Wishinsky, Elkhart, Ind., USA

Key words: Interferences
Simplified methods
Test strips

The early developers of spot tests were quite remarkable in their ability to blend a combination of art and science and achieve consistent results. Much the same can be said of the development of 'Simplified Tests'. Among the creators of art, there is a diversity of technique; among the viewers of art, there is even greater variability of interpretation. In science, one naturally strives to eliminate the problem of variability in technique which, of course, can lead to different results. To achieve similar results means the control of the variabilities of man. The basic concept behind diagnostic kits is to eliminate as many variables as possible and to develop systems that consistently yield the same or similar results. The simplest form of kit is the reagent-impregnated paper; the reagent area of a dip-and-read strip. Because of their format strip tests appear 'simple'. They are, however, far more complex than the usual liquid reagent test systems used in the laboratory. Perhaps one reason for their being referred to as 'simple' is that they are generally handled under less carefully controlled conditions in the laboratory than the more sophisticated procedures normally performed.

Who makes use of the strip tests?

1. The physician in his office, his nurse, or a technician.
2. In the hospital, the tests are performed occasionally by a trained laboratory technologist,but,perhaps,more often by the newest trainee in the department.

Urine strip tests are usually performed on random specimens. Therefore, quantitation such as that obtained on serum specimens is not usually required. Results are usually expressed in either qualitative or semiquantitative units.

Why perform qualitative or semiquantitative tests on random urine specimens? Primarily, because they serve a much needed purpose. A properly performed test results is a measurement that yields information to the physician. He may use the result to screen for some pathological problem, to guide him in therapy or to rule out an unknown factor. In other words, urine testing is another tool in the physician's armamentarium.

Urine strip systems presently marketed are designed to yield reliable results in uncontrolled and diverse environments. The uncontrolled variables include laboratory lighting, temperature and humidity, specimen variation, dietary variation, technician variability, as well as others. A scientist, in the laboratory, developing a urine strip test only for use in the laboratory has far fewer development problems than the manufacturer attempting to provide the same test to a broad spectrum of clinical-diagnostic test users. The laboratory scientist can adjust his test conditions for the pecularities of his environment, or his specimen. The manufacturer must adapt his test to a broader spectrum of variables over which he has little or no control. In order to illustrate the thinking and process that enters into the development, manufacture and marketing of a general use diagnostic test, I will take you step-by-step through the developmental highlights of one of our urine glucose tests – namely, *Diastix*®[1].

First, how does an industrial organization determine that it wants to market a new diagnostic test. The initial impetus derives from the recognition of the limitations of an existing test and the need for an improved one. The recognition of such a need is often expressed to the manufacturer by the user. Until recently, Ames Company marketed only two urine test systems for glucose, *Clinitest*® and *Clinistix*®. Clinitest requires a certain amount of user manipulation; e.g. sample dilution, to yield a semiquantitative reading. Furthermore, the test is based on a copper-salt reduction (non-specific) and is, therefore, subject to reaction in the presence of reducing sugars other than glucose. Clinistix, on the other hand, is an enzymatic analysis which, although more convenient to use and highly specific, yields only qualitative results. Thus, there was need for an improved system; i.e., a test that has the convenience and specificity of Clinistix, as well as the ability to yield the semiquantitative results of Clinitest.

At its inception, an industrial development project is no different from an analytical methods development project in a laboratory. After establishing need for a new procedure, one attempts to satisfy the need by bringing to bear background knowledge. In the case of glucose testing, Ames has developed knowledgeability about enzymatic methods through its Clinistix development and, in addition, determined that semiquantitation of test strips was possible through its development of *Dextrostix*® for the measurement of blood glucose. A project, therefore, was initiated which was based upon the use of the glucose oxidase-peroxidase redox indicator system for the semiquantitative measurement of glucose in urine.

The reactions involved in the enzymatic system are shown in fig. 1. Glucose oxidase is used to catalyze the oxidation of glucose in the urine to δ-gluconolactone and peroxide, the latter of which reacts with the indicator in the presence of peroxidase. Indicators traditionally used in this system have been either o-dianisidine or o-tolidine. It has recently become evident, for a number of reasons which need not be highlighted here, that better indicators would be desirable. As you can see from fig. 1, a potassium iodide-iodine indicator was finally developed and incorporated into a new urine glucose assay strip, Diastix.

[1] Covered by U.S. patent numbers 2, 981, 606, 3, 164, 534 and 3, 814, 668 and corresponding foreign patents and applications.

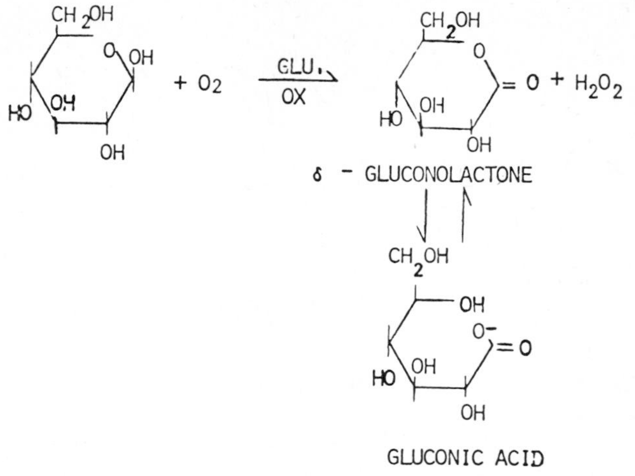

$$H_2O_2 + 2I^- + 2H^+ \xrightarrow{PEROX} I_2 + 2H_2O$$

$$I_2 + PVP \longrightarrow I_2 \cdot PVP \text{ (COLORED COMPLEX)}$$

Fig. 1.

Table 1 is a list of components used in the Diastix system. Incorporated into the formulation is a dye, Brilliant Blue FCF, which in conjunction with the color formation of the potassium iodide-iodine indicator yields better visualization of the various levels of glucose. Citric acid and sodium citrate serve as the system's buffer. The *Gantrez* and polyvinylpyrrolidone are incorporated as thickening agents; they serve to stabilize the two enzymes. However, the polyvinylpyrrolidone serves still another purpose. You will note, there is no starch in the system to form the intensely colored starch-iodine complex. We found that the iodine-polyvinylpyrrolidone complex is a good color-former for this test. It should be emphasized that this formulation did not, by itself, yield the semiquantitative characteristics required. In order to achieve a semiquantitative test system, it was necessary to overlay, on top of the previously impregnated paper, a hydrophobic film made from either ethyl cellulose or related hydrophobic film formers. The function of the film is still not fully understood. It may serve to limit the thickness of the sample film on the strip more so than the normally hydrophilic paper surface and, thus, allow for free oxygen permeation to the glucose oxidase, or it may, also, serve to diffusion limit glucose penetration into the strip. Diffusion control would yield a system in which color formation would depend directly upon the glucose concentration external to the film. Whatever the function of the film, it served to yield a semiquantitative system when used in conjunction with the formulation shown in table 1.

Table 1. Diastix® Formulation

Potassium iodide
Brilliant blue FCF
H_2O
Citric acid – citrate buffer
Gantrez AN-139
Polyvinylpyrrolidone
Peroxidase
Glucose oxidase
Impregnated paper overlayed with an ethyl cellulose film

At this point in a methods development project, an independent investigator would be nearly finished, needing only to identify the occasional aberrant sample and adjust it to fit this method. He has the ability to control most of the factors that may enter into the use of his formulation in his laboratory. The manufacturer, on the other hand, must develop the formulation further, to make it useful in all parts of the world under vastly different temperature and humidity conditions and under variable conditions of technological capabilities.

The industrial research and development laboratory, prior to release of a laboratory procedure to manufacturing, must take into consideration the following:

Interfering substances
Handling conditions
Manufacturing
Quality control
Storageability
Clinical efficacy

The first two will be covered in some detail later in this presentation, the next three are *must* aspects for any ethical manufacturer, since the product must meet a specific set of criteria in order to serve its intended purpose and obviously must have sufficient stability to meet rather diverse shipping and storage requirements. The last item, clinical efficacy, is the final consideration for any diagnostic test, whether qualitative, semiquantitative or quantitative. This, too, will be covered later in this presentation.

Table 2 is a list of items that might be expected to interfere with the enzymatic glucose test. The first five listed are metabolic factors that are more or less universally variable. Ascorbic acid might be expected to vary due to diet or fad.

Preservatives for urine specimens must be evaluated as to their possible interference in the Diastix reaction.

Since enzyme activities are pH dependent, one must be concerned with the pH ranges of urine specimens and the extent to which this range may influence the response of the

Table 2.

pH
Specific gravity
Protein
Uric acid
Acetone, acetoacetic acid, β-OH butyric acid
Ascorbic acid
Urine preservatives

system. Users of our test systems are not expected to adjust the specimen pH to satisfy the test. Therefore, the Diastix formulation is buffered to yield no significant variation in response over a urine pH range of 3 to 9. Figure 2 shows the effect of pH on glucose results.

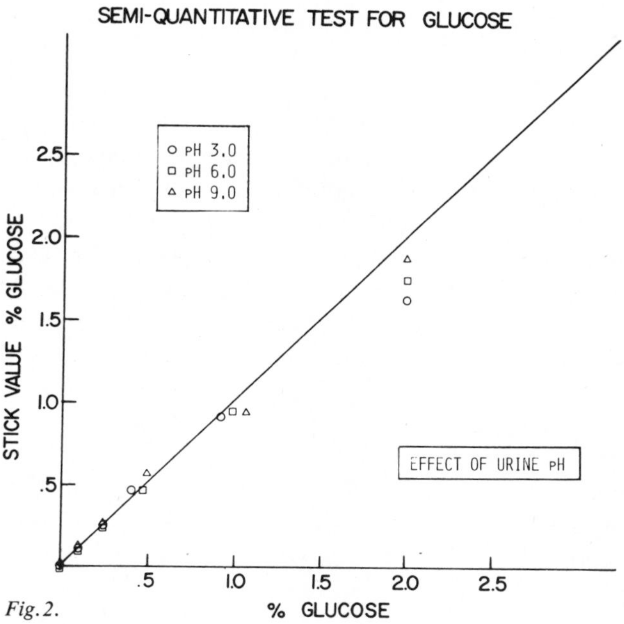

Fig. 2.

Urinary protein levels up to 1000 mg/dl have no significant effect upon the Diastix test system. Uric acid levels up to 1 gram per liter of urine had, essentially, no inhibitor effect. However, on high purine diets there is some inhibition at higher levels of glucose, fig. 3.

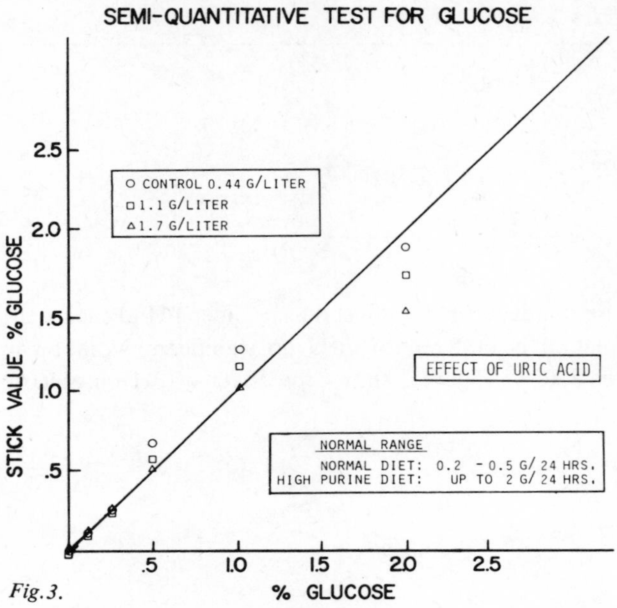

Fig. 3.

Acetone and β-hydroxybutyric acid at artificially high levels showed, essentially, no inhibition of the Diastix reaction. However, acetoacetic acid does have an effect upon the reaction. Figure 4 shows the effect of varying levels of acetoacetic acid and its inhibitory effect upon Diastix response. At what point does the inhibition create a possible problem. Our data indicate that at levels of 80–120 mg/dl acetoacetic acid in urine, results would drop one color block when read against the label color chart. Extensive research yielded no way in which the test could be reformulated to eliminate vulnerability to high levels of acetoacetic acid. Thus, the Diastix package insert cautions the user about the potential inhibitory effect of acetoacetic acid. Since the value of determining acetoacetic acid in diabetics with elevated glucose levels in both blood and urine is well recognized, a *Keto-Diastix®* test system was developed. The user of Keto-Diastix, therefore, has a method which can signal the validity of his glucose reading, by providing him with a measure of acetoacetic acid in the same sample.

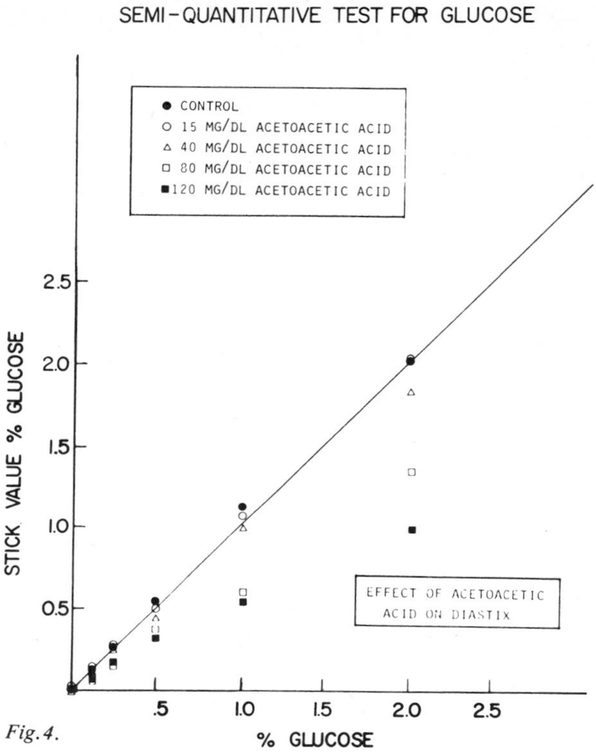

Fig. 4.

The increased use of ascorbic acid in foods, pills, etc. within the past few years has created problems in the analysis of a number of constituents in urine and has required readjustment of some established procedures. Ascorbic acid is a good reducing agent; as such it interferes with most redox indicators including the peroxide-peroxidase, potassium iodide reaction used in Diastix. The extent to which it interferes is illustrated in fig. 5. The ascorbic acid interference at the 30 mg/dl level is obviously minimal for a test of this type. Levels of 90 mg/dl ascorbic acid in urine would, at most, show a one color block shift downward. This level of ascorbic acid in urine is rarely found.

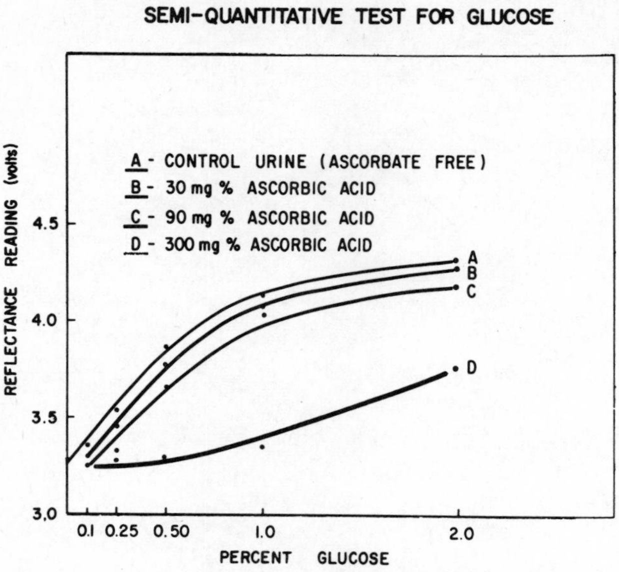

THE EFFECT OF ASCORBIC ACID INHIBITION
ON SEMI-QUANTATIVE GLUCOSE STRIPS

INHIBITION AS READ FROM ABOVE GRAPH

GLUCOSE	ASCORBIC ACID CONCENTRATION		
	30 MG/DL	90 MG/DL	300 MG/DL
NEGATIVE	-	-	-
0.1	0.07	0	0
0.25	0.2	0.1	0
0.50	0.4	0.3	0
1.0	0.8	0.7	0.1
2.0	1.7	1.0	0.4

Fig. 5.

Independent studies untertaken by the Ames Medical Department and Research and Development to determine ascorbic acid levels in several types of population groups, yielded the data shown in table 3. Of the total number of individuals (A, B and C) studied, 5.5% had ascorbic acid levels over 15 mg/dl; less than 2% had levels 40 mg/dl or over.

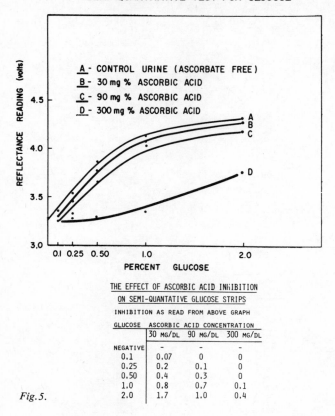

Table 3. Ascorbic Acid Levels in Random Urine Samples

AA mg/dl	A No. Tests	A %	B No. Tests	B %
0	822	49.5	346	73.8
1–5	516	31.1	68	14.5
10	212	12.8	17	3.6
10–15	18	1.1	14	3.0
20	52	3.1	8	1.7
20–40	10	.6	4	0.9
40	29	1.8	12	2.5
Total Tests	1659		469	

AA mg/dl	C No. Tests	C %
0	118	24.3
1–5	225	46.3
10	95	19.5
10–15	18	3.7
15 +	30	6.2
Total Tests	486	

It may be of interest to describe a specific approach that may be taken by a manufacturer when dealing with an interfering substance as contrasted to the method by which an individual laboratory investigator might approach the same problem. As a last resort, the manufacturer will insert a precautionary note. However, he will first attempt to formulate around the interfering substance. A good example is the effect of specific gravity on Diastix. Specific gravity is a measure of the concentration of dissolved components. It is related to ionic strength and, as is well known, the activity of an enzyme is dependent upon ionic strength. In urine, one would expect specific gravity to definitely affect the response of the enzyme system to the glucose determination. This problem does occur. During our early formulation studies, specific gravity effects were substantial. We obtained low color response at high glucose levels with increased specific gravity. At low glucose levels there appeared to be less specific gravity dependence. Extensive investigations were undertaken, but no simple way to overcome this effect was found.

The individual laboratory investigator, in developing a test of this type for his own use, could simply dilute his urines to some constant specific gravity and adjust enzyme concentrations to account for the reduced concentration of glucose. However, the user, who wishes convenience and does not wish to go through a dilution step and subsequent calculations, creates within the manufacturer's research and development group the proper stress that helps answer a problem. The approach we took was as follows.

A clinical study was undertaken to determine specific gravity and glucose levels in the urine of diabetics, the group this product was, primarily, designed to serve. Figure 6 shows the distribution. Urines containing higher glucose levels are more likely to have specific gravities in the range of 1.021–1.030 as represented by curves E, D, and F. Urines containing lower glucose levels are more likely to be in the range of 1.011–1.020 as represented by curves A, B, and C. In our experience, specific gravity effects at low glucose levels appear to be minimal. Based on such data, one can adjust formulations and optimize the test to yield maximum resolution within the specific gravity ranges most frequently encountered in diabetic urines. In addition, the color comparison chart provided with the test is calibrated so that combined high glucose, high specific gravity specimens which tend to inhibit color development may be properly interpreted. The combined optimized formulation and calibrated color chart then underwent extensive clinical studies and were varied, if necessary, to achieve a confidence level of approximately 95% for any measured value of glucose.

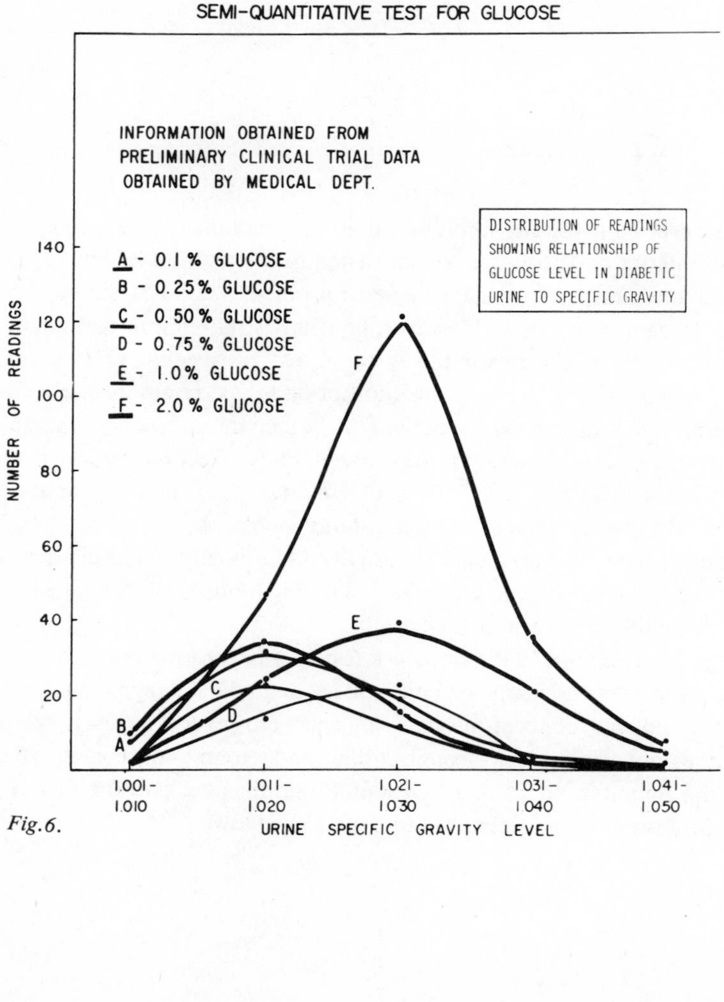

Fig.6.

The results of the revised formulation and color charts are seen in fig. 7. Specific gravities of 1.020 and 1.030 yield results within the desired experimental range. A urine specific gravity of 1.040 will lower the reading approximately one-half a color block. In addition, a precautionary note is included in the package insert stating that reactivity may be influenced by specific gravity.

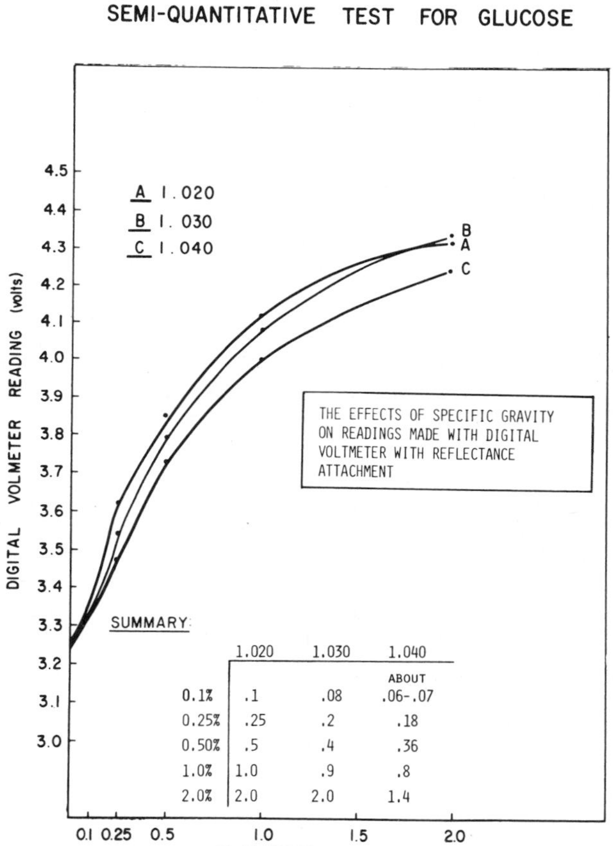

Fig. 7.

Since Diastix is dipped into a specimen, it is important to know the effect of immersion time on the result. Figure 8 shows that the formulation can be in contact with the specimen up to three seconds without significant change in response; all readings were performed at 30 seconds.

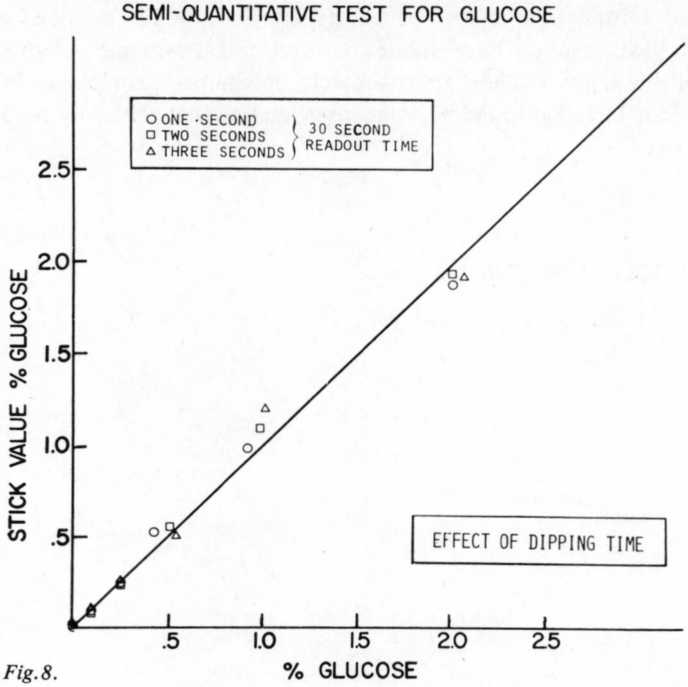

Fig. 8.

Readout time for Diastix is critical. This was verified by both our own studies and clinical studies performed in qualified laboratories. No way was found to allow for varying reading times. Readings made at 20 seconds were generally low (fig. 9). It appears that 30 and 40 seconds are, essentially, the same. However, urines of low specific gravity at the 0.5% and 1.0% glucose level, tend to read high at 40 seconds. Therefore, the recommended reading time of 30 seconds may not be significantly changed.

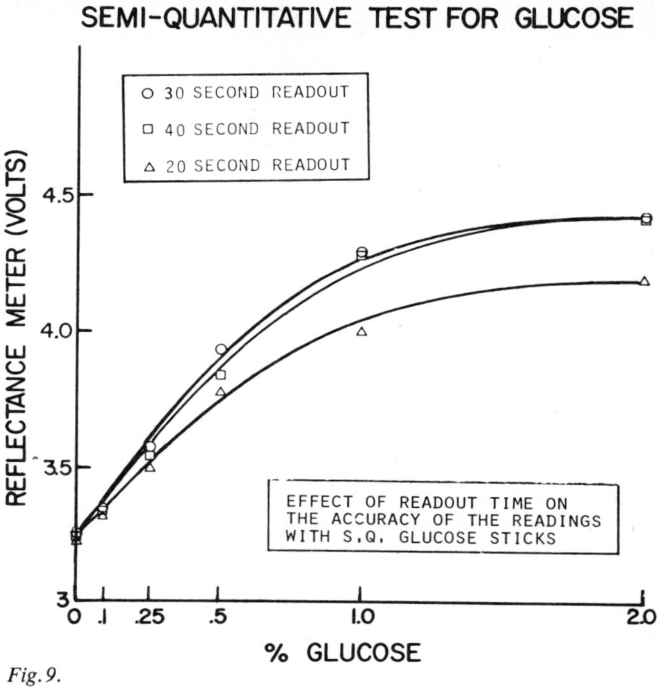

Fig. 9.

The influence of specimen temperature is illustrated in fig. 10. Between room temperature and 37 °C there is no effect upon Diastix. However, a refrigerated urine specimen tested with Diastix would, as expected, exhibit a low value.

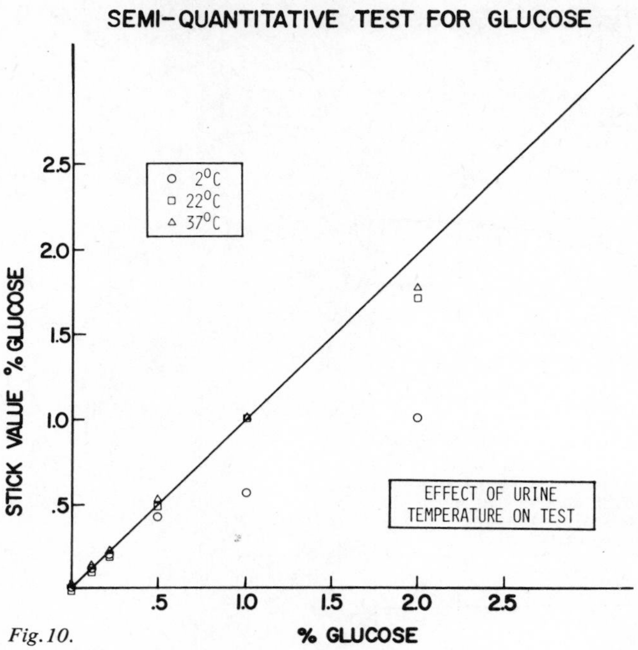

Fig. 10.

The development of color charts is a tedious, time-consuming problem. The colors on the chart make use of dyes different from those used in the reagent strip. The final color chart must be evaluated by taking into consideration the various light sources and intensities that are used in different laboratories. The problem of metamerism must be evaluated and eliminated, otherwise bizarre results may be obtained. The printing of such charts is a separate art and science unto itself.

Scaling up a bench process to production usually results in changes to the bench process which must be reevaluated as to their effect on the end result. An enzyme dried on a piece of paper will retain its activity for a considerable period of time. The same enzyme in an aqueous buffered solution often degenerates in a few hours. An enzyme solution used immediately after preparation may have a different activity to one used over a matter of hours. Therefore, a firm knowledge of the stability of raw materials, materials in process, etc. must be established. Methods must be developed and standards specified, in order to quality control not only the raw materials, but the working formula. In addition, the stability of the individual components in the finished strip must be determined along with the stability of the final product. Therefore, statistically valid stress tests must be designed. When a manufacturer labels his product stable for one year, he should have the stability data available.

Figure 11 is an example of the time degradation of peroxidase activity in Diastix stressed at varying temperatures. As might be expected, the higher the temperature the shorter the shelf life of the enzyme. Such data can be used to predict the room temperature life time of the final product. Peroxidase is the most unstable compound in our reaction mix. This type of data is available for each of the active ingredients in the test strip.

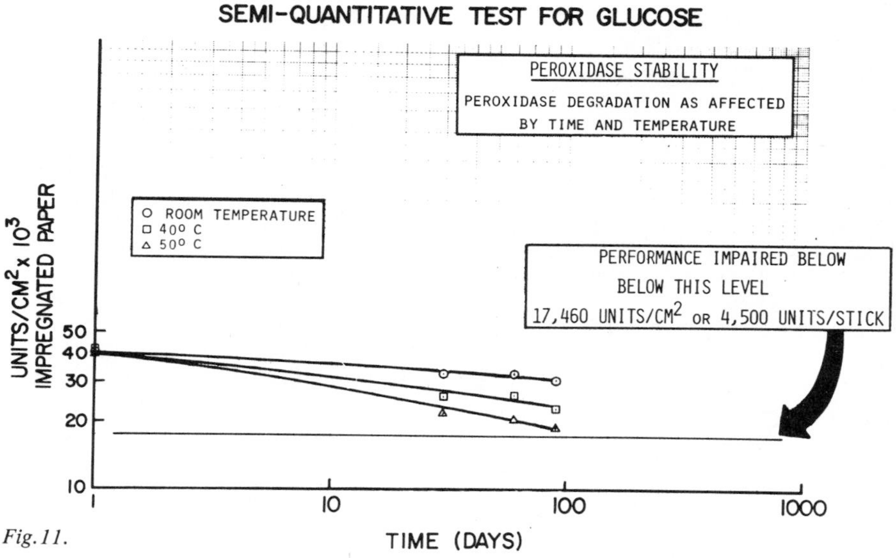

Fig. 11.

Perhaps the most critical test that the product must meet is clinical efficacy. Built into this requirement must be all of the factors previously mentioned, plus many more too numerous to discuss.

Table 4 gives some idea of the extensiveness of these trials to which these test strips are subjected. If the product does not meet the requirements of our Medical Department and of the clinical investigators, the entire experimental process just presented starts over again.

Table 4. Premarketing Clinical Study[1]-Diastix®

Purpose: To establish in a diabetic population[2] the effect of specific gravity, albumin, acetoacetic acid, pH and medications in urine specimens upon the determination of glucose using Diastix.
To compare Diastix against competitive urine glucose tests and determine area and investigator differences.

Number of investigators: 15

Countries involved in this study[3]

Australia	France
Columbia	Japan
England	United States

Number of specimens tested (only diabetics):

Negatives	788
Positives	1688
Total	2476

[1] Utility studies continued after marketing.
[2] Random population studies were performed separately.
[3] Countries selected where there were Ames Medical Directors. (After initial marketing and with the addition of new Area Medical Directors, the above studies were expanded to include Germany, Scandinavia, Italy, Canada, Mexico and Africa.)

In conclusion, I would like to reiterate this paper's original intent, to describe in some small way the real complexity of what often appears to the user to be a 'simple' test. Although they are simple to use, they are by no means simple to design or simple to make.

The Acceptability of Enzyme Methods

G. N. Bowers, Jr.[1], Hartford, Connecticut (USA)

Key words: Enzyme methods
Reagent materials
Reference materials
Reference methods

I. Introduction

The criteria for acceptability of an enzyme method for use in any one laboratory can be summarized as follows:

1. *applicability* to the clinical needs, and
2. *reliability* of the analytical performance.

However, the criteria for acceptability of an enzyme method for use by more than one laboratory calls into play yet another requirement –

3. *compatibility* of the results.

Compatibility between laboratories in the area of clinical enzymology means that each laboratory measuring the same enzyme containing material, be it a patient specimen, control material or reference enzyme material, reports the same numerical result, subject only to the limitation imposed by random error. Measurement compatibility cannot be expected when each person in charge of a laboratory chooses to go his own independent way. Achieving compatibility requires a serious commitment to establishing sound agreements on methods and materials and to seeing that these agreements are embodied in practice. Thus, when one attempts to discuss the criteria for the acceptability of enzyme methods for use in a large number of laboratories and in particular an international network of laboratories, this third criteria of compatibility becomes the overriding concern. It brings into clear perspective the essential reason why we must reach agreements through cooperative efforts within the international community.

This paper will review the efforts of various individuals and groups within several nations and at the international level to establish systems of more meaningful

[1] Dr. *Bowers* is now member and was formerly the chairman of the Expert Panel on Enzymes of the Committee on Standards, IFCC. Dr. D. Moss (London) is currently the EPE chairman and Drs. H. Bergmeyer (Tutzing) and M. Hørder (Arhus) are the other EPE members.

measurements in clinical enzymology. *Paul Cali* [1] of NBS has already discussed the critical role that reference *materials,* founded on accurate measurement, can play in achieving compatibility. In a subsequent presentation, Dr. *S. Brown* [2] of CRC has shown how the accuracy of routine and reference *methods* can be evaluated with the help of matrixed reference materials, when their value has been determined by a highly accurate definitive method and a certified reference material. My presentation will attempt to illustrate how knowledge of the interactions between the newer reference type enzyme methods, instruments meeting rigid specifications, and well characterized materials, can provide the objective information by which to reach sound agreements in enzymology. It will be suggested (similar to the experience with calcium and glucose), that a hierarchy of internationally accepted enzyme methods, devices and reference enzyme materials will be required to reach and maintain compatibility within any international network of clinical laboratories.

II. The problem – confusion

Figure 1 illustrates the rise in the physician-generated demand for enzyme measurements at Hartford Hospital, a 900-bed community hospital. A similar rise in demand for alkaline phosphatase determinations at Sydney Hospital in Australia suggests that the Hartford data may also be typical of the experience in many countries. We need not belabor the point that the measurement of an enzyme's activity in serum has become an accepted part of the modern practice of medicine to aid in the differential diagnosis

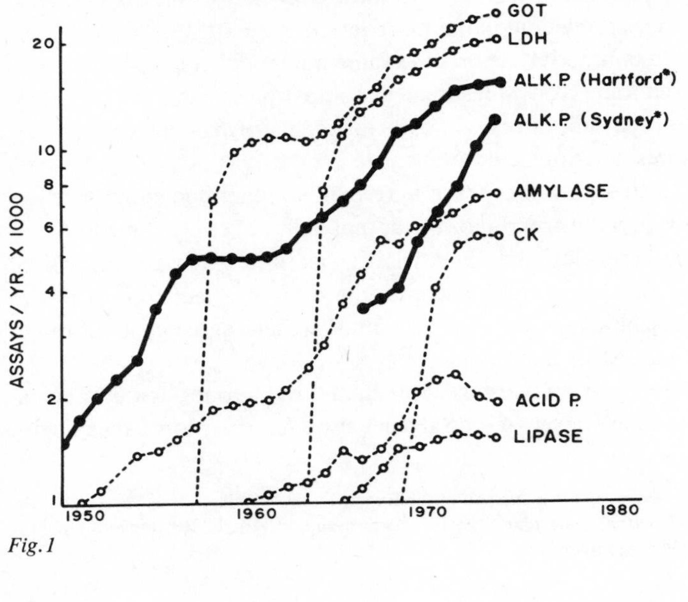

Fig. 1

and/or treatment of human diseases. There is no doubt that the pattern of enzyme changes with time provides much relevant information about disease processes to a physician, even though the underlying patho-physiologic mechanisms causing these changes are not always known.

Unfortunately, the lack of agreement on a uniform way of measuring and reporting the results of an enzyme activity measurement creates the potential for serious confusion in the physician's evaluation of this information and may actually do so far more often than we care to admit. Despite my special interest in clinical enzymology, I am sometimes confused by the numerical values given in case reports in the medical literature, especially when the reference intervals (normal limits) for the method employed are not given. Likewise, on numerous occasions, I have experienced first-hand the confusion created when a visiting medical professor or a new intern or resident house officer gives either too little or too much weight to an enzyme activity measurement made in our laboratory. Usually the problem can be traced to the fact that the physician was interpreting the result against another laboratory's reference intervals, not ours. As so often happens, this becomes just another 'Laboratory Error' to many clinicians. Yet from the standpoint of all concerned, be he patient, physician, laboratory scientist, government health official, or the manufacturer of enzyme reagents, controls, kits, or instruments, this situation can only be called 'chaotic' and must be rectified as soon as possible for the good of all.

If one turns to the literature for factual data from proficiency surveys and other studies which have objectively tested interlaboratory variability, one finds ample evidence that there is indeed confusion. For example, in a paper by Fasce, et al. [3], it was reported (see table 1) that in 336 laboratories taking part in a 1972 New York State testing program, a

Table 1. Enzyme Methods and Standardizations Used in Clinical Laboratories in New York State as of January 1972 [1]

Aspartate aminotransferase			Lactate dehydrogenase		
Method	No. laboratories	%	Method	No. laboratories	%
AutoAnalyzer colorimetric	51	14.9	AutoAnalyzer colorimetric	41	13.5
AutoAnalyzer '340 nm'	37	10.8	AutoAnalyzer '340 nm'	40	13.2
Reitman-Frankel	169	49.4	Cabaud-Wroblewski	121	39.9
Babson	28	8.2	Babson-Phillips	36	11.9
Kinetic	51	14.9	Kinetic	60	19.8
Standardization			Standardization		
Pyruvate	136	39.8	Pyruvate	99	32.7
Serum	153	44.7	Serum	141	46.5
Absorbance change (340 nm)	42	12.3	Absorbance change (340 nm)	49	16.2
Absorbance change (366 nm)	6	1.8	Absorbance change (360 nm)	8	2.6

[1] Methods and types of standardization used by fewer than 1.5% of the laboratories are not listed. (New York City not included.)

number of enzyme methods and standardization techniques were used for lactate dehydrogenase (LDH) and aspartate aminotransferase (ASAT) measurements. However, the startling fact to me was that 47 different units, methods and temperature combinations were used for LDH and 48 combinations were used for ASAT! There is ample evidence to support the view that a parallel situation exists in many other states and countries. In fact, there is no logical reason to expect uniformity in such a complex field as clinical enzymology, where independent decisions about the acceptability of an enzyme method have been the rule.

The manufacturers of enzyme-containing materials for calibration and/or control uses have long been familiar with this dilemma in clinical enzymology and have had to cope with many problems because of it. Their solution, due to the lack of a clear consensus amongst the clinical laboratory users of their products, has been pragmatic. They give the measured assay value for each of several methods in common use. Therefore, on the package insert which accompanies each new lot of assayed calibration and control materials, the assay value is given together with other information about each method, such as the appropriate reference interval and the manufacturer's suggested 'within control' limits. However, as I have attempted to show in the second column of table 2 for lactate dehydrogenase (LDH) and of table 3 for aspartate aminotransferase (ASAT), even the most carefully-determined assay values can also lead to confusion if the numerical result is separated from its appropriate reference interval. For example, for the 13 methods for LDH listed in table 2, the 'LDH units' (not further defined in the package insert and thus requiring additional special knowledge of the method for proper interpretation) range from 70 to 416, while the 13 methods for ASAT in table 3 range from 39 to 189 'ASAT units'. As one of my fellow AACC colleagues has recently written in respect to this number of assay values

> 'Granted, the units and methods differ, but this point may not always get through to the physician who visits different hospitals or who receives data from several laboratories.' [4]

Table 2. LDH Assay Values for A Control Material (Package insert information[1])

Method[2]	Assay[1] Value	Reference[1] Interval	Calculated Ratio Assay/upper limit
I. 340 nm ultraviolet			
A. Continuous, 30 °C, L to P	268	45–175	1.53
E. Continuous, 30 °C, L to P	135	30–110	1.22
M. Continuous, 30 °C, L to P	145	29– 92	1.57
B. Continuous, 25 °C, P to L	315	0–195	1.62
D. Continuous, 30 °C, P to L	416	125–270	1.54
K. End point, 37 °C, P to L	283	90–200	1.42
L. End point, 37 °C, P to L	301	90–200	1.51
II. Colorimetric			
H. Manual, end point, 37 °C	116	24– 78	1.49
I. Automated, end point, 37 °C	286	90–200	1.43
J. Automated, end point, 37 °C	282	90–200	1.41
III. Unknown by me			
C. (? colorimetric – 37 °C)	70	0– 48	1.46
F. ? UV, ? end point, 37 °C	220	20–186	1.18
G. Automated, ? colorimetric, 37 °C	140	46–124	1.13
Total range	70 to 416	–	1.1 to 1.6

[1] These values were taken exactly as given, with no corrections for different units; Lot # 0487052 Validate-A®, abnormal human serum content, general diagnostics, N.J. 07950.

[2] Re-arranged to group by chemical or technologic principle. A = Amador-Wacker 30 °C; B = BMC (Cat. # 15977) 25 °C; C = BMC (Cat. # 16119); D = Calbiochem-P, Stat-Pack 30 °C; E = Calbio-L, Stat-Pack 30 °C; F = Eskalab (Cat. # 82133) 37 °C; G = Hycel Mark X, H = LacDehystrate 37 °C; I = SMA 12/60 (Cal. Std.) Colorimetric 37 °C; J = SMA 12/60 (Tech. Std.) Colorimetric 37 °C; K = SMA 12/60 (Cal. Std.) 340 nm; L = SMA 12/60 (Tech. Std.) 340 nm; M = Worthington UV, Statzyme 30 °C.

Table 3. ASAT Assay Values for A Control Material (Package insert information[1]).

Method[2]	Assay[1] Value	Reference[1] Interval	Calculated Ratio Assay/upper limit
I. 340 nm ultraviolet			
B. Continuous, 25 °C	39	0–12	3.25
C. Continuous, 30 °C	48	5–20	2.40
G. Continuous, 30 °C	113	12–40	2.83
E. End point, manual, 37 °C	91	10–26	3.50
J. End point, automated, 37 °C	121	10–40	3.03
K. End point, automated, 37 °C	136	10–40	3.40
II. Colorimetric			
D. Manual, 37 °C	114	10–40	2.85
L. Manual, 37 °C	126	9–36	3.50
A. Automated, 37 °C	72	10–40	1.80
F. Automated, 37 °C	157	25–75	2.10
H. Automated, 37 °C	141	10–50	2.82
I. Automated, 37 °C	189	10–50	3.78
Total range	39 to 189		1.8 to 3.8

[1] These values were taken exactly as given, with no corrections for different units; Lot # 0487052 Validate-A®, abnormal human serum content, general diagnostics, N.J. 07950.

[2] Re-arranged to group by chemical or technologic principle. A = AutoAnalyzer; N-25b; B = BMC (Cat. # 15788) 25 °C; C = Calbiochem, Stal-Pack 30 °C, D = DADE (Reitman-Frankel) 37 °C; E = Eskalab (Cat. # 82043) 37 °C; F = Hycel Mark X; G = Karmen (Henry Modif) 30 °C; H = SMA 12/60 (Cal. Std.) Colorimetric 37 °C; I = SMA 12/60 (Tech. Std.) Colorimetric 37 °C; J = SMA 12/60 (Cal. Std.) 340 nm, 37 °C; K = SMA 12/60 (Tech. Std.) 340 nm; L = TransAc 37 °C; M = Worthington Statzyme 30 °C.

Unfortunately, the relatively simple manner of calculating the ratios between the assay value and the upper limit of the reference interval (column 4 of table 2 and 3) while reducing somewhat the spread of the data, still does very little to rectify the confusion. This is not particularly surprising when there are so many variables in both the method and the enzyme material which are still so poorly understood. I have the intuitive feeling that a full and open discussion between manufacturers and users on the problem of assigning an enzyme assay value to a calibration material for use with special types of automated instruments, such as the SMA 12/60, would provide yet another example of the deep confusion which exists, and could only give further support to the idea that there is an urgent need for agreements.

III. Efforts to establish compatibility

In response to the need to improve the reliability and interlaboratory compatibility of enzyme measurements used for patient care, several national organizations for clinical chemistry and the IFCC have commissioned groups of their members with expertise in enzymology to study the analytical aspects of the problem. As shown in table 4, several of these groups have already made recommendations which have appeared in published form [5–10]. Special enzyme committees have been, or are, at work in Australia, Canada, France, Italy, Japan and the United States; but to my knowledge, written recommen-

Table 4. Method Recommendations by Expert Groups.

Organization and Committee	Publication	Methods for:
German Society for Clinical Chemistry – Enzyme Commission (5)	Standardization Methods (1972)	1. Aspartate aminotransferase 2. Alanine aminotransferase 3. Creatine kinase 4. Glutamate dehydrogenase 5. Lactate dehydrogenase 6. Hydroxybutyrate dehydrogenase 7. Alkaline phosphatase
British Association of Clinical Biochemists – Working Party (6)	A Reference Method (1972)	1. Aspartate aminotransferase 2. Alanine aminotransferase 3. Alkaline phosphatase
Scandinavian Society for Clinical Chemistry and Clinical Physiology – Committee on Enzymes (7)	Recommended Methods (1972)	1. Aspartate aminotransferase 2. Alanine aminotransferase 3. Lactate dehydrogenase 4. Alkaline phosphatase
International Federation of Clinical Chemistry – Expert Panel on Enzymes, Committee on Standards (8, 9)	Draft Proposals for IFCC Methods to AM's, CS and EB (1972–1975)	1. General Considerations on Measurement (1974) (8) 2. Aspartate aminotransferase (1975) (9)
American Association of Clinical Chemists – Committee on Standard Methods (10)	Standard Methods of Clinical Chemistry, Academic Press 1953–1970	Volume I: Amylase, lipase, alk. & acid phos. Volume II: Lipase, alk & acid phosphatase Volume III: Aldolase, aspartate aminotransferase, cholinesterase, phosphohexase isomerase Volume IV: Cholinesterase, lactate dehydrogenase Volume V: Alkaline & acid phosphatase Volume VI: Transaminase (colorimetric)
Editorial Board of Selected Methods	Academic Press, N.Y. 1972	Volume VII: 5'-nucleotidase, lipase, CK

Table 5. Present Activities in the U.S.A. Related to Clinical Enzymology.

Organization and Committee	Activity	Goal
American Association of Clinical Chemists		
I. Editorial Board of Selected Methods	Publication of Volume VIII Selected Methods (probably 1976)	1. Alkaline phosphatase method 2. Aspartate aminotransferase method
II. Enzyme Subcommittee, Committee on Standards	Recommandations for reference type methods by AACC with substantial cooperative efforts with other professional and governmental organizations	1. Aspartate aminotransferase 2. Alkaline phosphatase 3. Lipase
National Committee for Clinical Laboratory Standards (NCCLS)		
I. Reference Enzyme Subcommittee of Area Committee on Clinical Chemistry	Reference enzyme materials	Create specifications for and testing of enzyme materials from all sources for their suitability as reference enzyme materials
II. Assay Conditions Subcommittee of Area Committee on Clinical Chemistry	Study assay conditions for enzyme methods, especially temperature	Recommendations on assay conditions for enzyme measurements
III. Subcommittee on Enzyme Kits Area Committee on Kits and Reagents	Reviewing kit methods and packaged reagents.	Specifications for kits and reagents
Pharmaceutical Manufacturers Association	Reaction temperature	Obtaining information, technical references, and monitoring the activities of other national and international bodies.
United States Department of Health, Education and Welfare		
Center for Disease Control	Interstate regulations – Clinical Laboratories Improvement Act of 1967 Laboratory standards, inspections and proficiency testing	Improvement of clinical laboratory performance in USA by scientific, educational, and legal means
	Development of scientific bases for FDA product class standards	Scientific technical support of FDA
Food and Drug Administration	Regulations – Product class standards in enzymology	Improvement in health laboratory services by use of its regulatory/legal authority
State Health Departments		
Usual functions	Accredit laboratories and administration of the Medicare Laws	Assuring that Federal and State standards are upheld

Table 5. (Continued). Present Activities in the U.S.A. Related to Clinical Enzymology.

Organization and Committee	Activity	Goal
Special functions – N.Y. State	Research into use of Reference enzyme materials for testing purpose	1. purified ASAT and LDH 2. matrixed ASAT 3. method evaluation

dations are not yet available. For example, in the United States several groups, as listed in table 5, are presently developing recommendations. I am sure there are similar efforts taking place in other countries, which will come to light during our discussion period.

Characteristically, the efforts of each country's group of experts started by reaching a consensus about the reaction temperature. The members then proceeded to select a well-accepted method or to develop one, in part from their prior experience and in part from new experimental observations. After extensive testing had proved the adequacy of the new method, the experts requested the parent organization to endorse its use by the laboratories of that country. Despite the arbitrary nature of many of the key decisions, there is now good evidence that compatibility can be improved within one nation and also between several countries when one of these newly recommended methods is used in the majority of service laboratories [11].

Table 6 gives a detailed listing of the parameters for each of the newly recommended ASAT methods versus the original *Karmen,* et al. [12] procedure, the earlier AACC Standard Method [10] and the modified *Karmen* method by *Henry,* et al. [13]. It becomes quite clear that each group of experts has been forced to make a number of subjective decisions which were 'trade-offs' between concepts of what would be ideal versus what is practical. Note that one group of experts favored 25 °C, while others picked 30 °C or 37 °C. Likewise, serum sample size varied from 0.15 to 0.50 ml, while the total volume ranged from 1.25 to 3.70 mls, giving ratios from 1 : 6 to 1 : 15.

Table 6. Recommendations for Aspartate Aminotransferase.

Parameter (Reference)	Karmen (12)	AACC (10)	Henry (13)	British (6)	German (5)	Scandin. (7)	IFCC (9)
Year Method introduced	1955	(1959, 1961)	1960	1972	1972	1974	1975
Reaction temperature (°C)	(23–28)	25	32	25	25	37	30
Sample volume, v (ml)	0.2	0.5	0.2	0.2	0.5	0.15–0.3	0.2
Total reaction volume, V (ml)	3.0	3.0	3.0	3.0	3.70	1.25–2.50	2.40
Ratio, v : V	1 : 15	1 : 6	1 : 15	1 : 15	1 : 7.4	1 : 8.3	1 : 12
Buffer type	phosphate	phosphate	phosphate	phosphate	phosphate	Tris/EDTA	Tris
Buffer concentration ($mmol \times l^{-1}$)	33	50	100	50	80	20	82
pH of final mixture	7.4	7.4	7.4	7.4	7.4 (25 °C)	7.7 (37 °C)	7.8 (30 °C)
L-aspartate ($mmol \times l^{-1}$)	33	33	125	125	200	200	200
2-oxoglutarate ($mmol \times l^{-1}$)	6.7	6.7	6.7	6.7	12	12	12
Reduced NAD ($mmol \times l^{-1}$)	0.16	0.16	0.18	0.24	0.18	0.15	0.20
[1]Pyridoxal phosphate ($mmol \times l^{-1}$)	–	–	–	–	–	(altern.)	0.10
Malate dehydrogenase ($mmol \times s^{-1} \times l^{-1}$)	1,000	1,000	5,000	2,800	10,000	10,000	10,000
[1]Lactate dehydrogenase ($nmol \times s^{-1} \times l^{-1}$)	–	–	–	–	20,000	3,000	15,000
[1]Preincubation (minutes)	5	–	10	10	10	5–15	6
[1]Reagent blank	–	–	–	?	?	?	required
Description of Method	Original	Standard	Mod. Karmen	Reference	Standard	Recommended	IFCC Method
Reporting units	ΔA/min	ΔA/min	ΔA/min	U/l	U/l	U/l	$mol \times s^{-1} \times l^{-1}$

[1] Arbitrary decisions or differences for which agreements must be found.

In fig. 2, I have tried, diagrammatically in the upper half, to show the spread of values obtained by each method in U/l under the stated conditions of temperature. How do we resolve these differences between 'the experts' by some sound means of reaching agreements that will in turn then be acceptable to the entire international community?

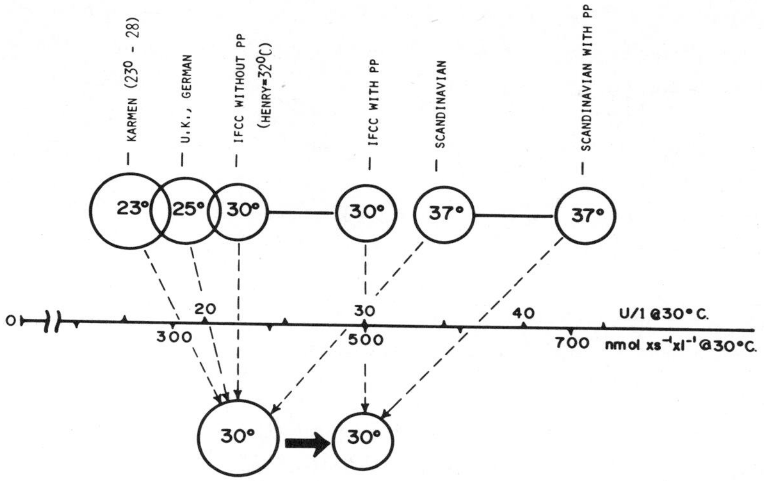

Fig. 2 **RECOMMENDATIONS FOR ASAT**

First, let me emphasize that fig. 2 and table 6 already represent substantially more agreement than may at first be apparent. For example, *all recommendations* utilize the same ultraviolet instrumental technique at 340 nm to continuously monitor the progress of the reaction. Furthermore, *all are based upon the same chemical reactions*. In many respects, as shown in the bottom half of fig. 2, the differences, except for pyridoxal phosphate supplementation, yes even those concerning the *reaction temperature,* and volume differences are relatively minor and can be reconciled by appropriate factors based upon well-understood principles to give reasonably compatible answers[2]. All that would be needed at this point is agreement to report these modified values in a unified manner as either $mol \times s^{-1} \times l^{-1}$, as the Expert Panel on Enzymes recommends [8], or as kat/l, as the Expert Panel on Quantities and Units recommends [8]. One might ask why the EPE members upset this possible chance for widespread agreement by deciding that pyridoxal phosphate supplementation was necessary, when no method in common use today in clinical laboratories includes this factor, with the possible exception of a few Swedish laboratories. In the *Introduction* of the EPE proposed recommendations, *'General Considerations'* document [8], the following was stressed,

> 'the selection of a method which is to serve as an internationally agreed method of reference to measure the catalytic activity of an enzyme must rest upon *experimental observations* which have been verified in many laboratories ...'
>
> 'The major aim of an IFCC Method is to achieve maximum reproducibility of analysis both within each laboratory and between laboratories throughout the world. Therefore, the sensitivity, precision, specificity and accuracy of the analytical measuring system must be of primary importance.'

---

[2] Dr. Raymond Vanderlinde of Albany has been able to convert nearly all ASAT values on several large U.S.A. surveys to one common answer by the use of such factors.

I know of no sure way to decide which of two or more methods in clinical enzymology is the more *accurate*. However, in the case of ASAT considerations, the *experimental observations* of numerous investigators as far back as *O'Kane* and *Gunsalus* [14] in 1947 have clearly established that pyridoxal phosphate is a required cofactor in ASAT measurements. Despite this knowledge and for reasons not altogether clear, this cofactor has been missing in nearly all ASAT measurements used in clinical enzymology. Yet in 1966 *Hamfelt* [15] reported an average increase in ASAT activity of 17% in the serum from healthy subjects when the specimen was supplemented with pyridoxal phosphate. He concluded that there was

> 'a fundamental error in the method for aminotransferase determination as currently used in clinical laboratories.'

Recently *Rej, Fasce* and *Vanderlinde* [16] have re-examined the role of pyridoxal phosphate supplementation. As shown in table 7 these workers noted a 16% increase in activity. Perhaps even more importantly, they demonstrated that pyridoxal phosphate had a protective effect against the loss of ASAT activity during the preincubation period with L-aspartate, particularly as the temperature of incubation was increased from 30 °C to 37 °C or even as high as 45 °C as shown in fig. 3. They also showed that lesser amounts of pyridoxal phosphate were needed, and shorter preincubation periods required, when the phosphate buffer which competitively inhibited the recombination of the coenzyme with apoenzyme was replaced by a Tris buffer. Similar to Hemfelt's conclusion, their report states,

> 'pyridoxal phosphate supplementation seems to be desirable in clinical and reference methods for the estimation of true aspartate aminotransferase activity in human serum.'

Table 7. Increase Effect in Aspartate Aminotransferase (AST) Activity of Human Serum by Added Pyridoxal Phosphate.

Population	AST activity, U/liter	No. specimens	Pyridoxal-supplemented/control[1]
Normal	9–22	16	1.16 ± 0.02
Hospital (normal serum AST)	4–24	97	1.18 ± 0.03
Hospital (moderately elevated serum AST)	25–40	16	1.15 ± 0.02
Hospital (elevated serum AST)	> 40	12	1.12 ± 0.03

[1] Mean ± std. error.

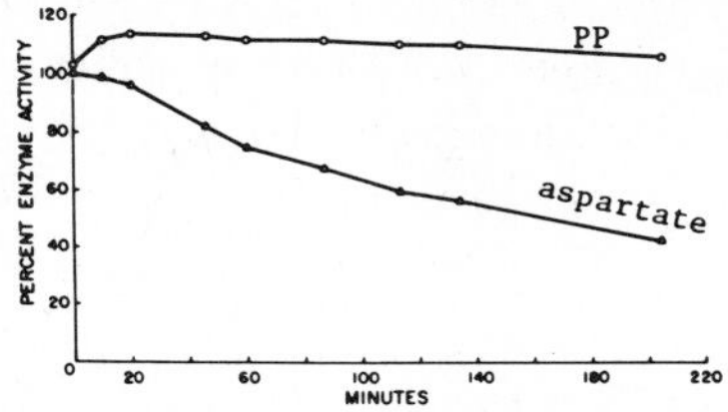

Fig. 3. Effects of pyridoxal phosphate and L-aspartate on preincubation

During various stages of the development of the present draft proposal for an IFCC Method for ASAT, the effect of the pyridoxal phosphate stimulation has been found to be $30 \pm 3\%$ [17, 18]. In Tris buffer with use of higher substrate concentrations of 12 mmol/l for 2-oxoglutarate and 200 mmol/l for L aspartate as called for in the final conditions of Draft 6 protocol [9], the average increase in stimulation has been found to be 38%, as

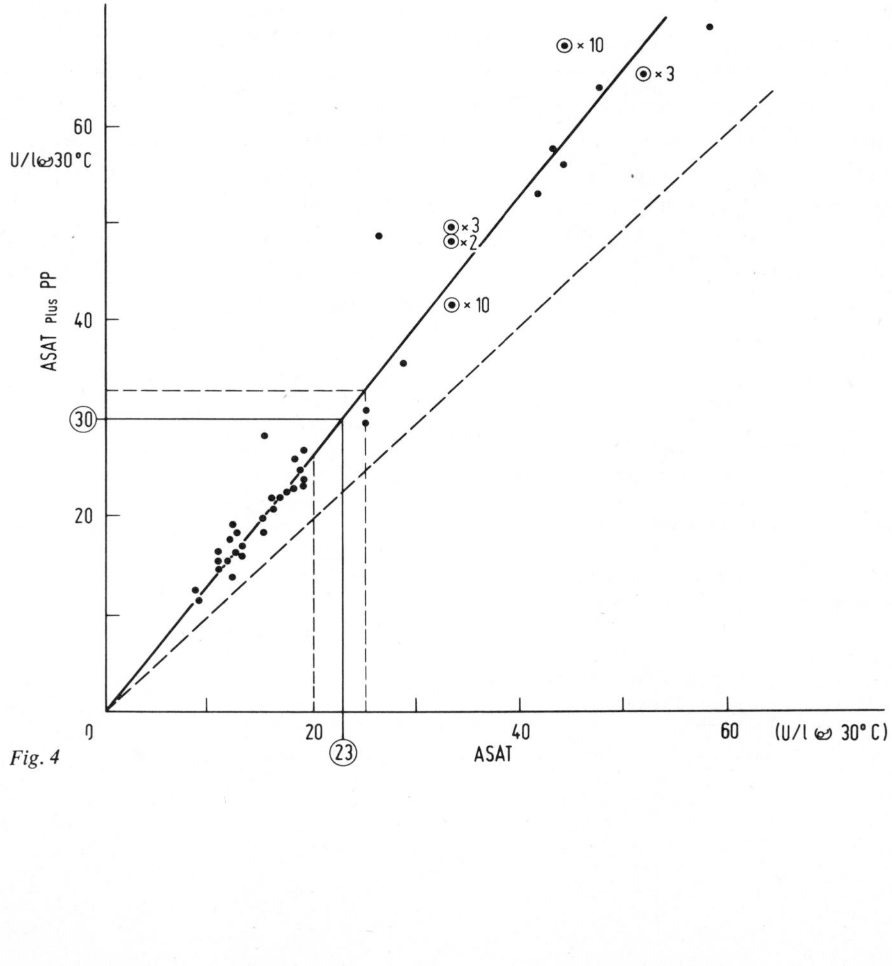

Fig. 4

shown in fig. 4 [19]. The coefficient of variation for the IFCC Methods of ASAT in our work at Hartford has been approximately 2% at the upper limit of the reference interval; this figure compares favorably with the other recommended methods for ASAT given in table 6[3]. The question therefore still remains, how do we decide which (if any) of two or more methods provides the more meaningful measurement?

IV. Reagent specifications and reliability

It is rather rare to find detailed reagent specifications in the description of a method in clinical enzymology; yet, we all know that poor quality reagents can be the cause of endless troubles. The EPE document recommends in section 5 the following:

> '*Reagents*
> Specifications for reagent chemicals, water and enzymes should refer to an authoritative source. these are not available or are found to be inadequate to insure the method's success, the needed additional specifications should be included.' [8]

Dr. *Robert McComb* and I have just submitted to *Selected Methods* an alkaline phosphatase method which is based upon our earlier work [20, 21]. The final assay conditions are given in table 8, but to my mind, the real addition has been in the development of reagent specifications. For example, the specifications for p-nitrophenol permit one to judge the purity of this product to better than 99%. This allows the user to calibrate instrumentation of almost any type with the absorbing species under the exact assay conditions of temperature, pH and buffer strength. We have been able to bring several different types of instruments (Cary 16, 3 Gilford 2000's, LKB and PE KA-150) into a compatible spectrophotometric network for alkaline phosphatase measurements using this high purity stable material. For such materials, the EPE has recommended the following in 5.4:

> '*Comparison Material ("Standard")*
> The composition and purity of the comparison material (usually a substrate, product or coenzyme, but not an enzyme material) must receive additional specifications which go beyond section 5.1. The absorption coefficient of the comparison material must be determined at several increasing concentrations under the conditions which prevail in the final reaction mixture.' [8]

Table 8. Alkaline Phosphatase: Final Reaction conditions.

Substrate – 15 mmol/l, p-nitrophenyl phosphate
Buffer – 0.8 mol/l, 2-amino-2-methyl-1-propanol, pH 30 °C = 10.30
Magnesium – 100 μmol/l, Mg^{++}
Temperature – 30.0 °C
Sample – 1 vol. sample is added to 26 vols. of buffer and 2 vols. of substrate (1 → 30 dilution)

[3] Experiments by Dr. *Mogens Hørder,* Visiting Scientist on leave from the University of Arhus, Denmark.

In our recent experiments,we have found that the use of specifications for the substrate based upon a) the molar (linear) absorption coefficient at 311 nm, b) the absorbance at 415 nm for p-nitrophenol content, and c) the measurement of the phosphorus content, have helped to differentiate acceptable lots from poor lots of p-nitrophenyl phosphate ($Na_2 \cdot NO_2C_6H_4OPO_3 \cdot 6\ H_2O$). Of 12 materials tested from 8 different commercial sources, the 5 meeting our specifications gave activity of 100 ± 0.5%. In contrast, the 7 unacceptable materials gave activity values of 83, 88, 98, 99, 100, 100, and 101% of the mean value of the acceptable materials.

Likewise, the source of the reagent used as the buffer may effect the reliability of an assay. In testing 7 lots of diethanolamine (DEA) buffer from 6 suppliers, activity was found to be from 87, 88, 93, 97, 97, and 100%. Identical testing of 6 lots of 2-amino-2-methyl-1-propanol (AMP) from 3 suppliers gave activity of 100 ± 0.5%. DEA has been the buffer chosen by both the German and the Scandinavian enzyme committees in their recommendations; however, this must be re-examined in the light of the above testing. If inhibitor-free DEA cannot be assured by specifications and testing, then AMP or other buffers should probably be utilized for alkaline phosphatase measurements. The EPE recommends the following in respect to buffers in section 5.5:

> '*Buffers*
> Buffers should be prepared by using an explicitely stated, easily reproduced technique with clearly-defined reagents of specified purity. The buffer capacity should be adequate to hold the pH of the reaction mixture to within pre-established limits. These limits should be such that the change in pH, from any source, during the period of measurement should not introduce relative changes in the measurements of catalytic activity exceeding 0.005 (0.5%). Storage time limits for the buffer should be established such that changes in pH or production-rate influencing decomposition products arising from storage will not introduce relative changes in catalytic activity measurements exceeding 0.005 (0.5%). Buffer substances should not react with any compound of the analytical system unless such a reaction is specifically described (e.g. transphorylation with some amino alcohol buffers in alkaline phosphatase methods).' [8]

In the present draft proposal of an IFCC Method for ASAT [9] considerable time and attention was also given to the specifications for reagent enzymes. The means of testing the lactic dehydrogenase (LDH) and malic dehydrogenase (MDH) to reduce the non-specificity due to aminotransferases and glutamic dehydrogenase were given in much detail. The EPE recommends the following in respect of reagent enzymes in section 5.3:

> '*Reagent Enzymes*
> Enzymes employed as reagents (indicator and auxiliary enzymes of section 1.2.7) must be of stated quality and meet specifications of authoritative sources. These reagents must be essentially free from contamination from other enzymes, metabolites and impurities which might alter the rate of the primary or secondary reaction being followed. If contaminants or side activities are unavoidable, they should be described.' [8]

There can be no doubt that detailed *reagent specifications* are an absolute requirement for meaningful measurements in clinical enzymology. Even reagent grade water must be shown to meet specifications as stated in section 5.2 of the EPE recommendations:

'Reagent Water
Water specifications must meet the requirements of an authoritative source. In addition, known inhibitors *of the enzyme in question* must, if present, be below the minimum inhibitory concentration. (These minimum levels should be given.) Sterile water (free of any additives) may be required for reagent solutions which are to be stored for any length of time.' [8]

V. The role of reference enzyme materials

For years, stable enzyme containing control and calibration materials have been commercially available and seem to have been used with reasonable success. However, it is a sorry fact that the average user of these materials does so on 'faith' and has little or no knowledge about the fundamental characteristics of the enzymes he uses. We became aware of this problem in 1966, when we were sent a New York State survey sample to test for its alkaline phosphatase activity by the method we had just published. Because of marked analytical problems with this test material, we became deeply concerned about how little was known about the complex interactions which occur between these enzyme materials and our routine assay methods [22]. We soon found out that the unknown enzyme in the N. Y. State testing material, known enzymes and also many of those added to commercially available quality control materials, frequently differed rather remarkedly from the enzyme(s) of human serum.

In fig. 5 and 6, alkaline posphatases from varied sources were studied by subjecting the enzyme-containing materials to various lengths of preincubation at 30 °C in the AMP buffer pH 10.15. The original problem of loss of activity with time in the unknown enzyme in the N. Y. material, only served to uncover for us a far more complex situation in which some alkaline phosphatase containing materials lost activity at this alkaline pH while others, including those in serum, gained. Heat denaturation and inhibition studies with phosphate, EDTA and L-phenylalanine were also used, but we could only conclude that there was

> 'an urgent need for establishing criteria of stability and chemical reactivity for enzymes utilized in reference samples and control materials.' [22]

We also suggested that

(A) 'Information concerning the species source, tissue of origin, isolation procedure, preservation technics, and the isoenzyme form of enzymes added to reference samples and control materials should be fully documented and made readily available to the user.'

(B) 'Critical evaluation of data on enzyme measurements obtained by survey reference sample or control technics must recognize the profound influence of the aforementioned conclusions on the final observed variability of enzyme tests (i.e., the marked sensitivity to alkaline denaturation of the unknown enzyme reported in this paper).'

(C) 'There is at present no laboratory evidence or body of scientific information which provides a sound basis for the labeling of any commercial control material as a standard for serum enzyme analyses.'

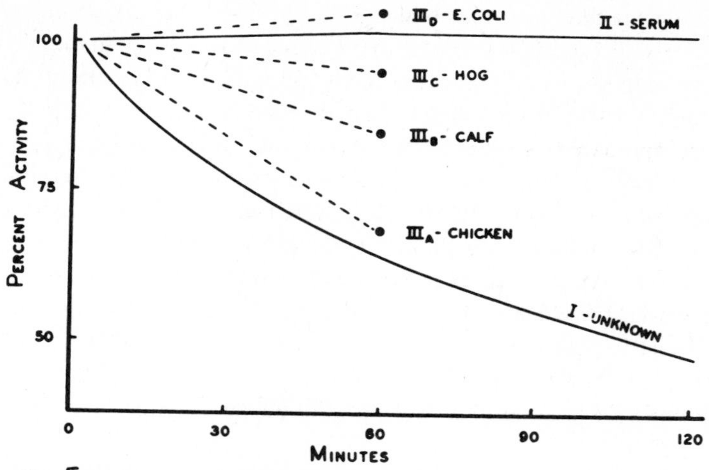

Fig. 5 Alkaline stability-denaturation studies on alkaline phosphatases preincubated in buffer at $pH_{30°} = 10.15$. I, unknown; II, human pooled frozen serum; III_A, III_B, III_C, and III_D: partially purified enzyme preparations.

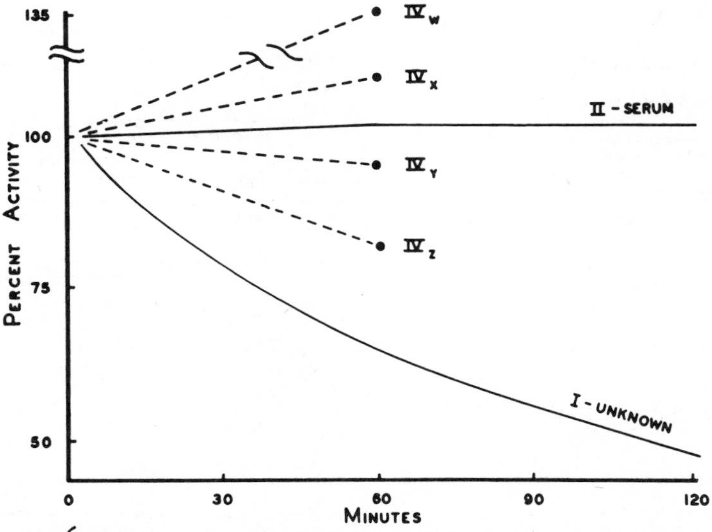

Fig. 6. Alkaline stability-denaturation studies on alkaline phosphatases preincubated in buffer at $pH_{30°} = 10.15$: I, unknown; II, human pooled frozen serum. Commercial serum enzyme control materials: IV_W, IV_X, IV_Y, and IV_Z.

Today, almost a decade after making the last statement (C), I believe there is experimental evidence and pragmatic testing experience to support the idea that an enzyme might become a standard reference material. Highly purified stable cytoplasmic L-aspartate: 2-oxoglutarate aminotransferase (ASAT) from human red blood cells [23], human liver [24] and pig heart [25] have been prepared specifically for use in clinical enzymology. Fortunately, each preparation is very similar to the other and each reacts in nearly parallel fashion to the 'native' serum ASAT(s) when added to and tested in serum. As shown in fig. 7 and 8, the variation in ASAT activity with changing concentrations of aspartate + 2-oxoglutarate respectively between the purified enzyme and the 'native' enzyme found in serum is nearly identical. Likewise, the effect of temperature change on activity is also identical (fig. 9). However, the most important characteristic of these potential reference enzyme materials is the stability as shown in fig. 10 when the proper stabilizing matrix and storage conditions were found. Perhaps at last we have found an enzyme 'standard' reference material.

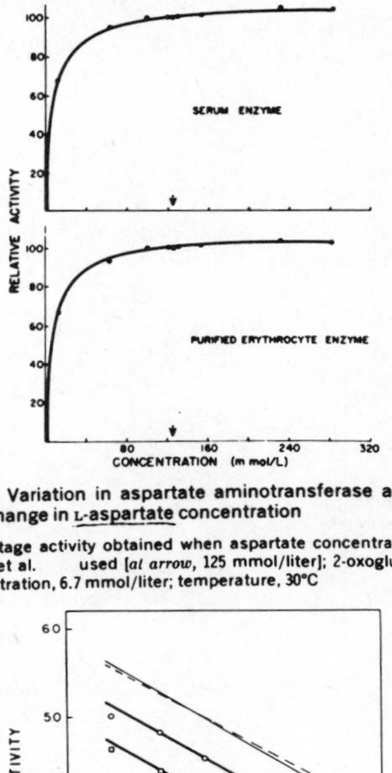

Fig. 7. **Variation in aspartate aminotransferase activity with change in L-aspartate concentration**

Percentage activity obtained when aspartate concentration of Henry et al. used [*at arrow*, 125 mmol/liter]; 2-oxoglutarate concentration, 6.7 mmol/liter; temperature, 30°C

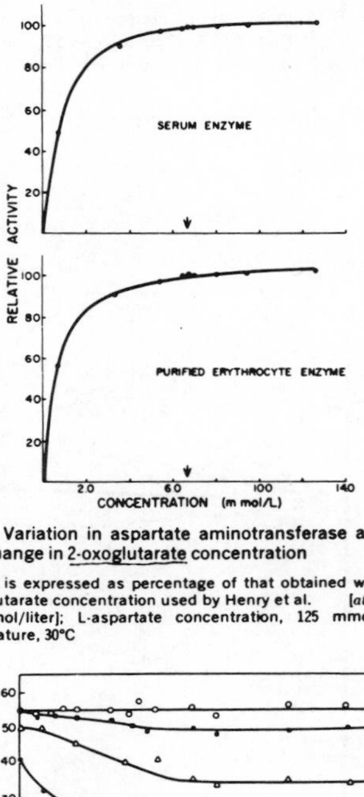

Fig. 8. **Variation in aspartate aminotransferase activity with change in 2-oxoglutarate concentration**

Activity is expressed as percentage of that obtained with the 2-oxoglutarate concentration used by Henry et al. [*at arrow*, 6.7 mmol/liter]; L-aspartate concentration, 125 mmol/liter; temperature, 30°C

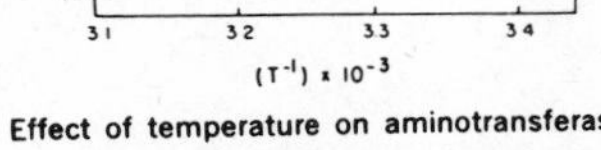

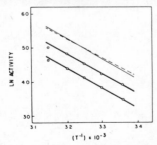

Fig. 9. **Effect of temperature on aminotransferase activity**

Arrhenius plot of ln enzyme activity vs. reciprocal of absolute temperature (K^{-1}). O-O-O purified erythrocyte enzyme (slope, -5.84×10^{-3}). □-□-□ human serum enzyme (slope, -5.95×10^{-3}). - - - - - Arrhenius slope of -5.78×10^{-3} found by Schneider and Willis (30). —— Arrhenius slope of -5.92×10^{-3} found by Henry et al. (23)

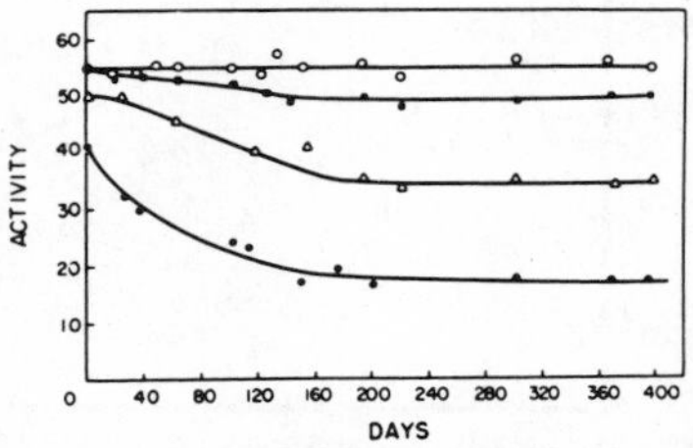

Fig. 10. **Stability of purified erythrocyte aminotransferase**

Activity in U/liter vs. time in days. Enzyme was lyophilized in: 0.1 mol/liter tris(hydroxymethyl)aminomethane buffer, pH 7.5(●); 1 mg/ml human serum albumin (fraction V), 0.1 mol/liter Tris pH, 7.5 (△); Preparation A_1 (■); Preparation A (O)

VI. Devices: The tie-point for reference methods and materials

Mr. *Cali* and Dr. *Brown* have reviewed the key role that reference materials and a hierarchy of methods must play in bringing compatibility based upon accuracy into being at the national level. I would like to add another ingredient to this scheme – an intermediate category of *devices* (instruments) as shown in table 9. In today's world, the instruments we employ are the critical tie-point between methods and materials. Without these unique devices, *accuracy,* as we know it today would be only an ideal rather than a reality. Yet in many survey type studies in clinical enzymology, instrumental sources of error have proven to be far too large. The members of the EPE have suggested that all critical measuring steps involving instruments should be safeguarded with rigid specifications.

Table 9. Meaningful Measurements in Clinical Chemistry

	CLINICAL LABORATORY	CALIBRATION LABORATORY	NATIONAL OR INTERNATIONAL LABORATORY
METHODS	ROUTINE	REFERENCE	DEFINITIVE
DEVICES	WORKING	SPECIFIED INSTRUMENT	MAXIMUM STATE OF THE ART
MATERIALS	PATIENT SAMPLES	MATRIXED SUBSTANCE	"PURE" SUBSTANCE

For example, table 10 gives the EPE Recommendations for Reaction Temperature. Although many will first focus their attention on the recommended reaction temperature set-point of 30 °C, I trust the critical specifications for the control (Item 1) and Accuracy (Item 2.1) of the reaction temperature and sensor will not be overlooked. In similar manner, table 11 gives the EPE recommendations on instruments and equipment. Note that the specifications for reference method work are designed to minimize systematic bias from these sources.

Table 10.

Reaction Temperature
The set point in degrees Celsius of the reaction temperature is to be assigned as a part of the method. Only one temperature should be endorsed for each method and its choice fully documented in the appendage. It is recommended that with as few exceptions as possible, the IFCC Methods be carried out at a uniform temperature of 30.00 °C.

1 *Temperature Control Specifications*
The methods, procedure and equipment used for controlling temperature, in mixing specimens with reagents, and in inserting them into the measuring device shall be such that during the entire actual time of observation of the reaction mixture, the *recorded* temperature of the *liquid* near its center varies by less than $\pm$ 0.05 °C from the nominal set-point temperature, expressed as the standard deviation of at least 16 measurements made following exactly the same procedures and using the same reagents as used in determining the catalytic activity.

2 *Temperature Sensor Specification*
The temperature sensing element used shall have the following characteristics:

2.1 *Accuracy*
The mean value of the set-point of the reaction temperature shall be traceable to the International Practical Temperature Scale of 1968.

2.2 *Thermal Mass, Self Heat, and Conductance*
The immersion element plus its leads shall have a heat capacity relative to that of the heat capacity of the volume of liquid reaction mixture into which it is immersed of less than 0.01 (1%).
The thermal conductance of the immersion element at the *most* extreme external environmental temperature difference to the liquid in the cuvette, and the self-heat generated, if any, shall be such that the change of temperature caused thereby shall be less than $\pm$ 0.05 °C during the specified observation time.

2.3 *Speed of Response*
To ensure that significant short-term transient temperature changes are observed, the response time of the immersion element and its recording system expressed as a time constant shall be less than 0.1 (10%) of the specified observation time during which the determination of the catalytic concentration is made.

Table 11.

Instrumentation and Equipment

The instruments and equipment employed should meet clearly-stated specifications to reduce measurement errors from laboratory to laboratory.

1 Spectrometers must meet spectral purity (wavelength, band pass and stray light) and photometric accuracy specifications which are to be stated for each method. Similar specifications should be given for other types of instruments not involving photometry.

Note: Photometric errors are often neglected, but can readily introduce systematic relative differences of 0.01 to 0.05 absorbance units. Errors due to fluorescent effects can be especially troublesome in measurements with reduced NAD.

2 Cuvettes should have parallel faces of optical glass or quartz which transmit light without significantly reducing the light intensity due to absorption, reflections or other scattering effects. The light beam should in no way be influenced by the walls of the cuvette or events on the wall's surfaces, and the internal path-length should be 10.00 mm and deviate less than $\pm$ 0.01 mm. If cuvettes with other dimensions are used, the performance specifications must be demonstrated to equal those for square cuvettes.

3 pH meters should be calibrated at the reaction temperature with reference buffers from an authoritative source (e.g., IUPAC or NBS).

Note: When the final pH must be adjusted with measurements from a pH meter, specifications to avoid slope errors, sodium ion errors at high pH and junction potential errors should be given.

4 All volumetric glassware should be calibrated to reduce inaccuracy to less than 0.001 from the nominal volume or meet stated specifications (NBS class A or other national equivalents). Corrections for cubic expansion of liquids must be made if calibrations of the glassware were at a temperature different from the reaction temperature.

5 Surfaces in contact with any part of the sample, reagents, or reaction mixture must be chemically clean and free from traces of acids, metals or detergents or other compounds known to interfere with enzyme activity measurement.

Turning to table 12, we can now easily see the importance of instruments in the case of calcium – atomic absorption spectrometers and mass spectrometers, in tying together the calcium hierarchy of methods and materials. Likewise in table 13 a similar function is given over to ultraviolet spectrophotometers at 340 nm and mass spectrometers for $^{13}C/^{12}C$ ratios for glucose. In table 14, I have attempted to show how, even in the enzyme measurement for L-aspartate 2-oxoglutarate aminotransferase (ASAT), specialized ultraviolet spectrophotometers with exacting temperature control (all carefully described with detailed specifications) must play a central role in relating the reference method(s) to the reference enzyme material(s).

Table 12. Meaningful Measurements in Clinical Chemistry

CALCIUM

	CLINICAL LABORATORY	CALIBRATION LABORATORY	NATIONAL OR INTERNATIONAL LABORATORY
METHODS	COLORIMETRIC AAS OTHERS	AAS REFERENCE METHOD NBS 260-36 (SELECTED METHOD)	ISOTOPE DILUTION (^{44}CA)
DEVICES	COLORIMETERS AA SPECTROMETERS OTHERS	AA SPECTROMETER (SPECIFICATIONS)	MASS SPECTROMETER
MATERIALS	PATIENT SAMPLES CONTROL MATERIALS CALIBRATORS STANDARDS	CALCIUM IN SERUM MATRIX (CERTIFIED ANALYSIS BY THE REFERENCE OR DEFINITIVE METHOD	CALCIUM CARBONATE NBS/SRM #915 (PURITY = 99.9%)

Table 13. Meaningful Measurements in Clinical Chemistry

GLUCOSE

	CLINICAL LABORATORY	CALIBRATION LABORATORY	NATIONAL OR INTERNATIONAL LABORATORY
METHODS	COLORIMETRIC ENZYMATIC	ENZYMATIC REFERENCE METHOD (HEXOKINASE)	ISOTOPE DILUTION (^{13}C GLUCOSE)
DEVICES	COLORIMETERS SPECTROPHOTOMETERS KINETIC ANALYZERS	SPECTROPHOTOMETER (SPECIFICATIONS)	MASS SPECTROMETER
MATERIALS	PATIENT SAMPLES CONTROL MATERIALS CALIBRATORS STANDARDS	GLUCOSE IN PLASMA MATRIX (CERTIFIED ANALYSIS BY THE REFERENCE OR DEFINITIVE METHOD)	D-GLUCOSE NBS/SRM #917 (PURITY $\cong$ 99.9%)

Table 14. Meaningful Measurements in Clinical Chemistry

ASPARTATE AMINOTRANSFERASE (ASAT)

	CLINICAL LABORATORY	CALIBRATION LABORATORY	NATIONAL OR INTERNATIONAL LABORATORY
METHODS	COLORIMETRIC ULTRAVIOLET, 340 "KITS"	ASAT/IFCC (GOT/W. GERMANY) (GOT/SCANDINAVIA)	?
DEVICES	COLORIMETERS SPECTROPHOTOMETERS KINETIC ANALYZERS	SPECTROPHOTOMETER (IFCC SPECS. FOR 340NM, 30.00°C, ETC.)	SPECTROPHOTOMETER 340NM, 30.00°C,
MATERIALS	PATIENT SAMPLES CONTROLS CALIBRATORS	ASAT IN PROTEIN MATRIX, ?SOURCE (CERTIFIED ACTIVITY VALUE BY REFERENCE METHOD)	"PURE," HUMAN ASAT. (RBC SOURCE)

Note, that even for the enzyme ASAT, it is possible that the only box in the 9 member grid which cannot be suggested at this time is the *definitive method.* I am confident that it is only a matter of a few more years until the interactions between the candidate reference methods for ASAT and the new ASAT reference enzyme materials have been extensively investigated and agreements reached on one international reference method and material. Already, several ways to study the specificity (or lack of it) of the reference method by altering the reagent initiation and preincubation sequences have been utilized. It may well be that numerous techniques will, in total, constitute the definitive method, each telling something of the specificity of the reference method.

VII. Meaningful measurements in clinical enzymology

Before closing this discussion, it is necessary that we ask the very difficult but central question of what theoretically is accuracy in clinical enzymology and how do you make pragmatic judgements concerning improvements in accuracy in this complex area? From my view, as a physician-clinical chemist, it is clear that this question of accuracy is not only a philosophical and an analytical one, but also one which must be answered with continued reference to our growing understanding of man's fundamental chemical nature. The medical rationale for making enzyme measurements in body fluids and tissues is to relate these changes in the internal body chemistry in some meaningful way to our clinical understanding of health and/or disease, particularly, but not exclusively, in man. Although we talk easily about the association between enzyme activity and disease, the complexity of this chemical-biological phenomenon is staggering. Is this association based upon the relative number of molecular events per unit time, or the relative index of the number of protein molecules present? Depending upon which we center our attention, it is possible to arrive at quite different conclusions about the 'accuracy' of an enzyme measurement. Is our activity-minded chemist who describes conditions giving more moles × seconds^{-1} × liters^{-1} necessarily increasing the fundamental chemical-biological significance of an enzyme measurement, or must he also account for them in a framework that includes yet another insight gained by the molecule-oriented chemist who estimates the number of molecules present by a non-enzymatic technique such as radio-immunoassay [26]? Obviously, each of these enzyme chemists can contribute to our understanding, but neither stands as great a chance of contributing to the understanding of the whole enzyme complex if he limits his insights. No single clinical or chemical approach, technique, instrument, method refinement, or pure material, will provide the answer to, *what is an accurate measurement in clinical enzymology?* However, I am confident that current experimental observations and pragmatic experience both in the laboratory and at the bedside will reduce the rather broad range of nearly incompatible answers which now suggest greater inaccuracy in clinical enzymology than may indeed exist, if we start emphasizing our agreements rather than our discords.

In summary, recognition of the confusion created by too many methods and units has brought about the clear need for greater compatibility in clinical enzymology. Cooperative efforts within nations have lead to national agreements which are the first step in bringing greater uniformity in results between nations. International agreements are now actively being considered, and the first IFCC Method for aspartate aminotransferase has recently been circulated in draft form. Interaction between reference-type methods, highly refined instruments and well-characterized reference enzyme materials will provide the information required to resolve the present differences between the various recommended national methods. We can expect to see, in parallel with other measurements in clinical chemistry, the development of Reference Methods and Reference Materials which will give a basis for acceptance of enzyme methods on the International level.

References

[1] *Cali, P.:* Acceptability of Standards. First paper of this IFCC Symposium.
[2] *Brown, S.:* Acceptability of Definitive, Reference and Routine Methods. Third paper of this IFCC Symposium.
[3] *Fasce, C.F., Jr., Rej, R., Copeland, W.H. and Vanderlinde, R.E.:* A discussion of enzyme reference materials: Applications and specifications. Clin. Chem. *19,* 5 (1973).
[4] *Peters, T.:* Recommendation to AACC Board of Directors from Standards Committee regarding *Calibration Materials and Controls,* dated August 22, 1974.
[5] Recommendations of the German Society for Clinical Chemistry. Z. Klin. Chem. Klin. Biochem. *6,* 37 (1972).
[6] *Wilkinson, J.H., Baron, D.N., Moss, D.W., and Walker, P.G.:* Standardization of clinical enzyme assays: A reference method for aspartate and alanine aminotransferase. J. Clin. Pathol. *25,* 940 (1972).

[7] Committee on Enzymes of the Scandinavian Society for Clinical Chemistry and Clinical Physiology. Recommended methods for the determination of four enzymes in blood. Scand. J. Clin. Lab. Invest. *33*, 291 (1974).
[8] IFCC proposal on enzyme standardization in clinical enzymology. Clin. Chem. *19*, 268 (1973). Draft 16 submitted to Committee on Standards, Oct. 1974 as recommendations of Expert Panel on Enzymes (EPE).
[9] IFCC Enzyme Method, Draft No. 6 of Aspartate Aminotransferase (ASAT) submitted to Associate Members EPE, February, 1975.
[10] *Friedman, M.M. and Taylor, T.H.:* Transaminase in *Standard Methods of Clinical Chemistry 3* (1961), Seligson, D., Editor, Academic Press, N.Y.
[11] *Hørder, M.:* Personal communication based upon experience on the Committee on Enzymes of the Scandinavian Society for Clinical Chemistry and Clinical Physiology.
[12] *Karmen, A.:* A note on the spectrophotometric assay of glutamic-oxalacetic transaminase in human blood serum. J. Clin. Invest. *34*, 131 (1955).
[13] *Henry, R.J., Chiamori, N., Golub, O.J., and Berkman, S.:* Revised spectrophotometric methods for the determination of glutamic-oxalacetic transaminase, glutamic-pyruvic transaminase, and lactic acid dehydrogenase. Am. J. Clin. Pathol. *34*, 381 (1960).
[14] *O'Kane, D.E. and Gunsalus, I.C.:* The resolution and purification of glutamic-aspartic transaminase. J. Biol. Chem. *170*, 425 (1974).
[15] *Hamfelt, A.:* The effect of pyridoxal phosphate on the aminotransferase assay in blood. Scand. J. Clin. Lab. Invest. *18* (Suppl. 99), 181 (1966).
[16] *Rej, R., Fasce, C.F., Jr., and Vanderlinde, R.E.:* Increased aspartate aminotransferase activity of serum after in vitro supplementation with pyridoxal phosphate. Clin. Chem. *19*, 92 (1973).
[17] *Bergmeyer, H.:* Personal Communication.
[18] *Rej, H.:* Personal Communication.
[19] *Hørder, M.:* Personal Communication
[20] *Bowers, G.N., Jr. and McComb, R.B.:* A continuous spectrophotometric method for measuring the activity of serum alkaline phosphatase. Clin. Chem. *12*, 70 (1966).
[21] *McComb, R.B. and Bowers, G.N., Jr.:* Study of optimum conditions for measuring alkaline phosphatase activity in human serum. Clin. Chem. *18*, 97 (1972).
[22] *Bowers, G.N., Jr., Kelley, M.L., and McComb, R.B.:* Precision estimates in clinical chemistry. 1. Variability of analytical results in a survey reference sample related to the use of a non-human serum alkaline phosphatase. Clin. Chem. *13*, 595 (1967).
[23] *Rej, R., Vanderlinde, R.E., and Fasce, C.F., Jr.:* An L-aspartate: 2-oxoglutarate aminotransferase reference material from human erythrocytes: Preparation and characterization. Clin. Chem. *18*, 374 (1972).
[24] *Rej, R.:* Personal Communication.
[25] *Gruber, W.:* Paper delivered at 1st European Conference on Clinical Chemistry, Munich, April 1974.
[26] *Ryan, J.P., Carballo, A.J., and Davis, R.H.:* Radio-immunoassay of serum pancreatic amylase in normal and pancreatectomized pigs. Proc. Soc. Exptl. Biol. & Med. *148*, 194 (1975).

Acceptability of Diagnostic Kits[1]

G. Vanzetti, Milano-Niguarda (Italy)

Key Words: Kit Labelling
Kit Validation
Licensing
Reagent Kits

Introduction

In clinical chemistry, reagents have long been prepared by analysts themselves. Now the situation has changed, due to an increasing need for special reagents, for instance, enzymatic and antibody preparations, which are difficult to prepare in the laboratory. In addition, ready-made reagent packages afford substantial time-saving: an important consideration, in view of the high cost of skilled labor in advanced countries. In smaller laboratories especially, kits account for only a fraction of total operating costs.

In a recent survey in Italy, we found that in hospital laboratories about 75% of current clinical chemical tests were performed with reagent kits. The same appears to be true in other western countries. Reagent kits are currently used for measuring enzymatic activities, and often also for the assay of common constituents such as glucose and urea. The use of reagent-kits is not only established, but still expanding; specific enzymatic methods are now available, for example, for the assay of cholesterol, creatinine and bicarbonate; and specific immunological methods are currently used for the assay of individual plasma proteins and of various drugs. Special packages are used in many laboratories for emergency tests, biochemical profiles, and for high-volume analyzers.

The use of ready-made analytical packages is even more widespread in allied laboratory fields, for serological, bacteriological, and in-vitro radioactive tests.

This being the situation, the reliability of laboratory tests does not depend totally on the analyst's skill: manufacturers of reagent packages and of diagnostic instruments must take their share of responsibility. Today, the manufacturer of diagnostic products is responsible not only for the quality of reagents, but also, at least to some extent, for the selection and validity testing of analytical methods.

Industry has made important contributions to progress in clinical chemistry. Practical

[1] This presentation is based on work done by a special group of NATO's Committee for the Challenges of Modern Society (CCMS) working on Automation of Clinical Laboratories. Members of this group are Prof. *Wootton* (Chairman) and Prof. *Whitby* of England, Prof. *Delbrueck* of Germany, Dr. *Mullertz* of Denmark, Dr. *Allen* of Canada, Dr. *Coelho* of Portugal, Dr. *Melville* of the US, Dr. *Raguet* of France and the author. The guidelines given in this report represent the view of the entire group, though not necessarily the official policy of CCMS.

diagnostic tests require, among other things, enzymatic preparations of certified activity; pure coenzymes and substrates; specific antisera, etc. If these essential materials are available on the market today, we owe it to the efforts not only of pure research scientists, but also of those working for industry.

On the other hand, we must acknowledge existing shortcomings. Analysts often complain about the quality and presentation of diagnostic reagents. At least some of these complaints are justified[2].

Here is a list of common complaints:

- in commercial diagnostic kits, the composition of individual reagents is not always given in detail – sometimes it is not given at all;
- reference to the original literature related to the analytical method is often omitted;
- the analytical procedure is often modified without warning and also without adequate testing of the modified method;
- reagents of insufficient purity, and enzymatic preparations of suboptimal activity are sometimes used;
- reagents are not always adequately tested for stability;
- unwarranted claims are often made by manufacturers about the reliability of an assay, and possible sources of error are not pointed out;
- low-cost reagents are often overpriced.

If we consider, in addition, the multitude of analytical procedures used for the assay of a given constituent, the frequent lack of reliable reference methods, and the scarcity of qualified technical personnel, we can easily understand the poor agreement between analytical results often found in cooperative surveys.

We all know that basic research in methodology and instrumentation, and widespread availability of well-controlled standard reference materials and methods, are indispensable for improvement in the quality of laboratory work.

For many constituents, however, this will require years of painstaking research. Meanwhile, steps must be taken, in the interest of the population's health, to secure diagnostic reagents of high quality, through the cooperative effort of analysts and manufacturers, and through enactment of adequate regulations.

With this in mind, our group has prepared a set of guidelines for the manufacture and supply of diagnostic reagents; these guidelines cover the preparation, control, storage, and labelling of reagents, adequate product information, including methodology, the selection and control of analytical methods, and the problems of documentation and licensing.

These guidelines are in keeping with the regulations already adopted in several countries, as well as with the recommendations of the International Conference on Standardization of

[2] In a recent quality control survey, we found that the spread of results from laboratories using reagent kits was about the same as from laboratories using home-made reagents.

Diagnostic Materials (Atlanta, May 1973), and of more recent W.H.O. meeting; they are meant to facilitate the selection of reliable diagnostic materials as well as the rejection of products of inferior quality.

Our proposed guidelines call for strict cooperation between scientific and professional associations, the manufacturers of diagnostic products, and government agencies. This co-operation is essential for making progress and ensuring the necessary flexibility in our rapidly developing field without getting stranded in bureaucratic quagmires.

We are the first to recognize that the enactment of such regulations would impose a burden upon the makers of diagnostic reagents. However, we believe that the expected gains in terms of laboratory performance and overall reliability would in time reflect favorably on the manufacturer's own prestige. We also realize that state licensing of diagnostic products may not be without certain drawbacks, and alternative solutions might be explored.

In this spirit, these guidelines are presented here as a contribution to general discussion.

Recommended guidelines for the manufacture and supply of diagnostic reagents

I – *Scope*

Prepacked diagnostic reagents and reagent kits are widely used today in clinical laboratories throughout the world, for manual analytical procedures as well as with automatic equipment. The quality of these products, however, is not always satisfactory, and the testing of recommended procedures is sometimes inadequate; this may lead to unreliable analytical results. Rigorous controls are needed during the manufacturing process, and validity testing of the analytical procedure is required, in the interest of the population's health. Accordingly, we suggest the following guidelines for the manufacture and supply of diagnostic products.

II – *Raw materials*

The manufacturer should test raw materials for purity, and make sure that impurities do not exceed proper limits. This would, of course, not be required for chemically pure products of certified composition. Storage of raw materials in conditions ensuring their stability should be the manufacturer's responsibility.

In the case of biologically active materials, the manufacturer should control activity by procedures recommended or accepted by official international agencies or by recognized experts in the field.

III – *Labelling and control of individual reagents, including calibration materials*

The composition of reagents should be stated on the label or in an accompanying sheet, not only in conventional units, but also in S.I. units, according to the recommendations of the International Federation of Clinical Chemistry. The nature and amount of additives should be stated. For calibration materials, the chemical formulae of additives should be given. For biological materials, the source (animal species and tissue, bacterial strain, etc.) should be specified. Biological materials should carry a batch number as well as indications of storage requirements and expiration date. For hazardous reagents, a warning should be prominently displayed and suitable handling precautions given.

Storage conditions and shelf life after opening of containers should always be specified.

The manufacturer should carry out suitable control procedures to ensure uniform quality for each reagent, assess its effectiveness in use, and control its stability and shelf life in field conditions.

IV – *Instructions for the use of prepacked reagent kits*

Every kit should contain a detailed description of the chemical, physical, or biological basis of the test procedure; also, the specificity, sensitivity, limitations, and interferences of the test should be clearly stated, and data concerning accuracy and precision given.

The analytical procedure should be described in detail, starting with sample collection and ending with calculation of results. Concentrations and quantities should be given in S.I. units, in keeping with the recommendations of the International Federation of Clinical Chemistry. For quantitative assays, a normal range should be indicated.

Calibration materials should be included in the package, with data on concentration and confidence limits; for qualitative tests, positive and negative controls should be supplied.

Adequate bibliography should be provided in all cases; changes in method or procedure should be reported and justified.

Unwarranted, unsupported or misleading claims should not be permitted.

V – *Validation of the analytical procedure*

The analytical procedure recommended by the manufacturer should be validated through field testing in one or more qualified clinical laboratories. The results should be compared by an appropriate statistical method with those of a reliable reference procedure. The outcome of the comparison should be published or made available to public authorities and prospective users.

VI – *Licensing*

The sale and distribution of ready-made reagents and prepacked reagent kits should be permitted only after evaluation of the products and of the analytical procedure by an independent, government-sponsored technical agency or control institution. We suggest that a special agency or division of an existing agency be set up, under government supervision and with the cooperation of the national scientific societies concerned with clinical laboratory work. The control agency should have the capability of evaluating diagnostic products and analytical procedures as required. In the case of new diagnostic products and procedures, the agency should carefully evaluate the evidence submitted by the manufacturer, and request additional data if necessary.

Products already on the market, however, could be approved on a temporary basis. Provision should be made for the collection and evaluation of complaints and other comments on such products; also, periodic revisions of licences should be provided for.

Materials and Methods for Health Testing

G. Siest, O. Houot, J. Henny, Vandœuvre-les-Nancy (France)

Key Words: Analytic variability
Biological variability
Frequent values
Methods
Preventive medicine
Reagents
Reference values
Standards

Laboratory tests were the basis for the development of preventive medicine as it is practised today, that is, a preventive medicine not geared toward research in microbic or parasitic diseases. Very often, in fact, health screening centers were, or are still, satisfied with a quick questionnaire and a series of laboratory tests.

The automatization of these laboratory tests was a determining factor, backed up by economic criteria. Unfortunately, the existing laboratory tests, as well as the corresponding automatic instruments, were conceived for use in curative medicine, whereas the only test that will represent an advance in preventive medicine is one that can define a state of health. As unbelievable as it may seem, there have been both methods and instruments which, although not designed for this goal, have in fact, made the field of preventive medicine progress nonetheless. Although manufacturers of automatic equipment have made some efforts to present these views to the general public and public health officials, the origin of the above phenomenon is essentially a lack of clarity, a more or less voluntary imprecision in the statement of goals. The detection of clinically defined diseases has been confused with prevention, or the maintenance of the state of health.

A laboratory test performed during an individual's life may have several values, corresponding to different states of health, or to various pathologies. One must admit, that a few years ago we were still fairly ignorant of the problems of physiological variations. Medical reasoning was largely responsible for this ignorance, for it sought to define disease, and the state of health merely represented an absence of disease. It is this way of thinking that must be radically changed both by informing health officials, and by educating patients. As *Claude Bernard* wrote: 'les maladies ne sont que des fonctions physiologiques dérangées', and we must, at the same time 'conserver la santé et guérir les maladies' [1].

The adjective 'clinical' (clinical chemistry, clinical pharmacology, etc. ...), in its general meaning, must be eliminated from the clinical chemist's vocabulary. Its Greek etymology 'lying' is indeed restrictive, when one wants to study the healthy man. To this effect, *Sanz* proposed the term 'anthropochemistry' [2].

Similarly, the term 'preventive medicine', used in different ways, is therefore ambiguous. The term 'preventive medicine' itself is directed toward pathology [3]. In order to facilitate this evolution, centers for preventive medicine should change their names to become health centers.

In addition, the success of molecular biology and medicine, particularly where inborn errors concerned, has overshadowed the less prestigious and common chronic diseases.

Clinical chemistry can and must contribute, here again, to a change in thinking. This discipline, provides quantitative values with defined reference intervals.

Progress must be made in two directions:

Improve the use of laboratory data currently being produced. This is the problem of reference values.

Find laboratory tests which are better suited for the definition of states of health.

This second part will not be developed here.

Use of current human chemistry data – the problem of reference values

In the investigation of individuals and of populations, laboratory tests provide data which are among the most elaborate and the most well-organized now available. It is for this reason that they are frequently criticized, the limits of their information content is often not well understood by users. This information content of human chemistry data can be improved considerably, if all the people involved in its production: that is, the patients, clinical chemists, manufacturers of materials or reagents, clinicians, statisticians, technicians, etc. ..., monitor the quality of these data. Their quality might vary as a function of the goals pursued. The quality of the data must, in all cases, be adapted to these goals. The reliability of classifications of subjects into one state of health group or another, or into a specific pathological group, strictly depends on this quality. This is particularly true in preventive medicine, where long-term, longitudinal variations are measured.

We feel that in the coming years, the number of systematic laboratory tests – be they in pathology or in the definition of health – should not be increased. Their information content must be increased, and thus, their use improved. This aim should take priority. During this time, well-programmed research should, nevertheless, continue, in order to find the laboratory tests which are best suited to the goals pursued, and which will be able to replace those whose information content proves insufficient.

1. The concept of reference values in human chemistry

Up until now, the clinical chemist's major role has been to study the chemical composition of the body during the course of various diseases, or following functional exploration. More recently, he has tackled measurements on supposedly healthy subjects, in order to evaluate physiological variations. Thus, the clinical chemist's fundamental task has been, and still is, to provide the most precise and accurate quantitative values possible, these values being used in the definition and observation of the state of health, in detection, in the diagnosis, the prognosis of diseases, and in the follow-up of treatments.

But more and more, the clinical chemist's duty is to play a fundamental role in the interpretation of the values he produces. The obtained values only have meaning if they are interpreted in comparison to similar values chosen in view of well-defined goals: *reference values* [4, 5].

There are two types of problems to be studied and defined:

1.1. The production of frequent values and of reference values

It will be necessary to define a methodology guiding, on one hand, the selection of reference populations – healthy or pathological – in order to produce the frequent values for a homogeneous group, and on the other hand, the values for a given individual.

The exclusion factors (physiological variations, for example) and inclusion factors (clinical criteria, for example), will have to be carefully specified in each case, taking the goals into account. The analytical variations will have to be known, controlled and measured.

1.2. The use and interpretation of reference values

We must know which reference values may be used to interpret the value observed. The choice can vary according to the goals, which are numerous:

Examples of goals necessitating specific references values:

- Definition of a state of health
- Detection of physiological variations
- Study of variations due to environment
- Pathological deviation from the state of health
- Aid to diagnosis
- Confirmation of diagnosis
- Aid to prognosis

- Follow-up of treatment or of disease's evolution
- Elimination of an inadequate treatment
- Epidemiological studies
- etc. ...

Finally, the presentation of these reference values is an important factor contributing to more comfortable relationships with clinicians and patients, facilitating the interpretation of these values, thereby furthering the two objectives which must be the basis of our work.

increase the health of each patient
decrease the cost to society.

2. Basic notions on biological and analytic variability

The relative importance of analytical and physiological variations, or environmental variations are essential factors to be considered both in the production of frequent values and in the interpretation of a value.

The overall objective is to control the important variation factors. To do so, one has to:

determine what these factors are
determine their relative importance
break them down, if possible, in order to control them more fully (analytical variation broken down into short and long term analytical variations).

This study must not be simply a descriptive one. The optimization and standardization of the relations between the different variation factors should result from the study, if certain basic considerations are taken into account:

the analytical error must not enlarge the spread of physiological values significantly (bearing in mind that the ratio analytical variation over spread of physiological values of
$^1/_{20}$ causes a 2% widening
$^1/_{12}$ causes a 5.4% widening [6]
¼ causes a 41.4% widening

Long-term analytical variations must represent about ⅓ to $^1/_5$ of the variations observed for a group of individuals (*Cotlove* suggested up to ½) [7].

Resolution of variation factors

Analytic variations

Long-term: variation in the same serum measurement on different days (short-term variation deduced)
Short-term: duplicate measurement of the same sample within a series
Short-term variation can itself be broken down into pre-instrumental, and instrumental variations [8].

Biological variations

Intra-individual: the same person gives a specimen at different times (includes biological rhythms and long-term analytic variations)
Inter-individual: variations between people due to biological (genetic) or environmental (dietetic) differences.

By accepting the hypothesis that the different components of the variance are cumulative and independent of mean values, one can establish certain relations between these components (thus calculating some of them using the estimation of others).

A look at table 1 indicates that only a detailed study of each of these variances can increase our knowledge of the global information content usually obtained 'S_T^2'.

TABLE 1 : RELATION BETWEEN THE DIFFERENT FACTORS OF VARIATION

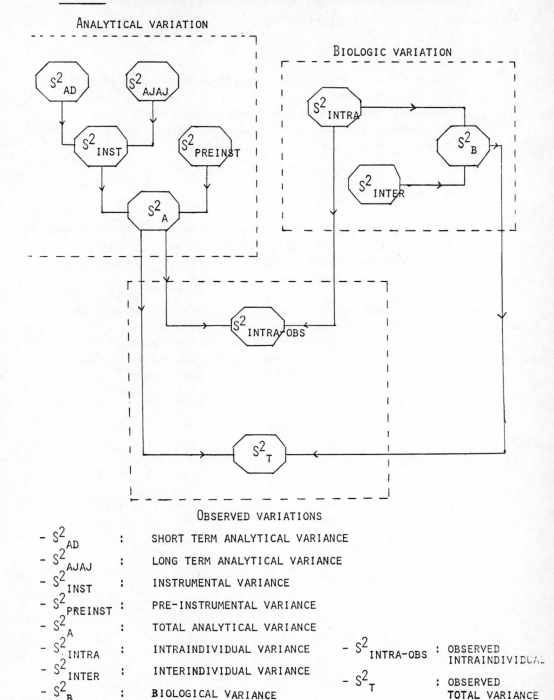

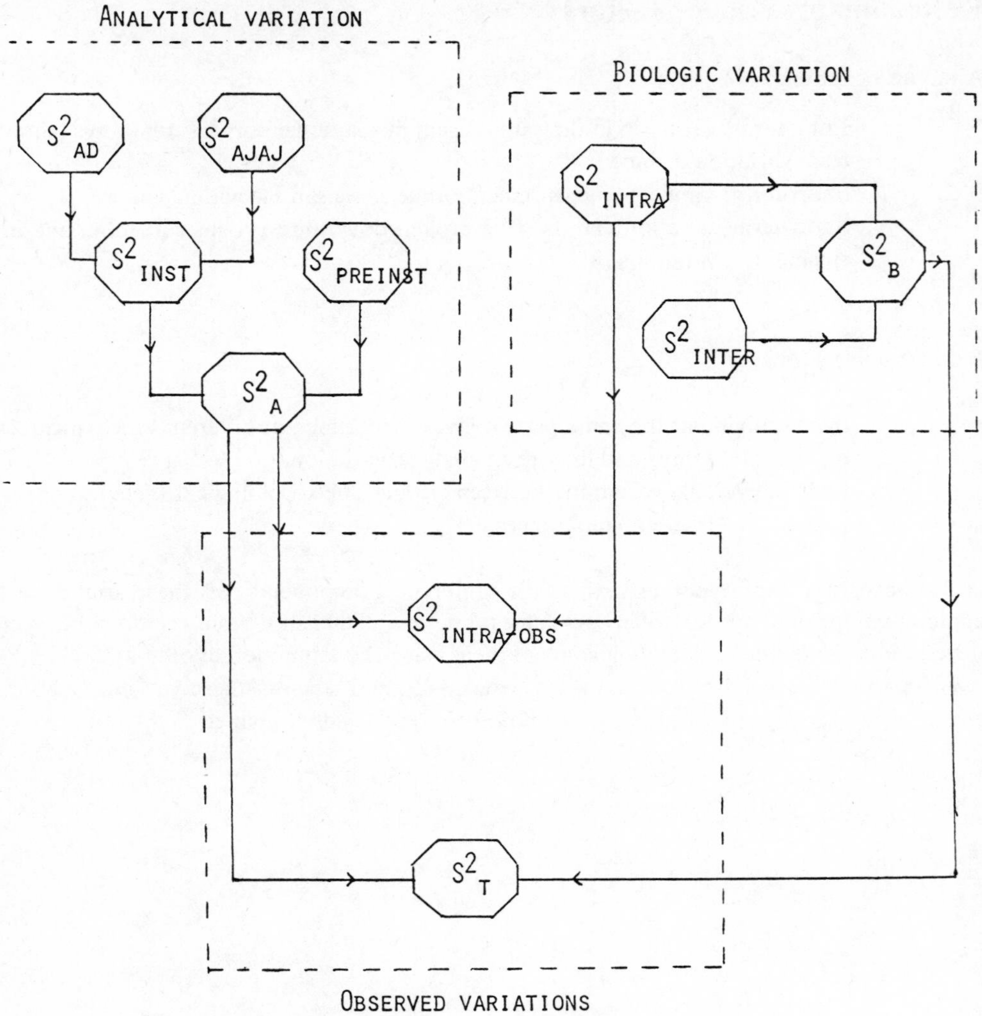

- S^2_{AD} : SHORT TERM ANALYTICAL VARIANCE
- S^2_{AJAJ} : LONG TERM ANALYTICAL VARIANCE
- S^2_{INST} : INSTRUMENTAL VARIANCE
- $S^2_{PREINST}$: PRE-INSTRUMENTAL VARIANCE
- S^2_{A} : TOTAL ANALYTICAL VARIANCE
- S^2_{INTRA} : INTRAINDIVIDUAL VARIANCE
- S^2_{INTER} : INTERINDIVIDUAL VARIANCE
- S^2_{B} : BIOLOGICAL VARIANCE
- $S^2_{INTRA-OBS}$: OBSERVED INTRAINDIVIDUAL
- S^2_{T} : OBSERVED TOTAL VARIANCE

Indeed, each analytical or physiological variance can itself be broken down into n factors: estimation of the variance of each factor can be made in the same study or in studies conducted simultaneously. One must, however, be very careful in the interpretation of observations, and consider the information obtained from descriptive, and not from a cumulative point of view. In fact, the variation factors are no doubt not linked so simply, and their contribution to the observed variance is not so easy to estimate. Using the theoretical scheme, only an elaborate protocol (choice of population, instruments, length of study ...) will enable us to know which are the sources of variations taken into account.

In all cases, respecting certain conditions contributes to the quality of the results:

Use of a suitable statistical model
Representative sample
Standardization
Verification of statistical application conditions (normality, eventual transformations ...)

3. Production of frequent values and of reference values for homogeneous groups

As we have just described, when laboratory tests are performed on a random population, frequent values corresponding to this population are obtained.

But we know little or nothing about the characteristics of this population, or about most of the variation factors which bring uncertainty to the contents and the limits of these values.

Frequent values will become reference values when:

the population is carefully described
the objectives are defined
the variation factors which are important for these objectives are controlled.

Producing frequent values and reference values therefore demands:

first, a thorough knowledge of analytical variations in order to have precise and accurate data
then, control of the samplings
last, selection of the populations, of homogeneous groups:

- by gathering information in order to know the intra and inter-individual variations
- by defining the clinical criteria with great precision
- by choosing, after description of distribution, the suitable statistical methods.

3.1. Knowledge of analytical variations

Until now, in preventive medicine, precision has been the dominant criteria, but it is time to emphasize accuracy, for if the methods are not accurate, it is impossible to compare measurements performed on subjects over intervals of several years.

3.1.1. The study of precision

Precision, measured using commercial lyophilized control serums, or laboratory-prepared serum pools, has already been widely studied. We will not discuss this here, as it is understood that this control is performed daily in the laboratory, being the laboratory technician's only way to validate his results immediately.

The duplicate analysis of each patient's specimen is another way of judging reproducibility [8]. Calculation of the variance between these two measurements gives a good picture of the analytic dispersion. Table 2 shows some examples. Let us point out, that the dispersion of the measurement of cholesterol by the enzymatic method is clearly reduced, compared to the dispersion of the measurement of cholesterol by the chemical method.

Table 2. Reproducibility with duplicate analysis

	m	s^2	s	CV
Uric acid µmoles/l	289.26	233.45	15.29	5.3%
Glucose mmoles/l	5.61	0.061	0.25	4.5%
Phosphates mmoles/l	0.99	0.00096	0.030	3.1%
Creatinine µmoles/l	73.4	56.27	7.6	10.3%
Cholesterol (chemical method) mmoles/l	6.20	0.38	0.59	9.6%
Cholesterol (enzymatic method) mmoles/l	5.42	0.023	0.15	2.8%

Can the quality of the results be improved through systematic duplicate measurements of each specimen, or rather, can duplicate measurements decrease the influence of the analytical variation on the physiological variations?

On a series of patient specimens ($50 < n < 100$) measured in duplicate, a correlation coefficient was calculated. A simple statistical test states that if the correlation is good, then the dispersion is not improved by using the average of these duplicate measurements.

Table 3 shows that the correlation is good for uric acid, phosphate and cholesterol (by the enzymatic method); the correlation is poor for creatinine and cholesterol (by the chemical method).

Table 3. Correlation coefficient (a) and regression curve (y = ax + b) between duplicate analyses

	r	a	b
Uric acid	0.97	0.99	0.30
Glucose	0.85	0.81	0.21
Phosphate	0.98	0.97	0.56
Creatinine	0.65	0.68	2.52
Cholesterol (chemical method)	0.51	0.53	0.96
Cholesterol (enzymatic method)	0.99	0.98	0.04

The slopes of the regression lines which link the two measurements are near one for well-correlated parameters.

After studying the correlation coefficients, the variance on single assay is calculated, then the variance on the average of duplicate assays. One observes (table 4) that the dispersion is smaller for cholesterol (by the chemical method) and creatinine when calculated on the average of the duplicate measurements. It is not improved for the other parameters, not even for glucose.

Table 4. Comparison of variances

	Single analyse s^2	Duplicate analyse s^2
Uric acid	5034.0 4956.1	4952.5
Glucose	0.574 0.549	0.546
Phosphate	0.0237 0.0233	0.0230
Creatinine	105.7 112.7	86.9
Cholesterol (chemical method)	1.03 1.06	0.767
Cholesterol (enzymatic method)	1.10 1.08	1.10

To conclude this first part, we can say that when a good level of reproducibility is reached, it does not seem necessary to perform duplicate measurements. On the other hand, the influence of analytic variation on physiological variations can be reduced by duplicate measurements, where reproducibility is not too good.

One can also consider a change in methodology: in the case of cholesterol, the enzymatic method yields better results than the chemical method and it is not necessary to perform duplicate measurements.

3.1.2. Study of accuracy

In the study of reference values, one must not satisfy himself with reproducible methods, the leitmotif that developed with the advent of automatic instruments. As *Annino* said [9], accuracy must be an important criterion in the choice of a method.

The accuracy of methods can be approached through a comparative study of different commercial control serums, or through participation in inter-laboratory quality controls. These are, then, either punctual controls or controls covering six months or a year. Comparative accuracy, on a longer-term basis, can be studied the way Williams does it, on control serums. It can also be studied by taking the monthly average of the patients (7.1).

Hoffmann [10] was the first to speak of using the patients' average as a means of controlling the reproducibility of measurement techniques. This technique may be used differently, by calculating not the daily average but the monthly average of the same patients. For this calculation, the extreme pathological or sub-pathological values should be eliminated, as well as certain sources of great physiological variations.

For example, the values of results obtained for children should not be used.

With this technique, different types of errors may be detected: errors due to a reference material, errors due to a problem of reagent stability.

3.1.2.1. Calibration problem

The use of automatic instruments, and particularly continuous flow instruments, practically imposes the use of commercial titrated lyophilized control serums to calibrate. These serums are available in bulk for one or two years of operation.

Two examples will demonstrate the danger of such use. Figure 1 represents the variation of the monthly average of calcium (complexon cresolphthaleine, method SMA 12/60) during the years 1971 to 1974. One observes a very clear break in March 1972, then another one – a little less distinct, in December 1973. These two breaks correspond to two changes in batches of calibration serum.

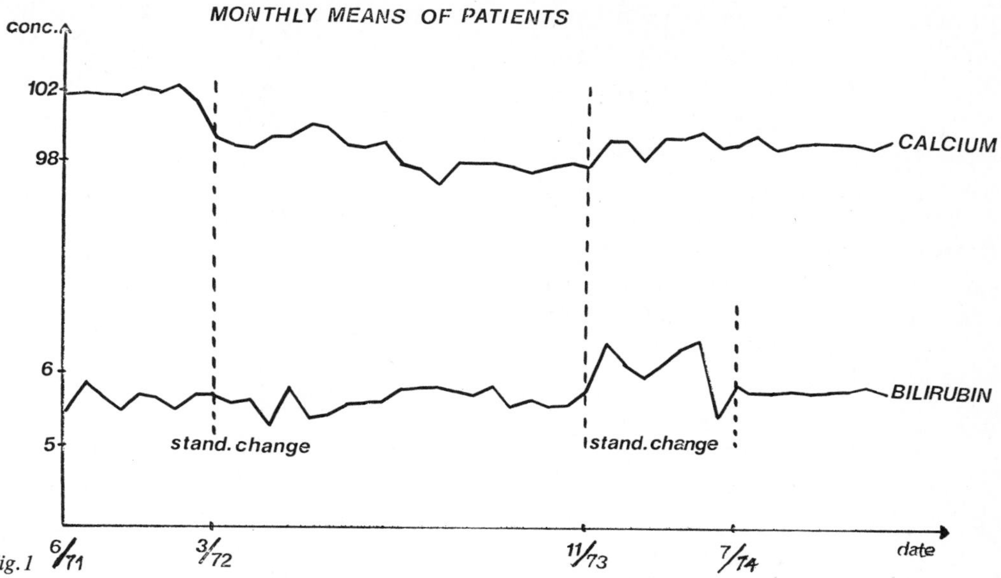

Fig. 1

In the same figure 1, one can follow the variations of the monthly average of total bilirubin (caffeine with benzoate – method SMA 12/60) over the same time period. No variation in this average is observed with the change in batches of serum in March 1972. However, in December 1973, one observes simultaneously a slight increase, and a greater dispersion of the results obtained. In July 1974, a standard in accordance with the CAP recommendations is used for bilirubin [11]. The stability of the monthly average has, since then, been remarkable.

Another error due to calibration is a bit different. It concerns the stability of the reconstituted lyophilized serum. The evolution of the alkaline phosphatase concentration in a reconstituted lyophilized serum has already been studied by a number of authors [12].

Each morning, the amount of serum necessary for the day's work is put into solution. Table 5 shows the significant variations obtained in the duplicate measurement of alkaline phosphatase, performed on patient specimens at two hour-intervals (paranitrophenyl-phosphate – method SMA 12/60). The difference between the measurements is small, but always in the same direction.

Table 5. Variation in the measurement of alkaline phosphatase, effect of time, 60 duplicate samples analyzed in a period of two hours

Mean of differences	1.52 mU/ml
Variance	3.12
Student test	$t = 6.74$

$t > 3.29$ $p = 0.001$

A serum put into solution the day before, and measured against a serum freshly put into solution, shows an increase in the level of alkaline phosphatase of between 10 and 20%.

3.1.2.2. Problem of the reagents

The monthly average of patients enables us to study the stability of the reagents. Phosphate (phosphomolybdate – stannous chloride – hydrazine sulfate – SMA 12/60) is one example shown in fig. 2. Until January 1972, stannous chloride in a hydrochloric solution was prepared once a month or more, according to the need for it. Only the mixture of stannous chloride and hydrazine sulfate was prepared daily.

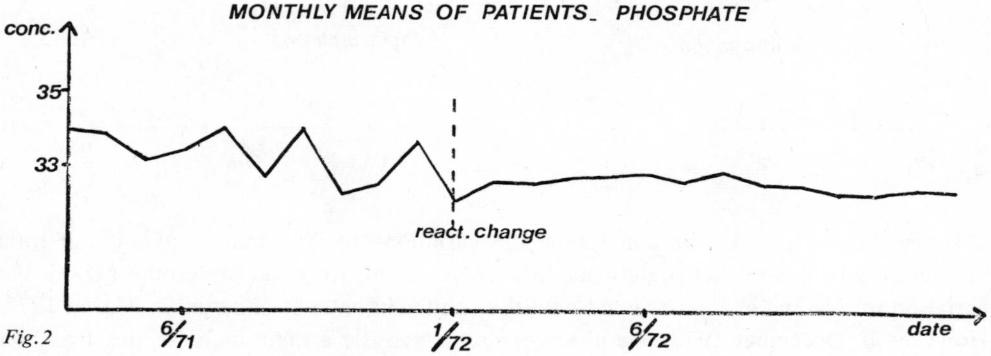

Fig. 2

From January 1972, the stannous chloride solution was prepared each week. One then observes a very good stability of the patients' monthly average.

An error in accuracy involving, this time, the purity of the reagents, can again be brought out, thanks to the patients' monthly average. Figure 3 shows the variation of the average of lactic dehydrogenase (kinetic at 37 °C – optimized reagents – Automate 5010 Eppendorf). A very clear break is observed for July 1974. It corresponds to a change in the batches of reagents, which causes an increase of about 10 mU/ml in the results. This variation is probably due to the purity of $NADH_2$, which can contain either inhibitors or activators. On the graph corresponding to the same period (fig. 3), we do not observe the same variations for alanine aminotransferase (ALT). They are probably hidden by the great physiological variations. It is indeed important to note that the monthly averages can be used correctly to study the variations in accuracy of different methodologies only if the physiological variations are not too great.

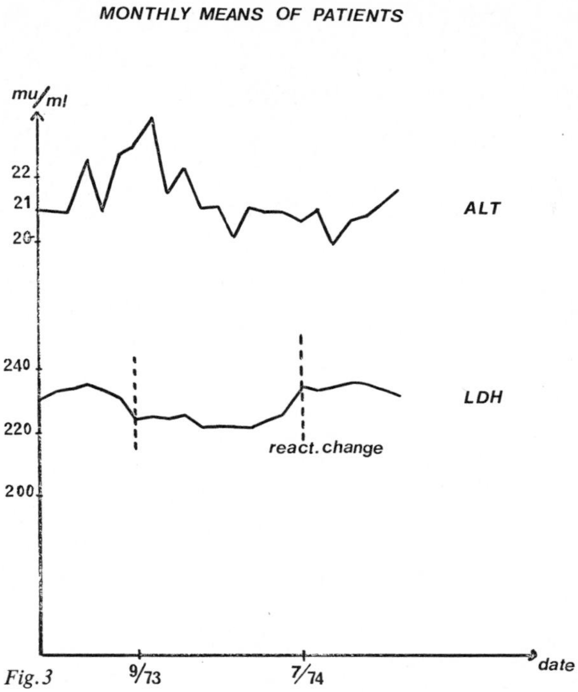

Fig. 3

Another error, which is not detected by taking the patient's monthly average, but which is nevertheless due to a problem of reagent stability, can be discussed here. This error is brought out by an analysis of variance performed on a daily duplicate measurement of a control serum. Table 6 shows that the values for aspartate aminotransferase (AST) differ significantly at the outset and at the end of a series of analyses ($F = 7.5$). The instrument cannot be questioned, since ALT is measured with the same instrument, and this type of error does not occur. It is, therefore, the stability of reagents put into solution each day, which is questionable.

Table 6. Variance analysis

AST

Origin of the variation	Squares sums	Degrees of freedom	Variance	'F' test
Total	19.24	39	0.49	
Between days	11.37	19	0.60	2.0
Between samples	2.25	1	2.25	7.5
Remainder	5.62	19	0.30	

ALT

Origin of the variation	Squares sums	Degrees of freedom	Variance	'F' test
Total	20.69	39	0.53	
Between days	8.81	19	0.46	0.74
Between samples	0.006	1	0.006	0.01
Remainder	11.86	9	0.62	

Significance levels

$F^{19}_{19} = 2.16 \ (p < 0.05)$

$F^{1}_{19} = 4.38 \ (p < 0.05)$

The problems of accuracy that have just been raised, are only problems of comparative accuracy. It is interesting, however, to try to attain real accuracy. In doing so, the problem of standards and especially of the choice of techniques, and their specificity, is raised.

3.1.2.3. Choice of standards

For a purist, there can be but one standard per compound to be measured. This standard must be clearly defined chemically. Unfortunately, in daily laboratory practice, with the development of automatic instruments, the technician must often call upon substitute solutions which prove to be more or less satisfying.

These problems have already been widely discussed, particularly at the International Conference in Atlanta [13]. We call to mind here the preceding example of bilirubin, whose analytical variations were reduced because a standard recommended by the NBS was used.

3.1.2.4. Choice of techniques

Numerous international authorities are presently studying one technique after another. For instance, the NBS has studied the measurement of calcium by atomic absorption [14], the F. D. A. has studied the measurement of glucose [15].

Specificity is as important in preventive medicine as in curative medicine.

For instance, for triglycerides, we preferred the Soloni technique to the enzymatic technique. Indeed, the interferences pointed out in the literature concerning the latter technique are much more numerous, in particular the influence of endogenous glycerol in the specimen, which is especially important in enzymatic techniques, since it is not eliminated (either by extraction or absorption) before analysis [16].

We can also mention the influence of alkaline phosphatases, whose high activity in children and adolescents can disturb the measurement of triglycerides. The predictive value of triglyceride measurements for these age groups is now recognized.

These were only some examples of analytical problems. It is also necessary to emphasize other controls, such as the specimen treatment, the water purity, the instrument control, the electricity stability and to mention the influence of the proportion of staff members, etc. ...

3.2. The prime role of blood sampling

The greatest efforts to attain precision and accuracy are in vain if the sample has not been taken properly. Errors at this stage of the analysis can be very important. For instance, certain parameters vary according to posture. Slight variations will have to be interpretable, and sampling conditions set up to reduce the causes of error at this level [17]. The following should be given particular attention:

Posture
The place and type of blood drawn
The sampling technique (tourniquet – desinfectant)
The material used: syringe or not – type of needle
Recipient for collecting the blood
Nature of the anticoagulant

Information concerning the subject is taken at the same time: the patient's identification and age, some clinical information (jaundice), treatment followed (anticoagulants, antibiotics), the time and date of the sampling, as well as the intake of a meal.

The information collected on the subject's condition, as well as on the sampling itself, will be useful in selecting homogeneous groups.

Since the purpose of describing a method is to be sure of mastering it, the condition of the subject prior to sampling must be described. The dialogue established with the patient (at the time of sampling) is important.

No one is in a better position than the clinical chemist to educate the patient and explain the precautions that are to be taken to avoid individual variations that would be too great.

This privileged moment conditions the quality of the analyses, and influences the evolution of our discipline. The clinical chemist must always remain accessible and available for patients and clinicians. This would avoid a tendency toward a 'general check-up' where samplings and analyses would be automatic, not controlled; the results, therefore, inprecise and useless.

3.3. Selection of homogeneous population or sub-groups

The criteria for selecting populations must be precise, easy to use and to control. These criteria can be gathered by means of questionnaires, or other measures.

Categories of information for the selection of homogeneous populations

1. Age – Sex
2. Selection based on questionnaires, surveys:
   general questionnaires
   specialized questionnaires
3. Selection based on morphological criteria:
   size
   weight
   skin foldsideness
   ...
4. Selection based on genetic factors:
   blood types
   isoenzymes
   tissue group
   ...
5. Selection based on physiological measurements:
   blood pressure
   respiratory capacity
   ...
6. Selection based on clinical criteria
7. Selection based on other biological tests.

These criteria will be developed at the forthcoming colloquium in Toronto [18].

Among the advantages and the usefulness of reference values for a clearly defined population, the standardization of methods and tests should be mentioned, since, as we have demonstrated, slight variations can be detected using the monthly averages of the population. This is particularly true and necessary for enzymatic and immunologic methods, for which reference materials are not available.

Finally, the study and the control of analytical and biological variations can be useful for choosing laboratory tests suited to the definition of states of health. The choice of these tests must be based not so much on acquired experience in pathology, as on the sensible physiological or environmental variations of human plasma or blood cells constituents. This will only be possible with accurate (and precise) reference methods.

References

[1] *Claude Bernard:* Introduction à la médecine expérimentale.

[2] *M.C.Sanz:* 2e colloque international 'Automatisation et Biologie Prospective' de Pont-à-Mousson, 1972 (communication orale).

[3] *E.Cheraskin and W.M.Rigsdorf:* Predictive medicine. A study in strategy. Mountain view, Pacific Press Publ., 1973, 182 p.

[4] *T.P.Whitehead (Birmingham): chairman, R.Gräsbeck (Helsinki), G.Siest (Nancy), G.Z.Williams (San Francisco):* International Federation of Clinical Chemistry, Expert Panel on Theory of Reference Values.

[5] *G.Siest (Nancy), président, J.P.Bretaudière (Paris), J.Dorche (Lyon), M.Nyssen (Lyon), C.Sachs (Paris), J.Buret (Liège), C.Heusghem (Liège), R.Zehnder (La Chaux-de-Fonds):* Société Française de Biologie Clinique, commission Valeurs de Référence.

[6] *H.Büttner:* Präzisierung von Normalwertbereichen. In: Optimierung der Diagnostik. *H.Land, W.Rick, L.Roka:* Springer Verlag Ed., 1973.

[7] Biological and analytic components of variation in longterm studies of serum constituents in normal subjects.

1. *G. Z. Williams, D. S. Young, M. R. Stein, E. Cotlove:* Objectives, subject selection, laboratory procedures and estimation of analytic deviation. Clin. Chem., 1970, *16,* 1016.
2. *E. K. Harris, P. Kanofosky, G. Shakarji, E. Cotlove:* Estimating biological components of variation. Clin. Chem., 1970, *16,* 1022.
3. *E. Cotlove, E. K. Harris, G. Z. Williams:* Physiological and medical implications. Clin. Chem., 1970, *16,* 1028.
4. *D. S. Young, E. K. Harris, E. Cotlove:* Results of a study designed to eliminate long-term analytic deviations. Clin. Chem., 1971, *17,* 403.

[8] *H.Bokelund, P.Winkel, E.Statland:* Factors contributing to intra-individual variation of serum constituents: 3. Use of randomized duplicate serum specimens to evaluate sources of analytical error. Clin. Chem., 1974, *20,* 1507.

[9] *J.S.Annino, L.A.Williams:* Clin. Chem., 1972, *18,* 488.

[10] *R.G.Hoffmann:* Establishing quality control and normal ranges in the clinical laboratory. Exposition Press, New York 1971.

[11] CAP: College of American Pathologists: Recommendation on a uniform bilirubin standard. Clin. Chem., 1962, *8,* 405.

[12] *G.Szasz:* Scand. J. Clin. Lab. Invest., 1972, *29,* 126.

[13] International conference on standardization of diagnostic materials sponsored by W.H.O. and C.D.C., Atlanta, 1973.

[14] National Bureau of Standards. Clinical chemistry interaction plan to develop reference methods.

[15] Food and drug administration. Federal register, 1974.
[16] *T. O. Tiffany, J. M. Morton, E. M. Holl, A. S. Garret:* Clin. Chem., 1974, *20,* 476.
[17] *B. E. Statland, H. Bokelund, P. Winkel:* Clin. Chem., 1974, *20,* 1513.
[18] *G. Siest:* Reference values in human chemistry. International congress on clinical chemistry, July 13–18, 1975, Toronto.

International Criteria for Diagnostic Methods

Discussions

G. Anido (U.S.A.): It has been our privilege to have a distinguished panel of clinical chemists give us their thoughts on what should be the international criteria for diagnostic methods.

I see my role here as that of a catalytic agent stimulating discussion to a series of problems the clinical laboratory faces as it applies to the subject of diagnostic methods. There is no question, that methods developed in one country are being used on an increasing frequency in other countries. The problem is compounded by the fact that new instrumentation specifically designed for given test procedures is being constantly offered to the chemistry laboratory.

During the past ten years, the clinical laboratory in general, and in particular the chemistry laboratory, has expanded in a geometric progression on the services it provides to the practicing physician. However, this expansion of tests has not resulted in an equally expanded acceptance of results by the same physician. To me this is most dramatically apparent in the area of the clinical diagnosis of myocardial infarcts. I am convinced the chemistry laboratory through a battery of enzyme and isoenzyme tests has a lot to offer to the internist; yet, most of the cardiologists with whom I have discussed this topic are more inclined to put their faith on the EKG tracing and only give a casual consideration to the chemistries. The explanation I get most often is that enzyme determinations are a jungle, where methods, units, normal values, sensitivity either too low or too high, and questionable specificity makes interpretation difficult.

The following are questions I wish to submit to you to get the discussion started:

1. Are we in the 70's living up to the claim that this would be the decade of accuracy?
2. What should we do at the international level about immunoassay procedures?
3. Should official publications of societies of clinical chemistry check on claims of performance of methods submitted for publication?
4. Should societies of clinical chemistry check on claims of performance of 'referee' methods?
5. Why is it there are so few on-going standardization programs?
6. Should societies of clinical chemistry check on the educational standards of the technical personnel?

I feel that a justification of the above questions is in line, so that the discussion may be more productive.

Q.1 Are we in the 70's living up to the claims that this would be the decade of accuracy?

The clinical chemist would have a hard time, in this day and age, trying to build up a case in favor of poor accuracy in an analytical procedure; yet, we do have to strike a happy medium as it applies to the information we are after, in terms of the medical significance a determination may provide.

I will not bring up at this time the question of accuracy in enzyme determinations. However, I will list the calcium concentrations of four specimens obtained by nine referee laboratories participating in the ASCP Clinical Chemistry Check, Sample No. CC-90 (1974).

	Calcium Concentration (mg/dl)	
Unknown	Mean	Range
A	9.50	9.1– 9.9
B	9.56	9.0– 9.9
C	10.03	9.4–10.5
D	8.01	7.5– 8.3

The accuracy of these values from a series of referee laboratories shows a rather wide range of values, well in excess of the 2% allowed by the referee method for calcium.

I consider this exercise quite revealing, in that all four unknowns contain calcium in aqueous solution and unknowns A and B were blind duplicates.

If we take unknown D, we notice that values range from 7.5 to 8.3 mg/dl. This represents a spread of 0.8 mg/dl. Would this be medically significant if we were dealing with a patient's serum? Would we make an error of clinical judgement if, for example, unknown D was actually from a patient and we were to have it reported as having a concentration of 7.5 mg/dl? Would it make any difference if the report came in as being 8.5 mg/dl? Should we have expected a wider range of values if the unknowns had been serum specimens rather than aqueous solutions?

Q.2 What should be done at the international level about immunoassay procedures?

Immunoassay procedures, of which radioimmunoassays constitute the great majority, are just becoming as complicated as the field of diagnostic enzymology. Practically every day there is a new method out, with a new set of normals based on the nature of the antibody.

I have recently reviewed the Digoxin values obtained from a series of patients, using three different methods with three different antibodies. The data clearly shows that each antibody reacts in a different manner, with results being biased accordingly. Similar situations apply practically to every radioimmunoassay procedure.

We are again creating a situation where the physician requesting a determination by RIA will end up getting widely divergent results, depending on the type of procedure followed by the laboratory.

Q.3 Should official publications of societies of clinical chemistry be required to check on claims of new methods submitted for publication?

I am sure that at one time or another some of you have tried to set up a procedure published in a journal and have found out that the method does not work as expected. This is frustration of the highest degree. Communication with the author may or may not provide the clue as to why the procedure did not work. We have heard Dr. Copeland's recent experience on this subject.

Since an increasing number of the procedures that are published are later on placed into the market as a 'kit', it would appear that some 'proof of claims' should be demanded from the author by the Editor of the Journal. In my mind, such action would result in a general improvement in the quality of new procedures and would eliminate practically all the sources of frustration in not being able to make a method work, based on its published description. In addition, if the new method should find its way into the market-place, we would have available a published reference as to the accuracy, precision, sensitivity and specificity of the method.

Q.4 What should be the role of the societies of clinical chemistry as it applies to claims of performance of 'referee' methods?

We may be having a series of 'referee' methods made available to us in the near future. It is hoped that a 'referee' method will solve problems related to the proper determination of a given constituent. However, we must have available to us information as to how the 'referee' method came to be. Before a 'referee' method is worked on, it would appear that the national society should first make available to their membership the proposed 'referee' method so that laboratory workers may know ahead of time what it is about. There is always the possibility that a better method may be suggested. Also, the proposed method should also be made available to the international forum, so that here again better methods may be submitted or improvements to the proposed method may be offered. Once the 'referee' method is worked out by the author and field tested by a select group of laboratories, it should be the responsibility of the national society of clinical chemistry of the country where it was developed to have it checked out by several laboratories at the international level. This applies specifically to the claims of performance of the 'referee' method. These should not only be closely scrutinized by a panel of members of the national society, but should also be confirmed by other laboratories at the international level. Not to do so would put the 'referee' methods down the same path to obscurity suffered by the so-called 'Standard Methods' in clinical chemistry of several years ago.

Q.5 Why is it there are so few on-going standardization programs?

It would appear that concerned clinical chemists would welcome standardization programs such as the Cholesterol and Triglycerides Standardization Program conducted by CDC – WHO and which was the subject of Dr. *G. Cooper's* award lecture. Our chemistry laboratory at DADE joined that program several years ago in the section dealing with triglycerides standardization. At the time we joined, there were over one hundred laboratories in the program. It is somewhat disappointing to notice that, not only did the number of participating laboratories not increase, but actually many laboratories have dropped out from the program. In my mind, the Triglycerides Standardization Program is an exciting exercise which induces a participating laboratory to take a good look at the method in use and make the necessary corrections in order to meet the demands for accuracy and precision established by the organizers of the program, on the basis of realistic goals.

We need more involvement along the lines of standardization programs and, perhaps, less rhetoric to cover up existing indifference toward an effective means of accomplishing good correlation at the national and the international levels.

Q.6 Should societies of clinical chemistry check on the education standards of the technical personnel?

It appears as if there is an increasing gap between what is known about clinical chemistry today and the educational preparation of the average clinical chemistry technologist. We must keep in mind that no matter how much government intervention there is as to how a kit is prepared, or an instrument is assembled, or a piece of glass is calibrated, in the last analysis the test is going to be performed by a technologist.

An example of what I mean may be found in the January 1975 issue of *Summary Report,* published by the American Society of Clinical Pathologists. Under the title 'Serious Error in UV Enzymes' we are told how a 17-year old girl with acute hepatitis was misdiagnosed as obstructive jaundice and operated upon, because of the reporting of normal values for SGOT and SGPT. In retrospect, she was found to have extremely high levels of SGOT and SGPT, which were missed entirely.

It appears that the U.V. kinetic procedures for SGOT and SGPT were changed in this particular laboratory, in that first, ten specimens were prepared at a time, with a zero time reading at 30-second intervals, in such a manner that the tenth specimen would be using up substrate for five minutes before it was read. Then, a second reading of the unknown was made five minutes after the zero time reading and linearity of reaction assumed. The fact that the initial absorbance ($t = 0$) was quite low did not appear to be significant to the laboratory worker and so when the second value ($t = 5$ minutes) showed only minimal change, resulting in a low delta absorbance, a report of a normal value was issued.

The points to be considered in this example are as follows:

1. How can a kinetic method be arbitrarily transformed into an end-point methodology?
2. Why was the low time zero absorbance accepted, not even questioned?
3. What useful purpose is there to be served by a government agency demanding the manufacturer to make endless specifications about his product if there is no check on the technical ability of the user? Please notice I have not used the word 'qualifications'. Most likely the changes in the method were made by a 'qualified' person by virtue of a diploma or a license.

The end of the sad story I have related is that based on the normal SGOT and SGPT results issued by the laboratory, the patient was operated on as having an obstructive jaundice and died several days afterwards as the result of an operation that should have never taken place.

Now I would like to open the discussion on the six questions I have put up to you.

P. Cali (U.S.A.): With regard to the question on checking reference methods. Certainly everything concerned with the issue of an official method should be subject to the most vigorous checking in every possible way. I would point out that the Calcium Reference Method has been not only checked, but utilized in the United Kingdom by Dr. *Mitchell's* laboratory at the CRC. There is now a potential proposal within EEC to check that method throughout Europe. I certainly encourage it. As a matter of fact, I think the answer is that you must follow the procedure of extensive checking. I would also like to point out that within the National Committee on Clinical Laboratory Standards (NCCLS) in the United States, the calcium reference method is now undergoing the consensus process, and beyond that through the World Health Organization. In summary, I am very much in favor of extensive testing of referee methods.

W. Gruber (Germany): I would like to try to answer one of the questions posed by Dr. *Brown*. This is the question, 'should definitive and reference methods be tested in the context of pathological or potentially interfering substances as well as normal ones?' I would like to say a few words on our philosophy of how we try to become aware of interferences with new methods. Interferences with new methods can not be evaluated by quality control with the usual accuracy controls. Special determinations are necessary to determine interferences by turbidity, anti-coagulants, bilirubin, hemoglobin, etc. But special determinations must also be done to establish interference by therapeutic agents, and now we have developed a way to do this. First of all, we classified the most important drugs according to their chemical composition. Then a list is made up of some 20 reactive groups of importance.

From this, the drug which is prescribed in the highest dosage is selected and added to a serum pool to determine its interference. If it interferes at all, in-vivo experiments with the same drug are carried out. In most cases, it has been found that interference in vivo is much lower than expected. Of course, there is one exception. This exception is found in the sera of uremic patients. We feel that the most stringent check of interferences is determination on sera of uremic patients, since in these sera we have found practically all the interferences that may be found under pathological conditions. The best way to do this is to have available a very specific method known to be free of interferences; then the new method is compared against the well established reference method and its correlation is calculated. If there is no such interference-free method, then recovery experiments are performed, by the addition of the constituent to the serum after first removing the internal constituent. That may be done adequately by using a carrier-bound enzyme which destroys the specific compound in the sample; then the enzyme is removed, and now you are ready to perform recovery experiments. We think this is the best way to determine what the interferences are, without a lot of work.

H. Büttner (Germany): May I add that the definition of reference methods to which Dr. *Brown* referred, says 'after exhaustive testing'. I think all these points are included under the heading of exhaustive testing.

H. Bergmeyer (Germany): I would like to make some remarks about Dr. Vanzetti's lecture. The members from the biochemical research industry present here must be quite amazed by the listing of possible complaints that Dr. *Vanzetti* has compiled. I am sure that the ethical and biochemical research industry does far more than this NATO Committee wants to be done. I would like to invite the members of this committee to our plant to show them what we do before a new kit is brought out. And I would like to ask Dr. Vanzetti whether his committee includes researchers from industry who are engaged in developing methods and kits? If the committee in question does not include this type of member, I cannot see how this paper could be accepted by industry, or by the IFCC for that matter.

G. Vanzetti (Italy): Our guidelines call for strict cooperation between scientists, professional associations, governmental agencies, and manufacturers of diagnostic products. I want to stress the need for cooperation: I think this is a most important point. Of course, I have listed many complaints, but this should not be interpreted as criticism of industry as a whole. In Italy, we are planning now to set up contacts between industry representatives and the Italian Society of Clinical Biochemistry in order to work on these problems. I believe that regulation by consensus is the best way to solve the problems; and I am quite aware of the problems which have to be solved by industry. I have also said that I recognize the importance of the contributions made by industry in our field. Therefore, I must stress the need for mutual understanding.

On the other hand, not seeing the difficulties and insisting that everything is alright would never help solve any problem.

On the question about the presence of representatives of industry on our committee, my answer is 'no', our committee is made up only of analysts. I realize that the viewpoint of analysts could perhaps not coincide with those of industry.

R. Wieme (Belgium): I should like to point out that in general all recommendations given by Dr. *Vanzetti* are listed in most kits on the market, but that does not mean that the given recommendations are true. For instance, in the case of enzyme determinations, the methodology and composition of the reagents are listed, but the control criteria at the production level in industry are not the same as the control criteria in your own laboratory. For example, buffer capacities may not be strong enough to balance serum capacities. And here I should like to point out something that is very important. Regarding control serum, Dr. *Louderback* spoke this morning about the fact that serum has a pH of 7.4. This is not so. Serum has a basic pH, between 8.5 and 9. So if you determine enzyme activity in control serum, which has a pH of 7.4, you do not have the same conditions as are found in serum from patients in your own laboratory.

I know by experience that most buffers which are produced in industry for CPK determinations are between 7 and 7.2. The optimum pH for CPK activity determination is at pH 7 or 6.95. Accordingly, the production criteria followed by industry of using a pH between 7 and 7.2 can make a difference.

P. Wilding (U.K.): I should like to comment on the series of questions raised by Dr. *Anido* which I think are really close to the vital issues which we should be considering. His first question raised was, 'How do we face the problem of accuracy in the 70's?'. I think our record, on the whole, shows that progress has been made, but that progress is far from satisfactory. It is because of this lack of progress that we have seen the introduction or arrival of governmental and international agencies on the scene. Furthermore, it is because of the failure of the profession. The arrival of those agencies is essential because they are the people with money, but if we lose our influence on those agencies, then I think the situation will not improve. The way to exert that influence, I think, is the way in which Dr. Anido perhaps posed his final question, and that is by education. Most of the organizations of which we are part, do have some mechanism of accredition or the awarding of higher qualifications, and it is only by that mechanism, that the influence that we have can be exerted. I would like to compliment Dr. Anido because I think it is these issues which really are important, not perhaps other small issues which are being overdiscussed.

S. Rosalki (U.K.): I should like to comment on Dr. *Gruber's* remarks on screening for interferences. While his aim is laudible, I think it is inadequate to screen reactive or potentially interfering groups *in-vitro*, and *then* to proceed to examine *in-vivo*, *only* those compounds which *in-vitro* screening shows might interfere. The reason I consider this inadequate, is simply that in many cases it may be the *metabolite* of the compound that interferes.

A. Rappoport (U. S. A.): The title of this symposium is called 'The Clinical Laboratory from an International Viewpoint' and, therefore, I would like to represent the clinical fraternity for a moment. May I point out that while we have heard extremely vital data and input about the technical area, let's not forget the medical arena in which we are working. I would like to emphasize that, in connection with accuracy and precision, you are in a clinical laboratory. For instance, the question of validating the clinical usefulness of cardiac enzymes obviously should go back either to a normal person or a sick patient. To review the chemical data without consideration of the clinical picture is, of course, a weak point. Most of the physicians in the audience are quite well acquainted with the fact that in many cases, the cardiac enzyme studies will show severe myocardial disease while the EKG will not. I think of the arrythmias, the bundle-branch blocks, the Wolff-Parkinson-White syndromes. It seems to me that we must never forget that we must return eventually to the patient, to establish the ultimate verity of our data. In a practical sense, there so often are discrepancies between what the bench laboratory data reveals and what the EKG will reveal.

Another clinically significant problem requires emphasis even though it's not directly concerned with quality control. It is the question of exposure to disease as a result of handling clinical material. I trust that most of you are acquainted with the hazards of such possibilities as hepatitis, and how we must control our methods of handling the serums and plasmas that come to us.

So, I repeat this plea, that we are not in a laboratory of pure, people-unrelated chemistry, but are dealing with living persons. We must constantly bear in mind, that in addition to quality control, appropriate environmental conditions must be established to produce highest clinical reliability, usefulness and safety.

H. Bergmeyer (Germany): I have a question for Dr. *Bowers*. I am referring to the standard reference material for enzymes which you mentioned. Earlier in the morning we heard the list of requirements for standard reference materials, given by Dr. *Louderback*. My question is, how do you intend to prepare such an enzyme standard reference material, how will you keep it constant, and how will you keep it stable?

G. Bowers (U. S. A.): I have specifically included the work that has come out of Albany by Vanderlinde and Rej because I believe they have answered this very well in their publications. I also know of the work that is going in your organization where ASAT from human source of similar degree of purity has been characterized and referenced against, I believe swine kidney ASAT. We have a primary human material which seems to have excellent characteristics of stability. It has been reproduced in several different batches now as a primary human material that would be a sort of a definitive material. This has now been transmitted, for comparison in several laboratories with a material from another species but shown to be extremely similar. What we cannot do, perhaps, is to put human material out all over the world, but we can translate it into equivalent animal material showing similar kinetics. In my mind, this has been the first example where we have a clear-cut indication that this route can go the same way it can with calcium. Now, there will have to be confirmation of this in many laboratories, but in a half-dozen laboratories I know who have worked with human ASAT, there seems to be a cluster of opinion that this material can be stabilized. This is a very exciting area.

H. Bergmeyer (Germany): I think there are fundamental differences between a reference standard material, like glucose, which can be a primary standard, and reference material consisting of enzymes.

In case of enzymes, you have to define the reference material by a method which later on should be checked against this reference material. I cannot understand the need to extend the good idea of a standard reference material to enzymes.

G. Bowers (U. S. A.): A standard reference material can, if necessary, be mud from the bottom of a swamp with some lead in it that's extremely homogenized, if it is prepared in such a format, in a very complex matrix, that everyone looking at it, with the proper technique, can come up with a similar answer. It does not have to have the property of being glucose, which is a fundamental, elemental type of thing that we can analyse in some other way. Now, I do think that with these highly purified materials, and the fact that batch after batch can be made in a very similar way (they have had a fair amount of work done now on their amino acid composition), there are ways to test them besides just for their enzymatic activity. I think we are getting to the point where they are approaching credence by other criteria than just activity. This will bear the test of time and I will stick my neck out and say that we have a model that can lead us into an interaction between material and methods, which we have not previously had. Previously, all we've done is run around and say, 'I've got a better method than you have', and we have had nothing to interact. Now, if you will look carefully at Rej's paper, you'll find that he has tested several methods and has shown they are biased because of protein related effects that we hadn't understood until we used the material to interact with it, I believe it's a model that could be pursued.

Earlier, we had a comment that somebody had suggested, I think it was Dr. *Louderback,* that maybe we had recommended placental alkaline phosphatase. There has been a great effort to study this constituent, but I do not know of anyone who has seriously proposed it as a standard in the same sense that is now being proposed for ASAT.

Session III

Topic: International Criteria for Clinical Laboratory Instrumentation

Session-Chairman: E. J. van Kampen, Holland
Discussion-Leader: G. Sims, USA

Opening Remarks

E.J. van Kampen, Holland

I am pleased to open this IFCC-session III, which is devoted to 'International Criteria for Clinical laboratory instrumentation'.

Instrumentation and Clinical Chemistry are more and more dependent on each other.

We even have the impression that, in some cases, so-called normal values have become *instrument-dependent* values and a so called normal range is determined more by method and instrument than by physiological considerations.

Analysing this inter-dependency – as we are supposed to do – often creates the impression that there exists a lack of communication.

This session will attempt to improve this situation and try to provide an answer to many of the questions confronting us.

National Committee for Clinical Laboratory Standards A Model for achieving International Clinical Laboratory Consensus Standards

R. G. Nadeau, Villanova, Pennsylvania (U.S.A.)

Key Words: Instrumentation
National Committee for Clinical Laboratory Standards
Standardization

Thank you for the opportunity to present my views on how to develop international criteria for clinical laboratory instrumentation. I come here not only as a representative of the American National Committee For Clinical Laboratory Standards, but also as a member of the clinical instrumentation manufacturing industry.

To develop a scientific instrument, the manufacturer must first search and analyze the market in hopes that he can identify a problem that needs to be solved, as well as one that he has the resources to solve. Too often because of inaccurate information, the manufacturer makes the fatal mistake at this very first step in the development process and sets out to solve the wrong problem. After making the product development selection, he immediately begins to share in the many problems presented by Dr. *Mitchell* and Mr. *Broughton.* These problems, which are extremely difficult, if not impossible, for the developer to cope with on a domestic basis, are still further complicated when he considers the international market with its language, terminology and environmental differences.

In 1968, a small group of individuals in the United States felt one answer was to have better communication between professional organizations, government agencies and the manufacturers of clinical laboratory products. As a result, the American National Committee For Clinical Laboratory Standards was organized to provide a forum and a mechanism through which these parties could work together to develop the consensus agreement essential for high quality clinical laboratory standards.

Today NCCLS' membership has grown to include 18 professional organizations, 7 governmental agencies and 58 companies. Each member organization has a voting delegate and an alternate (see fig. 1).

18	Professional Associations
7	Government Agencies
58	Industrial Organizations

Each member organization is represented by 1 voting delegate and 1 alternate delegate.

Fig. 1. Membership of the National Committee for Clinical Laboratory Standards (NCCLS)

The bylaws of NCCLS require that a balance between the industrial and the non-industrial segments exist on the Board of Directors (see fig. 2).

President	Nathan Gochman, Ph. D. Veteran's Administration
President Elect	Richard G. Nadeau, Ph. D. Du Pont Instruments
Secretary-Treasurer	John A. O'Malley, Ph. D. Oxford Laboratories
Executive Director	John N. McConnell NCCLS
Director	George N. Bowers, Jr., M. D. Hartford Hospital
Director	James E. French SAMA
Director	Helene Loux, Ph. D. Northeastern University
Director	Robert W. Pritchard, M. D. Bowman Gray School of Medicine
Director	Robert Schaffer, Ph. D. National Bureau of Standards
Director	Hariette D. Vera, Ph. D. BioQuest

Executive Office: 771 East Lancaster Avenue, Villanova, Pennsylvania, 19085 USA

Fig. 2. Officers and directors for the National Committee for Clinical Laboratory Standards

	Chairman
Clinical Chemistry	Theodore Peters, Ph. D.
Labeling	Alfred H. Free, Ph. D.
Hematology	Leonard S. Kaplow, M. D.
Immunohematology/Blood Banking	Chester M. Zmijewski, Ph. D.
Instrumentation	G. Phillip Hicks, Ph. D.
Kits and Reagents	James O. Westgard, Ph. D.
Microbiology	Albert Balows, Ph. D.
Ad hoc committees	
Product Class Standards	Alfred H. Free, Ph. D.
Task forces	
Radioactive Materials	William D. Odell, M. D., Ph. D.

Fig. 3. Area committees of the National Committee for Clinical Laboratory Standards

Reporting to the Board of Directors are 7 standing area committees, 1 task force and 1 ad hoc committee (see fig. 3). It is in these groups and in their subcommittees that the real consensus process begins. Again, the bylaws of NCCLS and the operating procedures require balanced input.

The consensus process begins with the selection of an existing source document or with the development of a new source document (see fig. 4). The area committee, through many hours of meetings and discussions, attempts to resolve misunderstandings and differences prerequisite to the agreement necessary to achieve a consensus. Once this is accomplished, the area committee submits its draft of the proposed standard to the Board of Directors for approval and submission to the membership. If the Board is satisfied that a basis for consensus appears to exist, then the proposed standard is submitted to the membership for review and comment for a period of 60 days. All comments and differences arising from this survey must be adequately resolved by the area committee before the proposed standard is again submitted to the membership for final review. If adopted, the proposed standard becomes a tentative standard and will remain as such for a period of 1 year. After this year, the tentative standard is submitted again to the membership for review and comment. Once all negative comments are resolved and all necessary revisions made, the standard reaches the approved status where it will remain as such for a period of 3 years. At this time, the area committee is asked to review and determine whether any changes of a significant nature have occurred to warrant further revision. Of course, the standard could be revised at any time if a significant objection arises, or changes in the state of the art occur.

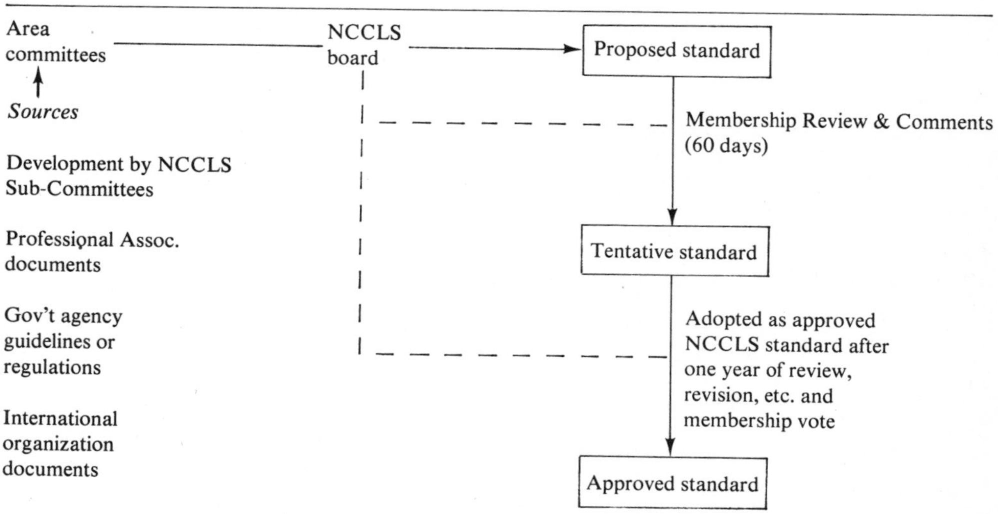

Fig. 4. Mechanism for development and adoption of clinical laboratory standards by NCCLS

In 1969, shortly after its formation, the NCCLS Area Committee on Instrumentation recognized that one of the most difficult problems facing the user of scientific equipment was the inadequacy of instruction manuals supplied by most manufacturers. Using a source document developed by the College of American Pathologists subcommittee, chaired by *Mathew M. Patton,* M. D., the NCCLS area committee developed an approved standard, 'The Preparation of Manuals for Installation, Operation and Repair of Laboratory Instruments'.

The Area Committee on Kits and Reagents has developed and recently submitted to the Board, a proposal for a standard on a protocol for the evaluation of major automated clinical chemistry systems. In addition, the membership has recently approved the Area Committee on Clinical Chemistry's standard for 'Calibrator Reference Materials and Control Products'. This document is being used as the primary source material in the development of the United States Food and Drug Administration's Product Class Standard on Calibrators. Copies of these and other NCCLS standards, which have been approved or are presently under development, may be obtained directly from NCCLS headquarters[1] (see fig. 5).

Approved

ACI-1/Preparation of Manuals for Installation, Operation and Repair of Laboratory Instruments.
ACC-1/Standardized Protein Solution (Bovine Serum Albumin).
ACM-1/Analysis of Fluorescein.
ACM-2/VDRL Antigen.
ACM-3/Buffered Saline.
ACH-1/Standard Method for the Human Erythrocyte Sedimentation Rate (E. S. R.) Test.
ACL-1/Labeling of Laboratory Reagents.
Standards for Calibration Reference & Control Materials.

Tentative Standards

Performance Standards for Antimicrobial Disc Susceptibility Tests.
Analysis of Proteins Labeled with Fluorescein Isothiocyanate.
Standards for Blood Banks and Transfusion Services.
PHS Regulation for the Manufacture of Biological Products.

Proposed Standards

A Referee Method for Determination of Total Calcium in Serum.
Reagent Water Specifications.

Fig. 5. Current status of NCCLS standards

The American NCCLS has shown that it is practical and desirable to develop widely accepted consensus standards through general agreement between various professional associations, governmental agencies and the industrial community. As Dr. *Mitchell* and

[1] National Committee For Clinical Laboratory Standards, 771 East Lancaster Avenue, Villanova, Pennsylvania 19085 USA.

Mr. *Broughton* have pointed out, there is no international mechanism for achieving this same kind of consensus. Ideally, an international body equivalent in scope and function to the American National Committee For Clinical Laboratory Standards needs to be established. At present, however, this appears to be a more long range goal. In the interim, it would seem that the expert panel, as outlined by my colleagues, could serve the international clinical laboratory instrumentation field in much the same way as NCCLS functions in America.

In order to achieve its goal, to effectively deal with the broad range of difficult problems, and to achieve general acceptance of their efforts, the expert panel should have not only geographical representation, but also from the various professional disciplines, the government sector, and industry. As an initial task, the expert panel might review, modify and seek international consensus agreement on those approved standards developed by the American NCCLS, or on other pertinent standards existing in other countries. There are no easy solutions to the problems discussed. Individual attempts to solve them have, for the most part, been unsuccessful. What is needed now, is the positive synergistic effect of mutual involvement.

International Requirements for Instrumentation in Clinical Chemistry

P.M.G.Broughton, Leeds, U.K. and *F.L.Mitchell,* Harrow (U.K.)

Key word: Instrumentation

During the last 30 years, the use of instruments in clinical chemistry has developed rapidly, and this is now a substantial and specialised market for scientific instrument manufacturers. Although many successful instruments were originally conceived by individual clinical chemists, the profession as a whole has exerted little influence on developments, either on a national or international basis. As a result, there is unnecessary duplication and competition on the world market – for example, with multichannel analysers – whereas suitable instrumentation for some areas of clinical chemistry is either inadequate or completely lacking. Although most laboratories have similar needs, there have been almost no attempts at standardisation of the design, quality or reliability of instruments. Recently, instrumentation has become increasingly complex and expensive (often unnecessarily), and the technical ingenuity and excitement of new machines has tended to obscure more fundamental issues, such as whether a new machine is really needed or economically justified.

In this paper an attempt is made to define some of the outstanding problems concerning instrumentation in clinical chemistry, and to outline possible solutions to them. The views expressed are those of the authors, not of IFCC, and are presented to stimulate discussion.

1. Terminology

There is no general agreement on terminology, so that manufacturers' specifications and users' requirements are often misunderstood because they use words in different senses. Terms such as accuracy, specificity, sensitivity, precision, resolution, etc. need to be clearly defined.

Currently, several national and international organisations are considering terminology. There is a need to bring together those terms and definitions relevant to instrumentation and make definitive recommendations for clinical chemistry. This is already being done in several areas by IFCC Expert Panels, and will be extended by the new Expert Panel on Instrumentation (see below).

2. Instrument evaluation

Users frequently need advice on selection of instruments. One method of obtaining this is by evaluating the instrument in the laboratory. This is often done rather haphazardly, so that the results cannot be repeated elsewhere, and, although some countries have comprehensive schemes for evaluating equipment, the information obtained is not generally available worldwide. Both users and manufacturers need advice on how evaluations should be made and which instrumental factors are important.

A protocol for the evaluation of instruments is required, similar to that published by *Broughton* et al. (1974), which could be accepted for use on an international basis. When an instrument is tested, it is important that there should be no obligation to the company concerned, and for this reason it is best for the instrument to be purchased as a production model, and the testing procedure carried out with only the normal service facilities provided by the manufacturer. Testing schedules for equipment should include long runs, usually in excess of 100,000 operations, aimed specifically to test the dependability of the equipment. Arrangements need to be made for evaluations to be carried out in different countries and under different environmental conditions. Unnecessary duplication of effort must be avoided, and the information gained must be made generally available by publication.

The disadvantage of this approach is the time and cost of evaluation work. An alternative would be for manufacturers to prepare precise specifications of the performance to be expected from their instruments, possibly in consultation with users. If published, this specification could then serve as a guarantee and the performance could be verified by any user. Provided that terminology was unambiguous, this might be a more rapid and realistic solution.

3. Instrumental quality

Since development has largely been in the hands of industry, commercial exploitation of the market has sometimes tended to override the primary concern for patient welfare. In some countries, commercial arguments also prevail in the laboratory where, to yield the highest financial return, the aim may be to produce the largest number of assays on a patient. Under these circumstances the quality of the work can suffer. This approach has undoubtedly stimulated the market for expensive analysers, where attention to a multichannel capability had had a higher priority than accuracy. Manufacturers are often unaware of the quality of performance required from instruments, and the profession needs to define its requirements and make these known. Manufacturers' literature should specify the performance which can be expected,in a manner which the user can understand and use.

The principles used in the calibration of some instruments, particularly multichannel analysers, are often questionable. These must be based on some absolute measurement. For example, if a colorimeter or spectrophotometer is calibrated with a pure substance weighed into solution, it must be remembered that the matrix of the material being assayed may have a profound effect upon the measurement. Allowance must be made for this by relating the measurement, where possible, to a definitive or reference method. For instruments which depend on single or two point calibration, the linearity of response must be carefully investigated. If instruments, such as multichannel analysers, require to be calibrated by a secondary standard, such as precalibrated serum, the standardisation of the secondary material must be done properly. Precalibrated material sold by manufacturers without providing details of the methods used for calibration, should not be accepted. When the accuracy of the result depends on instrumental readings or settings made by the manufacturer (e.g. temperature, absorbance, recorder chart speed), the user must be able to check these for himself.

4. Maintenance requirements

In the developed countries, the dependability (that is, freedom from breakdown) of instruments is not of prime importance, since expert knowledge, suitable equipment and spare parts are usually available to effect repairs. Consequently, manufacturers tend to develop instruments for the most lucrative market, where there are adequate servicing facilities, and do not give a sufficiently high priority to dependability. The profession has come to accept this situation, but it is possible to produce instruments which are guaranteed never to break down, and there is no reason why this should be limited to space technology. It is more an attitude of mind rather than a necessary state of affairs (*Halpin,* 1967).

Instrument manufacturers should be aware of the necessity to provide adequate maintenance facilities for their instruments in all circumstances and at all times. Users must realise the risks of purchasing a new instrument in a remote country, when the nearest maintenance engineer may be thousands of kilometers away. This aspect has probably been overlooked by manufacturers because of their unawareness of the problems and the unattractiveness of the market. There is a general need to delineate the maintenance and repairs which can be done by the user, and those which should be referred to the manufacturer. When instruments are required to operate considerable distances from the parent maintenance workshop or factory, it must be recognised that local operators or engineers will require more information and training. The maintenance manual provided by the manufacturer should be evaluated together with the equipment, and guidance given to manufacturers on the content of maintenance manuals. Manufacturers should be encouraged to provide full circuit-diagrams and repair instructions.

5. The development of foolproof machines for independent operation

There is a growing requirement for instruments which will carry out a complete assay and can be operated by non-scientifically skilled persons. These machines could be operated by nurses in wards or by doctors in their surgeries, and could also be used by a technically unskilled person in a developing country, with skilled supervision and maintenance provided on a long-term basis from, say, a central laboratory. The instruments could range from the highly sophisticated, with a repertoire of many tests, to one performing only blood glucose estimations. Instruments of this type are becoming available, but are at present expensive to buy and to operate. At the Copengagen International Congress of Clinical Chemistry in 1972 a working party met under Professor Magnus Hjelm to delineate requirements for such instruments, and the work of the group should be continued.

6. The needs of developing countries

Instrument development has proceeded entirely in the developed world in favourable environmental conditions, where there is an unlimited and stable electricity supply, where operators are highly trained and where the density of population and ease of communication favour rapid maintenance and repair. Where none of these prevail, as in most developing countries, modern instruments do not work. There is therefore a need to concentrate upon the 'indigenisation' of instrumentation.

At present, virtually no equipment has been developed specifically to meet the requirements of developing countries. Principles and systems developed for temperate lands with advanced technological economies, cannot be applied successfully in many of these countries without certain (often considerable) modification and rethinking. Though all branches of pathology are involved, the difficulties are particularly acute in clinical chemistry. Often the electricity supply is inadequate or extremely erratic, and under these circumstances a major feature in the design of equipment must be a minimum dependence on electricity, and some arrangement for independent supply. Non-temperate climatic conditions can ruin unprotected instruments; for example, the barrier-layer photoelectric cell in hot, humid conditions has a life of only weeks. Reliability is of particular importance when the operators are not mechanically or electrically minded and repair facilities not immediately available. Maintenance requirements are not thoroughly understood in many countries and often equipment is purchased from diverse manufacturers, none of which sell sufficient instruments in an area to enable them to provide an adequate maintenance service.

This problem is of paramount importance, and the difficulties need to be thoroughly investigated and solutions found. The market is potentially enormous, but commercial exploitation on its own will not necessarily achieve the best results. Industry needs advice about the types of instruments which are most suitable, and individual nations need information about the instruments which are most suited to their requirements and where they can be obtained. A large number of manufacturers selling in any one country will each be unable to obtain a large enough share of the market to provide adequate maintenance facilities, and for this reason, an element of selection or cooperation in any one country seems desirable.

7. Instrument standardisation

Some instruments and components which have been fully developed and accepted as satisfactory could now be selected for standardisation. Although this has already occurred to a limited extent in some countries, there are difficulties in extending it more widely. New developments might be inhibited, patent legislation could cause difficulties and competition between manufacturers reduced to the extent that monopolies developed.

Nevertheless, more could be done to ensure compatibility of components by encouraging the manufacturer of standard interchangeable modules. For example, there are now many common features in colorimeters, spectrophotometers and simple flame photometers which could be standardised and made interchangeable (e.g. cuvettes, lamps, recorders, photocells, rheostats, galvanometers, etc.). Similarly, with automated equipment it should not be difficult to specify dialysers, cuvettes and recorders.

8. Education and training

Few users get the best performance from their equipment, and this is generally due to poor understanding of general principles as well as inadequate techniqûe. More attention needs to be given to education in the principles, as well as the practical techniques of spectrophotometry, flame photometry, GLC, ion specific electrodes, etc. This could be done by placing a greater emphasis on instrumentation in the curriculae of qualifications in clinical chemistry, and by developing practical exercises, such as quality control methods, which can be carried out in the laboratory. Manufacturers can help by improving the standard of instruction manuals, which should be supplied in a language spoken in the country where the instrument is to operate. The American National Committee for Clinicaly Laboratory Standards has produced excellent guidelines for the production of instruction manuals, and these should be considered for international adoption. Manufacturers can also help by recommending appropriate quality control methods and sponsoring practical workshop courses.

9. Safety

Guidelines need to be drawn up and accepted internationally to ensure electrical, mechanical and microbiological safety in instruments. When instruments are evaluated, aspects of safety should be investigated as a high priority, and fully reported.

10. Communication between manufacturers and users

Manufacturers rarely consult national or international organisations for advice about the type and quality of instruments required by the profession, resulting in the inevitable failure of many instruments. Often they find it difficult to obtain information or advice as to which type of instrument is most suitable for different climates, national situations and medical requirements generally.

An independent survey from time to time of the instrumental needs of the profession would therefore be useful, with the findings reported in the scientific press. This would need to cover aspects such as safety, the requirements of commercial laboratories, the needs of developing countries, and any aspects of developments which may adversely affect accuracy. This information would be of use to manufacturers in making decisions about the design of an instrument, and which type of instruments to concentrate on. It would also help users to assess which type of instrument was most suitable for a certain set of circumstances.

11. IFCC Expert Panel on Instrumentation

The International Federation of Clinical Chemistry is setting up an Expert Panel on Instrumentation, and it is hoped that this will cover many of the problems discussed in this paper. Some of these are the primary concern of the profession, whereas others are the direct responsibility of manufacturers, and close cooperation between these groups will be necessary in reaching solutions.

The Panel will operate along the lines of the other Expert Panels of the IFCC, with members drawn from different countries and possibly from industry. The proposals of the Panel would be subjected to the detailed review mechanism used with all IFCC recommendations: that is, they are first considered by other committees and then published as draft recommendations. National Societies, independent experts and other interested persons are invited to submit comments on the draft. These are then reviewed, published and the draft amended as may be appropriate based upon comments from the scientific community. Final recommendations are presented to the Council of IFCC for approval, after which they are accepted as an international recommendation.

In addition to formulating specific recommendations, it is hoped that the Panel will be able to stimulate and co-ordinate work in different countries and gather together and distribute information. It is also intended that the Panel will promote the organisation of international conferences of instrument manufacturers and other interested bodies or persons, with the aim of providing a free discussion of problems, to suggest solutions and to monitor progress.

References

Broughton, P.M.G., Gowenlock, A.H., McCormack, J.J. and Neill, D.W.: A revised scheme for the evaluation of automatic instruments for use in clinical chemistry. Ann. clin. Biochem. 1974, *11*, 207.

Copeland, B.E.: Basic principles of acceptability of diagnostic instruments. Proc. Int. Conf. on Standardisation of Diagnostic Materials. U.S. Dept. of Health, Education and Welfare (1974).

Halpin, J.F.: Zero Defects. McGraw-Hill, New York, 1967.

National Committee for Clinical Laboratory Standards. Preparation of manuals for installation, operation and repair of laboratory instruments. Approved Standard A-Cl-1. Los Angeles, 1972.

Rand, R.N.: Practical spectrophotometric standards. Clin. Chem. 1969, *15*, 839.

International Criteria for determining the Acceptability of Laboratory Instrumentation

G. Sims, Fullerton, California (USA)

Key Word: Instrumentation

What criteria are necessary in determining the acceptability of clinical laboratory instruments? Who determines these criteria!'. The immediate response is, 'I, the laboratory worker, determine the necessary criteria!'. I would suggest that the laboratory user only determines if his personal criteria are met by the instrumentation under consideration. I would suggest that he has not defined his needs, rather he has left the definition up to industry to generate as many unique and novel approaches as technical capability and profitability will allow.

The choice of instrumental approaches is almost unlimited. For enzymes, one may select single beam, double beam or bichromatic; discrete, semi-discrete or continuous flow; ultraviolet or colorimetric; sample-initiated or substrate-triggered. But, can the general laboratory worker adequately discriminate and select the approach most suited to assist in providing optimal patient care? If the answer be yes, why then are 30 to 50% of laboratories performing sample initiated, two-point, colorimetric aminotransferase activity measurements?

To protect each new approach, if it should prove to be acceptable to a large enough segment of the clinical populous, the manufacturer will certainly cover his efforts with protective patents. This economic fact of industrial survival has made it increasingly difficult for any single manufacturer to design and manufacture instrumentation incorporating the maximal number of those criteria thought to be necessary for an acceptable instrumental approach.

Analytical procedures are designed for, and judged acceptable by, their precision, accuracy and specificity, while instruments are currently designed to meet the unwritten specifications for productivity, precision and versatility, in that order.

Most laboratory workers have submitted to the substitution of precision for accuracy, and allowed through-put and instrumental versatility to become the over-riding considerations in judging the acceptability of new instruments. The quantity of work required in the laboratory today and the rate at which it is increasing, certainly imposes a realistic productivity as a criterion for acceptability – but at what sacrifice in analytical excellence and ultimately in patient care?

Twenty years ago we began performing continuously monitored kinetic aminotransferase activity measurements in the clinical laboratory. Instead of improving this analytical approach and designing instrumentation to handle the increasing demand, we substituted faster, less accurate procedures. These less desirable and often grossly inaccurate approaches have become so precise, fast and inexpensive that these have become the dominant factors in justifying the relinquishment of accuracy and specificity. After twenty years of employing the kinetic approach to aminotransferase activity measurements, we are still trying to agree upon – not optimal, but mutually acceptable – reaction conditions.

I recently attended a panel discussion to consider temperature in enzyme activity measurements. After two hours of reverbalizing all the pros and cons of all the popular temperatures in use, the final conclusion was that no decision could, as yet, be reached as to the most acceptable temperature, and the entire dilemma was due to the fact that the Beckman DU, upon which the original work was done, had no temperature control. This occurred in 1954, before temperature was considered a factor and there is, as yet, no rational analytical agreement defining the optimal temperature for enzyme activity measurements. If the clinical chemists cannot determine the temperature requirements necessary, how then can industry design to meet this and other necessary criteria?

In a recent publication in a reputable journal, Dr. *Arthur Krieg* made a plea for the manufacturer and the clinical chemist to work together for standardization. Following this plea, the editor of the journal responded: 'The manufacturer, in the heat of competition, proliferates instruments too often not in the best interest of the patient'. The editorial response is a bit frightening as it suggests that the laboratory has relinquished its control over the release of diagnostically valuable information to the instrument manufacturer.

My points thus far, have been to emphasize the immediate need for definition, agreed upon criteria of acceptance, and encouraged compliance by both domestic and international societies involved in the enhancement of laboratory medicine. I would suggest that these societies seek the active participation of the chemical and analytical knowledge that has developed in industry, in formulating definitions and evaluating various analytical approaches. This is an invaluable resource that should not be overlooked.

The current approaches to quality control in the laboratory have come from industry. Many of the approaches used in evaluating new instrumentation have come from industry. If industry is to share the responsibility for poor patient care, then it should also participate in the definition of criteria for instrument acceptance.

For those of you unfamiliar with the evolution and maturation of clinical instrumentation, I would like to offer a brief insight into some of the problems.

The first step is to attempt to define the needs of the laboratory two to five years into the future, as it will take that period to bring an instrument to the market. This first step is the most critical and the most difficult, as no guidelines exist. The laboratory worker is faced with today's problems today – the manufacturer is faced with tomorrow's problems today.

The next step is to discuss the proposed instrumental concept with various pundits in the field, to determine the viability of the concept, its strengths and its weaknesses, and a judgement must be made as to the value of these inputs. How can the manufacturer, who is removed from the clinical laboratory, evaluate such information? Yet, it is on such sources of information that large sums of money, time and talent are committed.

Having established the path of development of a new instrument, a process of engineering, evaluation and re-engineering, begins until those making final analytical judgements deem the device acceptable. This judgement must be based upon available resource, the growth or decline of the market, the estimated return on investment, and the anticipated analytical superiority of the design approach. Here again an arbitrary decision is made, as no guidelines exist. During the process of development, instruments are shaken, dropped, heated, run in high-humidity environments, various components are exposed to caustic and corrosive atmospheres, evaluated as subsystems and as a total system and finally, exposed to the ultimate test, the laboratory technician, who invariably can stimulate malfunctions when none of the previous testing could.

How much evaluation should be done? When should it be done and by whom? I recently read a claim for a new analyzer whose evaluation data was based upon the assay of 1000 patient sera. Is this adequate? I have in my files evaluation data, for an instrument, which contains approximately 300,000 assays on patient sera. Is this necessary? What are the criteria of acceptability for evaluation? Depending upon the procedure under consideration, I would suggest 50 to 100 thousand assays carried out under defined and well controlled evaluation conditions, will provide the information necessary for the manufacturer to judge the performance level of his device. It should then only be necessary to verify the claimed performance on three carefully selected sample groupings: 100 randomly selected normal samples, 100 elevated samples and 100 samples from patients with known interferences, that is, drug therapy, other disease states, or metabolic disorders.

This data should be properly documented and made available to those interested, the goal being to offer sufficient information to allow the laboratory worker to make a judgement regrading acceptability without having to invest valuable time on re-evaluation. To accomplish this, agreed upon definitions and protocols must be developed on an international level. The evaluation should ideally be done prior to introduction of the device, by an independent testing laboratory. However, data generated at this time might prove to be invalid as it would not be performed on a production instrument, since the first 5 to 20 instruments are usually of a prototype nature, and actual production conditions may alter final instrument performance.

Several firms in the United States are currently participating in the College of American Pathologists verification of claims program. The claims verified are those agreed upon by the Committee on Evaluation and the manufacturer involved. Without active support from the clinical laboratories and all involved manufacturers, a program such as this runs the risk of losing its effectiveness.

It is unrealistic to expect a manufacturer to redesign, after final release, based upon evaluation conditions present in only small isolated areas where only a few instruments may be sold. These needs must be conveyed to industry early in the development and design process, and judgements made regarding the feasibility and practicability of meeting these unique needs.

Consider, if you will, the criteria of acceptability that industry places on the components used in instrument manufacturing. A component is selected based upon the raw material suppliers' test specifications. For example, the specification may indicate that failure occurs in only one-tenth of one percent (0.1%) of the items in question. If this level of acceptability is set as the standard for all involved components, then it can be assumed that if the instrument design calls for 1000 different components – all instruments will fail.

As this specification is tightened, the component cost rises logarithmically. The manufacturer must compromise between a reasonable cost and an acceptable failure rate. This compromise must again be arbitrarily determined,as no requirements for instrument backup, allowed failure rate, or allowed down-time have been established.

The definition of precision must also be viewed in a different light. As a manufacturer of parachutes, for example, I might be allowed a 5% failure rate. Does that imply that each parachute will be allowed to fail 5% of the time or 5% of the parachutes may fail each time used?

When the laboratory worker demands a precision at 100 milligrams per deciliter, plus or minus two standard deviations of 2 mgm/dl, what does that mean to the instrument manufacturer? Does it imply that 95% of the instruments manufactured recover 100 ± 2 mgm/dl or that all instruments recover 100 ± 2 mgm/dl 95% of the time? These are very different requirements dictating different design approaches.

A manufacturer must relate performance specifications to hundreds of instruments – while a laboratory technician thinks only in terms of a single unit.

The College of American Pathologists Summary Report on the survey data generated by its Chemistry Resource Committee, states that within-laboratory errors contribute 68% to the total analytical error seen, while between-laboratory errors contribute 32%. The Committee's conclusions were as follows:

1. Comparison of the size of the sources of analytical error suggests that the majority of analytical error arises from short and long term change within the individual laboratories.
2. The Survey findings suggest that laboratory improvement can be achieved by controlling these 'within-laboratory' factors and that attention should be directed toward the selection of methods with good precision, and close monitoring of internal quality control.

These factors as well as many others, make it imperative that the laboratory worker and the manufacturer interact in establishing definitions, design criteria and evaluation protocols.

If there are no formal criteria for acceptability, what then does the user have a right to expect? A comprehensive and usable manual. But, who defines usable? Proper maintenance requirements. But, who defines these requirements? Meaningful evaluation data. But, who defines meaningful? Anticipated performance characteristics, that is, spectral stability and linearity, pipetting precision, temperature accuracy and control. But, who defines the conditions under which these are determined?

The Scientific Apparatus Manufacturers Association Task Force on Instrument Definition in the U.S.A. has determined that it must begin formulating what we believe will be the most meaningful vocabulary necessary to define performance characteristics. This is an effort on the part of industry to remove the ambiguity from instrument claims in an effort to provide more meaningful information to the laboratorian.

The American Association of Clinical Chemists Subcommittee on Enzyme Standardization met last month with representatives from industry to discuss specifications and requirements for future enzyme activity analyzers.

The National Committee for Clinical Laboratory Standards has defined those components necessary in an acceptable instrument manual.

These are steps in the right direction, but require international coordination.

Most of the laboratory instrument industry is concerned with the achievement of one primary goal: the improvement of instrumental approaches for achieving molecular solutions to disease oriented problems. How can this goal be realized if you cannot agree whether diagnostic usefulness should dictate the necessary level of analytical achievement, or analytical excellence will dictate diagnostic significance?

The building blocks of enlightened self-interest are being cast, but we need rapid, decisive, well-founded international intervention and cooperation to build a lasting and firm foundation. There is currently a great deal of national activity, the fruits of which have an effect only domestically. Once legislated and accepted, these independent activities are difficult to modify. It thus becomes imperative that we all strive for and contribute to rapid international action consistent with domestic needs.

I challenge each individual and society to begin, in this discussion today, rechannelling their thoughts and efforts from defending their current stands, to negotiating the resolution of the analytical differences that are retarding the growth of laboratory medicine.

International Criteria for Clinical Laboratory Instrumentation

Discussion

E.J. van Kampen (Holland): Thank you, Dr. *Sims,* for giving your opinions and challenges about the international criteria for clinical laboratory instrumentation. I am certain that many of us do not agree and this opens the session for discussion from the floor.

W.E. Elion-Gerritzen (Holland): My comment concerns the establishment of criteria for acceptability. It has been mentioned repeatedly in this session and during the previous days, that precision and accuracy are different things. Reference materials, for example, can only be valuable in correcting for systematic bias, if variability in the laboratory is negligible.

How far are we on the road to good precision?

We should agree, in this meeting on Quality Control, that precision in the laboratory – particularly long-term precision – is a basic requirement. Firstly, because we can neither talk nor think about accuracy or comparability without precision and secondly, because for clinical reasons, this would have far reaching consequences.

- it would mean that many national quality control schemes should be redesigned to provide optimal information on intralaboratory performance
- it would mean that we should focus on different areas, such as training of technicians in the field of quality control
- it would mean that consistent performance of reagents and methods would be more important than accuracy:
  (stability on storage would then be as important as, or more important than absolute purity even though this may be against our scientific intuition: A buffer for which the manufacturer can guarantee low batch-to-batch variability would be preferable to an optimal buffer with production difficulties)
- also, for instrumentation, stability over long periods of time would be as important as good performance in a single quality check.

I would consider it a great achievement of this meeting if we could settle the essential question of priorities: precision or accuracy, since actions and criteria for acceptability of methods and reagents are often contradictory.

E. van Kampen (Holland): Can you formulate what you are suggesting in one or two sharp questions?

W. Elion-Gerritzen (Holland): My point is, we should establish priorities as to which is more important – precision or accuracy, particularly from the clinician's point of view. The answer to this question would dictate important criteria for materials and instruments.

E. van Kampen (Holland): Thank you. I believe that you cannot compare precision and accuracy since they are two entirely different things, as has been defined yesterday and this morning.

W. Elion-Gerritzen (Holland): I am just trying to point out that they are indeed two different things.

E. van Kampen (Holland): Yes, and therefore you cannot and should not make a choice between the two, nor can you establish a priority.

F. Mitchell (U.K.): I think we should really refer this question to the speakers in this morning's session. We could spend the rest of this afternoon answering it. I believe we should agree with the fundamental thoughts behind your question, Dr. *Gerritzen,* since they have worried many of us for a long time. At present, our quality control programs control only precision and this is a considerable worry. We are moving to a future where control will be in the realm of accuracy as well, by means of definitive and reference technology. But could we for a snap answer refer to somebody talking about this, this morning?

P. Cali (U. S. A.): I believe that the question that was asked is very valid and to the point, and I would answer in this way: Measurement networks must be looked at in their totality – one should not examine only the bits and pieces in isolation. Someone, somewhere must be concerned with the totality of the entire measurement network. In clinical chemistry today, this is only starting, in contrast to some industrial measurement networks which are indeed in very, very good control. For instance, in the metals industry in the USA a half billion (5×10^8) measurements are made with turnaround times of from 2 to 5 minutes, and with accuracies of 1 to 2%. If you could achieve that accuracy in clinical chemistry, I think we would agree that we were well on our way to having a good, reliable measurement network. I think that education and training must be two of the foremost factors in the building of the reliability of any measurement network, together with checking of routine methods, so that the totality of the entire system can be evaluated. It is a broad front approach that must be taken.

Th. Horne (UK): This being a discussion period, I would like to make some comments on the paper by Dr. *Mitchell* and Dr. *Broughton,* rather than pose questions. They refer to unnecessary duplication and competition in the field of clinical chemistry analyzers. Certainly, it is very true that the number of analyzers on the market is only exceeded by the number which has already appeared and failed. Sometimes, it appears that the clinical chemistry industry has taken over from the aerospace industry the responsibility for maintaining full employment amongst engineers. However, competition is a major factor in holding down the price of instrumentation, a point which I feel Dr. *Broughton* overlooks. It is the operation of the free market economy which prevents manufacturers from increasing their prices still further. In any event, the various fair trade acts and restrictive practices legislation in different countries would prevent much of the sort of cooperative effort which they described in their paper from being undertaken by manufacturers on their own. Might it nevertheless be possible for governments or international bodies to take the lead in initiating some such joint program? But let us at all costs avoid designs by committees. On the question of patents to which Dr. *Sims* referred, I would suggest that in the general field of the clinical laboratory, over the past 20 years, there are really only two advances which have exercised a major influence in the development of new equipments, and these two have been of great simplicity, but perhaps of major importance. I refer, of course, to the work of Dr. *Skeggs* on continuous flow analyzers, and the formulation by Wallis Coulter, of the Coulter principle. All other patents, I feel, really have not influenced the development or availability of instruments to any significant extent.

On the question of maintenance, and in order to maintain the ability of equipment, which Dr. *Broughton* refers to, I would say that industry regards this of major importance for all products in all markets. We in industry are providing a service to the clinician. We cannot be said to be doing that if our equipment breaks down frequently and we are unable to provide rapid service for it.

At these meetings, many speakers have stressed the importance of an agreed-upon, fully understood terminology, and this has been largely in the context of workers all within basically one discipline. I would suggest that it is even more essential for inter-disciplinary communication that the terminology be agreed upon. All too often, we find the clinician cannot express his requirements in the form that could be understood by the engineer. Similarly, engineers who are notorious for their inability to express themselves in words anyway, cannot formulate their questions so the clinicians can understand. One way in which this might be improved perhaps is for full membership of professional bodies, like the Association of Clinical Biochemists or the German Society for Clinical Chemistry, to be more freely available to properly qualified people from industry.

There is an obligation, I feel, on the user to publicize his requirements, as well as on the manufacturer to make himself aware of these needs. This extends, of course, to equipment after the development stage when it is in the field. You, yourself, Mr. Chairman, made reference yesterday to certain of the products of my company. We both, I feel, have an obligation to initiate and to maintain a constructive dialogue to clarify the situation to which you referred and to remedy any defects. No company wishes to produce equipment which is inaccurate, imprecise and difficult to calibrate. I suggest we must all keep reminding ourselves that our prime concern is the well-being of the patient; by working together (the manufacturer to provide relevent equipment and the clinician with respect to the use of that equipment) we can provide better patient care.

E. van Kampen (Holland): Thank you for your remarks. I think we are in position to give each other the benefit of the doubt. I believe that in order to open up communication channels it was appropriate to express my doubts yesterday. If we do this I am sure we can resolve our problem.

Unidentified Speaker: Very briefly, I would like to compliment the last speaker as being one of the few manufacturers I know who will persistently come and ask questions and say, 'What is it you fellows want?' And if many more manufacturers would do that more frequently, users would be thinking much more and try to clarify their own minds.

On the question of competition between manufacturers, my complaint is that they have all been competing, producing the same type of multichannel analyzers, doing the same analyses, but by different methods; whereas, I can think of many analyses I want to do in large numbers, but I cannot interest a manufacturer to take the risk and launch out on his own and do something different.

J. Henry (U.S.A.): I am very impressed with the topic of this afternoon's session, and the emphasis on instrumentation, particularly after this morning's review of materials and methods. If we look at the laboratory overall in terms of trends, it stands out, at least in the United States, that of the three primary functions of the clinical laboratory, production is critical in terms of the task before us today, the other two functions being the selection of chemical measurements and also their interpretation or translation. We are really focusing on production, and there is no question, I think, in the minds of many of us, that production does focus on technology and instrumentation. Both require defined criteria and priorities. The first priority is concerned with the analytical chemistry. The particular method must utilise sound materials, references and standards upon which accuracy and precision are dependent. The second priority is for sophisticated engineering, and computerisation to support the technology needed for production. It is also essential that the system be cost-effective. It is my opinion, that there is a trend from manual to semiautomated to automated methods. The development of instrumentation based upon excellence in analytical chemistry is the key to the future in the next five years. Adequacy for clinical utility is defined by the sensitivity and specificity of analytical methodology.

P. Akinaynju (Nigeria): I wish to make a few comments on Professor *Mitchell's* presentation. I am glad that he has highlighted some of the problems that clinical chemists in developing countries are faced with, but the problem is not only what we lack in terms of infra-structural facilities like water, light, etc., but another problem is the inadequacy of communication between manufacturers of equipment and control materials, and the clinical chemists in our environment. Usually, these big manufacturers are represented in developing countries, in Nigeria for example, by businessmen who know very little about instrument repairs, maintenance, or even use: so I would like to appeal to these manufacturers to open up generous communication lines with clinical chemists in these countries and to make known to us enough information about new developments and new products.

A. Rappoport (U.S.A.): Along these lines, there is an important problem in this discussion, and that is, are we talking about a suit which really fits the body for which it is being designed? And how much does it cost? For instance if you would walk along the road of automation, you will find the skeletons of some very handsome expensive instruments lying along the path. All of these we, the consumer, had to pay for. Consider such devices as the Robot Chemist, Mr. *Sim's* DAS (Beckman) which has succumbed, at least on the American market; the Vickers machine and a large number of other devices that might be mentioned. It would be interesting to wonder what was the environment in which these dinosaurs failed to survive. Furthermore why have other similar instruments that we know about flourished so well? Apparently in the marketplace, the final ultimate value is reached by the competitive forces which are effective, and the cost/benefit ratio is not the least of these. Now, are we carrying the financial burden of the tremendous investments that we were made and lost over the last 10 or 15 years on the instruments that we are buying today. Are we really correct in attempting to have a universal solution to a multi-faceted problem? I am thinking of the previous speaker's remarks about emerging nations – do they need this type of technology? I am thinking of institutions where the test volumes are so low that these instruments and the investments for those instruments may be entirely inappropriate. As my father used to tell me – 'when all else fails, consider the cost of the pleasure you desire'. Consequently let's consider the cost-effectiveness and the appropriateness of the investment to solve the particular problem that we are confronted with.

Session IV

Topic: National Regulations and International Recommendations

Session-Chairman: R. Dybkaer, Denmark
Discussion-Leader: H. Bergmeyer, Germany

The Regulation of Diagnostic Products in the United States

E. Eavenson, Rockville, Maryland (USA)

Key words: Diagnostic products
Regulations

The regulation of diagnostic products in the United States did not occur precipitously. There were many indications that such action was necessary. Attempts by voluntary groups to encourage the improvement of the quality of the materials used in the laboratory were of limited success. Although government agencies such as the Center for Disease Control, the National Institutes of Health and the National Bureau of Standards had programs which focused on one or more aspects of improvement in the quality of laboratory results, they were heavily dependent on the acceptance and cooperation of the clinical laboratory public. In many cases, these constructive attempts were frustrated by the marketing skills of the diagnostic products industry.

The Food and Drug Administration, in regulations written following the passage of the Federal Food, Drug and Cosmetic Act of 1938, considered that commercially prepared reagents used in the laboratory to obtain diagnostic results on specimens taken from human subjects were clearly subject to the provisions of that Act. This consideration was based on statutory definitions of 'drug' and 'device', both of which include 'articles intended for use in the diagnosis of disease'. Since the few such products available at that time derived from well-established formulations documented in the scientific literature, the regulations provided a labeling exemption for such products. This exemption continued with few exceptions until 1972, even though the number and types of reagent products increased many-fold in the ensuing years and basic information about their formulation and intended use became more difficult to find. In 1969, the United States Supreme Court, in recognition of the critical importance of laboratory diagnostic materials, found that anti-infective susceptibility discs containing antibiotic substances were subject to the provisions of the Food, Drug & Cosmetic Act that requires testing and certification of each manufactured batch prior to distribution. Performance standards for these discs are published in the form of testing monographs, and established appropriate and legally binding limits for product performance. In addition, the U.S. Public Health Service Act contains provisions for regulating materials of biologic origin, and under that authority the present Bureau of Biologics of the FDA (formerly, Division of Biologic Standards of the NIH) licenses some diagnostic products, principally those used in, or associated with, blood banking.

The following factors entered into the decision to establish a central regulatory program for *in vitro* diagnostic products manufactured and/or used in the United States.

1. Laboratories had become more dependent on external sources for materials. While in the mid-1960's many laboratories continued to prepare the reagents they used routinely, very few clinical laboratories had the facilities or expertise to synthesize, purify or analyze reagent components.
2. Physicians' demands for more complete laboratory workups on patients led laboratories to look to commercial sources for work-simplifying and cost-reducing materials.
3. The development of mechanized or automated instrumentation led manufacturers to develop compatible reagent systems. Laboratories became increasingly dependent on these systems, and the costs involved in changing from one system to another became prohibitive.
4. Increasing emphasis on health maintenance led to increasing use of screening procedures. Many of these procedures depended on assumptions which were not valid for individual specimens.

A number of attempts were made to improve the quality of diagnostic products in an orderly way. Professional associations developed voluntary guidelines for reference materials and methods, specifications for certain chemical and biological materials used in laboratory reagents, and for the labeling of reagents. The National Committee for Clinical Laboratory Standards was formed from industry, government and professional societies to develop consensus standards. The Center for Disease Control has now printed its fourth edition of *Specifications and Evaluation Methods for Immunological and Microbiological Reagents*. These specifications are the basis for the Center's voluntary testing of a large number of important reagents, an activity now widely accepted and respected among industry and laboratory scientists. The National Bureau of Standards provides a number of materials to laboratories and industry in its Standard Reference Materials (SRM) program.

Though these efforts are useful to the laboratory in its goal of self-improvement, most groups directly concerned with laboratory medicine concluded that mandatory regulations were needed. The nature of such regulations was of great concern, and many approaches were considered. Industry was wary of any regulations resembling those requiring premarket approval, mainly because of their experiences with getting approval of new drugs from FDA. They assumed that the time required to develop the data considered appropriate for pre-market approval of diagnostic products would eliminate smaller companies from the marketplace. Furthermore, they anticipated costly studies that would completely prohibit development of new products. The physician was concerned that he would be hampered in his practice of medicine and might no longer be able to use methodologies that he had found useful in the management of patients. The laboratory consumer wanted assurance that the materials he had come to rely on would continue to be available.

The regulatory approach that emerged from these considerations was a joint effort of the Food and Drug Administration and the Center for Disease Control, both agencies of the Department of Health, Education and Welfare. The Food and Drug Administration had authority under the provisions of the Food, Drug & Cosmetic Act to regulate all *in vitro* diagnostic products as either drugs or devices or as combinations of drugs and devices. The Center for Disease Control has been dedicated for a number of years to a program of clinical laboratory improvement, and has the expertise and facilities necessary to develop and evaluate specifications for products used in clinical laboratories. The combined efforts of the two Agencies should be complementary and should provide a total, united approach to assure quality materials in the marketplace.

Since the products of concern were numerous and had been marketed widely for many years, a regulatory approach was needed that would not be disruptive to patient care but that would result in steadily improving quality of results to the physician. Final regulations based on the authority of the Food, Drug and Cosmetic Act were published in March of 1973. These permit the regulation of all *in vitro* diagnostic products in the following manner:

1. *In Vitro* diagnostic products are defined as reagents, instruments and systems intended for use in the diagnosis of disease or in the determination of the state of health, and include products intended for use in the collection, preparation and examination of specimens taken from the human body.
2. General labeling requirements provide more consistent and useful information to the laboratory user about the nature of the product, its use and limitations, and any pertinent performance characteristics, permitting an informed selection of products to satisfy a particular laboratory need.
3. Each claim for the product must be supported by data that clearly substantiates the claim. There is no requirement that this data be supplied routinely to the FDA.
4. Every product must be manufactured in accordance with current good manufacturing practices and the process is subject to inspection by the FDA field staff.
5. All products are subject to review and evaluation by FDA to determine that they are in compliance with the requirements of the law.
6. 'Product Class Standards' may be developed for any product or group of products which require designations for performance limits, specifications of composition or purity necessary to obtain a particular quality of performance, more specific labeling requirements, or detailed testing or evaluation protocols.
7. The basis for determining the need for a product class standard includes consideration of the degree of risk or injury associated with the use of the product, the availability of information relating to the sciences upon which the products or their uses are based, the approximate number of products subject to the standard, the medical need for the products and the available means of achieving the objective of the standard with a

minimal disruption of supply and of reasonable manufacturing and other commercial practices.

8. Any interested person may propose that a standard be developed by one of the following: (a) an existing standard may be utilized, or (b) interested persons outside the Food and Drug Administration may develop a proposed standard, or (c) the Food and Drug Administration may develop the standard.
9. Any standard developed will ordinarily be published as a proposal subject to comment from all interested persons prior to its becoming an effective regulation.

The Diagnostic Products Advisory Committee was established to take advantage of the best advice available on the medical usefulness of various diagnostic procedures, current good laboratory practices and available methodologies. This Committee consists of members of the scientific community involved in clinical pathology, microbiology, chemistry, medical technology and related fields. The Committee is requested to determine which products require standards or some form of premarket clearance in addition to the general requirements already in effect, to develop priorities for product class standards, and to recommend reference materials and methodologies and testing protocols that would be adequate to assure quality products. The Advisory Committee also reviews proposals for standards and recommends product development and evaluation protocols for products requiring pre-market clearance. Several product class standards are in the process of being developed by the FDA, based on the priorities recommended by this Committee. These standards relate to the performance of products and do not restrict materials or methods. The FDA has published a proposed product class standard for products that detect or measure glucose, and has issued requests for data and information to determine the need for product class standards for calibrators for clinical chemistry procedures, products involved in the measurement of hemoglobin in human blood, and products used in non-treponemal tests for syphilis.

The need for standards that are meaningful and that will provide products that are useful requires input, not only from the professionals who use the products, but also from the manufacturers who develop and make the products. Many of their concerns, relating to proprietary information and trade secrets, the current status of manufacturing practices, and the costs involved in meeting certain performance requirements, are recognized by the Food and Drug Administration as being legitimate. Therefore, procedures have been established for relating these concerns early in the development of pertinent regulations.

The Advisory Committee has one non-voting member from industry, one representing consumer interests and several from other government agencies. The industry representative is an important link who presents the views of industry to the Committee and who transmits to industry the concerns of the Committee regarding the manufacture or use of particular diagnostic products.

All Committee meetings are announced in advance so that any interested parties may provide input into the deliberations. Any persons wishing to address the Committee on a subject relating to the announced agenda may petition to do so. Specific time periods are available during each meeting, to allow participation by any interested party; professional and consumer groups can make their concerns known to Committee members.

When the FDA has determined that a need may exist for a standard, an announcement is made declaring that a standard is anticipated for a particular group of products which they make or use. Particularly, information is requested which would indicate how the product is intended to be used, with supporting data for all claims made. FDA, with its Advisory Committee, must then relate this information to performance requirements based on the medical usefulness of the results to be obtained by the use of the product. A proposal for a product class standard is then published, with opportunity for comment by interested persons. Professional associations and industry are encouraged to review and comment on any aspects of the proposed standard. All comments are carefully reviewed by FDA with the assistance of its Advisory Committee, and the proposed Standard is then revised accordingly. This process continues until FDA has a standard which will serve to regulate the products in question.

Consensus standards developed by professional, technical or trade associations and subjected to a review process are very useful in the establishment of any regulations. Such standards serve to identify the important characteristics of products which must be controlled in order to obtain quality results, as well as the appropriate reference materials and reference methods by which to judge product performance. It is very important that information about such standards be available on a continuing basis. Not only is such information necessary for preparing regulatory standards, but it is often useful in evaluating product compliance with existing regulations on labeling and good manufacturing practices. Consensus standards, or parts of such standards, may be considered as guidelines for product evaluation in lieu of a regulatory standard.

The enforcement of these regulations requires a rather extensive surveillance effort. Most products are not approved in advance of their marketing. The marketing of the product implies that the applicable regulations are met. Although one would expect that the labeling requirements would assure uniformity of labeling of similar products, this may not always be the case. Certain variations will arise from differences in marketing approaches as well as differences in interpretations of the general requirements. The labeling information must, however, be adequate to provide the user with the information he needs to use the product in the way intended.

Similarly, product class standards will not assure that every product is the same. The limits are intended to establish minimal performance for a particular medical use. Differences in methodologies and in patient populations may cause certain laboratories to prefer one product over the others. Again, the labeling information provided for the product must provide the basis for a choice.

The desired effect of these regulations is to bring about laboratory improvement by providing more reliable products to the laboratory, and by providing the information necessary for the use of the products. The FDA recognizes that the quality of laboratory results depends on many factors other than reagents and instruments. Without reliable reagents and instruments, however, good laboratory quality control becomes impossible to achieve.

Appendix

Part 328 – in vitro diagnostic products for human use

Subpart A – General Provisions

Subpart B – Labeling

Subpart C – Requirements for Manufacturers and Producers

Subpart D – Administrative Procedures

Authority: Secs. 201, 501, 502 505, 508, 510, 701, 52 Stat. 1040–1042, as amended, 1049–1051, as amended, 1053, as amended, 1055, as amended, 1056, as amended (21 U.S.C. 321, 351, 352, 355, 358, 360, 371).

Source: 39 FR 11732, Mar. 29, 1974, unless otherwise noted.

Subpart A – General Provisions

§ 328.3 Definitions

(a) Data and information submitted pursuant to the provisions of § 328.30 or § 328.10 (c) and falling within diagnosis of disease or in the determination of the state of health in order to cure, mitigate, treat, or prevent disease or its sequelae. Such products are intended for use in the collection, preparation and examination of specimens taken from the human body. These products are drugs or devices as defined in section 201 (g) and 201 (h), respectively, of the Federal Food, Drug, and Cosmetic Act (the act) or are a combination of drugs and devices, and may also be a biological product subject to section 351 of the Public Health Service Act.

(b) A 'product class' is all those products intended for use for a particular determination or for a related group of determinations or products with common or related characteristics or those intended for common or related uses. A class may be further divided into subclasses when appropriate.

(c) A 'product class standard' is a statement describing performance requirements necessary to assure accuracy and reliability of results, specific labeling requirements necessary for the proper use of a particular class, and procedures for testing the product to assure its satisfactory performance.

(d) 'Act' means the Federal Food, Drug, and Cosmetic Act.

§ 328.4 Confidentiality of submitted information

(a) Data and information submitted pursuant to the provisions of § 328.30 or § 328.10 (c) and falling within the confidentiality provisions of 18 U.S.C. 1905 or 21 U.S.C. 331 (j) shall be treated as confidential by the Food and Drug Administration and any consultant to whom it is referred. Confidentiality of information will be determined in accordance with the provisions of Part 4 of this chapter.

(b) Data and information submitted pursuant to § 328.30 in connection with the establishment, amendment or repeal of a product class standard will be made publicly available at the office of the Hearing Clerk of the Food and Drug Administration 30 days after publication of a proposed product class standard, except for the identity of inactive ingredients, any quality control or other manufacturing data or information, or other data and information to the extent that the person submitting it has demostrated that it falls within the confidentiality provisions of 18 U.S.C. 1905 or 21 U.S.C. 331 (j).

Subpart B – Labeling

§ 328.10 Labeling for in vitro diagnostic products

(a) The label for an in vitro diagnostic product shall state the following information, except where such information is not applicable, or as otherwise specified in a standard for a particular product class. Section 201 (k) of the act provides that 'a requirement made by or under authority of this act that any word, statement, or other information appear on the label shall not be considered to be complied with unless such word, statement, or other information also appears on the outside container or wrapper, if any there be, of the retail package of such article, or is easily legible through the outside container or wrapper.'

(1) The proprietary name and established name (common or usual name), if any.

(2) The intended use or uses of the product.

(3) For a reagent, a declaration of the established name (common or usual name), if any, and quantity, proportion or concentration of each reactive ingredient; and for a reagent derived from biological material, the source and a measure of its activity. The quantity, proportion, concentration or activity shall be stated in the system generally used and recognized by the intended user (e.g., metric, international units, etc.).

(4) A statement of warnings or precautions for users as established in the regulations contained in 16 CFR Part 1500 and any other warnings appropriate to the hazard presented by the product; and a statement 'For In Vitro Diagnostic Use' and any other limiting statements appropriate to the intended use of the product.

(5) For a reagent, appropriate storage instructions adequate to protect the stability of the product. When applicable, these instructions shall include such information as conditions of temperature, light, humidity, and other pertinent factors. For products requiring manipulation, such as reconstitution and/or mixing before use, appropriate storage instructions shall be provided for the reconstituted or mixed product which is to be stored in the original container. The basis for such instructions shall be determined by reliable, meaningful, and specific test methods such as those described in § 133.13 of this chapter.

(6) For a reagent, a means by which the user may be assured that the product meets appropriate standards of identity, strength, quality and purity at the time of use. This shall be provided, both for the product as provided and for any resultant reconstituted or mixed product, by including on the label one or more of the following:

(i) An expiration date based upon the stated storage instructions.

(ii) A statement of an observable indication of an alteration of the product (e.g., turbidity, color change, precipitate) beyond its appropriate standards.

(iii) Instructions for a simple method by which the user can reasonably determine that the product meets its appropriate standards.

(7) For a reagent, a declaration of the net quantity of contents, expressed in terms of weight or volume, numerical count, or any combination of these or other terms which accurately reflect the contents of the package. The use of metric designations is encouraged, wherever appropriate. If more than a single determination may be performed using the product, any statement of the number of tests shall be consistent with instructions for use and amount of material provided.

(8) Name and place of business of manufacturer, packer, or distributor.

(9) A lot or control number, identified as such, from which it is possible to determine the complete manufacturing history of the product.

(i) If it is a multiple unit product, the lot or control number shall permit tracing the identity of the individual units.

(ii) For an instrument, the lot or control number shall permit tracing the identity of all functional subassemblies.

(iii) For multiple unit products which require the use of included units together as a system, all units should bear the same lot or control number, if appropriate, or other suitable uniform identification should be used.

(10) Except that for items in paragraph (a) (1) through (9) of this section: (i) In the case of immediate containers too small or otherwise unable to accommodate a label with sufficient space to bear all such information and which are packaged within an outer container from which they are removed for use, the information required by paragraph (a) (2), (3), (4), (5), (6) (ii) (iii) and (7) of this section may appear in the outer container labeling only.

(ii) In any case in which the presence of this information on the immediate container will interfere with the test, the information may appear on the outside container or wrapper rather than on the immediate container label.

(b) Labeling accompanying each product (e.g., package insert) shall state in one place the following information in the format and order specified below, except where such information is not applicable, or as specified in a standard for a particular product class. The labeling for a multiple-purpose instrument used for diagnostic purposes, and not committed to specific diagnostic procedures or systems, may bear only the information indicated in paragraph (b) (1), (2), (6), (14), and (15) of this section. The labeling for a reagent intended for use as a replacement in a diagnostic system may be limited to that information necessary to identify the reagent adequately and to describe its proper use in the system.

(1) The proprietary name and established name (common or usual name), if any.

(2) The intended use or uses of the product and the type of procedure (e.g., qualitative or quantitative).

(3) Summary and explanation of the test. Include a short history of the methodology, with pertinent references and a balanced statement of the special merits and limitations of this method or product. If the product labeling refers to any other procedure, appropriate literature citations shall be included and the labeling shall explain the nature of any differences from the original and their effect on the results.

(4) The chemical, physical, physiological, or biological principles of the procedure. Explain concisely, with chemical reactions and techniques involved, if applicable.

(5) Reagents. (i) A declaration of the established name (common or usual name), if any, and quantity, proportion or concentration of each reactive ingredient; and for biological material, the source and a measure of its activity. The quantity, proportion, concentration or activity shall be stated in the system generally used and recognized by the intended user (e.g., metric, international units, etc.). A statement indicating the presence of and characterizing any catalytic or nonreactive ingredients (e.g., buffers, preservatives, stabilizers).

(ii) A statement of warnings or precautions for users as established in the regulations contained in 16 CFR Part 1500 and any other warnings appropriate to the hazard presented by the product; and a statement 'For In Vitro Diagnostic Use' and any other limiting statements appropriate to the intended use of the product.

(iii) Adequate instructions for reconstitution, mixing, dilution, etc.

(iv) Appropriate storage instructions adequate to protect the stability of the product. When applicable, these instructions shall include such information as conditions of temperature, light, humidity, and other pertinent factors. For products requiring manipulation, such as reconstitution and/or mixing before use, appropriate storage instructions shall be provided for the reconstituted or mixed product. The basis for such instructions shall be determined by reliable, meaningful, and specific test methods such as those described in § 133.13 of this chapter.

(v) A statement of any purification or treatment required for use.

(vi) Physical, biological, or chemical indications of instability or deterioration.

(6) Instruments: (i) Use or function.

(ii) Installation procedures and special requirements.

(iii) Principles of operation.

(iv) Performance characteristics and specifications.

(v) Operating instructions.

(vi) Calibration procedures including materials and/or equipment to be used.

(vii) Operational precautions and limitations.

(viii) Hazards.

(ix) Service and maintenance information.

(7) Specimen collection and preparation for analysis, including a description of: (i) Special precautions regarding specimen collection including special preparation of the patient as it bears on the validity of the test.

(ii) Additives, preservatives, etc., necessary to maintain the integrity of the specimen.

(iii) Known interfering substances.

(iv) Recommended storage, handling or shipping instructions for the protection and maintenance of stability of the specimen.

(8) Procedure: A step-by-step outline of recommended procedures from reception of the specimen to obtaining results. List any points that may be useful in improving precision and accuracy. (i) A list of all materials provided (e.g., reagents, instruments and equipment) with instructions for their use.

(ii) A list of all materials required but not provided: Include such details as sizes, numbers, types, and quality.

(iii) A description of the amounts of reagents necessary, times required for specific steps, proper temperatures, wavelengths, etc.

(iv) A statement describing the stability of the final reaction material to be measured and the time within which it shall be measured to assure accurate results.

(v) Details of calibration: Identify reference material. Describe preparation of reference sample(s), use of blanks, preparation of the standard curve, etc. The description of the range of calibration should include the highest and the lowest values measurable by the procedure.

(vi) Details of kinds of quality control procedures and materials required. If there is need for both positive and negative controls, this should be stated. State what are considered satisfactory limits of performance.

(9) Results: Explain the procedure for calculating the value of the unknown. Give an explanation for each component of the formula used for the calculation of the unknown. Include a sample calculation, step-by-step, explaining the answer. The values shall be expressed to the appropriate number of significant figures. If the test provides other than quantitative results, provide an adequate description of expected results.

(10) Limitation of the procedure: Include a statement of limitations of the procedure. State known extrinsic factors or interfering substances affecting results. If further testing, either more specific or more sensitive, is indicated in all cases where certain results are obtained, the need for the additional test shall be stated.

(11) Expected values: State the range(s) of expected values as obtained with the product from studies of various populations. Indicate how the range(s) was established and identify the population(s) on which it was established.

(12) Specific performance characteristics: Include, as appropriate, information describing such things as accuracy, precision, specificity, and sensitivity. These shall be related to a generally accepted method using biological specimens from normal and abnormal populations. Include a statement summarizing the data upon which the specific performance characteristics are based.

(13) Bibliography: Include pertinent references keyed to the text.

(14) Name and place of business of manufacturer, packer, or distributor.

(15) Date of issuance of the last revision of the labeling identified as such.

(c) A shipment or other delivery of an in vitro diagnostic product shall be exempt from the requirements of paragraphs (a) and (b) of this section and from a standard promulgated pursuant to this part provided the following conditions are met:

(1) For a product in the laboratory research phase of development, and not represented as an effective in vitro

diagnostic product, all labeling bears the statement, prominently placed: 'For Research Use Only. Not for use in diagnostic procedures.'

(2) For a product being shipped or delivered for product testing prior to full commercial marketing (e.g., for use on specimens derived from humans to compare the usefulness of the product with other products or procedures which are in current use or recognized as useful), all labeling bears the statement, prominently placed: 'For Investigational Use Only. The performance characteristics of this product have not been established.'

(3) The person making a shipment or delivery under paragraph (c) (2) of this section shall submit to the FDA a notification that such shipments are being made.

(4) Within 30 days after the first commercial shipment of an in vitro diagnostic product, the person making such shipment shall submit the information required by the Drug Listing Act as provided in § 132.5 of this chapter.

(d) The labeling of general purpose laboratory reagents (e.g., hydrochloric acid) and equipment (e.g., test tubes and pipettes) whose uses are generally known by persons trained in their use need not bear the directions for use required by § 328.10 (a) and (b), if their labeling meets the requirements of this paragraph.

(1) The label of a reagent shall bear the following information:

(i) The proprietary name and established name (common or usual name), if any, of the reagent.

(ii) A declaration of the established name (common or usual name), if any, and quantity, proportion or concentration of the reagent ingredient (e.g., hydrochloric acid: Formula weight 36.46, assay 37.9 percent, specific gravity 1.192 at 60 °F.); and for a reagent derived from biological material, the source and where applicable a measure of its activity. The quantity, proportion, concentration or activity shall be stated in the system generally used and recognized by the intended user (e.g., metric, international units, etc.).

(iii) A statement of the purity and quality of the reagent, including a quantitative declaration of any impurities present. The requirement for this information may be met by a statement of conformity with a generally recognized and generally available standard which contains the same information (e.g., those established by the American Chemical Society, U.S. Pharmacopeia, National Formulary, National Research Council).

(iv) A statement of warnings or precautions for users as established in the regulations contained in 16 CFR Part 1500 and any other warnings appropriate to the hazard presented by the product; and a statement 'For Laboratory Use'.

(v) Appropriate storage instructions adequate to protect the stability of the product. When applicable, these instructions shall include such information as conditions of temperature, light, humidity, and other pertinent factors. The basis for such information shall be determined by reliable, meaningful, and specific test methods such as those described in § 133.13 of this chapter.

(vi) A declaration of the net quantity of contents, expressed in terms of weight or volume, numerical count, or any combination of these or other terms which accurately reflect the contents of the package. The use of metric designations is encouraged, wherever appropriate.

(vii) Name and place of business of manufacturer, packer, or distributor.

(viii) A lot or control number, identified as such, from which it is possible to determine the complete manufacturing history of the product.

(ix) In the case of immediate containers too small or otherwise unable to accommodate a label with sufficient space to bear all such information, and which are packaged within an outer container from which they are removed for use, the information required by paragraph (d) (1) (ii), (iii), (iv), (v), and (vi) of this section may appear in the outer container labeling only.

(2) The label of general purpose laboratory equipment (e.g., a beaker or a pipette) shall bear a statement adequately describing the product, its composition, and physical characteristics if necessary for its proper use.

Effective Date: § 328.10 (a), (b), and (d) become effective September 15, 1974; paragraph (c) became effective September 17, 1973. See 39 FR 8610, Mar. 6, 1974. The effective date for paragraphs (a) and (b) of this section, as applied to licensed blood grouping serum, was stayed. See 39 FR 2089, Jan. 17, 1974.

Subpart C – Requirements for Manufacturers and Producers

§ 328.20 General requirements for manufacturers and producers of in vitro diagnostic products

(a) *Registration and product listing.* Any person who owns or operates any establishment engaged in the manufacture, preparation, compounding, or processing of an in vitro diagnostic product should register such establishment and list such product(s) in accordance with the procedures established under Part 132 of this chapter; except that registration and listing is not required or requested at this time for general purpose laboratory reagents and equipment for which labeling requirements are specified in § 328.10 (d). Any such establishment not currently registered should register within 30 days of the effective date of this regulation. Any such establishment currently registered as a drug establishment shall at the next period for registration use the appropriate registration form indicating that it is a producer of in vitro diagnostic products. Registration forms may be obtained from the Department of Health, Education, and Welfare, Food and Drug Administration, 5600 Fishers Lane, Rockville, MD 20852, or at any Food and Drug Administration district office. Registration and listing do not constitute an admission or agreement or determination that a product is a 'drug' within the meaning of section 201 (g) of the act.

(b) *Compliance with good manufacturing practices.* In vitro diagnostic products shall be manufactured in accordance with current good manufacturing practices. The principles established in Part 133 of this chapter, 'Drugs; Current Good Manufacturing Practice in Manufacture, Processing, Packing, or Holding', should be followed as a guideline.

Subpart D – Administrative Procedures

§ 328.30 Procedure for establishing, amending or repealing standards

(a) *Basis for standards and available approaches to developing standards.* Whenever in the judgment of the Commissioner the establishment of a product class standard is necessary to reduce or eliminate unreasonable risk of illness or injury associated with exposure to or use of an in vitro diagnostic product and there are no other more practicable means to protect the public from such risk, he may propose such a standard. In proposing a product class standard he shall consider, and publish in the *Federal Register* findings on, the degree of risk or injury associated with the use of the product, the availability of information relating to the sciences upon which the products or their uses are based, the approximate number of products subject to the standard, the medical need for the products, and the probable effect of the standard upon the utility, cost, or availability of the product, and available means of achieving the objective of the standard with a minimal disruption of supply and of reasonable manufacturing and other commercial practices. Three procedures are available for developing product class standards and may be proposed on the initiative of the Commissioner or by petition of interested persons: (1) An existing standard may be utilized, (2) interested persons outside of the Food and Drug Administration may develop a proposed standard or (3) the Food and Drug Administration may develop the standard. If a petition is filed by an interested person, it shall be in the form prescribed in § 2.65 of this chapter with the number of copies specified therein.

(b) *Advisory committee.* An advisory committee of qualified experts shall be appointed to advise the Food and Drug Administration on the priorities for establishing product class standards, the scientific basis for in vitro diagnostic products, the selection of reference methodologies and reference materials, the adequacy and reasonableness of proposed standards and other related matters as determined by the Commissioner.

(c) *Request for information and comment.* Whenever a new standard is to be developed, the Commissioner will publish a notice in the *Federal Register* requesting the submission of all information, data, and views relevant to a specific product class for review and evaluation. Any interested person may submit comments and views on any matter relevant to the development of the standard, including the factors required by paragraph (a) of this section, to be considered by the Commissioner. The format for such submission may be determined by the nature of the information to be submitted. Any product performance information submitted shall relate to the performance of that product as marketed or intended for marketing. For information submitted by a manufacturer of a product which will be affected by the standard, the specific product information requested and the format for submission shall be as described below unless changed in the *Federal Register* notice. The time allotted for submission will ordinarily be 90 days. Four copies of the information and data on any product within the designated class shall be submitted, indexed, and bound.

(1) Name of product class and date of *Federal Register* statement.

(2) Proprietary name of product.

(3) Name of person responsible for submission.

(4) Intended use or uses of the product.

(5) A statement categorizing the procedure (e. g., qualitative or quantitative).

(6) Copies of label and all other labeling under which product is currently marketed or, for a proposed product, the label and all other labeling under which marketing is intended.

(7) Description of the product, as appropriate: For example, if the product is or includes a reagent, state the proprietary name and established name (common or usual name), if any, and quantity, proportion, or concentration of each reactive, catalytic, or inactive ingredient. If the product is a biological material, list the source and a measure of its activity. Include a statement of any purification or treatment required for use. If the product is or includes an instrument or equipment, describe as appropriate its use or functions, installation procedures and any special requirements, principle of operating instructions, calibration procedures including materials and/or equipment to be used, operation precautions and limitations, hazards, and service and maintenance instructions.

(8) Stability information: A description of, and data derived from, studies of the stability of the product. For any product that requires manipulation (e. g., reconstitution or mixing), stability data shall be described for the reconstituted or mixed product. Describe the means by which the information was developed. The data shall be for the product in the container in which it is marketed to assure, among other things, that the container is not reactive, additive, or absorptive to an extent that alters the product or its performance. Include any expiration period data which supports any expiration date which appears in the labeling of the product. Describe the storage conditions necessary for the product, such as temperature, light, humidity.

(9) Hazards to user: A statement of the principal hazards associated with the product. Include the result of tests conducted to determine the applicability of hazard warnings or cautions, including those established in the regulations contained in 16 CFR Part 1500.

(10) History of methodology: A brief history of the methodology, with pertinent references. All references to reports of adverse or unfavorable experience with the product or the procedure on which it is based shall be included. If the product procedure is the same as one which has been published, cite the reference. If the product is based on a modification of a published procedure, cite the reference, state the reason for and the nature of the modification and the effect such modification may have on the results of the procedure as compared to the original. Include data illustrating the comparison of the modified procedure to the original procedure.

(11) Principle of test: An explanation of the test procedure including the chemical, physical, physiological, or biological principle of the procedure with chemical reactions and techniques involved, if applicable.

(12) Specimen collection and preparation: A description of the specimen to be subjected to analysis: (i) Special precautions regarding specimen collections, including special preparation of the patient as it bears on the validity of the test.

(ii) Additives, preservatives, etc., necessary to maintain the integrity of the specimen.

(iii) Known interfering substances and their effect on the procedure and results.

(iv) Appropriate storage, handling or shipping instructions.

(13) Procedure: A detailed, step-by-step description of the test procedure from reception of the specimen to obtaining of results, including any points that may be useful in improving precision and accuracy. Give the exact details of calibration. Identify reference material. Describe preparation of reference sample, use of blanks, etc. Include a description of methods to be used in determining the standard curve.

(14) Results: Explain the procedure for calculating the value of the unknown. Give an explanation of each component of the formula used for the calculation of the unknown. Include a sample calculation, step-by-step, explaining the answer. Values should be expressed to the appropriate number of significant figures. Provide the basis for evaluation of non-quantitative test results.

(15) Limitation of the procedure: Include a statement of the limitations of the procedure and an explanation of extrinsic factors, if any, that may affect the results. Include statements regarding minimum training needed

by the user, special precautions, interfering substances, likelihood of obtaining false positive or false negative results, etc. Positive data showing a lack of interference by commonly occurring substances shall be supplied. If a more specific or more sensitive laboratory test is indicated in certain instances, the indication for the additional test shall be stated and data submitted to support its value.

(16) Support of claims: Include all available data, published or unpublished, which supports or is critical of the product or its procedure. Include data for both normal and abnormal subjects and a description of the population or populations studies. State, for each claim: (i) Labeling claim.

(ii) Background documentation: Provide a bibliography and reprints of all pertinent references.

(iii) Procedure used for collecting evidence for claim.

(iv) Description of statistical protocol.

(v) Description of sampling procedure.

(vi) Summary of raw results in tabular form.

(vii) Analysis of results.

(viii) Statement of interpretation of results.

(17) Summary of scientific basis of procedure: A summary of the data and views setting forth the scientific rationale and purpose of the product, and the scientific basis for the conclusion that the product has or has not been proven accurate and reliable for its intended uses. If here is an absence of controlled studies in the material submitted, an explanation as to why such studies are not considered necessary shall be included.

(18) If the submission is by a manufacturer, a statement signed by the person responsible for such submission, that to the best of his knowledge it includes unfavorable information as well as any favorable information, known to him pertinent to an evaluation of the performance of the product. Thus, if any type of scientific data is submitted, a balanced submission of favorable and unfavorable data must be submitted. The same would be true of any other pertinent data or information submitted, such as consumer surveys or marketing results.

(d) *Review and evaluation.* Any existing standard or petition for a product class standard, together with any information and comments submitted pursuant to a published notice, will be reviewed and evaluated by the Food and Drug Administration in consultation with its advisory committee and the Center for Disease Control.

(e) *Proposed product class standard.* When the Commissioner has concluded that the criteria in paragraph (a) of this section are met and the information available has been reviewed and found to justify the establishment of a product class standard, he shall publish in the *Federal Register* a proposed product class standard establishing conditions under which the products in the class are safe and effective and not adulterated or misbranded. The standard shall include a statement of the performance requirements necessary to assure accuracy and reliability of results, specific labeling requirements for the proper use of the products in the class, and procedures for testing the products to assure satisfactory performance at the time of marketing. The standard may include, where necessary to assure the accuracy and reliability of results, individual lot testing by or at the direction of the Food and Drug Administration, in addition to that normally required of the manufacturer; except that the Commissioner shall exempt any particular product from such a requirement upon a showing that the manufacturer has demonstrated such consistency in the production of that product, in compliance with the regulations, as is adequate to ensure the accuracy and reliability of results, and the Commissioner shall revoke the requirement of individual lot testing under the standard when it is no longer necessary to the accuracy and reliability of the results of the product class covered by the standard. Any interested person may, within 60 days after publication of the proposed standard in the *Federal Register,* file written comments on the proposal, in quintuplicate, with the Hearing Clerk, Food and Drug Administration, Room 6–86, 5600 Fishers Lane, Rockville, MD 20852. Comments may be accompanied by a memorandum or brief in support thereof. All comments may be reviewed at the office of the Hearing Clerk during regular working hours, Monday through Friday.

(f) *Referral to an independent advisory committee.* The Commissioner may, in his descretion, refer a proposal under paragraph (e) of this section to an independent advisory committee of experts qualified in the subject matter at issue, for a report and recommendations with respect to any matter involved in such proposal which involves the exercise of scientific judgment. The Commissioner shall designate the chairman of each panel. The independent advisory committee may consult any person in connection with the matter referred to it. Any interested person may request, in writing, an opportunity to present oral views to the committee. Any interested person may present written data and views which shall be considered by the committee. The full report(s) of the committee and summary minutes of its meetings shall be made available upon request after submission of the report(s) to the Commissioner.

(g) *Final product class standard.* After reviewing all comments received in response to the proposal and considering all available relevant information, the Food and Drug Administration, in consultation with its advisory committee and the Center for Disease Control, and after consideration of any report of an independent advisory committee if the matter involved has been so referred, will publish in the *Federal Register* a final order containing a product class standard. This order shall state the reasons for promulgating the product class standard and the date the standard will become effective.

(h) *Petition to amend or repeal standards.* The Commissioner may propose to amend or repeal any standard established pursuant to this procedure or any interested person may petition the Commissioner for such action. A petition shall set forth the action requested and a detailed statement in support of the action. After review of the petition, the Commissioner may deny the petition if he finds a lack of reasonable support or he may publish a proposed amendment of or proposed repeal of the established standard in the *Federal Register* if adequate support has been presented. The petition shall be in the form specified in § 2.65 of this chapter with the number of copies and other information as specified therein. A new drug application submitted for an in vitro diagnostic product which does not comply with an applicable effective product class standard will be considered as a petition to amend the standard. Petitions for repeal or amendment for which reasonable support has been furnished will be handled pursuant to the procedures established in paragraphs (e) through (g) of this section.

§ 328.34 Court appeal

The product class standard promulgated in the final order represents final agency action from which appeal lies to the courts. The Food and Drug Administration will request consolidation of all appeals in a single court. Upon court appeal, the Commissioner, at his discretion, may stay the effective date for part of all of the standard pending appeal and final court adjudication, and may establish a new effective date after final court adjudication.

§ 328.35 Regulatory action

Any in vitro diagnostic product is subject to regulatory action if it fails to conform to an applicable product class standard or the general labeling requirements of § 328.10. If the product is a device, it is adulterated in violation of section 501 and it is misbranded in violation of section 502 of the act. If the product is a drug, it is in violation of section 505 as well as sections 501 and 502 of the act. If the product is a biologic, it is in violation of sections 501, 502, and 505 of the Federal Food, Drug, and Cosmetic Act and section 351 of the Public Health Service Act. Deviations from an established standard may be justified only by an amendment to the standard. Compliance with this part shall be deemed to constitute compliance with the labeling and new drug requirements of the act and with the labeling and licensing requirements of section 351 of the Public Health Service Act, unless the Commissioner otherwise informs the manufacturer or distributor of an in vitro diagnostic product of additional requirements imposed pursuant to either statute in order to protect the public health.

Analysis of Regulations on Clinical Chemistry in the European Community

K. F. Lauer, Brussels (Belgium)[1]

Key Words: European Community
Health Care
Measurement Methods

1. General introduction

We shall try to show the situation concerning laws, regulations, standardization (normalization), codes of conduct and technical efforts of harmonization and improvement. Arguments on why and how the above mentioned should exist are well-known and have been treated excellently before [1].

This paper surely can not claim to cover the field exhaustively, as not all existing information could be obtained in time.

Some introductory words are needed on the general structures and possible principles that are applied in this field within the Member Countries. In principle we are discussing here *measurement methods* in the field of *health care*. We have, therefore, to look for laws, regulations, conventions and technical studies that can be applicable to the two fields: *Measurement* and *Health Care* separately or conjointly. Historically, both fields have developed independently and often differently from each other. A further complication is that even within one field, the development has been rather different as we go from country to country.

2. Possibilities

2.1. Laws and regulation

2.1.1. Legal Metrology

Every member country has a legislation on *weights and measures*. These laws have been made to assure that all measurements concerned would fit into a homogeneous, coherent and transferable national system which should allow commerce, industry and science to dispose of compatible measurements, and last but not least, to safeguard public interest and safety. Very rapidly this system has been applied internationally, and the International

---

[1] Commission of the European Communities, Directorate-General for Research, Science and Education Community Bureau of Reference

Organization of Legal Metrology (IOLM) provides recommendations in this field which can be adopted as laws in countries (a number of countries have set up their own National Measurement Laboratories, Calibration Services or similar systems).

The European Community issues directives to member countries in this field.

The countries have different approaches to the control of the application of such laws.

2.1.2. Other legal possibilities

All member countries have specific laws in the fields of Public Health Care and Public Safety. The European Community can legislate in certain cases.

Many international organisations, like the World Health Organization (WHO), can make recommendations to member countries for application on any level of legislation within their countries.

2.2. Access to Profession

Many countries have regulated, and this of course particularly applies in the Health Care field, the access to particular professions.

It is here that official organizations of professions can regulate for their compulsory members. In the case of voluntary membership, only recommendations can be given (see also 3.2).

2.3. Pharmacopeia

National Pharmacopoeias can regulate methods, reagents and products in a rather wide range. The European Pharmacopeia of the Council of Europe (18 member countries) is an example of a regional cooperation in this field.

2.4. Standardization (= Normalization)

In parallel with increasing commerce and industrialisation goes, always, a need for conventions that will allow easier and more economical identification and exchange of goods or technical *parts* and *equipment*. This is the purpose for which standardization (= normalization) is conceived.

It now not only concerns goods, materials and equipment, but also *measurement methods* in a very wide sense of the word and in a multitude of technical and scientific sectors.

National Standards Institutes exist in all member countries and cooperate with each other and other external countries in the framework of the Commission Européenne pour la Normalisation (CEN) or the International Standards Organization (ISO).

Both these organizations issue recommendations which can be adopted as national standards. National standards are always voluntary, if not adopted expressly by national or community legislation.

2.5. Technical efforts of harmonization and improvement

Since the very first beginning of science and technology, cooperation has been one of the most important factors for harmonization of methods and their improvement. Learned societies, professional and industrial associations have sprung up very early and nowadays we see even the public at large entering the discussions.

All the above bodies might organize cooperative studies, exchange information, adopt conventions or even create their own national research institutes.

Many national organizations are members of a respective international organization active in this field:

- International Association of Biological Standardization
- International Association of Microbiological Societies
- International Committee for Standardization in Hematology
- International Federation of Clinical Chemistry
- International Society of Blood Transfusion
- International Society of Endocrinology
- International Society of Thrombosis and Haemostasis
- International Union of Pure and Applied Chemistry (Section of Clinical Chemistry)
- World Association of Anatomic and Clinical Pathology Societies

3. European Communities

In order to carry out their task, the Council and the Commission make regulations, issue directives, take decisions, make recommendations, or deliver opinions.

A regulation has general application. It is binding in its entirety, and directly applicable in all Member States.

A directive is binding, as to the result to be achieved, upon each Member State to which it is addressed, but leaves to the national authorities the choice of form and methods.

A decision is binding in its entirety upon those to whom it is addressed.

Recommendations and opinions have no binding force.

3.1. Regulations: none

3.2. Directive

A Council Directive of the European Communities concerning the mutual recognition of diplomas, certificates and other evidence of formal qualifications in medicine, including measures to facilitate the effective exercise of the right of establishment and freedom to provide services, is in discussion by the Council of Ministers.

3.3. Decision: none

3.4. Recommendations and opinions: none

3.5. Technical efforts

Community Bureau of Reference

In the framework of the Scientific and Technological Policy Programme of the Commission, work is being undertaken in connection with public, scientific and technological services for the member countries. The Community Bureau of Reference (CBR) constitutes one of the actions in this field.

The programme is concerned with the multitude of problems encountered with measurement methods and instruments and their calibration with reference materials (RMs). The determination of intrinsic properties of materials, as executed on all levels of the commercial, industrial and scientific processes, has to be done in such a way that results of the measurements find their place in a homogeneous and coherent system.

In general, it can be said that this programme does support, group, dovetail and supplement the efforts of member countries in this field.

In the field of clinical analysis this could lead to the cooperation of all bodies concerned, and to the laying of the technical foundations of future national or supranational legal acts.

4. Council of Europe

Resolution AP (70) 4 of 16. September 1970.

Recommendation to bring national laws into conformity.

Subject: Manufacture and control of laboratory reagents for the rapid diagnostic of human diseases.

Literature

[1] *H. Büttner:* Proc. Int. Conf. Stand. Diag. Mat. 1973, 55–59. CDC, Atlanta, Georgia, 30333.
[2] France: G. Siest, B. Capolaghï, 1974. Clinical Chemistry in France (Tentative document).

Table 1.

	B	Dk	F	G	Irl	I	L	N	UK
Laws:									
Legal Metrology:	–	–	–	+ [6]	–	–	–	–	–
Others:	–	–	i.p.[3]	–	–	+ [10]	–	–	–
Access to profession:	phys. pharm.	phys. biol. chem.	pharm. phys. vet.	phys. biol. chem.	phys. others	phys. chem. biol.	phys.	phys. chem.	phys. others
Pharmocopoeia:	–	–	–	–	–	–	–	–	–
Standardization = Normalization:	–	–	+ [4]	+ [7]	–	–	–	+ [12]	–
Technical efforts:	+ [1]	+ [2]	+ [5]	+ [8]	+ [9]	+ [11]	–	+ [13]	+ [14]

i.p. = in preparation
phys. = physicians
pharm. = pharmacists
biol. = biologists
chem. = chemists
vet. = veterinaries

Specific Remarks to Table 1

1. – Société Belge de Chimie Clinique
   Belgische Vereniging voor Klinische Chemie
   – Association pour la Qualité des Analyses de Biologie Chimique
   Vereniging voor de kwaliteit van de Ontledingen der Klinischen Biologie

2. Dansk Selskab for Klinisk Kemi

3. Bill proposed in the Assembly (9th November 1973) on:
   – Need for greater competence
   – Exclusive practice of the profession
   – Obligatory control of analysis in medical biology

4. 2 Mixed working groups of AFNOR and S.F.B.C. have started work on – nomenclature
   – sampling tubes

   AFNOR = Association Française pour la Normalisation
   S.F.B.C. = Société Française de Biologie Clinique

5. Société Française de Biologie Clinique
   Clinical Biology covers: clinical chemistry, hematology, bacteriology, immunology, parasitology, etc.

6. Measurement of mass, volume, pressure, density and temperature.
   Any measurement involving the above principles is subject to the Calibration Act. As an exception, statistical quality control of the overall measurement process can be used.
   The medical order (Bundesärztekammer) issues guide lines for quality control for any measurement involving volume measurements with non-officially calibrated devices.
   3 Chief investigators for the organization of collaborative quality control surveys have been named at the present moment. It is intended to cover as soon as possible all practising laboratories and all currently applied methods.

7. The German Normalization Institute (Deutscher Normen Ausschuss) has a committee «Fachnormenausschuss Medizin» which in turn has a working group C «Laboratoriumsmedizin» (medical laboratory) having a sub-group C 2 «Medizinische Chemie» (medical chemistry) looking at:

- general methodology
- method interferences
- quality control
- electrophoresis
- analytical coagulation
- terminology and nomenclature
- job evaluation and costs

8. Deutsche Gesellschaft für Klinische Chemie e.V.
   Deutsche Gesellschaft für Laboratoriumsmedizin
   Arbeitsgemeinschaft der Fachärzte für Laboratoriumsmedizin.
9. Association of Clinical Biochemists
   Pathology Section of Irish Medical Association
10. A law on the organization of hospitals giving details of general and administrative nature
11. Societa Italiana di Biochimica
12. The Netherlands Normalisatie Instituut has a working group on methods in clinical chemistry, about 20 standards have been drawn up.
13. Nederlandse Vereniging voor Klinische Chemie
    Stichting Kwaliteitsbewaking
    Vereniging van Laboratoriumartsen
14. Association of Clinical Biochemists
    Royal College of Pathologists
    Association of Clinical Pathologists

National Regulations and International Recommendations in Laboratory Diagnosis in Socialistic Countries

J. Krawczynski, Warszaw (Poland)

Key Words: Education Programs
Laboratory Diagnosis
National Regulations
Quality Control AMS
Socialistic Countries
Staffing
Standard Methods

Laboratory diagnosis is considered by Health Service Authorities in all Socialistic Countries (S. C.) as one of the most important medical branches.

Actually, a very important problem is to accelerate the development and the modernization of laboratory services in all of these countries.

The way to realize this program on the one hand, is to create the proper organization of laboratory diagnostics by the help of reasonable and flexible legislation, and on the other hand, to develop conditions for close cooperation especially between Socialistic Countries having a similar economic, social and political basis. The possibilities of cooperation with other countries are, of course, not excluded.

In the last 10–12 years the organization of systems of laboratory diagnostics have been developed in Socialistic countries. These systems are in most important aspects similar to each other, but differ considerably in detail. These differences, although of seeming minor importance, may sometimes have a negative influence on the solution of important problems which demand international cooperation. Lastly, we observe in all Socialistic countries the increasing trends for further unification of national organization systems in laboratory diagnostics.

It, therefore, seems reasonable to present here the actual legislative situation in laboratory diagnostics in Poland, with comments concerning the situation in the German Democratic Republic and in the Soviet Union, as well as the program and perspectives of international cooperation in this field between Socialistic Countries.

National Regulations in Laboratory Diagnostics in Poland

In Poland, almost all problems concerning laboratory diagnostics are regulated by the Ministry of Health and Public Welfare.

The Ministry acts permanently by way of the S. C., Specialist Advisory Board consisting of 20 provincial specialists, the head of which is the country specialist who is designated as the President of the Country Advisory Board.

All specialists are nominated by the Ministry for a 4 year period. Since they are the most experienced and trained laboratory doctors, they play a very important and decisive role in laboratory diagnostic and practically regulate and control all laboratory activities in each province as well as in the whole country.

Until January 1, 1975 the S.C. 'Laboratory diagnostics' comprised the following subspecialities: clinical chemistry, laboratory hematology, immunohematology and microbiological diagnostics. Actually, microbiological diagnostics and, in some degree, immunohematology are separated from laboratory diagnostics as independent specialties having each their own Specialistic Advisory Board.

In 1968, the special order of the Ministry of Health and Public Welfare was published, concerning the organization and activities in the field of laboratory diagnostics at the present time.

The following problems are regulated by the order:

1. *Classification of all laboratories according to their size, location whether hospital or polyclinic laboratories/and service activity:* All routine laboratories were divided into 8 groups/classes/with a varied obligatory work spectrum.
   Actually, according to the new organization of the Health Service in Poland, the classification of diagnostic laboratories must be changed. The tendencies are to reduce the number of laboratory groups/classes/from 8 to 5, as well as the number of laboratories. This is to be achieved by closing of small laboratories, which would be replaced by the so called 'laboratory manual sets' enabling test performance of some of the simplest laboratory investigations, such as screening tests of urine and blood, and prelaboratory diagnostics by the physician or nurse.

2. *Standardization and unification of laboratory methods:* Two former orders concern this problem; Order from 1959 and 1967. The Ministry of Health and Social Welfare approved and modified two editions of the 'Manual of Standardized and Unified Laboratory Methods' of 1959 and 1967. These are obligatory or recommended for all routine laboratories. In addition, the edition of one supplement 1971 and further supplements since 1974 will be published yearly in the bimonthly journal 'Laboratory Diagnostics', edited by the Polish Society of Laboratory Diagnostics.
   Practically, the standardization and unification of laboratory methods is continuously performed by the Committee for Standardization of Laboratory Methods and Technical Progress. This Committee has existed since 1966 as a branch of the Scientific Advisory Board of the Ministry of Health and Public Welfare.

3. *Education of Laboratory Staff:* The order, or its supplements, regulates the principles of education of laboratory staff and selection of persons for leading positions.

a) *Undergraduate education in medical and pharmaceutical faculties:* In medical faculties there are only 45 hours designated for education in laboratory diagnostic/in the 6th semester. Since 1971, in all pharmaceutical faculties there have been special students, 15–30 in each faculty, who are prepared for work in clinical laboratories. This two year program is given after 3 years of general pharmaceutical education. In Poland, about 200 pharmacists have been educated in this way, and we consider them as very valuable and well trained personnel for laboratory work.

b) *Specialization studies in laboratory diagnostic programs and analytical procedures for physicians and pharmacists:* The laboratory doctors and pharmacists may obtain the titles of specialists in laboratory diagnostics. There are two degrees of specialization: 1st – after 3 years of practical education and 2nd – after a further two year education and state examination, according to the official obligatory program.

c) *Special Postgraduate education programs and organization:* In Poland, the special system of postgraduate medical education is directed and controlled by the Medical Center for Postgraduate Education, MCPE. There are two levels of education; One is a central program established by MCPE medical schools and Research Institutes. The education in laboratory diagnostic is provided on this level by the Department of Laboratory Diagnostics in MCPE and by analogous departments of medical and pharmaceutical faculties. The second curriculum is provided by provincial programs in provincial centers for Postgraduate Education, eg. local medical and pharmaceutical faculties, and by provincial hospitals, polyclinics etc. The laboratory personnel are trained on this level in departments of laboratory diagnostics of medical and pharmaceutical faculties and in larger routine laboratories.
The education at the central level is mainly specialized, while that at the provincial level is rather basic. Actually, it is possible to train about 20% graduate laboratory personnel each year.

d) *Education of Technicians, professionals and postgraduates:* The laboratory technicians are educated in special middle level medical-technical schools. There are 18 schools of this type in the country. A center for Postgraduate Education of Middle Medical Personal including laboratory technicians, is also established.

e) *Obligatory qualifications necessary for persons designated to work in leading positions in clinical laboratories:* It is necessary to have special qualifications to be designated to work in leading positions in clinical laboratories. For example, the head of a small laboratory, or the head of a department in a larger laboratory, must be a specialist of the 1st degree, and the head of the largest laboratories a specialist of the 2nd degree.

4. *Statistics and Evaluation of Laboratory Work:* Since 1968, the unified report system in laboratory diagnostics has been introduced. This report system is based on the classification of all routine laboratory tests into 5 groups, depending approximately on the time needed for their performance.

Each group is characterized by a number of arbitrarily defined units. The simplest tests by 1 unit, the most complicated by 15 units. It was possible to use the following coefficients for objective evaluation of laboratory activities:

a) of paid productivity
b) of real productivity
c) of laboratory results utilized
d) of test structure
e) of control and methodologic research

The optimal values for each coefficient are established experimentally. The evaluation of laboratory activity is based on the comparison of coefficients calculated for the laboratory under consideration, with the above mentioned optimal values as a basis.

5. *Quality Control in Diagnostic Laboratories:* The recommendations were prepared by the Expert Commission of Standardization of Laboratory Methods. They comprise the internal quality control which should be performed in each laboratory and consist of:

a) precision control, with animal non-assayed lyophilized control serum/Serostandard-Polish production. It is performed with each series of determinations and the results are plotted on the control card.

b) accuracy control, with human assayed lyophilized control serum/Serostandard – N/normal/and P/pathological/containing 15 parameters. In large laboratories the commercial control sera/Dade, Hyland, Godecke/are also used. The controls are performed with every fourth series of determinations and the results are plotted on the control card.

c) for determinations lacking control material, the use of unknown duplicates is obligatory. This is performed with each series of determinations and the results are plotted on he control card.
External interlaboratory control is not completely systematized and not performed in all provinces.
In the future, the interlaboratory control will be carried out on different levels: province every 2 weeks, regional each two months, and interregional 3–5 times in the year.
A special center for national control and international collaboration will be organized.
Anonymity of control results is strictly preserved.

6. *Regulations concerning the number of laboratory staff employed in diagnostic laboratories:* Recently, a program for establishing requirements of the laboratory staff was prepared. For this, special coefficients were introduced which are, of course, variable for different types of laboratories. These coefficients depend mainly on the number of hospital beds and the number of inhabitants living in the region or province.

According to the longtime experience, established proportions between different groups of laboratory personnel employed in diagnostic laboratories have become the norm, e.g. 1 graduate for 4 technicians.

7. *Regulations concerning the planning of new laboratories:* In the last two years, principles of planning for routine laboratories for new hospital and polyclinic buildings were established by collaboration with specialized architects. Our new system of planning is based on the so-called universal laboratory unit, which can be arbitrally replicated depending on the real requirements of the hospital or polyclinic. In a short time, this system will be obligatory for architects planning diagnostic laboratories in health service centers.
   In summary, it must be stated that the national regulations cover almost all problems concerning laboratory diagnostics and in this way create conditions for the rational and rapid development of this medical speciality in the country.

National Regulations in other Socialistic Countries

In general, the national regulations in all Socialistic Countries are very similar, although the legislation does not go as far as in Poland. Of course, there are local differences.

In the Soviet Union, since 1968 and independently of the Country Advisor System, the Soviet Union Coordination Center in Laboratory Diagnostics/director: Prof. Dr. *W. W.Menshikov,* has been established as the official branch office of the Soviet Ministry of Health. In the above mentioned Center, all organization and technical problems concerning laboratory services are controlled. The Coordination Center also coordinates all activities concerning standardization and unification of laboratory methods and laboratory equipment. The Center is also the general supervisor of quality control performance in the whole country. The Coordination Center has paid special attention to this last problem and has stimulated industry to undertake the production of control material, standard and control sera.

In May 1975, The Presidential Committee of the Soviet Society of Laboratory Diagnosis will finally approve the quality control system, which will then be obligatory for all laboratories in the country.

In addition, the problems of quality control will be introduced as part of the official program of postgraduate education of laboratory personnel.

The Soviet Coordination Center cooperates, on the one hand, with the Soviet Ministry of Health for which it is the expert board, preparing orders and recommendations for official approval, and, on the other, with equipment and chemical industry as well as with various technical commissions.

Similar Coordination Centers exist also in the German Democratic Republic and in Hungary.

The general opinion is that such a Coordination Center plays very important roles in the development of laboratory diagnostics. There are very strong tendencies to organize such Centers in the other Socialistic Countries.

It should be mentioned, that in the GDR, the standardization and unification of laboratory methods is included in the German Pharmacopie, DAB 7 D. L. In this way, the standardization and unification of laboratory methods has the character of governmental order. A similar situation exists in Czechoslovakia.

In the development of laboratory diagnostics in all Socialistic Countries, a very important role is played by the National Societies of Laboratory Diagnostics or Societies of Clinical Chemistry. These Societies organize expert groups and collectives which very efficiently assist in the solution of organization and scientific problems.

International Recommendations

Since 1966, regular conferences of the Expert Group for Standardization of Laboratory Methods of Socialistic Countries have been held. In these conferences, from the start, representatives of Bulgaria, Czechoslovakia, GDR, Hungary, Poland and the Soviet Union and, most recently, the representatives of the Mongolian Socialistic Republic, became full members of the Expert Group.

The meetings of the Expert Group will now be organized each three years. The permanent coordination of Expert Group activity in the period between conferences will be performed by the Soviet Coordination Center. Till now, the following recommendations have been made and sent to the National Ministries of Health for official approval. These will then become obligatory for all countries who are members of the expert group:

1. General rules of standardization and unification of laboratory diagnostic methods.
2. Principles of unified characteristics of laboratory diagnostic methods.
3. Principles of unified procedures of laboratory method comparison.
4. Principles for the preparation of calibration curves.

In the near future the following important problems should be resolved:

1. Unified principles of intra- and interlaboratory quality control.
2. Multilanguage terminology and vocabulary for laboratory diagnostics.
3. Reference Methods.
4. Unified system of objective evaluation of diagnostic laboratory activities.
5. Principles of unified evaluation of usefulness of laboratory equipment as well as of diagnostic products/e. g. reagents, kits, standard and control sera etc.

The actual results of international cooperation between Socialistic Countries should be considered as very promising. It seems that this cooperation will not only stimulate the process of modernization of laboratory diagnostics in all cooperating countries, but will also contribute to the general acceptance of the efforts to solve the most important problems of laboratory diagnostics on a wide international basis.

National Regulations and International Recommendations

Discussions

H. Bergmeyer (Germany): We have heard the situation of governmental regulations or non-regulations of diagnostic products on both sides of the Atlantic and it is obvious there are big differences as to how this is being approached. At least one big difference is that in the large country of the United States uniformity is possible, whereas this is hardly possible at the time being in Europe. I had not thought about how big the differences were until today when they were explained to us. In my opinion, differences also exist in the philosophy of how to ensure high quality laboratory results. These differences in philosophy become evident if one looks into laboratories of Europe and America, or even in Japan. Since we all have the same goal, namely, to raise the quality of laboratory performance worldwide, governmental regulations or those of other national authorities, such as scientific associations, should follow the recommendations of the international federations. These international federations, like IFCC or WHO, must be actively creative. Their sources are the national scientists from the scientific societies, governmental organizations, and industry. To reach a common goal, several points have to be considered.

1. The creation of a uniform common philosophy on how to ensure high quality laboratory results.
2. The establishment of standardized international methods and reagent materials.
3. To raise the level of education of laboratory personnel, as well as that of the physicians who use laboratory data for their diagnosis.
4. Establishment of standards for the requirements of instrumentation which are adequate to the mean methods and reagents.

Let me state briefly what I understand under these topics. Perhaps you will allow me to summarize here a few remarks in Sessions I, II and III of this IFCC day. In order to explain this uniform philosophy, let me give you an example.

To point 1: I think it is a matter of fact that the American Clinical Chemists, supported by the government authorities and vice-versa, would like to have a standard substance for each parameter which is to be measured in biological fluids, including enzymes. That may have a historical background. How profound the differences are, we saw in the short discussion this morning. It is true also that the Europeans prefer to go to the physical constants wherever possible, namely, the molar absorption coefficient in photometry. For the calibration of a method, the standard substance must be measured just like the unknown. The accuracy and precision of this measurement depends on the method and equipment used. Now it may happen that one single measure of a standard will give a result outside the confidence limits. Relating the sample measurement to such a falsely determined standard will also yield, of course, false unknown values. I have nothing against standards or reference materials wherever they are necessary, but I would like to caution against the over-estimation of their value. Physical constants, like epsilon (ε), can, in principle, be determined with high accuracy and precision. I think this example shows clearly the task of international organizations, like IFCC with its commissions and expert panels, to create a worldwide valid philosophy for clinical chemistry.

Now, let's move to point 2 on standardized methods and reagent materials. The importance of the standardized method and reagent materials is unquestionable. IFCC has already done a lot of work in this field and I think that within a few years, say 1980, the four or five most commonly used and important methods will be worked out. For reagents and reagent kits, the same is true. The question arises as to how important international or national regulations consider the following points: a) the cost of highly sophisticated reagents and reagent kits, b) how the development of analytical biochemistry is influenced, and c) the consequences of these regulations on industrial competition, and their effect on prices.

The development of practical methods and reagents is the result of a good partnership between clinical chemists from industry and from professionals. No individual scientist today will be in the position to have the necessary funds available for the extended development and broad evaluation of a new method and kit. The costs are extremely high and the required time is extremely long. Regulations from national or international authorities should keep in mind that their limitations should be within the framework which covers the necessities of a good laboratory practice, but should not contain any over-estimated requirements; otherwise, the products of industry would become unnecessarily expensive.

As far as the effect on further developments in analytical bio-chemistry is concerned, I also think that all the well-founded reasons for regulations must give space for further advance in analytical sciences. All authorities must be flexible enough also to cancel an adopted method in favor of another, if the adopted method is proved to be unsatisfactory compared with a new one. For example, consider the advantages of the new fully enzymatic method for the determination of cholesterol. The former chemical method, according to Abel and Kendall, has been considered somewhat as a standard method in several parts of the world; today, it has been superseded by a better method. Governmental regulations should not only *not* inhibit progress in analytical chemistry, but should stimulate it. This can be done by flexible regulations and by efforts in eliminiating inferior material.

It is the aim of governmental regulations to also survey the quality of methods and material brought into the market by the manufacturers. The setting up of quality requirements for reagent materials by all participants, including industry, is highly appreciated. It will help to identify and eliminate diagnostic material of inferior quality manufactured by dubious companies. On the other hand, the keen and often zealous competitive atmosphere among reagent manufacturers is another major contributory factor to raising the quality of diagnostic materials to an even greater extent than government regulations can achieve. The pre-requisite for this, however, is a well-educated laboratory staff able to recognize dubious preparations. These demands on the knowledge of the laboratory worker lead me to my third point 'level of education'.

Not only is it necessary to educate the laboratory personnel in thinking according to a common philosophy of clinical chemistry, but it is equally important for the physician who uses the laboratory values for diagnosis to share this philosophy. He must be able to decide how far he should force the clinical chemistry laboratory to deliver accurate and precise values. Modern methods for the determination of enzyme activities can deliver a great amount of diagnostic information, but the values must be accurate and precise, and the physician must be trained to be able to handle these values. In my opinion, there has been greater progress in methodology and the quality of reagents than there has been in education and laboratory equipment in certain countries. There must be a real concerted effort to improve all that is needed for gaining highly accurate and precise results – and the method, reagents, equipment, and knowledge to handle them.

And now to the fourth point – 'the level of equipment'. In this sense, I understand the paper by Dr. Sims, and I agree it is necessary also to standardize the requirements for the instruments. It is a strange situation if, for instance, in the leading laboratories in Japan aminotransferase activities are measured according to Reitman and Frankel, on highly sophisticated automated equipment, yielding fantastic precision, but completely insufficient accuracy. It is no less strange if in our country aminotransferases are measured using UV methods on instruments without any temperature adjustment or control. The manufacturers of photometers and automated equipment also must have guidelines from an international level on how to build their instruments so that they can fulfill the requirements derived from our highly sophisticated methods and materials.

R. Dybkaer (Denmark): Thank you very much, Prof. *Bergmeyer*. You have beautifully summarized the complexity of our goals, but we will have no chance of achieving them unless industry and professions work together, and then advise government how they should regulate.

H. Büttner (Germany): I should like to say a few words about governmental regulation of methods. I think this is one of the most important points for clinical chemists, because such regulations could restrict the free decision of the clinical chemist, as a scientist, as to which methods he would like to use. Therefore, it is very much a problem for us. On the other hand, I can understand a government being interested in having comparable results throughout the whole country, and so national regulations and governmental regulations are under consideration. It is very simple to get those regulations, by just looking around the country to establish which method is being used in most laboratories and then prescribe that method. That is one way, the extreme way. A little bit better, but not really much better, is to ask a few experts what they think is the best method and then prescribe that method. All these ways, I think, are contrary to the scientific effort of clinical chemists. And so, I think, we cannot really recommend that government gives us regulations for methods.

In my opinion, there is only one way to solve this problem, and this way has two approaches, which we have discussed here today. One approach is from the top, that is: definitive methods and reference methods. This must be an international effort; we cannot develop these on a national level, and I am very happy that NBS, for example, represents a crystalization point for such efforts. The other way (I am very happy to say that a lot of scientific societies in clinical chemistry will follow us here) is that of selected methods, which means, to select methods for routine use by a special mechanism, utilizing the experience of experts, and reaching a consensus.

I think these two approaches, definitive methods and reference methods on one hand, and a selected methods concept on the other hand, are the ways the clinical chemist should go now, and not the way of certain prescribed methods in national or governmental regulations.

R. Dybkaer (Denmark): I will now ask Prof. *Martin Rubin,* President of IFCC, to close today's activities.

M. Rubin, U.S.A.: Thank you Dr. *Dybkaer.* The presentations and discussion today have provided ample evidence of the critical need for international agreement on many important facets of clinical laboratory function. Clearly this can only be achieved when the problems of language, of communication, of differing viewpoints, of national interests and of corporate objectives can be merged by the accomodations achieved in full, frank, vigorous, reasoned and open review. This meeting has been a major step toward this objective.

On behalf of all of us, I would like to express our thanks and appreciation to the Chairmen of these sessions, to the speakers who have been so generous of their time and efforts and to the discussion leaders and contributors. We are especially indepted to the Nestle Foundation, Hoffman La Roche, the Ames Company, and, of course, to the Dade Company who have supported this effort, not only by their financial contributions, but also by the provisions of many other organizational facilities. Indeed without the continuous and dedicated labors of Mrs. Divernois-Merz this meeting would not have been possible. And finally, may I add a personal note of thanks to my colleagues in the International Federation of Clinical Chemistry for their responsivenesss and help during the months of preparation for this Symposium.

Speakers

Prof. H. Adlercreutz
Department of Clinical Chemistry
University of Helsinki
Meilahti Hospital
00290 Helsinki / Finland

Prof. H. Aebi
Medizinisch-Chemisches Institut der Universität
Bühlstrasse 28
3012 Berne / Switzerland

Dr. G. Anido
Dade Division
American Hospital Supply Corporation
P. O. Box 520672
Miami, Florida 33152 / USA

Dr. O. W. van Assendelft
Laboratory of Chemical Physiology
University of Groningen
Bloemsingel 10
Groningen / Holland

Dr. A. L. Babson
Warner Lambert Company
201 Tabor Road
Morris Plains, New Jersey 07950 / USA

Prof. M. Bailly
Laboratoire de Biochimie A
Hôpital Necker
149, Rue de Sèvres
75730 Paris Cedex 15 / France

Prof. H. U. Bergmeyer
Direktor Boehringer Mannheim GmbH
Brahmsweg 6
8132 Tutzing / West Germany

Dr. G. N. Bowers, Jr.
Clinical Chemistry Laboratory
Department of Pathology
Hartford Hospital
Hartford, Connecticut 06115 / USA

Mr. P. M. G. Broughton
University Department of Chemical Pathology
General Infirmary
Leeds, LS1 3EX / U.K.

Dr. S. S. Brown
Clinical Research Centre
Division of Clinical Chemistry
Watford Road
Harrow, Middlesex HA1 3UJ / U.K.

Prof. Th. Bücher
Institut für Physiologische Chemie,
Physikalische Biochemie und
Zellbiologie der Universität München
Goethestrasse 33
8000 München 2 / West Germany

Dr. W. Bürgi
Zentrallaboratorium
Kantonsspital
5001 Aarau / Switzerland

Prof. J. Büttner
Medizinische Hochschule
Abt. Klinische Chemie
Postfach 180
3000 Hannover-Kleefeld / West Germany

Dr. J. P. Cali
Office of Standard Reference Material
National Bureau of Standards
Washington, D. C. 20234 / USA

Prof. G. Ceriotti
Laboratoire Centrale di Analisi
Ospedale Civile e Policlinico Universitario
Via Ospedale 1
35100 Padova / Italy

Dr. G. R. Cooper
Chief, Metabolic Biochemistry Branch
Clinical Chemistry Division
Bureau of Laboratories
Center for Disease Control
Atlanta, Georgia 30333 / USA

Dr. B. E. Copeland
Laboratory of Pathology NEDH
New England Deaconess Hospital
185 Pilgrim Road
Boston, Massachusetts 02215 / USA

Mr. G. M. Darnell
Dade Division of AHSC
P. O. Box 520672
Miami, Florida 33152 / USA

Dr. R. Dybkaer
Department of Clinical Chemistry
Geriatric Unit, De Gamles By
Nørre Allé 41
2200 Copenhagen N / Denmark

Dr. E. Eavenson
Acting Director
Division of Diagnostic Product Standards
and Research
Department of Health, Education and Welfare
5600 Fisher Lane
Rockville, Maryland 20852 / USA

Dr. W. Gerhardt-Hansen
Department of Clinical Chemistry A
Rigshospitalet
2011 Copenhagen Ø / Denmark

Dr. J. L. Giegel
Dade Division of AHSC
P. O. Box 520672
Miami, Florida 33152 / USA

Dr. M. Härkönen
Department of Clinical Chemistry
University of Helsinki
Meilahti Hospital
00290 Helsinki 29 / Finland

Dr. L. Havelec
Institut für Medizinische Statistik und
Dokumentation der Universität Wien
Schwarzspanierstrasse 17
1090 Wien / Austria

Prof. J. B. Henry
Department of Pathology
State University of New York
Upstate Medical Center
750 East Adams Street
Syracuse, New York 13210 / USA

Dr. A. Hyvärinen
City Hospital
Koljontie 3
33500 Tampere 50 / Finland

Dr. A. P. Jansen
St. Radboud Ziekenhuis
Laboratorium voor inwendige Geneeskunde
Geert Grooteplein Zuid 16
Nijmegen / Holland

Dr. E. J. van Kampen
Laboratory of Clinical Chemistry
Diakonessenhuis
Groningen / Holland

Prof. T. Kawai
Jichi Medical School
Department of Clinical Pathology
Minami-kawachi-machi
Tochigi / Japan 329-04

Prof. M. J. Krawczynski
Zaklad Doskonaleinia Lekarzy
Cegtowska 80
01 809 Warszawa / Poland

Mr. H. Küffer
Biochemistry R & D
Greiner Electronic Ltd.
Gaswerkstrasse 33–35
4900 Langenthal / Switzerland

Dr. D. Kutter
14, Rue Beck
Luxembourg

Dr. K.-F. Lauer
Commission of the European Communities
Directorate General for Research Science
and Education
Rue de la Loi 200
1049 Bruxelles / Belgium

Dr. R. Leclercq
Avenue des Frères Becqué 17
1080 Bruxelles / Belgium

Dr. A. L. Louderback
Clinical Chemistry Consultants
P. O. Box 761
Temple City, California 91780 / USA

Prof. A. Martinez
Ciudad Sanitaria de la Seguridad Social
'1° Octubre'
Carretera Andalucia 5.5.
Madrid / Spain

Dr. F. L. Mitchell
Clinical Research Centre
Division of Clinical Chemistry
Watford Road
Harrow, Middlesex HA1 3UJ / U. K.

Dr. R. G. Nadeau
Marketing Manager
Automatic Clinical Analyzer
E. I. Du Pont De Nemours & Co.
Instruments Products Division
Wilmington, Delaware 19898 / USA

Dr. A. E. Rappoport
Department of Laboratories
The Youngstown Hospital Association
Youngstown, Ohio 44501 / USA

Dr. S. B. Rosalki
St. Mary's Hospital
Praed Street
London W2 / U. K.

Prof. M. Rubin
Director of Clinical Chemistry
Georgetown Medical School
3800 Reservoir Road
Washington, D. C. 20007 / USA

Dr. S. Schwartz
Analisis Clinicos
Ciudad Sanitaria de la Seguridad Social
'Francisco Franco'
Travesera de Dalt 73/75, 4.°, 2.ª
Barcelona 12 / Spain

Prof. G. Siest
Centre de médecine préventive
2, Avenue de Doyen Jacques Parisot
54500 Vandœuvre-les-Nancy / France

Mr. G. M. Sims
Beckman Instruments, Inc.
2500 Harbor Blvd.
Fullerton, California 92634 / USA

Dr. H. E. Solberg
Institute of Clinical Biochemistry
University of Oslo
Rikshospitalet
Oslo 1 / Norway

Prof. D. Stamm
Max-Planck-Institut für Psychiatrie
Kraepelinstrasse 10
8 München 40 / West Germany

Prof. G. Vanzetti
Laboratorio di Biochimica
dell'Ospedale Maggiore
Ca'Granda
Milano / Italy

Prof. C.-H. de Verdier
Department of Clinical Chemistry
University Hospital
750 Uppsala 14 / Sweden

Prof. T. P. Whitehead
Department of Clinical Chemistry
Queen Elizabeth Medical Center
Edgbaston
Birmingham B15 2TH / U. K.

Dr. H. Wishinsky
Vice President
Research and Development
Division Miles Laboratories
Elkhart, Indiana 46514 / USA

Dr. R. Zender
Chef du Laboratoire de l'Hôpital
2300 La Chaux-de-Fonds

Dr. J. Ziegenhorn
Boehringer Mannheim GmbH
Bahnhofstrasse 5
8132 Tutzing / West Germany

International Federation of Clinical Chemistry

President	Prof. M. Rubin Director of Clinical Chemistry Georgetown Medical School 3800 Reservoir Road Washington, D.C. 20007 / USA
Vice-President	Dr. R. Dybkaer Department of Clinical Chemistry Geriatric Unit, De Gamles By Nørre Allé 41 2200 Copenhagen N / Denmark
Treasurer	Mr. P. M. G. Broughton University Department of Chemical Pathology General Infirmary Leeds, LS1 3EX / U.K.
Secretary	Prof. J. Frei Laboratoire Central de Chimie Clinique Hôpital Cantonal 1011 Lausanne / Switzerland
Associate Secretary	Prof. G. Siest Centre de médecine préventive 2, Avenue de Doyen Jacques Parisot 54500 Vandœuvre-les-Nancy / France